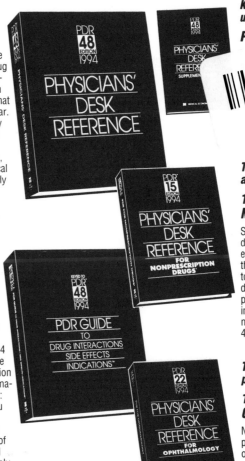
■ MEDICAL ECONOMICS DATA

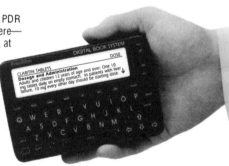
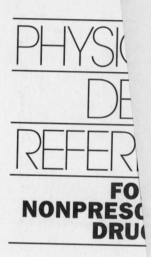

PHYSI
DE
REFER

FO
NONPRESC
DRU

Medical Consultant
Ronald Arky, MD, Charles S. Davidson Professor of Medicine
and Master, Francis Weld Peabody Society, Harvard Medical

Product Manager: Stephen B. Greenberg
Sales Manager: James R. Pantaleo
Account Managers:
Dik N. Barsamian
Jeffrey M. Keller
Michael S. Sarajian
Commercial Sales Manager: Robin B. Bartlett
Direct Marketing Manager: Robert W. Chapman
Manager, Professional Data: Mukesh Mehta, RPh
Manager, Database Administration: Lynne Handler

Edit
Direc
Assis
Produ
Produ
Forma
Index
Art Ass
Manag
Digital

FOREWORD

Welcome to the fifteenth edition of *Physicians' Desk Reference For Nonprescription Drugs*. This companion volume to the main edition of *PDR* provides detailed information on nearly 700 over-the-counter remedies, as well as a number of home diagnostic tests and other medical aids for consumers. As the trend to self-medication accelerates and the number of Rx-to-OTC conversions grows, we feel certain you'll find the book to be an ever more important part of your working reference library.

Together, *Physicians' Desk Reference, PDR For Nonprescription Drugs*, and *PDR's* special compendium for eye-care professionals, *PDR For Ophthalmology,* form America's most authoritative, comprehensive, and reliable database of precise, product-specific drug information. In turn, this core database is fully indexed in the 1,400 page *PDR Guide to Drug Interactions • Side Effects • Indications™*. An invaluable addition to the *PDR* library of drug references, the *PDR Guide* permits fast, easy identification of an adverse reaction's probable source — and the approved alternatives for the problem medication.

- Information from all four of these printed references is also available in a variety of electronic formats:

- *Pocket PDR™* — A handheld personal database of key information from each prescription-drug listing in PDR.

- *PDR Library on CD-ROM™* — Complete prescribing information from all PDR volumes on one convenient disc, for use on all IBM-compatible PC networks and individual PCs. Also available with the full text of The Merck Manual.

- *PDR Drug Interactions/Side Effects/ Indications Diskettes™* — A powerful screening program for patient regimens of up to 20 drugs.

- *PDR Database Tapes* — A preformatted text file suitable for integration in large mainframe-based information systems.

For more information on any of these printed and electronic references, please call, toll-free, 1-800-232-7379 or fax 201-573-4956.

PDR For Nonprescription Drugs is published annually by Medical Economics Data in cooperation with participating manufacturers. The function of the publisher is the compilation, organization, and distribution of product information obtained from manufacturers. Each product description has been prepared by the manufacturer, and edited and approved by the manufacturer's medical department, medical director, and/or medical consultant. During compilation of this information, the publisher has emphasized the necessity of describing products comprehensively, in order to provide all the facts necessary for sound and intelligent decision making. The descriptions seen here include all information made available by the manufacturer.

In organizing and presenting this material in *Physicians' Desk Reference For Nonprescription Drugs*, the publisher does not warrant or guarantee any of the products described, or perform any independent analysis in connection with any of the product information contained herein. *Physicians' Desk Reference For Nonprescription Drugs* does not assume, and expressly disclaims, any obligation to obtain and include any information other than that provided to it by the manufacturer. It should be understood that by making this material available the publisher is not advocating the use of any product described herein, nor is the publisher responsible for misuse of a product due to typographical error. Additional information on any product may be obtained from the manufacturer.

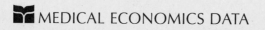
MEDICAL ECONOMICS DATA

CONTENTS

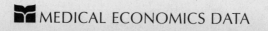

SECTION 1

MANUFACTURERS' INDEX

Listed in this index are all manufacturers that have supplied information in this edition. Each company's entry includes the address, phone, and fax number of its headquarters and regional offices, as well as contacts for inquiries, orders, and emergency information. A list of the company's major over-the-counter products is also included.

The ◆ symbol marks drugs shown in the Product Identification Guide. If a company has two page numbers, the first refers to its photographs in the Product Identification Guide, the second to its prescribing information.

ADVOCARE INTERNATIONAL, ... 502
L.L.C.
4100 Alpha, Suite 200
Dallas, TX 75244
Address Inquiries to:
Ruth Ann Box:
(214) 386-7782
FAX: (214) 386-6744

OTC Products Available:
ActoTherm
LipoTrol
Skin Secrets Advanced Liposome Therapy Mist
Skin Secrets Facial Sun Protection
Skin Secrets Glycolic Renewal
Skin Secrets Prepare Plus
Skin Secrets Ultimate Protection
Skin Secrets Youthful Eye Gel

B. F. ASCHER & 403, 502
COMPANY, INC.
15501 West 109th Street
Lenexa, KS 66219
Mailing Address:
P.O. Box 717
Shawnee Mission, KS 66201-0717
Address Inquiries to:
Joan F. Bowen: (913) 888-1880

OTC Products Available:
◆ Ayr Saline Nasal Drops
◆ Ayr Saline Nasal Mist
◆ Cough-X
◆ Itch-X Gel
◆ Mobigesic Analgesic Tablets
◆ Mobisyl Analgesic Creme
◆ Pen•Kera Creme

Unilax Stool Softener/Laxative Softgel Capsules

ASTRA USA, INC. 403, 503
50 Otis Street
Westboro, MA 01581-4500
Address Inquiries to:
Roy E. Hayward, Jr.: (508) 366-1100
For Medical Emergencies Contact:
Medical Information Services
(800) 225-6333

OTC Products Available:
◆ Xylocaine Ointment 2.5%

AU PHARMACEUTICALS, INC. 504
P.O. Box 131835
Tyler, TX 75713-1835
Address Inquiries to:
Christopher Burda, M.D.:
(800) 568-2873
For Medical Emergencies Contact:
Christopher Burda, M.D.:
(800) 568-2873

OTC Products Available:
Aurum Analgesic Lotion
Feminine Gold Analgesic Lotion
MAXIMRELIEF
PEDIGOLD
Theragold Analgesic Lotion
Therapeutic Gold Analgesic Lotion

AYERST LABORATORIES 504
Division of American Home Products Corporation
685 Third Avenue
New York, NY 10017-4071

For information for Ayerst's consumer products, see product listings under Whitehall Laboratories.
Please turn to Whitehall Laboratories, page 754

BAKER CUMMINS 403, 504
DERMATOLOGICALS, INC.
1950 Swarthmore Avenue
Lakewood, NJ 08701
Address Inquiries to:
(908) 905-5200
FAX: (908) 905-7726
For Medical Emergencies Contact:
Medical Department: (305) 590-2254
(800) 842-6704
FAX: (908) 905-7726

OTC Products Available:
Acno Cleanser
Acno Lotion
Acticort Lotion 100
Aqua-A Cream
◆ Aquaderm Cream
◆ Aquaderm Lotion
◆ Aquaderm Sunscreen Moisturizer (SPF 15 Formula)
Baker's Biopsy Punch (sizes 2, 3, 3.5, 4, 5 and 6 mm)
Baker's DTM
P&S HC Gel
P&S HC Liquid
◆ P&S Liquid
P&S Plus Tar Gel
◆ P&S Shampoo
Panscol Medicated Lotion
Panscol Medicated Ointment
Phacid Shampoo

PAGE   PAGE   PAGE

Fostex Medicated Cleansing Bar
Fostex Medicated Cleansing Cream
KeriCort-10 Cream
Keri Facial Soap
◆ Keri Lotion - Original Formula
◆ Keri Lotion -Silky Smooth with Vitamin E
◆ Keri Lotion - Silky Smooth Fragrance Free
   with Vitamin E
Minit-Rub Analgesic Ointment
Mum Antiperspirant Cream Deodorant
Chewable NODOZ Tablets
◆ No Doz Maximum Strength Caplets
Backache Caplets from Nuprin Analgesic
◆ Nuprin Ibuprofen/Analgesic Tablets &
   Caplets
Pazo Hemorrhoid Ointment &
   Suppositories
PreSun Active 15 and 30 Clear Gel
   Sunscreens
PreSun for Kids Lotion
PreSun 23 and PreSun For Kids, Spray
   Mist Sunscreens
PreSun 15 Moisturizing Sunscreen with
   KERI
PreSun 25 Moisturizing Sunscreen with
   KERI Moisturizer
PreSun 15 and 29 Sensitive Skin
   Sunscreens
PreSun 46 Moisturizing Sunscreen
Theragran Liquid
◆ Theragran Stress Formula
◆ Theragran Tablets
◆ Theragran-M Tablets with Beta Carotene
◆ Therapeutic Mineral Ice, Pain Relieving
   Gel
◆ Therapeutic Mineral Ice Exercise Formula,
   Pain Relieving Gel
Therapeutic Mineral Ice Plus Moisturizers
Tickle Roll-On Antiperspirant/Deodorant

W.K. BUCKLEY INC.......... 405, 531
P.O. Box 5022
Westport, CT 06880
Address Inquiries to:
Customer Service Office:
(203) 454-5966
FAX: (203) 454-8625
For Medical Emergencies Contact:
Customer Service Office
(203) 454-5966
FAX: (203) 454-8625

OTC Products Available:
◆ Buckley's Mixture

BURROUGHS WELLCOME ... 405, 531 CO.
3030 Cornwallis Road
Research Triangle Park, NC 27709
(800) 722-9292
For Medical or Drug Information:
Contact Drug Information Service,
Business hours only
(8:15 AM to 4:15 PM EST):
(800) 443-6763
**For 24-hour Medical Emergency
Information, Call:**
(800) 443-6763
For Sales Information:
Contact Sales Distribution
Department
Address Other Inquiries to:
Consumer Products Division

OTC Products Available:
◆ Actifed Allergy Daytime/Nighttime Caplets
   (Daytime)
◆ Actifed Allergy Daytime/Nighttime Caplets
   (Nighttime)
◆ Actifed Plus Caplets
◆ Actifed Plus Tablets
◆ Actifed Sinus Daytime/Nighttime Caplets
   (Daytime)

◆ Actifed Sinus Daytime/Nighttime Caplets
   (Nighttime)
◆ Actifed Sinus Daytime/Nighttime Tablets
   (Daytime)
◆ Actifed Sinus Daytime/Nighttime Tablets
   (Nighttime)
◆ Actifed Syrup
◆ Actifed Tablets
◆ Borofax Skin Protectant Ointment
◆ Empirin Aspirin
◆ Neosporin Ointment
◆ Neosporin Plus Maximum Strength Cream
◆ Neosporin Plus Maximum Strength
   Ointment
◆ Nix Creme Rinse
◆ Polysporin Ointment
◆ Polysporin Powder
◆ Sudafed Children's Liquid
◆ Sudafed Cold and Cough Liquidcaps
◆ Sudafed Cough Syrup
◆ Sudafed Plus Liquid
◆ Sudafed Plus Tablets
◆ Sudafed Severe Cold Formula Caplets
◆ Sudafed Severe Cold Formula Tablets
◆ Sudafed Sinus Caplets
◆ Sudafed Sinus Tablets
◆ Sudafed Tablets, 30 mg
◆ Sudafed Tablets, Adult Strength, 60 mg
◆ Sudafed 12 Hour Caplets

CAMPBELL LABORATORIES ..... 540 INC.
Address Inquiries to:
Richard C. Zahn, President
P.O. Box 812, FDR Station
New York, NY 10150-0812
(212) 688-7684

OTC Products Available:
Herpecin-L Cold Sore Lip Balm

CARE-TECH LABORATORIES...... 541
3224 South Kingshighway Boulevard
St. Louis, MO 63139
Address Inquiries to:
Sherry L. Brereton: (314) 772-4610
FAX: (314) 772-4613
For Medical Emergencies Contact:
Customer Service: (800) 325-9681
FAX: (314) 772-4613

OTC Products Available:
Barri-Care Antimicrobial Barrier Ointment
CC-500 Antibacterial Skin Cleanser
Care Creme
Clinical Care Dermal Wound Cleanser
   Concept
Formula Magic Antibacterial Powder
Just Lotion - Highly Absorbent Aloe Vera
   Based Skin Lotion
Loving Lather II Antibacterial Skin
   Cleanser
Loving Lotion Antibacterial Skin & Body
   Lotion
Orchid Fresh II Perineal/Ostomy Cleanser
Satin Antimicrobial Skin Cleanser
Skin Magic - Antimicrobial Body Rub &
   Emollient
Soft Skin Non-greasy Bath Oil with Rich
   Emollients
Swirlsoft Whirlpool Emollient for Dry Skin
   Conditions
Techni-Care Surgical Scrub
Velvet Fresh Non- Irritating Cornstarch
   Baby Powder

CHESEBROUGH-POND'S USA .... 542 CO.
33 Benedict Place
Greenwich, CT 06830
Address Inquiries to:
Consumer Affairs: (800) 243-5804

For Medical Emergencies Contact:
(800) 243-5804

OTC Products Available:
Dermasil Dry Skin Concentrated
   Treatment
Dermasil Dry Skin Treatment Cream
Dermasil Dry Skin Treatment Lotion
Vaseline Intensive Care Lotion Extra
   Strength
Vaseline Intensive Care Moisturizing
   Sunblock Lotion
Vaseline Petroleum Jelly Cream
Vaseline Pure Petroleum Jelly Skin
   Protectant

CHURCH & DWIGHT CO., INC. 543
469 North Harrison Street
Princeton, NJ 08543
Address Inquiries to:
Cathy Marino (609) 683-7015
For Medical Emergencies Contact:
HIS (800) 228-5635
Extension 7

OTC Products Available:
Arm & Hammer Pure Baking Soda

CIBA CONSUMER .... 407, 544 PHARMACEUTICALS
Division of CIBA-GEIGY Corporation
581 Main Street
Woodbridge, NJ 07095
Address Inquiries to:
Douglas Brownstone:
(908) 602-6000
FAX: (908) 602-6612
For Medical Emergencies Contact:
(908) 277-5000

OTC Products Available:
◆ Acutrim 16 Hour Steady Control Appetite
   Suppressant
◆ Acutrim Late Day Strength Appetite
   Suppressant
◆ Acutrim Maximum Strength Appetite
   Suppressant
Allerest Children's Chewable Tablets
Allerest Eye Drops
Allerest Headache Strength Tablets
Allerest Maximum Strength Tablets
Allerest No Drowsiness Tablets
Allerest Sinus Pain Formula
Allerest 12 Hour Caplets
Allerest 12 Hour Nasal Spray
◆ Americaine Hemorrhoidal Ointment
◆ Americaine Topical Anesthetic First Aid
   Ointment
◆ Americaine Topical Anesthetic Spray
   Bacid Capsules
◆ Caldecort Anti-Itch Hydrocortisone Cream
◆ Caldecort Anti-Itch Hydrocortisone Spray
◆ Caldecort Light Cream
◆ Caldesene Medicated Ointment
◆ Caldesene Medicated Powder
   Cholan HMB
◆ Cruex Antifungal Cream
◆ Cruex Antifungal Powder
◆ Cruex Antifungal Spray Powder
   Desenex Antifungal Cream
◆ Desenex Antifungal Ointment
◆ Desenex Antifungal Powder
   Desenex Antifungal Spray Liquid
◆ Desenex Antifungal Spray Powder
   Desenex Foot & Sneaker Deodorant
   Powder Plus
◆ Desenex Foot & Sneaker Deodorant
   Spray Powder
   Desenex Soap
◆ Doan's Extra-Strength Analgesic
◆ Extra Strength Doan's P.M.
◆ Doan's Regular Strength Analgesic

PAGE	**PAGE**	**PAGE**

◆ Dulcolax Suppositories
◆ Dulcolax Tablets
◆ Efidac/24
Emul-O-Balm
◆ Eucalyptamint Arthritis Pain Reliever
   (External Analgesic)
◆ Eucalyptamint Muscle Pain Relief Formula
Fiberall Chewable Tablets, Lemon Creme
   Flavor
◆ Fiberall Fiber Wafers - Fruit & Nut
◆ Fiberall Fiber Wafers - Oatmeal Raisin
◆ Fiberall Powder, Natural Flavor
◆ Fiberall Powder, Orange Flavor
Isoclor Liquid
Isoclor Tablets
Isoclor Timesule Capsules
Kondremul
Kondremul with Phenylphthalein
◆ Myoflex External Analgesic Creme
◆ Nõstril 1/4% Mild Nasal Decongestant
◆ Nõstril 1/2% Regular Nasal Decongestant
Nõstrilla Long Acting Nasal Decongestant
◆ Nupercainal Hemorrhoidal and Anesthetic
   Ointment
◆ Nupercainal Hydrocortisone 1% Cream
◆ Nupercainal Pain Relief Cream
Nupercainal Suppositories
◆ Otrivin Nasal Drops
◆ Otrivin Pediatric Nasal Drops
◆ Privine Nasal Solution and Drops
Privine Nasal Spray
Q-vel Muscle Relaxant/Pain Reliever
Sinarest Tablets
Sinarest Extra Strength Tablets
Sinarest No Drowsiness Tablets
Sinarest 12 Hour Nasal Spray
◆ Slow Fe Tablets
◆ Sunkist Children's Chewable Multivitamins
   - Complete
◆ Sunkist Children's Chewable Multivitamins
   - Plus Extra C
◆ Sunkist Children's Chewable Multivitamins
   - Plus Iron
◆ Sunkist Children's Chewable Multivitamins
   - Regular
◆ Sunkist Vitamin C - Chewable
◆ Sunkist Vitamin C - Easy to Swallow
◆ Ting Antifungal Cream
◆ Ting Antifungal Powder
◆ Ting Antifungal Spray Liquid
◆ Ting Antifungal Spray Powder
Vitron-C Tablets
Vitron-C Plus Tablets

COLUMBIA **408, 557**
LABORATORIES, INC.
2665 South Bayshore Drive
Miami, FL 33133
Address Inquiries to:
Professional Services Department
For Medical Emergencies Contact:
(305) 964-6666

OTC Products Available:
◆ Diasorb Liquid
◆ Diasorb Tablets
◆ Legatrin Tablets
Vaporizer in a Bottle Nasal Decongestant

COPLEY **408, 557**
PHARMACEUTICAL INC.
25 John Road
Canton, MA 02021
Address Inquiries to:
Copley Pharmaceutical Inc.:
(617) 821-6111
For Medical Emergencies Contact:
Dr. Antoon: (617) 821-6111

OTC Products Available:
Alum-Boro Effervescent Tablets and
   Powder Packets

Bromatapp Extended Release Tablets
Brompheril Extended Release Tablets
Diphenhydramine Hydrochloride Spray 2%
Doxylamine Succinate 25 mg Tabs
Hydrocortisone 0.5% Aerosol and 1.0%
   Aerosol
Miconazole Cream 2% and Spray Powder
◆ Miconazole Nitrate Vaginal Cream 2%
Saliv-Aid Oral Lubricant
Simethicone Drops
Tolnaftate 1% Liquid Aerosol
Tolnaftate 1% Powder Aerosol

DEL PHARMACEUTICALS, . . . 408, 559
INC.
A Subsidiary of Del Laboratories, Inc.
163 East Bethpage Road
Plainview, NY 11803
Address Inquiries to:
Peter Liman, V.P. Marketing:
(516) 293-7070
FAX: (516) 293-9018
For Medical Emergencies Contact:
Dr. John Schmermund:
(516) 293-7070, Ext. 3545

OTC Products Available:
ArthriCare Pain Relieving Rubs
Auro-Dri Ear Drops
Auro Ear Wax Removal Aid
Boil-Ease Antiseptic Drawing Salve
Dermarest Anti-Itch Gels
◆ Dermarest DriCort Anti-Itch Creme
◆ Dermarest Plus Gel
DeTane Desensitizing Lubricant
Diaper Guard Skin Rash Ointment
Exocaine Analgesic Rubs
Off-Ezy Corn Remover
Off-Ezy Wart Remover
Baby Orajel Nighttime Formula
◆ Baby Orajel Teething Pain Medicine
◆ Baby Orajel Tooth & Gum Cleanser
Denture Orajel Denture Pain Medicine
◆ Orajel Maximum Strength Toothache
   Medication
◆ Orajel Mouth-Aid for Canker and Cold
   Sores
◆ Pronto Lice Killing Shampoo &
   Conditioner in One Kit
◆ Pronto Lice Killing Spray
Propa pH Acne Medication Cleansing
   Lotion
Skin Shield Liquid Bandage
Stye Ophthalmic Ointment
◆ Tanac Medicated Gel
◆ Tanac No Sting Liquid
Tanac Mouth and Lip Sore Medicines
TripTone for Motion Sickness

EFFCON LABORATORIES, . . . 409, 561
INC.
P.O. Box 7509
Marietta, GA 30065-1509
Address Inquiries to:
Leigh Ann Buice: (800) 722-2428
FAX: (404) 499-0058
For Medical Emergency Contact:
Ed R. Burklow: (800) 722-2428
FAX: (404) 499-0058

OTC Products Available:
◆ Pin-X Pinworm Treatment
Pyrazinamide Tablets 500 mg.

FISONS CORPORATION **562**
PRESCRIPTION PRODUCTS
755 Jefferson Road
Rochester, NY 14623
Mailing Address:
P.O. Box 1766
Rochester, NY 14603

Address Inquiries to:
Professional Services Department
P.O. Box 1766
Rochester, NY 14603
(716) 475-9000

OTC Products Available:
Delsym Extended-Release Suspension

FLEMING & COMPANY **562**
1600 Fenpark Dr.
Fenton, MO 63026
Address Inquiries to:
John J. Roth, M.D.: (314) 343-8200
For Medical Emergencies Contact:
John R. Roth, M.D.: (314) 343-8200

OTC Products Available:
Chlor-3 Condiment
Impregon Concentrate
Magonate Tablets and Liquid
Marblen Suspension Peach/Apricot
Marblen Tablets
Nephrox Suspension
Nicotinex Elixir
Ocean Nasal Mist
Purge Concentrate

GEBAUER COMPANY **409, 563**
9410 St. Catherine Avenue
Cleveland, OH 44104
Address Inquiries to:
(800) 321-9348
FAX: (216) 271-5335
For Medical Emergencies Contact:
(800) 321-9348
FAX: (216) 271-5335

OTC Products Available:
Dr. Caldwell Senna Laxative
◆ Salivart Saliva Substitute

GLENBROOK LABORATORIES . . . . .
See STERLING HEALTH, page 725

HERALD PHARMACAL, INC. . . **409, 563**
6503 Warwick Road
Richmond, VA 23225
Address Inquiries to:
Gary Palmer, Marketing Director:
(804) 745-3400
(800) 253-9499
Fax: (804) 745-1963
For Medical Emergencies Contact:
Joseph A. Lewis, II
Executive Vice President:
(804) 745-3400
(800) 253-9499
FAX: (804) 745-1963

OTC Products Available:
◆ Aqua Glycolic Face Cream
◆ Aqua Glycolic Lotion
◆ Aqua Glycolic Shampoo & Body Cleanser
◆ Aqua Glyde Astringent & Cleanser
◆ Aqua Glyde Shave & Aftershave
Aqua Lacten Lotion
Aquamed Lotion
Aquaray Sunscreen
Cam Lotion
Herald Tar Shampoo
Mapo Bath Oil

INTER-CAL CORPORATION **564**
533 Madison Avenue
Prescott, AZ 86301
Address Inquiries to:
Gerald W. Elders: (602) 445-8063

OTC Products Available:
Ester-C Tablets, Caplets and Powder

PAGE

JOHNSON & JOHNSON 409, 565
CONSUMER PRODUCTS, INC.
Grandview Road
Skillman, NJ 08558
Address Inquiries: to:
Customer Information Services:
(800) 526-3967
For Medical Emergency Contact:
Customer Information Services:
(800) 526-3967

OTC Products Available:
Clean & Clear Blemish Fighting Stick
   Maximum Strength
Clean & Clear Facial Cleansing Bar
   (Sensitive Skin)
Clean & Clear Foaming Facial Cleanser
   (Sensitive Skin)
Clean & Clear Invisible Blemish Treatment
   Maximum Strength (Sensitive Skin)
Clean & Clear Oil Controlling Astringent
   (Sensitive Skin)
Clean & Clear Skin Balancing Moisturizer
   (Sensitive Skin)
Johnson's Baby Diaper Rash Relief
Johnson's Baby Sunblock, SPF 30+
Johnson's No More Burn Antiseptic Spray
Johnson's No More Germies Antibacterial
   Liquid Soap and Pre-Moistened
   Towelettes
Johnson's No More Itchies
Johnson's No More Ouchies First Aid
   Antiseptic Anesthetic Pump Spray
◆ K-Y Jelly Personal Lubricant
◆ K-Y Plus Spermicidal Lubricant
Purpose Dual Treatment
   Mositurizer-Fragrance Free, SPF15
Purpose Gentle Cleansing Bar
Purpose Gentle Cleansing Wash

JOHNSON & JOHNSON • 409, 565
MERCK CONSUMER PHARMACEUTICALS CO.
Camp Hill Road
Fort Washington, PA 19034
Address Inquiries to:
Consumer Affairs Department:
(215) 233-7000
For Medical Emergencies Contact:
(215) 233-7000

OTC Products Available:
◆ ALternaGEL Liquid
◆ Dialose Tablets
◆ Dialose Plus Tablets
◆ Ferancee Chewable Tablets
◆ Ferancee-HP Tablets
◆ Mylanta Gas Tablets-40 mg
◆ Mylanta Gas Tablets-80 mg
◆ Maximum Strength Mylanta Gas
   Tablets-125 mg
◆ Mylanta Gelcaps Antacid
◆ Mylanta Natural Fiber Supplement
◆ Mylanta Soothing Lozenges
◆ Mylanta Double Strength Liquid
◆ Mylanta Double Strength Tablets
◆ Infants' Mylicon Drops
◆ The Stuart Formula Tablets
◆ Stuartinic Tablets

KONSYL PHARMACEUTICALS, ... 570
INC.
4200 South Hulen
Ft. Worth, TX 76109
Address Inquiries: to:
Bill Steiber: (817) 763-8011
FAX: (817) 731-9389

OTC Products Available:
Konsyl Powder
Konsyl-D Powder
Konsyl-Orange Powder

PAGE

LACTAID INC. 411, 571
Pleasantville, NJ 08232
Address Inquiries to:
Alan E Kligerman: (609) 645-5100

OTC Products Available:
◆ Lactaid Caplets
◆ Lactaid Drops

LAVOPTIK COMPANY, INC. .. 572, 767
661 Western Avenue North
St. Paul, MN 55103
Address Inquiries to:
661 Western Avenue North
St. Paul, MN 55103-1694
(612) 489-1351
For Medical Emergencies Contact:
B. C. Brainard: (612) 489-1351
FAX: (612) 489-0760

OTC Products Available:
Lavoptik Eye Cup
Lavoptik Eye Wash

LEDERLE CONSUMER 410, 572
HEALTH
Division of American Cyanamid Co.
One Cyanamid Plaza
Wayne, NJ 07470
Address Inquiries to:
Consumer Affairs Department
(8:30 AM - 4:30 PM Eastern time):
(800) 282-8805
For Medical Emergencies Contact:
Consumer Affairs Department
(8:30 AM - 4:30 PM Eastern time):
(800) 282-8805
For After Hours Emergencies Contact:
(914) 732-5000
Distribution Centers:
ATLANTA
Contact EASTERN (Philadelphia)
Distribution Center
CHICAGO
Bulk Address:
1100 East Business Center Drive
Mt. Prospect, IL 60056
Mail Address:
P.O. Box 7614
Mt. Prospect, IL 60056-7614
(800) 533-3753
(708) 827-8871
DALLAS
Bulk Address:
7611 Carpenter Freeway
Dallas, TX 75247
Mail Address:
P.O. Box 655731
Dallas, TX 75265
(800) 533-3753
(214) 631-2130
WESTERN
Bulk Address:
16218 Arthur Street
Cerritos, CA 90701
Mail Address:
P.O. Box 6042
Artesia, CA 90702-6042
(800) 533-3753
(310) 802-1128
EASTERN (Philadelphia)
Bulk and Mail Address:
202 Precision Drive
P.O. Box 993
Horsham, PA 19044
(800) 533-3753
(215) 672-5400

PAGE

OTC Products Available:
◆ Caltrate 600
◆ Caltrate 600 + Iron & Vitamin D
◆ Caltrate 600 + Vitamin D
◆ Centrum
◆ Centrum, Jr. (Children's Chewable) +
   Extra C
◆ Centrum, Jr. (Children's Chewable) +
   Extra Calcium
◆ Centrum, Jr. (Children's Chewable) + Iron
◆ Centrum Liquid
◆ Centrum Silver
◆ Ferro-Sequels
◆ FiberCon Caplets
Gevrabon Liquid
Gevral T Tablets
Incremin with Iron Syrup
◆ Protegra Antioxidant Vitamin & Mineral
   Supplement
◆ Stresstabs Advanced Formula
◆ Stresstabs + Iron, Advanced Formula
◆ Stresstabs + Zinc Advanced Formula
◆ Zincon Dandruff Shampoo

LEVER BROTHERS.......... 411, 579
390 Park Avenue
New York, NY 10022
Address Inquiries to:
(212) 688-6000

OTC Products Available:
◆ Dove Bar
◆ Liquid Dove Beauty Wash
◆ Lever 2000
Liquid Lever 2000
Unscented Lever 2000

3M PHARMACEUTICALS 411, 579
3M Center Bldg. 275-4W-02
St. Paul, MN 55144-1000
For Medical Information Write:
Medical Services Department
3M Pharmaceuticals
3M Center Bldg. 275-4W-02
St. Paul, MN 55144-1000
Call: (612) 736-4930
(Outside 612 Area): (800) 328-0255
For Medical Emergencies: Call:
(612) 736-4930 (all hours)
Customer Service and Other Services:
Call: (800) 423-5197
(Outside of CA): (800) 423-5146
(CA Residents): (818) 341-1300
Pharmacy Returns:
(800) 447-4537
Address Inquiries to:
Customer Service: (612) 737-6587

OTC Products Available:
◆ Titralac Antacid Regular
◆ Titralac Antacid Extra Strength
◆ Titralac Plus Liquid
◆ Titralac Plus Tablets

MARLYN HEALTH CARE.......... 579
14851 North Scottsdale Road
Scottsdale, AZ 85254 USA
(800) 462-7596
(602) 991-0200
Address Inquiries to:
Kelly Easton: (602) 991-0200
FAX: (602) 991-0551

OTC Products Available:
4-Hair
4-Nails
Hep-Forte Capsules
Marlyn Formula 50 Capsules
Marlyn PMS
Osteo Fem

PAGE	PAGE	PAGE

Pro-Skin-E (Face Capsule)
Wobenzym N

**McNEIL CONSUMER 411, 580
PRODUCTS CO.**
Division of McNeil-PPC, Inc.
Camp Hill Road
Fort Washington, PA 19034
(215) 233-7000
Address Inquiries to:
Consumer Affairs Department
Fort Washington, PA 19034
Manufacturing Divisions:
Fort Washington, PA 19034
Southwest Manufacturing Plant
4001 N. I-35
Round Rock, TX 78664

OTC Products Available:
◆ Imodium A-D Caplets and Liquid
◆ PediaCare Cold Allergy Chewable Tablets
◆ PediaCare Cough-Cold Chewable Tablets
◆ PediaCare Cough-Cold Liquid
◆ PediaCare Infants' Decongestant Drops
◆ PediaCare Night Rest Cough-Cold Liquid
◆ Sine-Aid Maximum Strength Sinus
  Headache Gelcaps, Caplets and
  Tablets
◆ Tylenol acetaminophen Children's
  Chewable Tablets, Elixir, Suspension
  Liquid
◆ Children's Tylenol Cold Multi Symptom
  Chewable Tablets and Liquid
◆ Children's Tylenol Cold Plus Cough Multi
  Symptom Liquid
◆ Tylenol Hot Medication, Cold & Flu
  Packets
◆ Tylenol Cold Medication, Effervescent
  Tablets
◆ Tylenol Cold Medication No Drowsiness
  Formula Caplets and Gelcaps
◆ Tylenol Cold Night Time Medication Liquid
  Tylenol, Extra Strength, acetaminophen
  Adult Liquid Pain Reliever
◆ Tylenol, Extra Strength, acetaminophen
  Gelcaps, Caplets, Tablets
◆ Tylenol Extra Strength Headache Plus Pain
  Reliever with Antacid Caplets
◆ Tylenol, Infants' Drops and Infants'
  Suspension Drops
◆ Tylenol, Junior Strength, acetaminophen
  Coated Caplets, and Chewable
  Tablets
◆ Tylenol Maximum Strength Allergy Sinus
  Medication Gelcaps and Caplets
◆ Tylenol Maximum Strength Cough
  Medication
◆ Tylenol Maximum Strength Cough
  Medication with Decongestant
◆ Tylenol Maximum Strength Flu Medication
◆ Tylenol Multi Symptom Cold Medication
  Caplets and Tablets
◆ Tylenol, Maximum Strength, Sinus
  Medication Gelcaps, Caplets and
  Tablets
◆ Tylenol No Drowsiness Cold & Flu Hot
  Medication, Packets
◆ Tylenol, Regular Strength, acetaminophen
  Caplets and Tablets
◆ Tylenol PM Extra Strength Pain
  Reliever/Sleep Aid Gelcaps, Caplets,
  Tablets

MEAD JOHNSON PEDIATRICS 599
Mead Johnson & Company
A Bristol-Myers Squibb Company
2400 W. Lloyd Expressway
Evansville, IN 47721
(812) 429-5000
Address Inquiries to:
Scientific Information Section
Medical Department

OTC Products Available:
Enfamil Human Milk Fortifier
Enfamil Infant Formula
Enfamil Infant Formula Nursette
Enfamil With Iron Infant Formula
Enfamil Premature Formula
Enfamil Premature Formula With Iron
Fer-In-Sol
HIST 1
HIST 2
HOM 1
HOM 2
LYS 1
LYS 2
Lofenalac Iron Fortified Low Phenylalanine
  Diet Powder
Low Methionine Diet Powder (Product
  3200K)
Low PHE/TYR Diet Powder (Product
  3200AB)
MSUD Diet Powder
MSUD 1
MSUD 2
Mono- and Disaccharide-Free Diet Powder
  (Product 3232A)
Nutramigen Hypoallergenic Protein
  Hydrolysate Formula
OS 1
OS 2
PKU 1
PKU 2
PKU 3
Phenyl-Free Phenylalanine-Free Diet
  Powder
Poly-Vi-Sol Vitamins, Chewable Tablets
  and Drops (without Iron)
Poly-Vi-Sol Vitamins, Peter Rabbit Shaped
  Chewable Tablets (without Iron)
Poly-Vi-Sol Vitamins with Iron, Peter Rabbit
  Shaped Chewable Tablets
Poly-Vi-Sol Vitamins with Iron, Drops
Pregestimil Iron Fortified Protein
  Hydrolysate Formula with Medium
  Chain Triglycerides
ProSobee Soy Formula
ProSobee Soy Formula Nursette
Protein-Free Diet Powder (Product
  80056)
Ricelyte Oral Electrolyte Maintenance
  Solution Made With Rice Syrup Solids
Special Metabolic Diets
Special Metabolic Modules
TYR 1
TYR 2
Tempra 1 Acetaminophen Infant Drops
Tempra 2 Acetaminophen Toddlers Syrup
Tempra 3 Chewable Tablets, Regular or
  Double-Strength
Trind
Trind-DM
Tri-Vi-Sol Vitamin Drops
Tri-Vi-Sol Vitamin Drops with Iron
UCD 1
UCD 2

**MILES INC. 414, 600
CONSUMER HEALTHCARE
PRODUCTS**
1127 Myrtle Street
Elkhart, IN 46514
Address Inquiries to:
Director, Consumer Relations:
(800) 800-4793

For Medical Emergency Contact:
Professional Services - Miles (West
Haven):
(800) 468-0894

OTC Products Available:
Alka-Mints Chewable Antacid
◆ Alka-Seltzer Effervescent Antacid and Pain
  Reliever
◆ Alka-Seltzer Extra Strength Effervescent
  Antacid and Pain Reliever
◆ Alka-Seltzer Gold Effervescent Antacid
◆ Alka-Seltzer Lemon Lime Effervescent
  Antacid and Pain Reliever
◆ Alka-Seltzer Plus Cold Medicine
◆ Alka-Seltzer Plus Cold & Cough Medicine
◆ Alka-Seltzer Plus Night-Time Cold
  Medicine
◆ Alka Seltzer Plus Sinus Allergy Medicine
◆ Bactine Antiseptic/Anesthetic First Aid
  Liquid
◆ Bactine First Aid Antibiotic Plus Anesthetic
  Ointment
◆ Bactine Hydrocortisone Anti-Itch Cream
◆ Bugs Bunny Complete Children's
  Chewable Vitamins + Minerals with
  Iron and Calcium (Sugar Free)
◆ Bugs Bunny With Extra C Children's
  Chewable Vitamins (Sugar Free)
◆ Bugs Bunny Plus Iron Children's Chewable
  Vitamins (Sugar Free)
  Domeboro Astringent Solution
  Effervescent Tablets
◆ Domeboro Astringent Solution Powder
  Packets
◆ Flintstones Children's Chewable Vitamins
◆ Flintstones Children's Chewable Vitamins
  Plus Extra C
◆ Flintstones Children's Chewable Vitamins
  Plus Iron
◆ Flintstones Complete With Calcium, Iron &
  Minerals Children's Chewable
  Vitamins
◆ Flintstones Plus Calcium
◆ Miles Nervine Nighttime Sleep-Aid
◆ Mycelex OTC Cream Antifungal
◆ Mycelex OTC Solution Antifungal
◆ Mycelex-7 Vaginal Cream Antifungal
◆ Mycelex-7 Vaginal Inserts Antifungal
◆ One-A-Day Essential Vitamins with Beta
  Carotene
◆ One-A-Day Extras Antioxidant
◆ One-A-Day Extras Garlic
◆ One-A-Day Extras Vitamin C
◆ One-A-Day Extras Vitamin E
◆ One-A-Day Maximum
◆ One-A-Day Men's
  One-A-Day Women's

MURO PHARMACEUTICAL, INC.... 610
890 East Street
Tewksbury, MA 01876-1496
Address Inquiries to:
Professional Service Dept.:
(800) 225-0974
(508) 851-5981

OTC Products Available:
Bromfed Syrup
Guaifed Syrup
Guaitab Tablets
Salinex Nasal Mist and Drops

NATREN INC. 611
3105 Willow Lane
Westlake Village, CA 91361
Address Inquiries to:
Professional Services Department:
(800) 992-3323
FAX: (805) 371-4742
For Medical Emergency Contact:
Professional Services Department:

PAGE

(800) 992-3323
FAX: (805) 371-4742

OTC Products Available:
Bifido Factor
Bulgaricum I.B.
Life Start
M.F.A.
Pro-Bifidonate Powder
Pro-Bionate
Superdophilus

NATURE'S BOUNTY, INC..... 415, 612
90 Orville Drive
Bohemia, NY 11716
Address Inquiries to:
Professional Service Department:
(516) 567-9500
(800) 645-5412
FAX: (516) 563-1623

OTC Products Available:
ABC to Z
Acidophilus
Antioxidant 4000
B-Complex +C (Long Acting) Tablets
B-6 50 mg., 100 mg., 200 mg.
B-12 1000 mcg. Tablets
B-12 and B-12 Sublingual Tablets
B-50 Tablets
B-100 Tablets-Ultra B Complex
Beta-Carotene Capsules
Bounty Bears (Children's Chewables)
C-500 mg., C-1000 mg., C-1500 mg. &
    Time Release Formulas
Calcium Magnesium-Chelated Tablets
E-Oil 25,000 I.U.
◆ Ener-B Vitamin B$_{12}$ Nasal Gel Dietary
    Supplement
EnerVite (High Performance Nutrition)
Ferrous Sulfate Tablets
Garlic Oil 15 gr. & 77 gr.
KLB6 Capsules
l-Lysine 500 mg. Tablets & 1000 mg.
    Tablets
Lecithin 1200 mg. Capsules
M-KYA (For Leg Cramps)
Niacin 50 mg., 100 mg., & 250 mg.
Oat Bran 850 mg.
Odor Free Garlic
Oystercal-500 & Oystercal 500 + D
Shark Cartilage
Ultra Vita-Time Tablets
Vitamin A 10,000 I.U. & 25,000 I.U.
Vitamin E (Natural d-alpha tocopheryl)
Water Pill (Natural Diuretic)
Zinc 10 mg., 25 mg., 50 mg. Tablets

NICHE PHARMACEUTICALS, ... 612
INC.
300 Trophy Club Drive, #400
Roanoke, TX 76262
Address Inquiries to:
Steve F. Brandon: (817) 491-2770
FAX: (817) 491-3533
For Medical Emergencies Contact:
Gerald L. Beckloff, M.D.:
(817) 491-2770
FAX: (817) 491-3533

OTC Products Available:
MagTab SR Caplets

OHM LABORATORIES, INC....... 612
P.O. Box 279
Franklin Park, NJ 08823
Address Inquiries to:
Arun Heble: (908) 297-3030
For Medical Emergencies Contact:
(908) 297-3030

PAGE

OTC Products Available:
Bisacodyl Tablets 5 mg.
Cramp End Tablets
Docusate Potassium Capsules
Docusate Potassium with Casanthranol
    Capsules and Caplets
Ibuprohm Ibuprofen Caplets
Ibuprohm Ibuprofen Tablets
Loperamide Hydrochloride Caplets
Ohmni-Scon Chewable Tablets, Extra
    Strength
Pseudoephedrine Hydrochloride Tablets
    30mg and 60mg
Senna Tablets
Tribuffered Aspirin
Trisudrine Tablets

P & S LABORATORIES 614
210 West 131st Street
Los Angeles, CA 90061

See STANDARD HOMEOPATHIC
COMPANY.

PRN LABORATORIES, INC. 614
1275 Bennett Drive
Suite 122
Longwood, FL 32750
Address Inquiries to:
(407) 260-2225
FAX: (800) 761-1210
For Medical Emergency Contact:
(407) 260-2225
FAX: (800) 761-1210

OTC Products Available:
Dia Scan Gel
Pain Free Aloe Vera Gel with Capsaicin
Pain Free Natural with Capsaicin
Pain Freeze Menthol Gel
Pain Stop Extra Strength Lotion
Thera Scan Gel
Top Skin Multi-Purpose Skin Care Lotion

PARKE-DAVIS 415, 614, 767
Consumer Health Products Group
Division of Warner-Lambert Company
201 Tabor Road
Morris Plains, New Jersey 07950
See also Warner-Lambert Company
(201) 540-2000
For Product Information Call:
(800) 524-2624
(800) 223-0182
For Medical Information Call:
(800) 524-2642
(800) 223-0182

OTC Products Available:
Agoral, Marshmallow Flavor
Agoral, Raspberry Flavor
Alcohol, Rubbing (Lavacol)
Alophen Pills
◆ Anusol Hemorrhoidal Suppositories
◆ Anusol Ointment
◆ Anusol HC-1 Ointment
◆ Benadryl Allergy Sinus Headache Formula
◆ Benadryl Cold/Flu Tablets
◆ Benadryl Decongestant Elixir
◆ Benadryl Decongestant Tablets
◆ Benadryl Elixir
◆ Benadryl Itch Relief Cream, Children's
    Formula and Maximum Strength 2%
◆ Benadryl Spray, Maximum Strength 2%
◆ Benadryl Spray Children's Formula
Benadryl 25 Kapseals
Benadryl 25 Tablets
◆ Benylin Adult Formula
◆ Benylin Expectorant

PAGE

◆ Benylin Multisymptom
◆ Benylin Pediatric
◆ Caladryl Clear Lotion
◆ Caladryl Cream For Kids, Caladryl Lotion
◆ e.p.t. Early Pregnancy Test
◆ Gelusil Liquid & Tablets
    Lavacol (Rubbing Alcohol)
◆ Myadec
    Proxacol-Hydrogen Peroxide Solution
◆ Replens
◆ Sinutab Sinus Allergy Medication,
        Maximum Strength Caplets
    Sinutab Sinus Allergy Medication,
        Maximum Strength Tablets
◆ Sinutab Sinus Medication, Maximum
        Strength Without Drowsiness Formula,
        Tablets & Caplets
◆ Sinutab Sinus Medication, Regular
        Strength Without Drowsiness Formula
◆ Tucks Premoistened Pads
    Tucks Take-Alongs

THE PARTHENON COMPANY, ... 623
INC.
3311 West 2400 South
Salt Lake City, UT 84119
Address Inquiries to:
(801) 972-5184
FAX: (801) 972-4734
For Medical Emergency Contact:
Nick G. Mihalopoulos: (801) 972-5184

OTC Products Available:
Devrom Chewable Tablets

PFIZER CONSUMER 417, 623
HEALTH CARE DIVISION
Division of Pfizer Inc.
100 Jefferson Road
Parsippany, NJ 07054
Address Inquiries to:
Research and Development Dept.:
(201) 887-2100

OTC Products Available:
Ben-Gay External Analgesic Products
Bonine Tablets
◆ Daily Care from DESITIN
◆ Desitin Ointment
    Rheaban Maximum Strength Fast Acting
        Caplets
    Rid Lice Control Spray
    Rid Lice Killing Shampoo
◆ Maximum Strength Unisom Sleepgels
◆ Unisom Nighttime Sleep Aid
◆ Unisom With Pain Relief-Nighttime Sleep
        Aid and Pain Reliever
◆ Visine L.R. Eye Drops
◆ Visine Maximum Strength Allergy Relief
◆ Visine Moisturizing Eye Drops
◆ Visine Original Eye Drops
    Wart-Off Wart Remover

PHARMA-SINGER INC. 628
23201 Via Celeste
Coto de Caza, CA 92679
Home Offices:
Windeggstrasse 1, 8867 Niederurnen,
Switzerland
Telephone: +41-58-21 26 21
FAX: +41-58-21 23 02
Address Inquiries to:
Consumer Affairs: (714) 858-5250
FAX: (714) 858-3095

OTC Products Available:
Perskindol Liniment, Spray & Gel

PHARMAVITE 417, 629
CORPORATION
15451 San Fernando Mission Blvd.
Mission Hills, CA 91345

PAGE

Address Inquiries to:
PHARMAVITE
ATTN: Customer Service
P.O. Box 9606
Mission Hills, CA 91346-9606
(800) 423-2405

OTC Products Available:
Essential Balance Multivitamins
◆ Nature Made Antioxidant Formula
◆ Nature Made Essential Balance
Nutra E Skin Care Products
Private Label Vitamins
Sunny Maid Brand Vitamins

PLOUGH, INC.

See SCHERING-PLOUGH HEALTHCARE
PRODUCTS

POLYMEDICA 630
PHARMACEUTICALS (USA),
INC.

Subsidiary of PolyMedica Industries, Inc.
2 Constitution Way
Woburn, MA 01801
Address Inquiries to:
Dr. Arthur Siciliano: (617) 933-2020
FAX: (617) 933-7992
For Medical Emergencies Contact:
Dr. Arthur Siciliano: (617) 933-2020
FAX: (617) 933-7992

OTC Products Available:
Alconephrin Nasal Decongestant
Azo-Standard
Neopap Pediatric Suppositories

PREMIER, INC. 630
Greenwich Office Park One
Greenwich, CT 06831
Address Inquiries to:
Robert Albus: (203) 622-1211
FAX: (203) 622-0773
For Medical Emergency Contact:
Sergio Nacht, Ph.D.: (415) 366-2626
FAX: (415) 368-4470
Branch Office:
3696 Haven Avenue
Redwood City, CA
(415) 366-2626
FAX: (415) 368-4470

OTC Products Available:
Every Step Foot Deodorant
Exact Tinted Cream
Exact Vanishing Cream

PROCTER & GAMBLE 631
P.O. Box 5516
Cincinnati, OH 45201
Address Inquiries to:
Karen D. Kohlan (800) 358-8707
For Medical Emergencies Contact:
Call Collect: (513) 558-2085

OTC Products Available:
Children's Chloraseptic Sore Throat
Lozenges
Vicks Children's Chloraseptic Sore Throat
Spray
Chloraseptic Sore Throat Lozenges
Chloraseptic Sore Throat Spray and
Gargle
Head & Shoulders Intensive Treatment
Dandruff Shampoo
Head & Shoulders Intensive Treatment
Dandruff Shampoo 2-in-1 plus
Conditioner
Metamucil Effervescent Sugar Free,
Lemon-Lime Flavor

PAGE

Metamucil Effervescent Sugar Free,
Orange Flavor
Metamucil Powder, Orange Flavor
Metamucil Original Texture
Metamucil Smooth Texture, Citrus Flavor
Metamucil Smooth Texture Regular Flavor
Sugar Free
Metamucil Smooth Texture, Sugar Free,
Citrus Flavor
Metamucil Smooth Texture Powder,
Orange Flavor
Metamucil Smooth Texture Powder, Sugar
Free, Orange Flavor
Metamucil Wafers, Apple Crisp
Metamucil Wafers, Cinnamon Spice
Oil of Olay Daily UV Protectant SPF 15
Beauty Fluid-Original and Fragrance
Free (Olay Co. Inc.)
Pepto Diarrhea Control, Oral Solution &
Caplets
Pepto-Bismol Liquid & Tablets
Maximum Strength Pepto-Bismol Liquid
Percogesic Analgesic Tablets
Vicks Children's NyQuil Nighttime
Cold/Cough Medicine
Vicks Cough Drops
Extra Strength Vicks Cough Drops
Vicks DayQuil Allergy Relief 4 Hours
Tablets
Vicks DayQuil Allergy Relief 12 Hour
Extended Release Tablets
Children's Vicks DayQuil Allergy Relief
Vicks DayQuil Liquid
Vicks DayQuil LiquiCaps
Vicks DayQuil SINUS Pressure &
CONGESTION Relief
Vicks DayQuil SINUS Pressure & PAIN
Relief
Vicks Formula 44 Non-Drowsy Cold &
Cough Liquicaps
Vicks Formula 44 Maximum Strength
Cough
Vicks Formula 44D Cough & Head
Congestion
Vicks Formula 44E Cough & Chest
Congestion
Vicks Formula 44M Cold, Flu & Cough
Liquicaps
Vicks Formula 44M Cough, Cold & Flu
Vicks Nyquil Hot Therapy Adult
Vicks NyQuil LiquiCaps
Vicks NyQuil Liquid Original & Cherry
Vicks Pediatric Formula 44 Cough
Medicine
Vicks Pediatric Formula 44d Cough &
Head Congestion
Vicks Pediatric Formula 44e Cough &
Chest Congestion
Vicks Pediatric Formula 44m Cough &
Cold
Vicks Sinex Regular Decongestant Nasal
Spray
Vicks Sinex Regular Decongestant Nasal
Ultra Fine Mist
Vicks Sinex Long-Acting Decongestant
Nasal Spray
Vicks Sinex Long-Acting Decongestant
Nasal Ultra Fine Mist
Vicks Vapor Inhaler
Vicks VapoRub Cream
Vicks VapoRub Ointment
Vicks VapoSteam
Vicks Vatronol Nose Drops

REED & CARRNICK 417, 646
Division of Block Drug Company, Inc.
257 Cornelison Avenue
Jersey City, NJ 07302
Address Inquiries to:
Consumer & R&C Professional Affairs:
(201) 434-4000 X1821
FAX: (201) 434-3032

PAGE

For Medical Emergencies Contact:
Reed & Carnrick Medical Dept.:
(800) 568-6133 X1993

OTC Products Available:
Dura Screen
◆ Phazyme Drops
◆ Phazyme Tablets
◆ Phazyme-125 Chewable Tablets
◆ Phazyme-125 Softgels Maximum Strength
◆ Phazyme-95 Tablets
ProctoFoam-NS (Non-Steroid)
Proxigel
R&C Lice Treatment Kit
R&C Shampoo
R&C Spray
Trichotine Liquid Vaginal Douche
Trichotine Powder Vaginal Douche

THE REESE CHEMICAL 418, 647
COMPANY
10617 Frank Avenue
Cleveland, OH 44106
Address Inquiries to:
George W. Reese, III: (216) 231-6441
FAX: (216) 231-6444
For Medical Emergencies Contact:
Thomas J. Reese: (216) 231-6441
FAX: (216) 231-6444

OTC Products Available:
Bi-Zet Throat Lozenges
Cold Control+ Intense Cold Medicine
Colicon Drops
Dentapaine Gel
Licide Lice Control Kit
Licide Lice Control Shampoo
Pediatric Formula Cough & Cold Liquid
Pediatric Plus Cough & Cold Liquid
RE-AZO
◆ Recapsin Creme
Red Hearts Vitamin Tonic Tablets
Redacon DX Pediatric Drops
Reese's Pinworm Medicine
Sleep-ettes-D Tablets
Theracof Cough & Cold Liquid

REQUA, INC. 648
Box 4008
1 Seneca Place
Greenwich, CT 06830
Address Inquiries to:
J. Geils: (203) 869-2445
(800) 321-1085
FAX: (203) 661-5630

OTC Products Available:
CharcoAid
CharcoAid 2000
Charcoal Tablets
Charcocaps

RHÔNE-POULENC RORER ... 418, 649
PHARMACEUTICALS INC.
Consumer Pharmaceutical Products
500 Arcola Road
Collegeville, PA 19426-0107
**For Medical Emergencies/
Product Information Contact:**
Drug Product Safety and Product
Information: (215) 454-8870
For Regulatory Questions Contact:
Margaret Masters
Assoc. Director, Regulatory Control:
(215) 628-6085

OTC Products Available:
◆ Arthritis Pain Ascriptin
◆ Maximum Strength Ascriptin Caplets
◆ Regular Strength Ascriptin Tablets

SANOFI WINTHROP 683
PHARMACEUTICALS
Main Office
90 Park Avenue
New York, NY 10016
(212) 907-2000
Address Medical Inquiries to:
Product Information Services:
(800) 446-6267
All Other Information:
Customer Relations/Orders:
(800) 223-5511

OTC Products Available:
Anti-Rust Tablets
Breonsin Capsules
Drisdol
pHisoDerm (See Sterling Health)
Pontocaine Cream
Pontocaine Ointment
Zephiran Chloride Aqueous Solution
Zephiran Chloride Concentrate Solution
Zephiran Chloride Spray
Zephiran Chloride Tinted Tincture
Zephiran Towelettes

SCHERING CORPORATION

See SCHERING-PLOUGH HEALTHCARE
PRODUCTS

SCHERING-PLOUGH 422, 686
HEALTHCARE PRODUCTS
110 Allen Road
Liberty Corner, NJ 07938
Address Product Requests to:
Public Relations: (908) 604-1969
For Medical Emergencies Contact:
Clinical Department:
(901) 320-2998

OTC Products Available:
◆ A and D Medicated Diaper Rash Ointment
◆ A and D Ointment
◆ Afrin Cherry Scented Nasal Spray 0.05%
◆ Afrin Children's Strength Nose Drops
   0.025%
◆ Afrin Extra Moisturizing Nasal Spray
◆ Afrin Menthol Nasal Spray, 0.05%
◆ Afrin Nasal Spray 0.05% and Nasal Spray
   Pump
◆ Afrin Nose Drops 0.05%
◆ Afrin Saline Mist
◆ Aftate for Athlete's Foot
◆ Aftate for Jock Itch
  Aspergum
◆ Chlor-Trimeton Allergy Decongestant
   Tablets
◆ Chlor-Trimeton Allergy-Sinus Headache
   Caplets
◆ Chlor-Trimeton Allergy Tablets
◆ Chooz Antacid Gum

PAGE

◆ Complex 15 Therapeutic Moisturizing
   Face Cream
◆ Complex 15 Therapeutic Moisturizing
   Lotion
◆ Coricidin 'D' Decongestant Tablets
◆ Coricidin Tablets
◆ Correctol Extra Gentle Stool Softener
◆ Correctol Laxative Tablets & Caplets
  Cushion Grip Denture Adhesive
◆ Di-Gel Antacid/Anti-Gas
◆ Drixoral Cold and Allergy Sustained-Action
   Tablets
◆ Drixoral Cold and Flu Extended-Release
   Tablets
◆ Drixoral Cough Liquid Caps
◆ Drixoral Non-Drowsy Formula
◆ Drixoral Sinus
◆ DuoFilm Liquid
◆ DuoFilm Patch
◆ DuoPlant Gel
◆ Duration 12 Hour Nasal Spray
◆ Duration 12 Hour Nasal Spray Pump
◆ Feen-A-Mint Gum
  Feen-A-Mint Laxative Pills
◆ Femcare Vaginal Cream
◆ Femcare Vaginal Inserts
◆ Gyne-Lotrimin Vaginal Cream Antifungal
◆ Gyne-Lotrimin Vaginal Cream with 7
   Disposable Applicators
◆ Gyne-Lotrimin Vaginal Cream in Prefilled
   Applicators
◆ Gyne-Lotrimin Vaginal Inserts
◆ Gyne-Lotrimin Vaginal Inserts with External
   Vulvar Cream
◆ Gyne-Moistrin Vaginal Moisturizing Gel
◆ Lotrimin AF Antifungal Cream, Lotion and
   Solution
  Lotrimin AF Antifungal Spray Liquid, Spray
   Powder, Powder and Jock Itch Spray
   Powder
  Muskol Insect Repellent Aerosol Liquid
  Muskol Insect Repellent Lotion
  Muskol Insect Repellent Pump Spray
  Muskol Insect Repellent Roll-on
◆ Shade Gel SPF 30 Sunblock
◆ Shade Lotion SPF 45 Sunblock
  Shade UVAGUARD
◆ St. Joseph Adult Chewable Aspirin
   (81 mg.)
  St. Joseph Aspirin-Free Fever Reducer for
   Children Chewable Tablets
  St. Joseph Cold Tablets for Children
  St. Joseph Cough Suppressant for
   Children
◆ Tinactin Aerosol Liquid 1%
◆ Tinactin Aerosol Powder 1%
◆ Tinactin Antifungal Cream, Solution &
   Powder 1%
  Tinactin Deodorant Powder Aerosol 1%
◆ Tinactin Jock Itch Cream 1%
◆ Tinactin Jock Itch Spray Powder 1%

SCOT-TUSSIN PHARMACAL 699
CO., INC.
50 Clemence Street
Cranston, RI 02920-0217 (USA)
Mailing Address: P.O. Box 8217
Cranston, RI 02920-0217
Address Inquiries to:
(401) 942-8555
(401) 942-8556
(800) 638-SCOT (7268)
FAX: (401) 942-5690
For Medical Emergency Contact:
Dr. S. G. Scotti:
(800) 638-SCOT (7268)
FAX: (401) 942-5690

OTC Products Available:
Chlorpheniramine Maleate
Febrol SF and DF
Hayfebrol Allergy Relief Formula SF & DF

PAGE

  Romilar DM Pediatric Syrup
  Romilar Infant Decongestant Syrup
  Scot-Tussin Allergy Relief Formula
   Sugar-Free and Dye-Free
  Scot-Tussin DM Cough Chasers Lozenges
   Sugar-Free & Dye-Free
  Scot-Tussin DM Sugar-Free
  Scot-Tussin DM-2 Syrup USP
  Scot-Tussin Expectorant Sugar-Free,
   Dye-Free, Alcohol-Free
  Scot-Tussin Original Syrup
  Scot-Tussin Sugar-Free Original

SMITHKLINE BEECHAM 424, 699
CONSUMER
HEALTHCARE, L.P.
Unit of SmithKline Beecham, Inc.
P.O. Box 1467
Pittsburgh, PA 15230
Address Inquiries to:
Professional Services Department:
(800) BEECHAM
(412) 928-1050

OTC Products Available:
◆ A-200 Lice Control Spray and Kit
◆ A-200 Pediculicide Shampoo
◆ Cēpacol Anesthetic Lozenges (Troches)
◆ Cēpacol/Cēpacol Mint Mouthwash/Gargle
◆ Cēpacol Dry Throat Lozenges, Cherry
   Flavor
◆ Cēpacol Dry Throat Lozenges,
   Honey-Lemon Flavor
◆ Cēpacol Dry Throat Lozenges,
   Menthol-Eucalyptus Flavor
◆ Cēpacol Dry Throat Lozenges, Original
   Flavor
◆ CĒPASTAT Cherry Flavor Sore Throat
   Lozenges
◆ CĒPASTAT Extra Strength Sore Throat
   Lozenges
◆ CITRUCEL Orange Flavor
◆ CITRUCEL Sugar Free Orange Flavor
◆ Clear by Design Medicated Acne Gel
◆ Contac Continuous Action Nasal
   Decongestant/Antihistamine 12 Hour
   Capsules
◆ Contac Day Allergy/Sinus Caplets
◆ Contac Day & Night Cold/Flu Caplets
  Contac Maximum Strength Continuous
   Action Decongestant/Antihistamine
   12 Hour Caplets
◆ Contac Night Allergy/Sinus Caplets
◆ Contac Severe Cold and Flu Formula
   Caplets
◆ Contac Severe Cold & Flu Non-Drowsy
◆ Debrox Drops
◆ Ecotrin Enteric Coated Aspirin Maximum
   Strength Tablets and Caplets
◆ Ecotrin Enteric Coated Aspirin Regular
   Strength Tablets and Caplets
◆ Feosol Capsules
◆ Feosol Elixir
◆ Feosol Tablets
◆ Gaviscon Antacid Tablets
◆ Gaviscon-2 Antacid Tablets
◆ Gaviscon Extra Strength Relief Formula
   Antacid Tablets
◆ Gaviscon Extra Strength Relief Formula
   Liquid Antacid
◆ Gaviscon Liquid Antacid
  Geritol Complete Tablets
  Geritol Extend Caplets
  Geritol Liquid - High Potency Vitamin &
   Iron Tonic
◆ Gly-Oxide Liquid
◆ Massengill Disposable Douches
  Massengill Liquid Concentrate
◆ Massengill Medicated Disposable Douche
  Massengill Medicated Liquid Concentrate
◆ Massengill Medicated Soft Cloth
   Towelette
  Massengill Powder

For Medical Emergencies Contact:
(800) 942-2009

OTC Products Available:
MG 217 Medicated Tar Shampoo
MG 217 Medicated Tar-Free Shampoo
MG 217 Psoriasis Ointment and Lotion
ProTech First-Aid Stik
Retro G Medicated Cold Sore Gel
Skeeter Stik Insect Bite Medication

WAKUNAGA OF AMERICA .. 429, 746 CO., LTD.
Subsidiary of Wakunaga Pharmaceutical Co., Ltd.
23501 Madero
Mission Viejo, CA 92691
Address Inquiries to:
(714) 855-2776

OTC Products Available:
◆ Kyolic
  Kyo-Dophilus, Capsules: Acidophilus, Bifidus, S. Faecium
  Kyo-Green, Powder: Barley & Wheat Grass, Chlorella, Brown Rice, Kelp
  Kyolic Formula 106 Capsules: Aged Garlic Extract Powder (300 mg) & Vitamin E
  Kyolic Super Formula 104 Capsules: Aged Garlic Extract Powder (300 mg)
  Kyolic Super Formula 105 Capsules: Aged Garlic Extract Powder (200 mg)
  Kyolic Super Formula 100 Capsules & Tablets: Aged Garlic Extract Powder (300 mg)
  Kyolic Super Formula 100 Tablets: Aged Garlic Extract Powder (270 mg)
  Kyolic-Aged Garlic Extract Flavor & Odor Modified Enriched with Vitamins B_1 and B_{12}
◆ Kyolic-Aged Garlic Extract Flavor & Odor Modified Plain
  Kyolic-Aged Garlic Extract Liquid Enriched with Vitamin B & Vitamin B_{12}
  Kyolic-Aged Garlic Extract Liquid Plain
◆ Kyolic-Formula 101 Capsules: Aged Garlic Extract (270 mg)
  Kyolic-Formula 103 Capsules: Aged Garlic Extract Powder (220 mg)
  Kyolic-Formula 101 Tablets: Aged Garlic Extract Powder (270 mg)
  Kyolic-Super Formula 104, Aged Garlic Extract Powder (300 mg) with Lecithin
  Kyolic-Super Formula 103, Capsules: Aged Garlic Extract Powder (220 mg) with Vitamin C, Astragalus, Calcium
  Kyolic-Super Formula 105, Capsules: Aged Garlic Extract Powder (250 mg) with Selenium, Vitamins A & E
  Kyolic-Super Formula 106, Capsules: Aged Garlic Extract Powder (300 mg) with Vitamin E, Cayenne Pepper, Hawthorn Berry
◆ Kyolic-Super Formula 101 Garlic Plus Tablets & Capsules: Aged Garlic Extract Powder (270 mg) with Brewer's Yeast, Kelp & Algin
  Kyolic-Super Formula 102, Tablets & Capsules: Aged Garlic Extract Powder (350 mg) with Enzyme Complex

WALLACE LABORATORIES .. 429, 746
Half Acre Road
Cranbury, NJ 08512

Address Inquiries to:
Wallace Laboratories
Div. of Carter-Wallace, Inc.
P.O. Box 1001
Cranbury, NJ 08512
(609) 655-6000

For Medical Emergencies:
(800) 526-3840

OTC Products Available:
◆ Maltsupex Liquid, Powder & Tablets
◆ Ryna Liquid
◆ Ryna-C Liquid
◆ Ryna-CX Liquid
◆ Syllact Powder

WARNER-LAMBERT .... 429, 749 COMPANY
Consumer Health Products Group
201 Tabor Road
Morris Plains, NJ 07950
Address Inquiries to:
Consumer Affairs:
(800) 223-0182 Or (800) 524-2854
For Medical Emergencies Call:
Same as above

OTC Products Available:
Bromo-Seltzer
Corn Husker's Lotion
Efferdent Antibacterial Denture Cleanser
◆ Halls Mentho-Lyptus Cough Suppressant Tablets
◆ Maximum Strength Halls Plus Cough Suppressant Tablets
◆ Halls Vitamin C Drops
Listerex Lotion
◆ Listerine Antiseptic
◆ Cool Mint Listerine
◆ Listermint with Fluoride
Lubriderm Bath and Shower Oil
Lubriderm Body Bar
◆ Lubriderm Lotion
◆ Rolaids Antacid Tablets
◆ Rolaids (Calcium Rich/Sodium Free) Antacid Tablets
◆ Extra Strength Rolaids Antacid
◆ Soothers Throat Drops

WATER-JEL TECHNOLOGIES, ... 751 INC.
243 Veterans Boulevard
Carlstadt, NJ 07072
Address Inquiries to:
Bob Daniels:
(201) 507-8300
FAX: (201) 507-8325
For Medical Emergencies Contact:
Bob Daniels:
(201) 507-8300
FAX: (201) 507-8325

OTC Products Available:
Water-Jel Burn Jel
Water-Jel Burn Wrap
Water-Jel Fire Blanket Plus
Water-Jel Sterile Burn Dressings
Water-Jel Unburn (Sunburn Topical)

WELLNESS PHARMACEUTICAL, .. 752 INC.
3840 S. 103 E. Ave., Ste. 200
Tulsa, OK 74146
(418) 622-1226

OTC Products Available:
Physician's Health & Diet Program

WHITEHALL .... 430, 753, 768 LABORATORIES INC.
American Home Products Corporation
Five Giralda Farms
Madison, NJ 07940-0871
Address Inquiries to:
Consumer Affairs
Professional Samples:
(800) 343-0856

Other Information:
(800) 322-3129

OTC Products Available:
◆ Advil Cold and Sinus Caplets and Tablets (formerly CoAdvil)
◆ Advil Ibuprofen Tablets and Caplets
Anacin Caplets and Tablets (See A.H. Robins Consumer)
Maximum Strength Anacin (See A.H. Robins Consumer)
Aspirin Free Anacin, Maximum Strength (See A.H. Robins Consumer)
Baby Anbesol
Grape Baby Anbesol
Anbesol Gel - Regular Strength
Anbesol Gel - Maximum Strength
Anbesol Liquid - Regular Strength
Anbesol Liquid - Maximum Strength
Arthritis Pain Formula, Maximum Strength Analgesic Caplets
Bronitin Mist and Tablets
◆ Clearblue Easy
◆ Clearplan Easy
Compound W Gel
Compound W Liquid
Denorex Medicated Shampoo and Conditioner
Denorex Medicated Shampoo, Extra Strength
Denorex Medicated Shampoo, Extra Strength With Conditioners
Denorex Medicated Shampoo, Regular & Mountain Fresh Herbal Scent
Dermoplast Anesthetic Pain Relief Lotion
Dermoplast Anesthetic Pain Relief Spray
Dristan Allergy
Dristan Cold
Dristan Cold, Maximum Strength Multi-Symptom Formula
Maximum Strength Dristan Cold No Drowsiness Formula
Dristan Inhaler
Dristan Juice Mix-In
Dristan Nasal Decongestant Spray, Regular
Dristan Nasal Spray, Menthol
Dristan Saline Spray
Dristan Sinus
Dristan 12-hour Nasal Spray, Menthol
Dristan 12-hour Nasal Decongestant Spray
Freezone Corn Remover
Heet Liniment and Spray
InfraRub Analgesic Cream
Kerodex Cream 51 (for dry or oily work)
Kerodex Cream 71 (for wet work)
Momentum Backache Formula
Outgro Solution
Oxipor VHC Psoriasis Lotion
Posture 600 mg
Posture-D 600 mg
Preparation H Cleansing Tissues
◆ Preparation H Hemorrhoidal Cream
◆ Preparation H Hemorrhoidal Ointment
◆ Preparation H Hemorrhoidal Suppositories
◆ Preparation H Hydrocortisone 1% Cream
◆ Primatene Dual Action Formula
◆ Primatene Mist
◆ Primatene Mist Suspension
◆ Primatene Tablets
Riopan Suspension
Riopan Plus Suspension
Riopan Plus 2 Suspension
◆ Semicid Vaginal Contraceptive Inserts
Sleep-eze 3 Tablets
Today Personal Lubricant
Today Vaginal Contraceptive Sponge
Viro-Med Tablets

PAGE **PAGE** **PAGE**

WINTHROP CONSUMER PRODUCTS
Division of Sterling Winthrop Inc.
90 Park Avenue
New York, NY 10016
See STERLING HEALTH, page 725

WYETH-AYERST .... 431, 757 LABORATORIES
Division of American Home Products
Corporation
P.O. Box 8299
Philadelphia, PA 19101

Address Inquiries to:
Professional Service: (215) 688-4400
For EMERGENCY Medical Information,
Day or night call: (215) 688-4400

WYETH-AYERST DISTRIBUTION CENTERS
(Do not use freight addresses
for mailing orders.)
Atlanta, GA—P.O. Box 1773
Paoli, PA 19301-1773
(800) 666-7248

Freight Address:
100 Union Court
Kennesaw, GA 30144
Mail DEA order forms to:
P.O. Box 4365
Atlanta, GA 30302
Boston MA—P.O. Box 1773
Paoli, PA 19301-1773
(800) 666-7248

Freight Address:
7 Connector Road
Andover, MA 01810
Mail DEA order forms to:
P.O. Box 9776
Andover, MA 01810-0976
Chicago, IL—P.O. Box 1773
Paoli, PA 19301-1773
(800) 666-7248

Freight Address:
745 N. Gary Avenue
Carol Stream, IL 60188

Mail DEA order forms to:
P.O. Box 140
Wheaton, IL 60189-0140
Dallas, TX—P.O. Box 1773
Paoli, PA 19301-1773
(800) 666-7248
Freight Address:
11240 Petal Street
Dallas, TX 75238
Mail DEA order forms to:
P.O. Box 650231
Dallas, TX 75265-0231
Hawaii—P.O. Box 1773
Paoli, PA 19301-1773
(800) 666-7248
Mail DEA order forms to:
96-1185 Waihona Street, Unit C1
Pearl City, HI 96782
Kansas City, MO—P.O. Box 1773
Paoli, PA 19301-1773
(800) 666-7248
Freight Address:
1340 Taney Street
North Kansas City, MO 64116
Mail DEA order forms to:
P.O. Box 7588
North Kansas City, MO 64116-0288
Los Angeles, CA—P.O. Box 1773
Paoli, PA 19301-1773
(800) 666-7248
Freight Address:
6530 Altura Blvd.
Buena Park, CA 90622
Mail DEA order forms to:
P.O. Box 5000
Buena Park, CA 90622-5000
Philadelphia, PA—P.O. Box 1773
Paoli, PA 19301-1773
(800) 666-7248
Freight Address:
31 Morehall Road
Frazer, PA 19355
Mail DEA order forms to:
P.O. Box 61
Paoli, PA 19301
Seattle, WA—P.O. Box 1773
Paoli, PA 19301-1773
(800) 666-7248

Freight Address:
19255 80th Ave. South
Kent, WA 98032
Mail DEA order forms to:
P.O. Box 5609
Kent, WA 98064-5609

OTC Products Available:
◆ Aludrox Oral Suspension
◆ Amphojel Suspension (Mint Flavor)
◆ Amphojel Suspension without Flavor
◆ Amphojel Tablets
◆ Basaljel Capsules
◆ Basaljel Suspension
◆ Basaljel Tablets
◆ Cerose DM
◆ Collyrium for Fresh Eyes
◆ Collyrium Fresh
◆ Donnagel Liquid and Donnagel Chewable
   Tablets
◆ Nursoy, Soy Protein Isolate Formula for
   Infants, Concentrated Liquid,
   Ready-to-Feed, and Powder
◆ SMA Iron Fortified Infant Formula,
   Concentrated, Ready-to-Feed and
   Powder
◆ SMA Lo-Iron Infant Formula,
   Concentrated, Ready-to-Feed, and
   Powder
◆ Stuart Prenatal Tablets
◆ Wyanoids Relief Factor Hemorrhoidal
   Suppositories

ZILA PHARMACEUTICALS, .. 432, 763 INC.
5227 North 7th Street
Phoenix, AZ 85014-2817

Address Inquiries to:
Ed Pomerantz,
Vice President, Marketing:
(602) 266-6700

OTC Products Available:
DermaFlex Topical Anesthetic Gel
PeriGel Oral Care System
◆ Zilactin Medicated Gel
   Zilactin-L Liquid

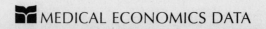
MEDICAL ECONOMICS DATA

SECTION 2

PRODUCT NAME INDEX

This index includes all entries in the "Product Information" and "Diagnostics, Devices, and Medical Aids" sections. Products are listed alphabetically by brand name.

If two page numbers appear, the first refers to the product's photograph, the second to its prescribing information.

- **Bold page numbers** indicate full prescribing information.

- *Italic page numbers* signify partial information.

- The ◆ symbol marks drugs shown in the Product Identification Section.

◆ Shown in Product Identification Guide

Italic Page Number Indicates Brief Listing

◆ **Shown in Product Identification Guide**   *Italic Page Number* Indicates Brief Listing

◆ *Shown in Product Identification Guide*

Italic Page Number Indicates Brief Listing

◆ Shown in Product Identification Guide   *Italic Page Number* Indicates Brief Listing

◆ **Shown in Product Identification Guide**   *Italic Page Number* Indicates Brief Listing

SECTION 3

PRODUCT CATEGORY INDEX

This index cross-references each brand by prescribing category. Entries in both the "Product Information" and "Diagnostics, Devices, and Medical Aids" sections are included. In each category, all fully described products are listed first, followed by those with only partial descriptions.

If two page numbers appear, the first refers to the product's photograph, the second to its prescribing information.

- **Bold page numbers** indicate full prescribing information.

- *Italic page numbers* signify partial information.

The categories employed in this index were established by the OTC Review process of the United States Food and Drug Administration. Classification of products within these categories has been determined in cooperation with the products' manufacturers or, when necessary, by the publisher alone.

A

ACNE PRODUCTS
(see ANTIBIOTICS, SYSTEMIC & DERMATOLOGICALS, ACNE PREPARATIONS)

ALLERGY RELIEF PRODUCTS
(see COLD & COUGH PREPARATIONS, NASAL SPRAYS & OPHTHALMIC PREPARATIONS)

AMEBICIDES & TRICHOMONACIDES
(see ANTIPARASITICS)

ANALGESICS
ACETAMINOPHEN & COMBINATIONS
Actifed Plus Caplets
(Burroughs Wellcome) **405, 531**
Actifed Plus Tablets
(Burroughs Wellcome) **405, 534**
Bayer Select Head Cold
(Sterling Health) **427, 732**
Bayer Select Headache Pain
Relief Formula (Sterling
Health) **427, 733**
Bayer Select Menstrual
Multi-Symptom Formula
(Sterling Health) **427, 733**
Bayer Select Night Time Pain
Relief Formula
(Sterling Health) **427, 733**
Bufferin AF Nite Time
Analgesic/Sleeping Aid Caplets
(Bristol-Myers Products) **514**
Aspirin Free Excedrin Analgesic
Caplets
(Bristol-Myers Products) **404, 521**

Aspirin Free EXCEDRIN Dual Caplets
(Bristol-Myers Products) **521**
Excedrin Extra-Strength Analgesic
Tablets & Caplets
(Bristol-Myers Products) **404, 522**
Excedrin P.M. Analgesic/Sleeping
Aid Tablets, Caplets
(Bristol-Myers Products) **404, 523**
Maximum Strength
Multi-Symptom Formula Midol
(Sterling Health) **428, 738**
PMS Multi-Symptom Formula
Midol (Sterling Health) **428, 737**
Teen Multi-Symptom Formula
Midol (Sterling Health) **428, 739**
Children's Panadol Chewable
Tablets, Liquid, Infant's Drops
(Sterling Health) **428, 740**
Junior Strength Panadol
(Sterling Health) **428, 740**
Percogesic Analgesic Tablets
(Procter & Gamble) **636**
Sominex Pain Relief Formula
(SmithKline Beecham
Consumer) **426, 719**
Tylenol acetaminophen Children's
Chewable Tablets, Elixir,
Suspension Liquid
(McNeil Consumer) **412, 582**
Tylenol, Extra Strength, acetaminophen
Adult Liquid Pain Reliever
(McNeil Consumer) **587**
Tylenol, Extra Strength,
acetaminophen Gelcaps,
Caplets, Tablets (McNeil
Consumer) **412, 589**
Tylenol Extra Strength Headache
Plus Pain Reliever with
Antacid Caplets
(McNeil Consumer) **413, 587**
Tylenol, Infants' Drops and
Infants' Suspension Drops
(McNeil Consumer) **412, 582**

Tylenol, Junior Strength,
acetaminophen Coated
Caplets, and Chewable
Tablets
(McNeil Consumer) **412, 591**
Tylenol Maximum Strength Flu
Medication
(McNeil Consumer) **413, 594**
Tylenol, Regular Strength,
acetaminophen Caplets and
Tablets (McNeil Consumer).... **412, 598**
Tylenol PM Extra Strength Pain
Reliever/Sleep Aid Gelcaps,
Caplets, Tablets
(McNeil Consumer) **413, 588**
Unisom With Pain Relief-Nighttime
Sleep Aid and Pain Reliever
(Pfizer Consumer) **417, 626**
Vanquish Analgesic Caplets
(Sterling Health) **429, 742**

ACETAMINOPHEN WITH ANTACIDS
Aspirin Free EXCEDRIN Dual Caplets
(Bristol-Myers Products) **521**
Tylenol Extra Strength Headache
Plus Pain Reliever with
Antacid Caplets
(McNeil Consumer) **413, 587**

ASPIRIN
Bayer Children's Chewable
Aspirin (Sterling Health) **427, 726**
Genuine Bayer Aspirin Tablets &
Caplets (Sterling Health)........ **427, 726**
Maximum Bayer Aspirin Tablets &
Caplets (Sterling Health)........ **427, 728**
Extended-Release Bayer 8-Hour Aspirin
(Sterling Health) **728**
Adult Low Strength Bayer Enteric
Aspirin Tablets (81 mg)
(Sterling Health) **427, 729**
Extra Strength Bayer Enteric
Aspirin (Sterling Health) **427, 729**

Italic Page Number **Indicates Brief Listing**

Italic Page Number **Indicates Brief Listing**

Italic Page Number **Indicates Brief Listing**

Italic Page Number **Indicates Brief Listing**

Italic Page Number **Indicates Brief Listing**

Italic Page Number **Indicates Brief Listing**

Italic Page Number **Indicates Brief Listing**

Italic Page Number **Indicates Brief Listing**

Italic Page Number **Indicates Brief Listing**

Italic Page Number **Indicates Brief Listing**

W

WART REMOVERS
  (see DERMATOLOGICALS, WART
  REMOVERS)

WEIGHT CONTROL PREPARATIONS
  (see APPETITE SUPPRESSANTS OR
  FOODS)

WET DRESSINGS
  (see DERMATOLOGICALS, WET
  DRESSINGS)

SECTION 4

ACTIVE INGREDIENTS INDEX

This index cross-references each brand by its generic ingredients. Entries in both the "Product Information" and "Diagnostics, Devices, and Medical Aids" sections are included. Under each generic heading, all fully described products are listed first, followed by those with only partial descriptions.

If two page numbers appear, the first refers to the product's photograph, the second to its prescribing information.

- **Bold page numbers** indicate full prescribing information.

- *Italic page numbers* signify partial information.

Classification of products under these headings has been determined in cooperation with the products' manufacturers or, if necessary, by the publisher alone.

Italic Page Number **Indicates Brief Listing**

Italic Page Number **Indicates Brief Listing**

Italic Page Number **Indicates Brief Listing**

Italic Page Number **Indicates Brief Listing**

Italic Page Number **Indicates Brief Listing**

Italic Page Number **Indicates Brief Listing**

Italic Page Number **Indicates Brief Listing**

Italic Page Number **Indicates Brief Listing**

Italic Page Number **Indicates Brief Listing**

Italic Page Number **Indicates Brief Listing**

Italic Page Number **Indicates Brief Listing**

Italic Page Number **Indicates Brief Listing**

Italic Page Number **Indicates Brief Listing**

Italic Page Number **Indicates Brief Listing**

Italic Page Number **Indicates Brief Listing**

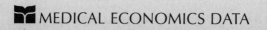

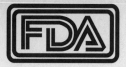

U.S. FOOD AND DRUG ADMINISTRATION

Medical Product Reporting Programs

MedWatch (24 hour service) **800-332-1088**
  Reporting of problems with drugs, devices, biologics (except vaccines), medical foods, dietary supplements.

Vaccine Adverse Event Reporting (24 hour service)................................**800-822-7967**
  Reporting of vaccine-related problems.

Mandatory Medical Device Reporting...**301-427-7500**
  Reporting required from User facilities regarding device-related deaths and serious injuries.

Veterinary Adverse Drug Reaction Program **301-594-0749**
  Reporting of adverse drug events in animals.

Medical Advertising Information (24 hour service)................................**800-238-7332**
  Inquiries from health professionals regarding product promotion.

Information for Health Professionals

Center for Drugs Executive Secretariat **301-594-1012**
  Information on human drugs including hormones.

Center for Biologics Executive Secretariat **301-594-1800**
  Information on biological products including vaccines and blood.

Center for Devices and Radiological Health..**301-443-4190**
  Automated request for information on medical devices and radiation-emitting products.

Office of Orphan Products Development **301-443-4718**
  Information on products for rare diseases.

Office of Health Affairs Medicine Staff **301-443-5470**
  Information for health professionals on FDA activities.

General Information

General Consumer Inquiries...**301-443-3170**
  Consumer information on regulated products/issues.

Freedom of Information **301-443-6310**
  Request for publicly available FDA documents.

Office of Public Affairs...**301-443-1130**
  Interviews/press inquiries on FDA activities.

Breast Implant Inquiries (24 hour service) **800-332-3541**
  Prerecorded message/request information.

Seafood Hotline (24 hour service)...**800-332-4010**
  Prerecorded message/request information (English/Spanish).

All numbers accessible 8:00 a.m. to 4:30 p.m. eastern time, except where otherwise noted.

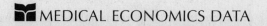

PRODUCT IDENTIFICATION GUIDE

To aid in quick identification, this section provides full-color, actual-size photographs of tablets and capsules. A variety of other dosage forms and packages are shown at less than actual size. In all, the section contains a total of more than 1,000 photos.

Products in this section are arranged alphabetically by manufacturer. In some instances, not all dosage forms and sizes are pictured. If others are available, a † symbol precedes the product's name. Letters or numbers representing the manufacturer's identification code are followed by an asterisk.

For more information on any of the products in this section, please turn to the "Product Information" or "Diagnostics, Devices, and Medical Aids" sections, or check directly with the manufacturer. For easy reference, the page number of each product's text entry appears with its photographs.

While every effort has been made to guarantee faithful reproduction of the photos in this section, changes in size, color, and design are always a possibility. Be sure to confirm a product's identity with the manufacturer or your pharmacist.

Manufacturer's Index

ASCHER & CO., INC.

B.F. Ascher & Co., Inc.
P. 502

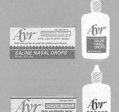

Saline Nasal Drops and Nasal Mist
Ayr®

B.F. Ascher & Co., Inc.
P. 502

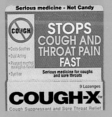

Cough Suppressant and
Sore Throat Relief Lozenges
COUGH-X™

B.F. Ascher & Co., Inc.
P. 502

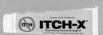

Available in: 35.4 g (1.25 oz) tube gel
ITCH-X®

B.F. Ascher & Co., Inc.
P. 503

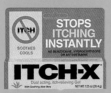

Analgesic Tablets
Available in: 18's, 50's & 100's
Mobigesic®

B.F. Ascher & Co., Inc.
P. 503

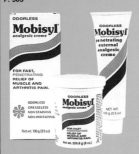

Analgesic Creme
Also available: 1.25 oz.
Mobisyl®

B.F. Ascher & Co., Inc.
P. 503

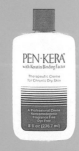

Therapeutic Creme for
Chronic Dry Skin
Available in: 8 oz. bottle
PEN·KERA®

ASTRA

Astra USA, Inc.
P. 503

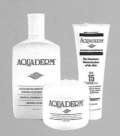

2.5% Ointment
Available in 35 gram Tube
Xylocaine®

BAKER CUMMINS

Baker Cummins Dermatologicals, Inc.
P. 505

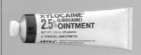

Lotion, Cream and
Sunscreen Moisturiser (SPF 15)
Aquaderm®

Baker Cummins Dermatologicals, Inc.
P. 505

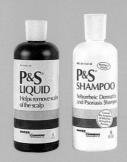

Liquid and Shampoo
P & S®

Baker Cummins Dermatologicals, Inc.
P. 505

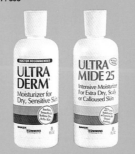

Moisturizer
**Ultra Derm®/
Ultra Mide 25®**

Baker Cummins Dermatologicals, Inc.
P. 506

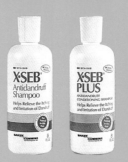

Shampoo
X-Seb®/X-Seb® Plus

Baker Cummins Dermatologicals, Inc.
P. 506

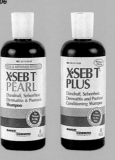

Shampoo
**X-Seb T® Pearl/
X-Seb T® Plus**

BEIERSDORF

Beiersdorf Inc.
P. 507

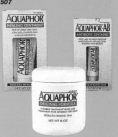

Healing Ointments For Dry Skin,
Minor Cuts and Burns
Aquaphor®

Beiersdorf Inc.
P. 507

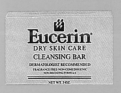

Cleansing Bar
Eucerin®

Beiersdorf Inc.
P. 508

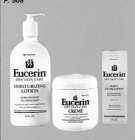

Sensitive Solutions For
Dry Skin Problems
Moisturizing Lotion,
Creme and Daily Facial Lotion
Eucerin® Dry Skin Care

BOCK

Bock Pharmacal
P. 512

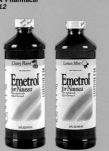

Emetrol®

BOIRON

Boiron Laboratories
P. 512

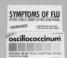

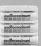

Homeopathic remedy for the natural relief of flu-like symptoms. Now also available in new family value pak. (6 doses)

Oscillococcinum®

BRISTOL-MYERS PRODUCTS

Bristol-Myers Products
P. 525

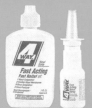

Regular available in: 1/2 oz. Metered Spray Pump and 1/2 oz. and 1 oz. Atomizers Mentholated also available

4-Way® Fast Acting Nasal Spray

Bristol-Myers Products
P. 526

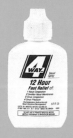

1/2 oz. Atomizers

4-Way® Long Acting Nasal Spray

Bristol-Myers Products
P. 512

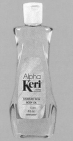

Shower and Bath Products 4, 8, 12 and 16 oz.

Alpha Keri®

Bristol-Myers Products
P. 515

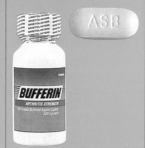

Bottles of 40 and 100 coated caplets

Bufferin® Arthritis Strength

Bristol-Myers Products
P. 513

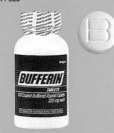

Bottles of 12, 30, 50, 100, 200 and vials of 10 tablets
Hospital and Institutional packs of 150 x 2 tablets in foil packets

Bufferin® Coated Analgesic

Bristol-Myers Products
P. 516

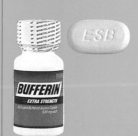

Bottles of 30, 50 and 100 coated tablets

Bufferin® Extra Strength

Bristol-Myers Products
P. 517

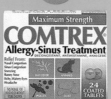

Available in blister packs of 24 and bottles of 50

Comtrex® Allergy-Sinus

Bristol-Myers Products
P. 518

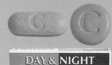
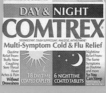

Multi-Symptom Cold Reliever
Blister packs of 24 & 48

Day & Night Comtrex®

Bristol-Myers Products
P. 516

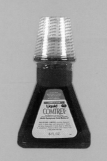

Bottles of 6 oz. Cherry Flavor

Liquid Comtrex®

Bristol-Myers Products
P. 516

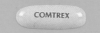
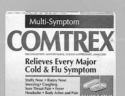

Blister packs of 24 and 50

Comtrex® Liqui-Gel Multi-Symptom Cold Reliever

Bristol-Myers Products
P. 516

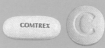
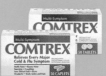

Caplets: Blister packs of 24 and bottles of 50. Tablets: Blister packs of 24, bottles of 50

Comtrex® Multi-Symptom Cold Reliever

Bristol-Myers Products
P. 519

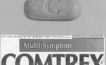

Multi-Symptom Cold Reliever Caplets
Blister packs of 24 and bottles of 50

Non-Drowsy Comtrex®

Bristol-Myers Products
P. 523

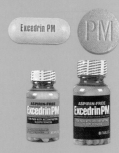

Bottles of 10, 24, 50 and 100 and vials of 10

Excedrin PM®

Bristol-Myers Products
P. 521

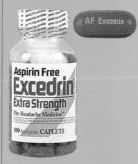

Bottles of 24, 50 and 100 caplets

Aspirin Free Excedrin®

Bristol-Myers Products
P. 522

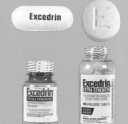

Bottles of 12, 24, 50, 100, 175 and 275, metal tins of 12 and vials of 10 tablets

Extra Strength Excedrin®

Bristol-Myers Products
P. 524

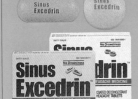

Available in blister packs of 24 and
bottles of 50 caplets and tablets

Sinus Excedrin®

Bristol-Myers Products
P. 526

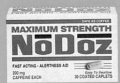

For Dry Skin Care
6.5, 11 and 15 oz. 20 oz. size
for Original Formula
Silky Smooth and Fragrance Free

Keri® Lotion

Bristol-Myers Products
P. 526

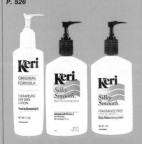

Maximum Strength
Blister packs of 16 caplets
Bottles of 36's and 60's

No Doz®

Bristol-Myers Products
P. 526

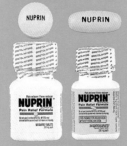

Bottles of 24, 50, 100, 150
and vials of 10 tablets

Nuprin®

Bristol-Myers Products
P. 529

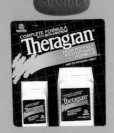

Complete Formula with Beta Carotene
High Potency Multivitamin Formula

Theragran®

Bristol-Myers Products
P. 529

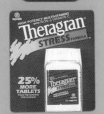

Complete Formula with Antioxidants
High Potency Multivitamin
Formula with Minerals

Theragran-M®

Bristol-Myers Products
P. 529

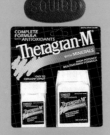

High Potency Multivitamin Formula
with Iron and Vitamin C

**Theragran® Stress
Formula™**

Bristol-Myers Products
P. 530

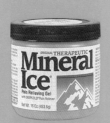

Available in: 3.5 oz., 8 oz.
and 16 oz. Pain Relieving Gel

Therapeutic Mineral Ice®

Bristol-Myers Products
P. 530

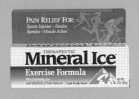

Tubes of 3 oz. Pain Relieving Gel

**Therapeutic Mineral Ice®
Exercise Formula**

W.K. BUCKLEY, INC.

W.K. Buckley, Inc.
P. 531

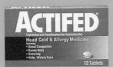

8 Fl. oz. and 4 Fl. oz.

Buckley's® Mixture

BURROUGHS WELLCOME

Burroughs Wellcome
P. 534

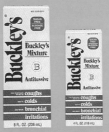

Available in 12, 24, 48 tablets
and bottles of 100

Actifed®

Burroughs Wellcome
P. 531

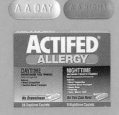

**Actifed® Allergy
Daytime/Nighttime**

Burroughs Wellcome
P. 533

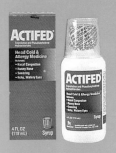

4 fl. oz.
Also available in pints

Actifed® Syrup

Burroughs Wellcome
P. 531

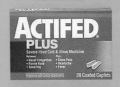

Available in 20 and
40 tablets and caplets

Actifed® Plus®

Burroughs Wellcome
P. 532

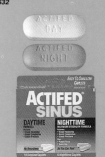

**Actifed® Sinus
Daytime/Nighttime**

Burroughs Wellcome
P. 533

**Actifed® Sinus
Daytime/Nighttime**

Burroughs Wellcome
P. 534

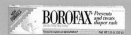

Skin Protectant Ointment
Available in 1.8 oz (50g) tube
Borofax®

Burroughs Wellcome
P. 535

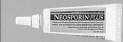
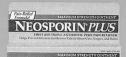

Maximum Strength Ointment
Available in 1/2 oz. (14.2g)
and 1 oz. (28.4g) tubes
Neosporin® Plus

Burroughs Wellcome
P. 538

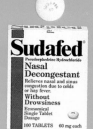

60 mg Tablets
Available in 100
Sudafed®

Burroughs Wellcome
P. 537

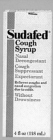

4 fl. oz. (118 mL)
Sudafed® Cough Syrup

Burroughs Wellcome
P. 535

Available in 50 and 100 tablets
Empirin® Aspirin

Burroughs Wellcome
P. 536

Lice Treatment Creme Rinse
2 fl. oz. (59 mL)
Also available in:
2-bottle family pack
Nix®

Burroughs Wellcome
P. 540

12 Hour Caplets
Available in 10 and 20 caplets
Sudafed® 12 Hour

Burroughs Wellcome
P. 538

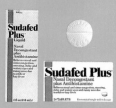

Available in 4 fl. oz liquid
and 24 and 48 tablets
Sudafed® Plus

Burroughs Wellcome
P. 535

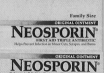

First Aid Antibiotic Ointment
Available in 1/2 oz. (14.2g)
and 1 oz. (28.4g) tubes
Neosporin®

Burroughs Wellcome
P. 536

First Aid Antibiotic Powder & Ointment
Powder, 0.35 oz. (10g) Ointment,
1/2 oz. (14.2g) and 1 oz. (28.4g)
Polysporin®

Burroughs Wellcome
P. 536

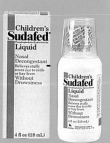

4 fl. oz.
**Children's Sudafed®
Liquid**

Burroughs Wellcome
P. 539

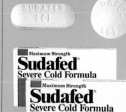

Available in 10 and 20
caplets and tablets
**Sudafed®
Severe Cold Formula**

Burroughs Wellcome
P. 535

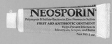
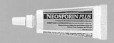

Maximum Strength Cream
Available in 1/2 oz. (14.2g) tubes
Neosporin® Plus

Burroughs Wellcome
P. 537

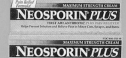

30 mg Tablets
Available in 24, 48 and 100
Sudafed®

Burroughs Wellcome
P. 537

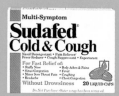

Available in 10's or 20's Liquid Caps
Sudafed® Cold & Cough

Burroughs Wellcome
P. 539

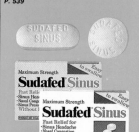
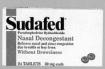

Available in 24 and 48
caplets and tablets
Sudafed® Sinus

CIBA CONSUMER

Ciba Consumer
P. 544

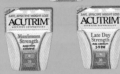

Appetite Suppressants
Caffeine Free/Works all Day

Acutrim®

Ciba Consumer
P. 546

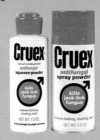

Antifungal Spray and Squeeze
Powder & Cream
Relieves Itching, Chafing, Rash
Cures Jock Itch

Cruex®

Ciba Consumer
P. 548

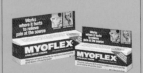

15 minutes to 1 hour
Fast Predictable Relief
Dulcolax
LAXATIVE
8 SUPPOSITORIES

Overnight Relief
Gentle and Predictable
Dulcolax
The original brand (bisacodyl USP)
LAXATIVE
SODIUM FREE
10 TABLETS

Tablets & Suppositories

Dulcolax® Laxative

Ciba Consumer
P. 551

MYOFLEX

External Analgesic Cream
Available in 2 oz. and 4 oz. tubes,
8 oz. and 16 oz. jars

Myoflex®

Ciba Consumer
P. 545

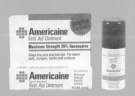

Ointment 3/4 oz. and Spray 2 oz.
Also available in
Hemorrhoidal Ointment 1 oz.

Americaine®

Ciba Consumer
P. 546

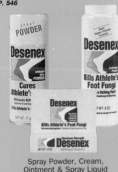

Spray Powder, Cream,
Ointment & Spray Liquid
Cures Athlete's Foot

Desenex®

Ciba Consumer
P. 549

EFIDAC/24
pseudoephedrine hydrochloride extended-release tablets
NASAL DECONGESTANT
24 HOUR RELIEF
• COLDS
• UPPER RESPIRATORY ALLERGIES
• NASAL & SINUS CONGESTION
No Drowsiness

Nasal Decongestant

Efidac/24®

Ciba Consumer
P. 551

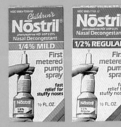

Children's & Regular
Metered Pump Spray
Also available in Nostrilla®
12 Hour Metered Pump Spray

Nóstril®

Ciba Consumer
P. 545

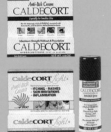

Caldecort and Caldecort Light® Cream
1.5 oz. Spray

Caldecort®

Ciba Consumer
P. 547

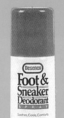

Foot & Sneaker Deodorant
Soothes, Cools, Comforts
and Absorbs Moisture

Desenex®

Ciba Consumer
P. 549

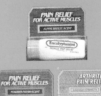

Alpine Breeze, Powder Fresh
and Arthritis Pain External Analgesics

Eucalyptamint®

Ciba Consumer
P. 552

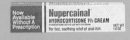

For fast, soothing relief of anal itch.

Nupercainal®

Ciba Consumer
P. 546

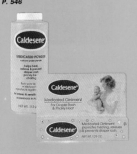

Medicated Powder and Ointment
Also available in 2 oz. and 4 oz. powder

Caldesene®

Ciba Consumer
P.547

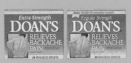

Backache Analgesic
Relieves Backache
Regular/Extra Strength/Nighttime

Doan's® & Doan's® P.M.

Ciba Consumer
P. 550

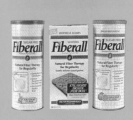

Powder and Wafers

Fiberall®

Ciba Consumer
P. 552

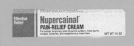

1 1/2 oz. Pain Relief Cream
Prompt, temporary relief of painful
sunbum, minor bums, scrapes, scratches,
and nonpoisonous insect bites.

Nupercainal®

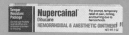
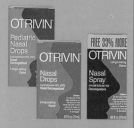
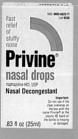
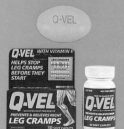
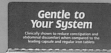
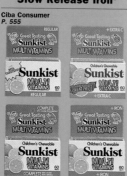
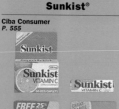
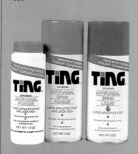

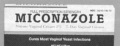

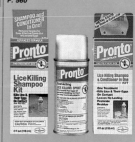

EFFCON

Effcon Laboratories
P. 561

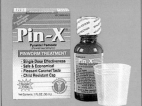

50 mg.

Pin-X®

GEBAUER

Gebauer Company
P. 563

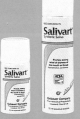

25 mL and 75 mL
Synthetic Saliva

Salivart®

HERALD

Herald Pharmacal Inc.
P. 563

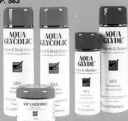

AHA Alpha Hydroxy
Acid Skin Care Products

**Aqua Glycolic®
and Aqua Glyde®**

JOHNSON & JOHNSON

Johnson & Johnson Consumer Products
P. 565

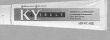

Available in 2 and 4 oz. tubes and
convenient sized 3-packs. Water
soluble for general lubricating needs

**K-Y® BRAND Jelly
Personal Lubricant**

Johnson & Johnson Consumer Products

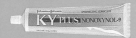

113g (4 oz.)
Spermicidal Lubricant
Safe to use with or without condoms
Clear, non-greasy, water soluble

**K-Y® Plus BRAND
Spermicidal lubricant
with Nonoxynol-9**

J&J-MERCK CONSUMER

J&J-Merck Consumer
P. 565

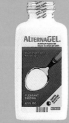

12 fl oz and 5 fl oz
High potency aluminum
hydroxide antacid

AlternaGel®

J&J-Merck Consumer
P. 566

100 mg / 65 mg   100 mg
Bottles of 36 & 100 tablets

**Dialose®
Dialose® Plus**

J&J-Merck Consumer
P. 566

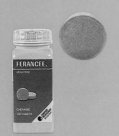

**Ferancee®
Chewable Tablets**

J&J-Merck Consumer
P. 566

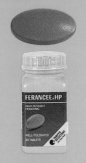

Bottles of 60 tablets
High potency hematinic ferrous

Ferancee® HP

J&J-Merck Consumer
P. 567

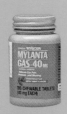

40 mg/0.6 mL
Available in 0.5 oz and 1.0 oz bottles

Infants' Mylicon® Drops

J&J-Merck Consumer
P. 568

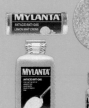

40 mg
Bottles of 100 tablets

Mylanta® Gas 40

J&J-Merck Consumer
P. 568

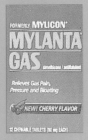

80 mg
12 & 30 tablet convenience packs
Bottles of 60 and 100

Mylanta® Gas

J&J-Merck Consumer
P. 568

MAXIMUM STRENGTH

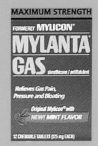

125 mg
12 & 24 tablet convenience packs

**Maximum Strength
Mylanta® Gas**

J&J-Merck Consumer
P. 569

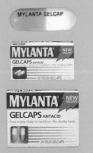

311 mg / 232 mg

**Mylanta® Gelcaps
Antacid**

J&J-Merck Consumer
P. 567

Tablets in 48 & 100 count bottles
& liquid bottles of 5, 12, 24 oz. 12
tablet rollpack

Mylanta®

J&J-Merck Consumer
P. 567

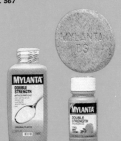

Bottles of 30 & 60 tablets & 8 tablet
rollpack/5 or 12 & 24 oz. liquid

**Mylanta®
Double Strength**

J&J-Merck Consumer
P. 569

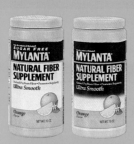

Orange flavor Available in
10 oz and 13 oz

**Mylanta® Natural
Fiber Supplement**

J&J-Merck Consumer
P. 569

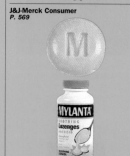

Bottles of 100 and
Boxes of 18 Lozenges

**Mylanta® Soothing
Lozenges**

J&J-Merck Consumer
P. 570

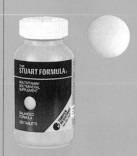

Bottles of 100 and 250 tablets

Stuart Formula®

J&J-Merck Consumer
P. 570

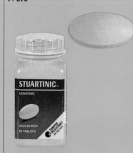

100 mg
Bottles of 60 tablets

Stuartinic®

LEDERLE

***LEDERMARK®
Product
Identification Code**

Many Lederle tablets and capsules bear an identification
code, and these codes are
listed with each product pictured. A current listing
appears in the Product
Information Section of the
1994 Physicians' Desk
Reference.

Lederle Laboratories
P. 573

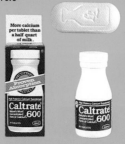

*C600
Bottles of 60
High Potency Calcium Supplement

Caltrate® 600

Lederle Laboratories
P. 573

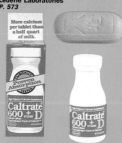

*C40
Bottles of 60
High Potency Calcium Supplement

**Caltrate® 600
+ Vitamin D**

Lederle Laboratories
P. 573

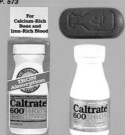

*C45
Bottles of 60
High Potency Calcium Supplement

**Caltrate®
600 + Iron + Vitamin D**

Lederle Laboratories
P. 573

Bottles of 100, 60 and 30
High Potency Multivitamin/
Multimineral Formula

Centrum®

Lederle Laboratories
P. 573

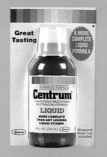

High Potency
Multivitamin/Multimineral Formula

Centrum® LIQUID

Lederle Laboratories
P. 574

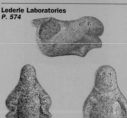

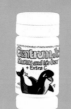

60 Tablets Children's
Chewable Vitamin/Mineral Formula
with beta carotene

**Centrum, Jr.® Shamu and
his Crew® + Extra C**

Lederle Laboratories
P. 574

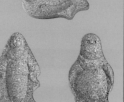

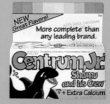

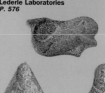

60 Tablets Children's
Chewable Vitamin/Mineral Formula
with beta carotene

**Centrum, Jr.®
Shamu and his Crew®
+ Extra Calcium**

Lederle Laboratories
P. 576

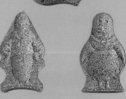

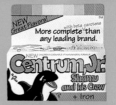

60 Tablets Children's
Chewable Vitamin/Mineral Formula
with beta carotene

**Centrum, Jr.®
Shamu and his Crew®
+ Iron**

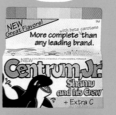

Lederle Laboratories
P. 576

*C511
Bottles of 60 and 100
Specially Formulated
Multivitamin/Multimineral
For adults 50+
Centrum® SILVER

Lederle Laboratories
P. 576

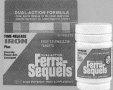

*F2
Available in blister packs of
30 and bottles of 30 and 100
High Potency Iron Supplement with
Proven Anti-Constipant
Ferro-Sequels®
Dual-Action

Lederle Laboratories
P. 576

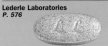

*F66
Available in boxes of
36 and 60 and bottles of 90
FiberCon®

Lederle Laboratories
P. 577

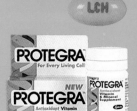

Bottle of 50 Softgels Antioxidant
Vitamin & Mineral Supplement
PROTEGRA™

Lederle Laboratories
P. 578

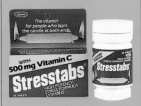

*S1
Bottles of 60 Advanced Formula
High Potency Stress Formula Vitamins
Stresstabs®

Lederle Laboratories
P. 578

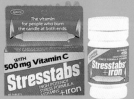

*S2
Bottles of 60 Advanced Formula
High Potency Stress Formula Vitamins
Stresstabs® with Iron

Lederle Laboratories
P. 578

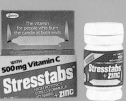

*S3
Bottles of 60 Advanced Formula
High Potency Stress
Formula Vitamins
Stresstabs® with Zinc

Lederle Laboratories
P. 578

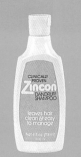

Bottles of 4 fl. oz. and 8 fl. oz.
Dandruff Shampoo
Zincon®

Lever Brothers
P. 579

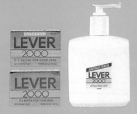

Antibacterial Soap
Available in Bar and Liquid
Lever 2000®

Lever Brothers
P. 579

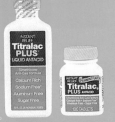

Available in Bar & Liquid
Dove®

3M
P. 579

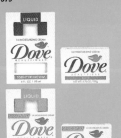

Antacid with Simethicone
Available in:
100 Tablets and 12 Fl. oz. liquid
Titralac™ Plus Antacid

3M
P. 579

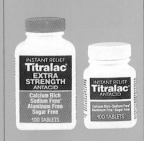

Available in: Regular Strength 40,
100, 1000 Tablets and Extra Strength
100 Tablets only
Titralac™ Antacid

McNeil Consumer Products
P. 580

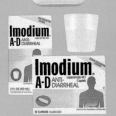

Available in 2, 3 and 4 fl. oz. bottles
with a convenient dosage cup, and
caplets in 6's, 12's and 18's
Imodium® A-D

**Lactaid Inc. Marked By
McNeil Consumer Products**
P. 571

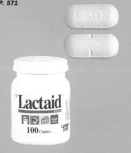

Caplets available in vials of 12 and
bottles of 50's and 100's
Lactaid® Caplets

**Lactaid Inc. Marked By
McNeil Consumer Products**
P. 572

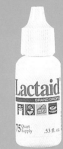

Available in 30 qt. and 75 qt. supply
Lactaid® Drops

McNeil Consumer Products
P. 580

Blister packs of 16
PediaCare® Cold-Allergy
Chewables

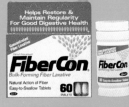

McNeil Consumer Products
P. 580

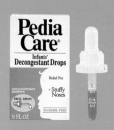

Available in 1/2 fl. oz. bottle with
child-resistant safety cap and
calibrated dropper

**PediaCare® Infants'
Decongestant Drops**

McNeil Consumer Products
P. 580

Pedia Care®
Cough-Cold
Chewables

Blister Packs of 16 Chewable Tablets
Liquid available in 4 fl. oz. bottle
with child-resistant safety cap and
convenient dosage cup

PediaCare® Cough-Cold

McNeil Consumer Products
P. 580

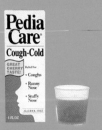

Available in 4 fl. oz. bottle with
child-resistant safety cap and
convenient dosage cup

**PediaCare® NightRest
Cough-Cold Liquid**

McNeil Consumer Products
P. 598

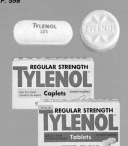

Tablets and Caplets available in:
24's, 50's, 100's and 200's

**Regular Strength
TYLENOL®**

McNeil Consumer Products
P. 589

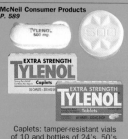

Caplets: tamper-resistant vials
of 10 and bottles of 24's, 50's,
100's, 175's and 250's

Tablets: tamper-resistant vials
of 10 and bottles of 30's,
60's, 100's and 200's

Liquid: tamper-resistant
bottles of 8 fl. oz.

Extra Strength TYLENOL®

McNeil Consumer Products
P. 589

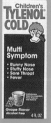

Geltabs available in tamper-resistant
bottles of 24's, 50's and 100's

Gelcaps available in tamper-resistant
bottles of 24's, 50's, 100's, 150's
and 225's

Extra Strength TYLENOL®

McNeil Consumer Products
P. 582

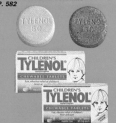

Fruit Flavor: bottles of 30 with
child-resistant safety cap and
blister-packs of 48

Grape Flavor: bottles of 30 with
child-resistant safety cap

**Children's TYLENOL®
80 mg Chewable Tablets**

McNeil Consumer Products
P. 582

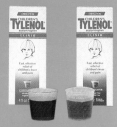

Available in cherry and grape flavors
in 2 and 4 fl. oz. bottles with
child-resistant safety cap and
convient dosage cup. Alcohol
Free, 80 mg. per 1/2 teaspoon

**Children's
TYLENOL® Elixir**

McNeil Consumer Products
P. 583

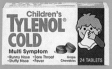

Available in bottles of 24 chewable
tablets with child-resistant safety cap

Children's TYLENOL® Cold

McNeil Consumer Products
P. 583

Multi-Symptom Formula
Available in 4 fl. oz. bottle with
child-resistant safety cap and
convenient dosage cup

**Children's TYLENOL®
Cold Liquid**

McNeil Consumer Products
P. 584

Multi-Symptom Plus Cough Formula
Available in 4 fl. oz. bottle with
child-resistant safety cap and
convenient dosage cup.

**Children's TYLENOL®
Cold Plus Cough Liquid**

McNeil Consumer Products
P. 582

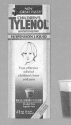

Available in rich cherry flavor in 2 and
4 fl. oz. bottles with child-resistant
safety cap and convenient dosage cup.
Alcohol Free, 80 mg per 1/2 teaspoon

**Children's TYLENOL®
Suspension Liquid**

McNeil Consumer Products
P. 582

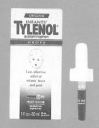

Available in 1/2 and 1 fl. oz. bottle
with child-resistant safety cap and calibrated dropper. Fruit Flavor, Alcohol
Free, 80 mg. per 0.8 mL

Infant's TYLENOL® Drops

McNeil Consumer Products
P. 582

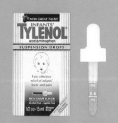

Available in 1/2 oz. bottle with child-
resistant safety cap and calibrated
dropper. Rich Grape Flavor, Alcohol
Free, 80 mg per 0.8 mL

**Infants' TYLENOL®
Suspension Drops**

McNeil Consumer Products
P. 591

Fruit Flavored Chewable tablets
available in blister pack of 24

**Junior Strength
TYLENOL®**

McNeil Consumer Products
P. 591

Swallowable Caplets: 160 mg
blister packs of 30
Chewable Tablets: 160 mg
grape flavor blister packs of 24

**Junior Strength
TYLENOL®**

McNeil Consumer Products
P. 590

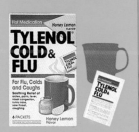

Available in cartons of 6 individual
packets. Hot Liquid Medication

TYLENOL® Cold & Flu

McNeil Consumer Products
P. 598

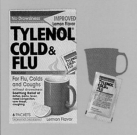

Available in cartons of 6 individual
packets. Hot Liquid Medication
No Drowiness Formula

TYLENOL® Cold & Flu

McNeil Consumer Products
P. 596

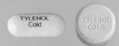

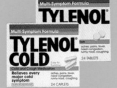

Caplets and Tablets available in
blister-packs of 24 and bottles of 50

**TYLENOL® Cold
Medication**

McNeil Consumer Products
P. 597

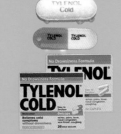

Tablets and Caplets available in
blister-packs of 24 and bottles of 50
No Drowsiness Formula

**TYLENOL® Cold
Medication**

McNeil Consumer Products
P. 585

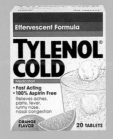

Available in cartons of 20
Effervescent Formula

**TYLENOL® Cold
Medication**

McNeil Consumer Products
P. 586

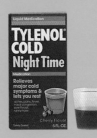

Liquid Medication available in 5 fl. oz.
bottle with child-resistant safety cap
and convenient dosage cup

TYLENOL® Cold NightTime

McNeil Consumer Products
P. 592

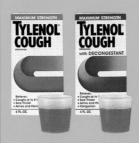

Available in 4 fl. oz. bottles

**Maximum Strength
TYLENOL® Cough**

McNeil Consumer Products
P. 594

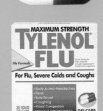

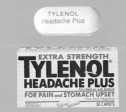

Blister packs of 10's, and 20's
No Drowsiness Formula

**Maximum Strength
TYLENOL® Flu**

McNeil Consumer Products
P. 587

Caplets available in 24's,
50's and 100's

TYLENOL® Headache Plus

McNeil Consumer Products
P. 588

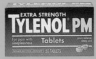

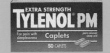

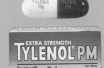

Tablets available in tamper-resistant
bottles of 24's and 50's
Caplets available in tamper-resistant
bottles of 24's, 50's and 100's
Gelcaps available in tamper-resistant
bottles of 20's and 40's

TYLENOL® PM

McNeil Consumer Products
P. 591

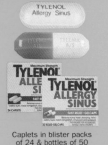

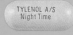

Caplets in blister packs
of 24 & bottles of 50
Gelcaps in blister packs
of 20 & bottles of 40

**Maximum Strength
TYLENOL® Allergy Sinus**

McNeil Consumer Products

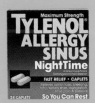

Caplets 24's

**Maximum Strength
TYLENOL® Allergy Sinus
NightTime**

McNeil Consumer Products
P. 582

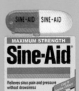

Tablets and Caplets in blister packs
of 24 & bottles of 50
Gelcaps in blister packs
of 20 & bottles of 40

**Maximum Strength
Sine-Aid®**

McNeil Consumer Products
P. 595

Caplets in blister packs
of 24 & bottles of 50
Gelcaps in blister packs
of 20 & bottles of 40

**Maximum Strength
TYLENOL® Sinus**

MILES

**Miles Inc.
Consumer Healthcare Products**
P. 600

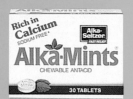

Chewable Antacid
Alka-Mints®

**Miles Inc.
Consumer Healthcare Products**
P. 600

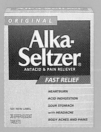

Effervescent Antacid & Pain Reliever
Alka-Seltzer®

**Miles Inc.
Consumer Healthcare Products**
P. 601

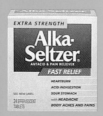

Extra Strength Effervescent
Antacid & Pain Reliever
Alka-Seltzer®

**Miles Inc.
Consumer Healthcare Products**
P. 602

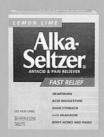

Lemon Lime Flavored Effervescent
Antacid & Pain Reliever
Alka-Seltzer®

**Miles Inc.
Consumer Healthcare Products**
P. 602

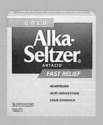

Effervescent Antacid
Alka-Seltzer® Gold

**Miles Inc.
Consumer Healthcare Products**
P. 604

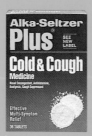

Cold & Cough Medicine
Nasal Decongestant Antihistamine
Analgesic Cough Suppressant
Alka-Seltzer Plus®

**Miles Inc.
Consumer Healthcare Products**
P. 603

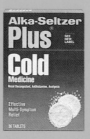

Cold Medicine Nasal Decongestant
Antihistamine Analgesic
Alka-Seltzer Plus®

**Miles Inc.
Consumer Healthcare Products**
P. 603

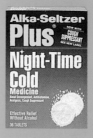

Night-Time Cold Medicine
Nasal Decongestant Antihistamine
Analgesic Cough Suppressant
Alka-Seltzer Plus®

**Miles Inc.
Consumer Healthcare Products**
P. 604

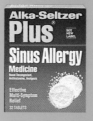

Sinus Allergy Medicine
Nasal Decongestant
Antihistamine Analgesic
Alka-Seltzer Plus®

**Miles Inc.
Consumer Healthcare Products**
P. 605

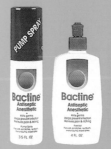

Antiseptic/Anesthetic
First Aid Spray and Liquid
Bactine®

**Miles Inc.
Consumer Healthcare Products**
P. 605

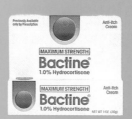

Anti-Itch Cream Maximum Strength
Bactine®

**Miles Inc.
Consumer Healthcare Products**
P. 605

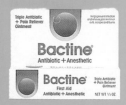

First Aid Antibiotic Ointment
Bactine®

**Miles Inc.
Consumer Healthcare Products**
P. 605

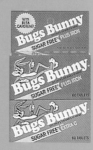

Sugar Free Children's Chewable
Vitamins with Extra C and Plus Iron
Bugs Bunny™

**Miles Inc.
Consumer Healthcare Products**
P. 606

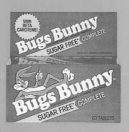

Sugar Free Children's Complete
Chewable Vitamines + Minerals
Bugs Bunny™

**Miles Inc.
Consumer Healthcare Products**
P. 607

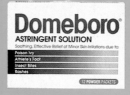

Astringent Solution
Also available:
100 Powder Packets and 12's &
100's Effervescent Tablets
Domeboro®

Miles Inc.
Consumer Healthcare Products
P. 606

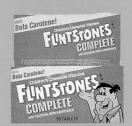

Complete Children's Chewable
Vitamins with Iron, Calcium & Minerals
Flintstones®

Miles Inc.
Consumer Healthcare Products
P. 605

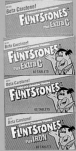

Children's Chewable Vitamins with
Extra C, Regular and Plus Iron
Flintstones®

Miles Inc.
Consumer Healthcare Products
P. 606

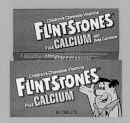

Children's Chewable Vitamins
Flintstones® Plus Calcium

Miles Inc.
Consumer Healthcare Products
P. 607

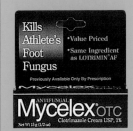

Also available: Mycelex OTC Solution
Kills Athlete's Foot Fungus
Mycelex® OTC

Miles Inc.
Consumer Healthcare Products
P. 608

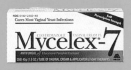

Clotrimazole (Antifungal)
Vaginal Cream 1%
Also available: Mycelex-7 Vaginal
Inserts 100 mg
Mycelex®-7

Miles Inc.
Consumer Healthcare Products
P. 607

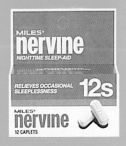

Nighttime Sleep-Aid
Nervine

Miles Inc.
Consumer Healthcare Products
P. 609

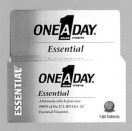

Essential Vitamins
One-A-Day® Essential

Miles Inc.
Consumer Healthcare Products
P. 609

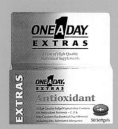

**One-A-Day®
Extras Antioxidant**

Miles Inc.
Consumer Healthcare Products
P. 609

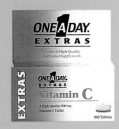

**One-A-Day®
Extras Vitamin C**

Miles Inc.
Consumer Healthcare Products
P. 609

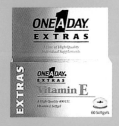

**One-A-Day® Extras
Vitamin E**

Miles Inc.
Consumer Healthcare Products
P. 609

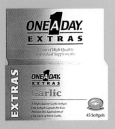

One-A-Day® Extras Garlic

Miles Inc.
Consumer Healthcare Products
P. 609

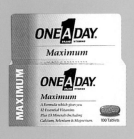

The Most Complete One-A-Day® Brand
One-A-Day® Maximum

Miles Inc.
Consumer Healthcare Products
P. 610

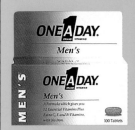

Multivitamin Supplement
One-A-Day® Men's

Miles Inc.
Consumer Healthcare Products
P. 610

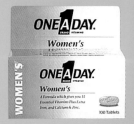

Multivitamin Supplement with
Extra Iron and Calcium Plus Zinc
One-A-Day® Women's

NATURE'S BOUNTY

Nature's Bounty
P. 612

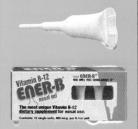

Vitamin B-12 Nasal Gel
Ener-B®

PARKE-DAVIS

Parke-Davis
P. 614

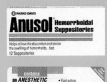

Suppositories available
in boxes of 12, 24 and 48
Ointment available in 1 oz. tubes
Anusol®

Parke-Davis
P. 615

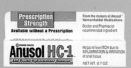

Anti-Pruritic Hydrocortisone Ointment
Anusol HC-1™

Parke-Davis
P. 618

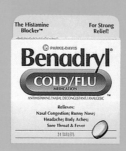

Available in boxes of 24 Tablets
Benadryl® Cold/Flu

Parke-Davis
P. 615

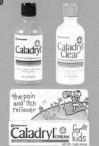

Children's Formula & Maximum Strength
Topical Antihistamine
**Benadryl® Itch
Relief Cream**

Parke-Davis
P. 619

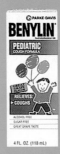

Available in 4 oz. bottles
Benylin® Pediatric

Parke-Davis
P. 617

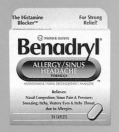

Available in boxes of 24 Caplets
**Benadryl® Allergy
Sinus Headache**

Parke-Davis
P. 616

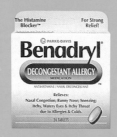

Available in boxes of 24 Tablets
**Benadryl®
Decongestant Allergy**

Parke-Davis
P. 618

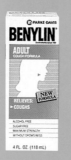

Available in 4 oz. bottles
Benylin® Adult

Parke-Davis
P. 620

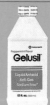

Itch Relief Plus Drying Action.
Available in Lotion, Clear Lotion
and Cream for Kids
Caladryl®

Parke-Davis
P. 617

Kapseals and Tablets
Available in boxes of 24 and 48
Benadryl® Allergy

Parke-Davis
P. 616

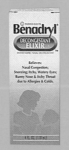

Available in 4 oz. bottles
**Benadryl®
Decongestant Elixir**

Parke-Davis
P. 620

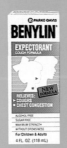

Available in 4 oz. bottles
Benylin® Expectorant

Parke-Davis
P. 620

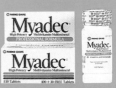

Antacid-Anti-gas Sodium Free
Available in boxes of 100 and as
a liquid in 12 Fl. oz. bottles
Gelusil®

Parke-Davis
P. 618

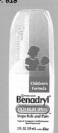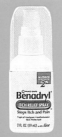

Children's Formula & Maximum Strength
Topical Antihistamine
**Benadryl® Itch
Relief Spray**

Parke-Davis
P. 616

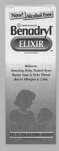

Available in 4 oz. and 8 oz. bottles
Benadryl® Elixir

Parke-Davis
P. 619

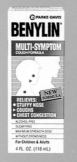

Available in 4 oz. bottles
Benylin® Multi-Symptom

Parke-Davis
P. 621

Multivitamin/Multimineral Supplement
Available in bottles of 130 Tablets
Myadec®

Parke-Davis
P. 621

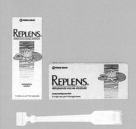

Vaginal Moisturizer
Available in boxes of 3 and 8
single-use applicators
Replens®

Parke-Davis
P. 621

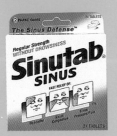

Regular Strength
Without Drowsiness Formula
Sinutab® Sinus

Parke-Davis
P. 622

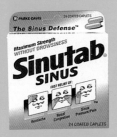

Maximum Strength
Without Drowsiness Formula
Available in Caplets or Tablets
Sinutab® Sinus

Parke-Davis
P. 622

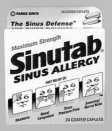

Maximum Strength Formula
Available in Caplets or Tablets
Sinutab® Sinus Allergy

Parke-Davis
P. 623

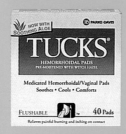

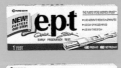

Pre-Moistened Pads
Available in 40 and 100 pad packages
Tucks®

Parke-Davis
P. 767

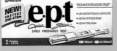

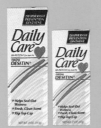

1 and 2 Test Kits Available
One Step. Easy to read.
Lab Accurate results.
e.p.t® Quick Stick®

Pfizer Consumer Health Care
P. 624

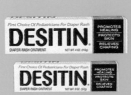

Diaper Rash Prevention Ointment
**Daily Care™
from DESITIN®**

Pfizer Consumer Health Care
P. 624

DESITIN®

Diaper Rash Ointment
DESITIN®

Pfizer Consumer Health Care
P. 626

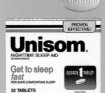

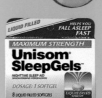

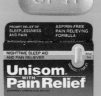

MAXIMUM STRENGTH
**Unisom®
SleepGels**
NIGHTTIME SLEEP AID
DOSAGE: 1 SOFTGEL
8 LIQUID FILLED SOFTGELS

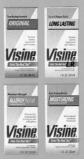

**Unisom
with
Pain Relief**
8 TABLETS

Unisom®

Pfizer Consumer Health Care
P. 627

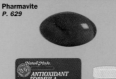

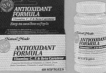

Original, Long Lasting,
Allergy Relief and Moisturizing
Visine®

Pharmavite
P. 629

Vitamins C, E and Beta Carotene
Package of 60 Softgels
**Nature Made®
Antioxidant Formula**

Pharmavite
P. 629

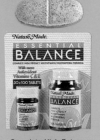

Complete High Potency
Multivitamin Multimineral
Bottles of 100 + 30
**Nature Made®
Essential Balance®**

Reed & Carnrick
P. 646

Available in bottles of 50's and 100's
An antiflatulent to alleviate or relieve
the symptoms of gas.
Phazyme® 95
(95 mg simethicone)

Reed & Carnrick
P. 646

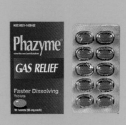

95 mg Coated Tablet
New Fast Dissolving Formula
Available in Packs of 10
Phazyme® 95
(95 mg simethicone)

Reed & Carnrick
P. 647

Maximum Strength 125 mg
Available in bottles of 50's
An antiflatulent to alleviate or relieve
the symptoms of gas.
Phazyme® 125
(125 mg simethicone)

Reed & Carnrick
P. 647

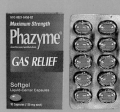

125 mg Softgel Capsule
Easy To Swallow
Available in Packs of 10
Phazyme® 125
(125 mg simethicone)

Reed & Carnrick
P. 647

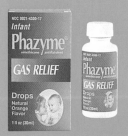

125 mg chewable tablet
Fresh mint taste
Packs of 10's and 50's
Phazyme® Chewables
(125 mg simethicone)

Reed & Carnrick
P. 647

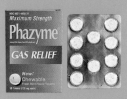

Available in 1 oz. and 1/2 oz. bottles
A liquid antiflatulent suitable for
relieving infant gas symptoms and for
those who prefer liquid dosage forms.
Phazyme® Drops

REESE

Reese Chemical Co.
P. 647

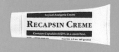
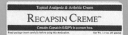

Topical Analgesic & Arthritic Cream
0.025% Capsaicin
with English & Spanish Instructions
1.5 oz (45 grams)
Recapsin Creme™

RHÔNE-POULENC RORER

Rhône-Poulenc Rorer Consumer Division
P. 649

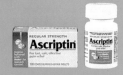

Bottles of 60, 100, 160,
225 & 500 Tablets
**Regular Strength
Ascriptin®**

Rhône-Poulenc Rorer Consumer Division
P. 650

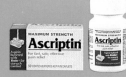

Bottles of 36, 50 & 85 Caplets
**Maximum Strength
Ascriptin®**

Rhône-Poulenc Rorer Consumer Division
P. 650

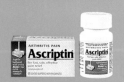

Bottles of 60, 100,
225 & 500 Caplets
**Arthritis Pain
Ascriptin®**

Rhône-Poulenc Rorer Consumer Division
P. 651

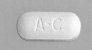
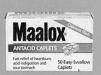

Blister Packs of 24's and Bottles of
50's Antacid Caplets
Maalox® Antacid Caplets

Rhône-Poulenc Rorer Consumer Division
P. 651

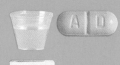
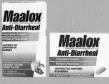

Available in 2 oz. and 4 oz. liquid
(cherry flavored) w/dosage cup
6 and 12 Caplets
Maalox® Anti-Diarrheal

Rhône-Poulenc Rorer Consumer Division
P. 654

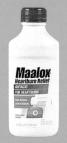
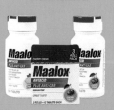

10 oz. Cool Mint Flavor Liquid
**Maalox®
Heartburn Relief®**

Rhône-Poulenc Rorer Consumer Division
P. 655

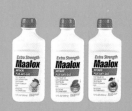

Lemon Creme & Cherry Creme Flavors
3 Roll Pack 50 & 100 Tablets
**Maalox® Antacid
Plus Anti-Gas**

Rhône-Poulenc Rorer Consumer Division
P. 655

Mint Creme, Cherry Creme and Lemon
Creme All available in 12 & 26 oz.
**Extra Strength Maalox®
Plus Anti-Gas**

Rhône-Poulenc Rorer Consumer Division
P. 655

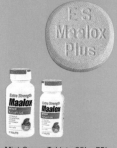

Mint Creme Tablets 38's, 75's
**Extra Strength Maalox®
Antacid Plus Anti-Gas**

Rhône-Poulenc Rorer Consumer Division
P. 654

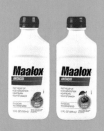

Mint & Cherry Creme
Available in 12 & 26 oz.
Maalox® Antacid

Rhône-Poulenc Rorer Consumer Division
P. 652

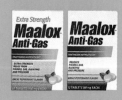

Regular Strength 12's & 48's
Extra Strength 10's
Maalox® Anti-Gas

Rhône-Poulenc Rorer Consumer Division
P. 653

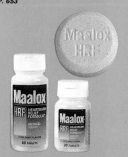

Heartburn Relief Formula Cool Mint
Bottles of 30 and 60 Tablets
Maalox® HRF

Rhône-Poulenc Rorer Consumer Division
P. 652

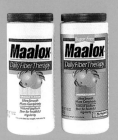

Orange and Citrus Flavors
Bulk-Producing Psyllium Fiber
Regular & Sugar Free
**Maalox® Daily
Fiber Therapy**

Rhône-Poulenc Rorer Consumer Division
P. 656

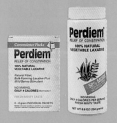

100% Natural Vegetable Laxative
100 mg and 250 mg
6-6gm packets and 20-6gm packets
Perdiem®

Rhône-Poulenc Rorer Consumer Division
P. 657

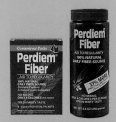

100% Natural
Daily Fiber Source
100 gm and 250 gm
6-6gm packets and 20-6gm packets
Perdiem® Fiber

ROBERTS

Roberts Pharmaceutical Corp.
P. 658

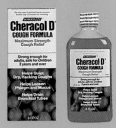

2 oz., 4 oz., 6 oz. Cough Formula
Also available in Cheracol Plus
Head Cold/Cough Formula 4 oz., 6 oz.
Cheracol D®

Roberts Pharmaceutical Corp.
P. 659

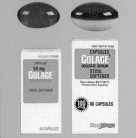

Stool softener – 50mg/100mg
100 mg available: Two tone color 30, 250
50 mg available: 30, 60, 250
Available in Liquid and Syrup
Colace®

Roberts Pharmaceutical Corp.
P. 660

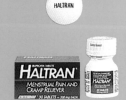

Bottles of 30 200 mg Tablets
Haltran®

Roberts Pharmaceutical Corp.
P. 661

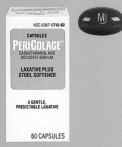

Bottles of 30, 1000
Laxative and Stool Softener
Available in Syrup
Peri-Colace®

Roberts Pharmaceutical Corp.
P. 661

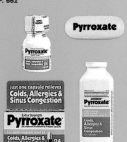

Nasal Decongestant/
Antihistamine/Analgesic
Bottles of 24 and 500 Caplets
Pyrroxate®

Roberts Pharmaceutical Corp.
P. 662

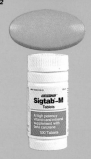

Bottles of 100 Tablets
High Potency Vitamin Supplement
Also Available in Sigtab
Sigtab®-M

A.H. ROBINS

A.H. Robins
P. 663

Extentabs® in: 12's, 24's,
48's, 100's and 500's
Grape Elixir in: 4 oz., 8 oz.,
12 oz., 16 oz. and 128 oz.
Dimetapp®

A.H. Robins
P. 666

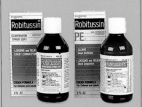

Original and PE
Robitussin® Syrup

A.H. Robins
P. 666

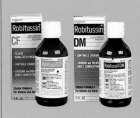

CF and DM
Robitussin® Syrup

A.H. Robins
P. 665

Severe Congestion and Cough & Cold
Available in: 12's and 20's
**Robitussin®
Liqui-Gels®**

ROSS

Ross Products
P. 669

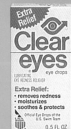

Lubricating Eye Redness Reliever
Eye Drops
Available in: 0.5 and 1.0 Fl. oz.
Clear Eyes®

Ross Products
P. 670

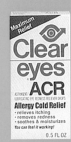

Astringent/Lubricating
Eye Redness Reliever Drops
Available in: 0.5 and 1.0 Fl. oz.
Clear Eyes® ACR

Ross Products
P. 670

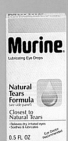

Lubricating Eye Drops
Natural Tears Formula
Closest to Natural Tears
Available in: 0.5 and 1.0 Fl. oz.
Murine®

Ross Products
P. 671

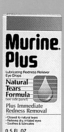

Lubricating Redness Reliever Eye Drops
Natural Tears Formula
Closest to Natural Tears
Available in: 0.5 and 1.0 Fl. oz.
Murine® Plus

Ross Products
P. 670

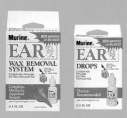

Ear Wax Removal System
and Ear Drops
Murine®

Ross Products
P. 671

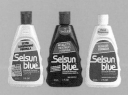

Extra Conditioning, Regular, Medicated
Treatment Dandruff Shampoo
Available in: 4, 7 and 11 Fl. oz.
Selsun Blue®

Ross Products
P. 672

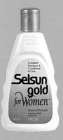

Dandruff Shampoo
Available in: 4, 7 and 11 Fl. oz.
Selsun Gold for Women®

Ross Products
P. 672

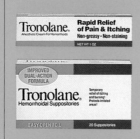

Hemorrhoidal Cream and Suppositories
Available in: Cream 1 and 2 oz. tubes;
Suppositories 10's and 20's
Tronolane®

RYDELLE

Rydelle Laboratories
P. 673

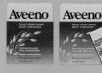

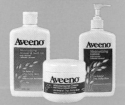

Bath Treatment: Regular and Dry Skin.
Cleansing Bar: For Combination
Skin, Dry and Acne.
Moisturizing: Cream and Lotion.
Shower & Bath Oil.
All With Colloidal Oatmeal For the
Relief of Dry, Itchy Skin
Aveeno®

Rydelle Laboratories
P. 673

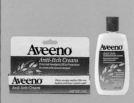

Anti-Itch Cream and Concentrated
Lotion External Analgesic Skin
Protectant Enriched with Oatmeal
Aveeno®

Rydelle Laboratories
P. 674

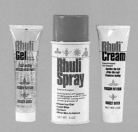

4 oz. Spray, 2 oz. Cream, 2 oz. Gel
Fast Cooling Relief of Itching
Rhuli®

SANDOZ

Sandoz Consumer Division
P. 674

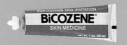
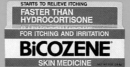

Cream 1 oz. (28.4 g)
Bicozene®

Sandoz Consumer Division
P. 675

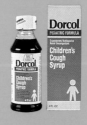

Children's Cough Syrup 4 oz., 8 oz.
Dorcol®

Sandoz Consumer Division
P. 676

Chocolated Laxative
Tablets 18's, 48's and 72's
Ex-lax®

Sandoz Consumer Division
P. 676

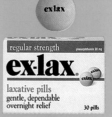
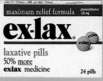

Regular Strength 8's, 30's, 60's
Maximum Relief Formula 24's, 48's
Extra Gentle 24's
Gentle Nature™ 16's
Ex-lax®

Sandoz Consumer Division
P. 677

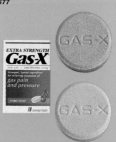

Extra-Strength Cherry 18's, 48's
Extra-Strength Peppermint 18's, 48's
(125 mg simethicone)
Gas-X®

Sandoz Consumer Division
P. 677

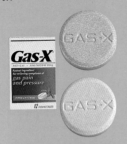

Cherry 12's, 36's
Peppermint 12's, 36's
(80 mg simethicone)
Gas-X®

Sandoz Consumer Division
P. 677

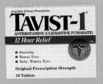

8's, 16's, 32's
Tavist-1®

Sandoz Consumer Division
P. 677

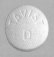

8's, 16's, 32's, 50's
Tavist-D®

Sandoz Consumer Division
P. 682

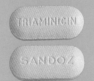

12's, 24's, 48's, 100's
Triaminicin®

Sandoz Consumer Division
P. 677

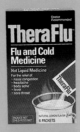

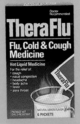

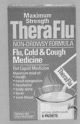

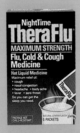

Flu and Cold Medicine
Flu, Cold & Cough Medicine
Maximum Strength Nighttime Flu,
Cold & Cough Medicine
Maximum Strength, Non-Drowsy Flu,
Cold & Cough Medicine
All available in 6's & 12's
TheraFlu®

Sandoz Consumer Division
P. 681

Sustained Release 10's, 20's
Triaminic-12®

Sandoz Consumer Division
P. 679

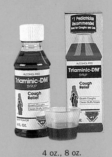

24's
Triaminic® Cold Tablets

Sandoz Consumer Division
P. 681

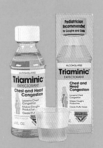

4 oz., 8 oz.
**Triaminic-DM®
Cough Relief**

Sandoz Consumer Division
P. 680

4 oz., 8 oz.
Triaminic® Expectorant

Sandoz Consumer Division
P. 680

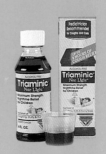

4 oz., 8 oz.
Triaminic® Nite Light®

Sandoz Consumer Division
P. 680

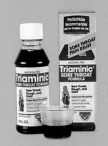

4 oz., 8 oz.
**Triaminic®
Sore Throat Formula**

Sandoz Consumer Division
P. 681

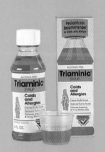

4 oz., 8 oz.
Triaminic® Syrup

Sandoz Consumer Division
P. 682

24's
**Triaminicol®
Multi-Symptom
Cold Tablets**

Sandoz Consumer Division
P. 682

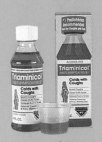

4 oz., 8 oz.
**Triaminicol®
Multi-Symptom Relief**

SCHERING-PLOUGH

Schering-Plough HealthCare
P. 686

Regular and Medicated
A and D® Ointment

Schering-Plough HealthCare
P. 686

Regular and Children's 12 Hour
Safety Sealed
Afrin® Nose Drops

Schering-Plough HealthCare
P. 687

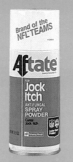

Also available in 1.5 oz.
shaker powder and 0.5 oz. gel
Aftate® for Jock Itch

Schering-Plough HealthCare
P. 687

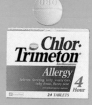

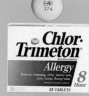

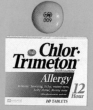

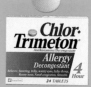

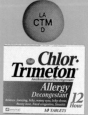

4 Hour Allergy Tablets
8 Hour Allergy Tablets
12 Hour Allergy Tablets
4 Hour Allergy Decongestant Tablets
12 Hour Allergy Decongestant Tablets
6 Hour Allergy Sinus Headache Tablets
Chlor-Trimeton®

Schering-Plough HealthCare
P. 686

Extra-Moisturizing 12 Hour
Afrin® Extra
Moisturizing Nasal Spray

Schering-Plough HealthCare
P. 687

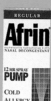

Non Medicated
Safety Sealed
Afrin® Saline Mist

Schering-Plough HealthCare
P. 688

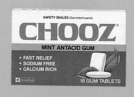

16 Antacid Gum Tablets
Chooz®

Schering-Plough HealthCare
P. 686

Regular 12 Hour
Safety Sealed
Afrin® Nasal Spray

Schering-Plough HealthCare
P. 686

Regular 12 Hour
Safety Sealed
Afrin® Spray Pump

Schering-Plough HealthCare
P. 688

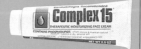

Phospholipid Therapeutic Moisturizing
Face Cream and Lotion
Complex 15®

Schering-Plough HealthCare
P. 686

Cherry Scented and Menthol 12 Hour
Safety Sealed
Afrin® Nasal Spray

Schering-Plough HealthCare
P. 687

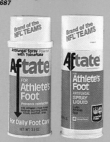

Also available in:
2.25 oz. shaker powder
and 0.5 oz. gel
Aftate®
for Athlete's Foot

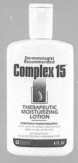

Schering-Plough HealthCare
P. 689

For Relief Of Cold & Flu Symptoms
Coricidin®

Schering-Plough HealthCare
P. 689

For Relief Of Cold, Flu
& Sinus Symptoms
Coricidin-D®

Schering-Plough HealthCare
P. 690

Laxative Tablets and Capsules
and Stool Softener Soft Gels
Correctol®

Schering-Plough HealthCare
P. 690

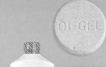

Liquid and Tablets
Mint, Lemon and Orange Flavors
6 fl. oz. liquid plus
30 and 90 tablets sizes.
Di-Gel®

Schering-Plough HealthCare
P. 690

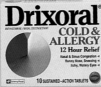

12 Hour Sustained-Action Tablets
**Drixoral®
Cold & Allergy**

Schering-Plough HealthCare
P. 691

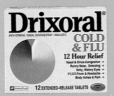

12 Hour Extended-Release Tablets
Drixoral® Cold & Flu

Schering-Plough HealthCare
P. 690

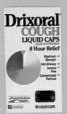

8 Hour Liquid Caps
Drixoral® Cough

Schering-Plough HealthCare
P. 691

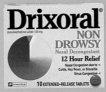

12 Hour
Extended-Release Tablets
Drixoral® Non-Drowsy

Schering-Plough HealthCare
P. 692

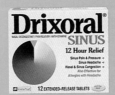

12 Hour Extended-Release Tablets
Drixoral® Sinus

Schering-Plough HealthCare
P. 692

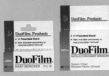

Wart Remover
and Plantar War Remover
DuoFilm®/DuoPlant®

Schering-Plough HealthCare
P. 693

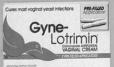

Nasal Spray and Pump
Available in 1/2 oz., 1 oz. and 1/2 oz.
measured dosage pump spray
Duration®

Schering-Plough HealthCare
P. 693

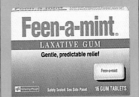

Laxative gum
Also available in Laxative
plus softener pills
Feen-a-mint®

Schering-Plough HealthCare
P. 693

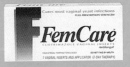

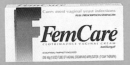

Antifungal Inserts and Cream
FemCare™

Schering-Plough HealthCare
P. 694

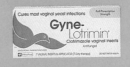

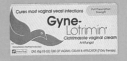

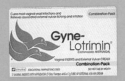

Clotrimazole Vaginal Antifungal
Inserts, Cream, Combination-Pack
and Pre-filled Applicators
Gyne-Lotrimin®

Schering-Plough HealthCare
P. 695

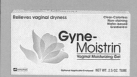

Vaginal Moisturizing Gel
Relieves Vaginal Dryness
Available in 1.5 and 2.5 oz. sizes

Gyne-Moistrin™

Schering-Plough HealthCare
P. 695

Antifungal for Athlete's Foot
and Jock Itch

Lotrimin® AF

Schering-Plough HealthCare
P. 696

Also available:
SPF 15 Gel, SPF 30 Lotion and Stick

Shade® Sunblock

Schering-Plough HealthCare
P. 697

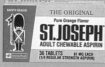

**St. Joseph®
Adult Chewable Asprin**

Schering-Plough HealthCare
P. 698

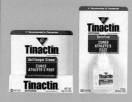

Cream and Solution for Athlete's Foot

Tinactin®

Schering-Plough HealthCare
P. 698

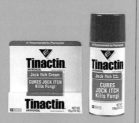

Cream and Spray Powder for Jock Itch

Tinactin®

Schering-Plough HealthCare
P. 698

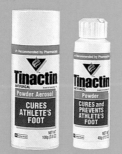

Powder Aerosol and Powder for
Athlete's Foot

Tinactin®

Schering-Plough HealthCare
P. 698

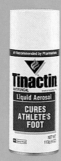

Liquid Aerosol for Athlete's Foot

Tinactin®

**SmithKline Beecham
Consumer HealthCare, L.P.**
P. 699

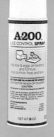
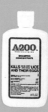

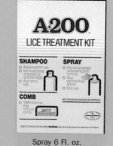

Spray 6 Fl. oz.
Pediculicide Shampoo
Special Comb Included
Also available: A-200® Shampoo 2 Fl. oz.
and Gel Concentrate 1 oz.
Lice Treatment Kit
Includes Shampoo, Spray & Comb

A-200®

**SmithKline Beecham
Consumer HealthCare, L.P.**
P. 700

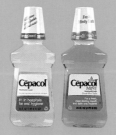

Gold and Mint
Mouthwash/Gargle
Available in 4, 12, 18, 24
and 32 Fl. oz. bottles

Cepacol®

**SmithKline Beecham
Consumer HealthCare, L.P.**
P. 701

Anesthetic Lozenges
18 lozenges per pack

Cepacol®

**SmithKline Beecham
Consumer HealthCare, L.P.**
P. 700

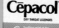

Dry Throat Lozenges
Original, Honey Lemon,
Cherry and Menthol Flavor
18 lozenges per pack

Cepacol®

**SmithKline Beecham
Consumer HealthCare, L.P.**
P. 701

Sore Throat Lozenges
Extra Strength and Cherry
18 lozenges per package

Cepastat®

**SmithKline Beecham
Consumer HealthCare, L.P.**
P. 701

Fiber Therapy for Regularity
Sugar Free Orange available in:
8.6 oz. and 16.9 oz.
Regular Orange available in:
16 oz. and 30 oz. containers

Citrucel®

SmithKline Beecham
Consumer HealthCare, L.P.
P. 702

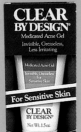

Medicated Acne Gel
1.5 oz. tube
Clear By Design®

SmithKline Beecham
Consumer HealthCare, L.P.
P. 704

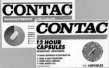

Continuous Action
Nasal Decongestant Antihistamine
Packages of 10, 20 and 40
capsules and caplets
Contact® 12 Hour

SmithKline Beecham
Consumer HealthCare, L.P.
P. 702

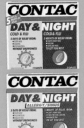

Contact® Day & Night
Cold & Flu and
Allergy/Sinus

SmithKline Beecham
Consumer HealthCare, L.P.
P. 705

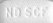

Non-Drowsy Formula
Packages of 16 and 30 caplets
**Contact® Severe
Cold & Flu**

SmithKline Beecham
Consumer HealthCare, L.P.
P. 706

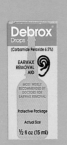
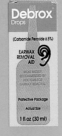

Drops
1/2 Fl. oz. 1 Fl. oz.
Debrox®

SmithKline Beecham
Consumer HealthCare, L.P.
P. 706

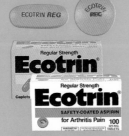

Regular Strength Tablets
in bottles of 100, 250, 500 and
1000 and Caplets in bottles of 100
Ecotrin®

SmithKline Beecham
Consumer HealthCare, L.P.
P. 706

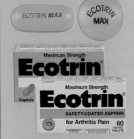

Maximum Strength Tablets
in bottles of 60, 150 and 300 and
Caplets in bottles of 100
Ecotrin®

SmithKline Beecham
Consumer HealthCare, L.P.
P. 708

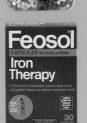

Packages of 30 and 60 capsules
Feosol®

SmithKline Beecham
Consumer HealthCare, L.P.
P. 709

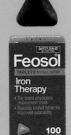

Bottles of 100 and 1000 tablets
Feosol®

SmithKline Beecham
Consumer HealthCare, L.P.
P. 709

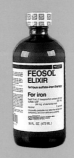

16 oz. bottle
Feosol® Elixir

SmithKline Beecham
Consumer HealthCare, L.P.
P. 709

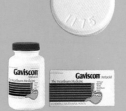

100-Tablet bottles
30-Tablet box (foil-wrapped 2s)
Gaviscon® Antacid

SmithKline Beecham
Consumer HealthCare, L.P.
P. 710

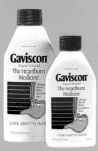

12 Fl. oz. 6 Fl. oz.
Gaviscon® Liquid Antacid

SmithKline Beecham
Consumer HealthCare, L.P.
P. 710

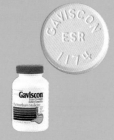

Extra Strength Relief Formula
100-Tablet bottles
**Gaviscon® Extra
Strength Antacid**

SmithKline Beecham Consumer
HealthCare, L.P.
P. 710

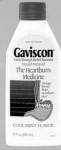

Extra Strength Relief Formula
**Gaviscon® Extra Strength
Liquid Antacid**

SmithKline Beecham
Consumer HealthCare, L.P.
P. 710

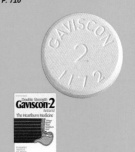

Box of 48 foil-wrapped tablets
Gaviscon®-2 Antacid

SmithKline Beecham
Consumer HealthCare, L.P.
P. 711

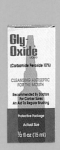
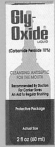

1/2 Fl. oz. 2 Fl. oz.
Gly-Oxide® Liquid

SmithKline Beecham
Consumer HealthCare, L.P.
P. 713

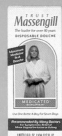

Medicated Disposable Douche
With Povidone-iodine
Available in single or twin packs
Massengill®

SmithKline Beecham
Consumer HealthCare, L.P.
P. 716

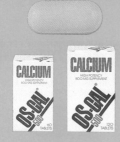

Bottles of 60 and 120 tablets
Os-Cal® 500

SmithKline Beecham
Consumer HealthCare, L.P.
P. 717

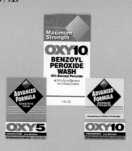

Acne Medication and
Benzoyl Peroxide Wash
Oxy5® and Oxy10®

SmithKline Beecham
Consumer HealthCare, L.P.
P. 720

Timed-Release Capsules
Packages of 12, 24 and 48 capsules
Teldrin®

SmithKline Beecham
Consumer HealthCare, L.P.
P. 713

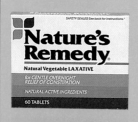

Laxative tablets available in:
boxes of 12's and 30's
Nature's Remedy®

SmithKline Beecham
Consumer HealthCare, L.P.
P. 716

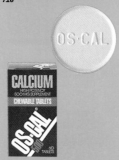

Bottle of 60 tablets
Os-Cal® 500 Chewable

SmithKline Beecham
Consumer HealthCare, L.P.
P. 717

Maximum Strength
No Drowsiness Formula Caplets
Sine®-Off

SmithKline Beecham
Consumer HealthCare, L.P.
P. 720

Throat Lozenges Box of 60
Throat Discs®

SmithKline Beecham
Consumer HealthCare, L.P.
P. 714

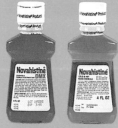

Cough/Cold Formula & Decongestant
and Cold & Hay Fever Formula
**Novahistine®
DMX & Elixir**

SmithKline Beecham
Consumer HealthCare, L.P.
P. 716

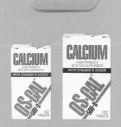

Bottles of 60 tablets
Os-Cal® 500+D

SmithKline Beecham
Consumer HealthCare, L.P.
P. 718

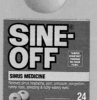

Regular Strength
Packages of 24, 48 and 100 Tablets
Sine®-Off

SmithKline Beecham
Consumer HealthCare, L.P.
P. 720

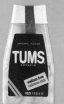
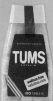

Original and
Assorted Flavors
Tums®

SmithKline Beecham
Consumer HealthCare, L.P.
P. 716

Bottles of 100 and 240 tablets
Os-Cal® 250+D

SmithKline Beecham Consumer
HealthCare, L.P.
P. 716

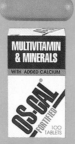

Multivitamin and Minerals
With Added Calcium
Bottles of 100 tablets
Os-Cal® Fortified

SmithKline Beecham
Consumer HealthCare, L.P.
P. 719

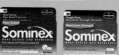

Night-Time Sleep Aids
Original Tablets, Maximum Strength
Caplets, Pain Relief Tablets
Sominex®

SmithKline Beecham Consumer
HealthCare, L.P.
P. 720

Peppermint, Cherry,
Wintergreen and Assorted Flavors
Tums E-X®

**SmithKline Beecham
Consumer HealthCare, L.P.**
P. 721

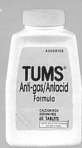

60 Tablets
Assorted Flavors
Tums® Anti-gas/Antacid

While every effort has been made to reproduce products faithfully, this section is to be considered a Quick-Reference identification aid.

For more detailed information on the products illustrated in this section, consult the Product Information Section or manufacturers may be contacted directly.

STERLING HEALTH

Sterling Health
P. 726

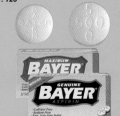

Genuine 325 mg, Maximum 500 mg
Toleraid® Micro-Thin Coating
Sodium Free and Caffeine Free
BAYER® Aspirin

Sterling Health
P. 726

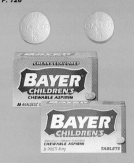

36's
Chewable Aspirin
BAYER® Children's

Sterling Health
P. 729

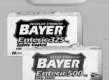

Regular 325 mg
Extra Strength 500 mg
Delayed Release Enteric Aspirin
Sodium Free and Caffeine Free
BAYER® Enteric

Sterling Health
P. 729

120's
Adult Low Strength 81 mg.
Delayed Release Enteric Aspirin
BAYER® Enteric

Sterling Health
P. 725

24's, 50's, 100's,
Effective Pain Relief
Plus Stomach Protection
Coated For Easy Swallowing.
BAYER® Buffered

Sterling Health
P. 732

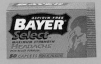

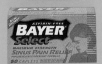
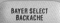
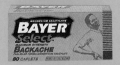

Headache 24's, 50's, 100's
Menstrual 24's, 50's
Night Time Pain Relief 24's, 50's
Pain Relief 24's, 50's, 100's
Sinus Pain Relief 24's, 50's
Backache 24's, 50's
**Aspirin-Free
Maximum Strength
BAYER® Select®**

Sterling Health
P. 731

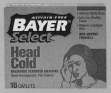

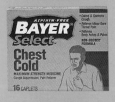
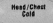
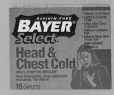

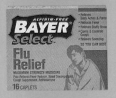
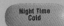
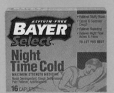

Head Cold 16's
Chest Cold 16's
Head & Chest Cold 16's
Flu Relief 16's
Night Time Cold 16's
**Aspirin-Free
Maximum Strength
BAYER® Select®**

Sterling Health
P. 731

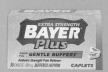

30's, 60's
Aspirin Plus Gentle Buffers
Extra Strength Pain Relief plus
Stomach Protection

**Extra Strength
BAYER® Plus**

Sterling Health
P. 734

Mist and Tablets
Asthma Remedy
Available in 15 cc Inhaler Units
and 15cc and 22.5 cc Refills
Tablets: 24's, 60's

Bronkaid®

Sterling Health
P. 736

Maximum Strength
First Aid Antibiotic Pain Reliever
Ointment 5 oz tube
and Cold Sore Gel .23 oz, .5 oz

Campho-phenique®

Sterling Health
P. 736

Pain Relieving Antiseptic Gel & Liquid

Campho-phenique®

Sterling Health
P. 740

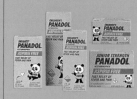

Chewable Tablets, Caplets,
Liquid and Drops

Children's Panadol®
(acetaminophan)

Sterling Health
P. 736

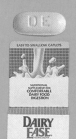

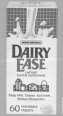
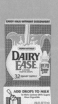

Caplets: 40's
Tablets: 12's, 36's, 60's and 100's
Drops: 32 quart size

Dairy Ease®

Sterling Health
P. 737

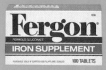

100's
Ferrous Gluconate
Iron Supplement

Fergon®

Sterling Health
P. 737

Cramp Relief Formula 24's, 50's
Maximum Strength 8's, 16's, 32's
PMS 8's, 16's, 32's
Teen 16's, 32's

Midol®

Sterling Health
P. 739

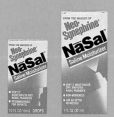

15 mL and 30 mL
Nasal Moisturizer Spray and Drops

NaSal®

Sterling Health
P. 739

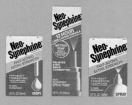

Nasal Decongestant Drops, Spray
Pump or Spray Bottle

Neo-Synephrine®

Sterling Health
P. 741

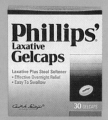

Laxative Plus Stool Softener
Also available in 60 gelcaps

Phillips'® Gelcaps

Sterling Health
P. 741

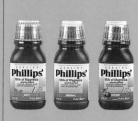

Available in mint, original,
and cherry flavors
4 oz, 12 oz, and 16 oz plastic bottles

**Phillips'®
Milk of Magnesia**

Sterling Health
P. 742

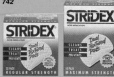

32's
Regular, Maximum,
Sensitive Skin with Aloe and
Super Scrub Oil Fighting Formulas

Stri-Dex®

Sterling Health
P. 741

Maximum Strength Clear Gel 1 oz
Acne Medicated and Anti-Bacterial
Cleansing Bar with Glycerin 3.5 oz

Stri-Dex®

Sterling Health
P. 742

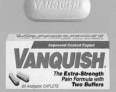

30's, 60's and 100's
Extra-Strength Pain Formula
with Two Buffers
Vanquish®

THOMPSON

Thompson Medical Co., Inc.
P. 743

Available in 1 oz. and 2 oz. creme
and 1 oz. ointment
Kids available in 1/2 oz.
and 1 oz. creme
Cortizone-5®

Thompson Medical Co., Inc.
P. 743

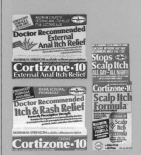

Creme: 1 oz., 2 oz. Ointment: 1 oz.
Liquid: 1.5 fl. oz. Creme with Aloe: 1 oz.
Cortizone-10™

Thompson Medical Co., Inc.
P. 744

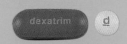
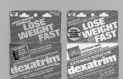

Available in 10, 20, and 40 caplet sizes
also in 20 and 40 tablet sizes.
**Maximum
Strength Dexatrim®**

Thompson Medical Co., Inc.
P. 745

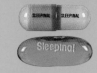

Available in 16 and 32
Softgel and Capsule sizes
Sleepinal®

Thompson Medical Co., Inc.
P. 745

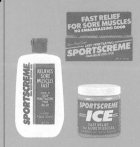

External Analgesic
Available in 1 1/4 oz., 3 oz. and
5 oz. creme; 6 oz. lotion; 8 oz. ice
Sportscreme®

Thompson Medical Co., Inc.
P. 745

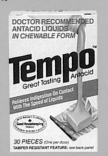

Soft Antacid
Available in 10, 30 and 60 tablet sizes
Tempo®

WAKUNAGA

Wakunaga
P. 746

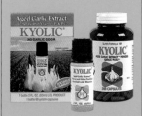

Aged Garlic Extract® with B1 and B12
Super Formula 101-Capsules
Kyolic®

WALLACE

Wallace Laboratories
P. 746

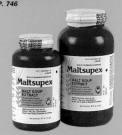

8 Fl. oz. (1/2 pt) and 16 Fl. oz. (1 pt)
Maltsupex® Liquid
(malt soup extract)

Wallace Laboratories
P. 746

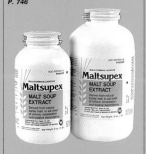

8 oz. (1/2 lb) and 16 oz. (1 lb)
Maltsupex® Powder
(malt soup extract)

Wallace Laboratories
P. 746

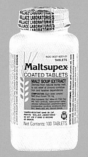

100 Tablets
Maltsupex® Tablets
(malt soup extract)

Wallace Laboratories
P. 748

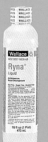

1 Pint (473 mL)
Also available: 4 Fl. oz. (118 mL)
Ryna® Liquid
(antihistamine/decongestant

Wallace Laboratories
P. 748

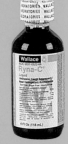

1 Pint (473 mL)
Also available: 4 Fl. oz. (118 mL)
Ryna-C® Liquid
(antitussive/antihistamine/
decongestant)

Wallace Laboratories
P. 748

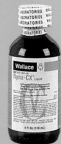

1 Pint (473 mL)
Also available: 4 Fl. oz. (118 mL)
Ryna-CX® Liquid
(antitussive/decongestant/
expectorant)

Wallace Laboratories
P. 748

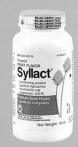

Syllact®
(powdered psyllium seed husks)

WARNER-LAMBERT

Warner-Lambert Co.
P. 749

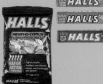

Cough Suppressant Tablets
Spearmint, Mentho-Lyptus, Ice Blue,
Honey-Lemon and Cherry Flavors
Halls® Mentho-Lyptus

Warner-Lambert Co.
P. 749

Cough Suppressant Tablets with
Soothing Syrup Centers
Honey-Lemon, Mentho-Lyptus and Cherry

**Maximum Strength
Halls® Plus**

Warner-Lambert Co.
P. 749

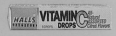
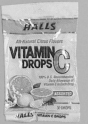

Assorted Citrus

Halls® Vitamin C Drops

Warner-Lambert Co.
P. 749

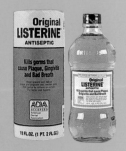

Listerine® Antiseptic

Warner-Lambert Co.
P. 750

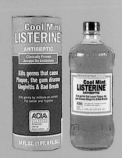

**Cool Mint
Listerine® Antiseptic**

Warner-Lambert Co.
P. 750

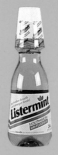

Anticavity Dental Rinse & Mouthwash

**Listermint®
with Fluoride**

Warner-Lambert Co.
P. 750

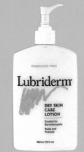

Fragrance and Fragrance Free Lotion
For Dry Skin Care

Lubriderm® Lotion

Warner-Lambert Co.
P. 750

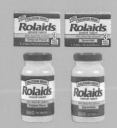

Original and Spearmint Flavors
Fast, Safe, Lasting Relief from
Heartburn, Sour Stomach or Acid
Indigestion and Upset Stomach
Associated with these Symptoms

Rolaids®

Warner-Lambert Co.
P. 751

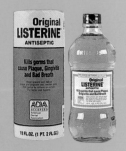

Fruit and Cherry Flavors
Calcium Rich, Sodium free Relief from
Heartburn, Sour Stomach or Acid
Indigestion and Upset Stomach
Associated with these Symptoms

**Calcium Rich,
Soduim Free Rolaids®**

Warner-Lambert Co.
P. 751

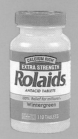

Wintergreen Flavor
Extra Strength Calcium, Sodium Free
Relief from Heartburn, Sour Stomach
or Acid Indigestion and Upset Stomach
Associated with these Symptoms

Extra Strength Rolaids®

Warner-Lambert Co.
P. 751

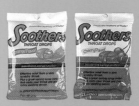

Throat Drops
From the makers of Hall's

Soothers™

WHITEHALL

Whitehall Laboratories
P. 754

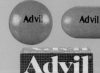

Coated Tablets in Bottles of
4, 8, 24, 50, 100, 165, 250
Coated Caplets in Bottles of
24, 50, 100, 165, 250

Advil®

Whitehall Laboratories
P. 755

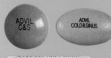
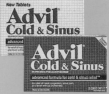

Coated Caplets and Tablets in
Packages of 20 and Bottles of 40

Advil® Cold & Sinus

Whitehall Laboratories
P. 768

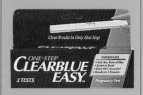

One-Step Pregnancy Test

CLEARBLUE EASY®

Whitehall Laboratories
P. 768

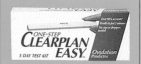

One-Step Ovulation Predictor

CLEARPLAN EASY™

Whitehall Laboratories
P. 755

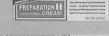
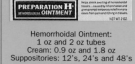

Hemorrhoidal Ointment:
1 oz and 2 oz tubes
Cream: 0.9 oz and 1.8 oz
Suppositories: 12's, 24's and 48's

Preparation H®

Whitehall Laboratories
P. 756

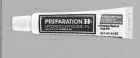

**Preparation H®
Anti-Itch Cream**

(hydrocortisone 1%)

Whitehall Laboratories
P. 756

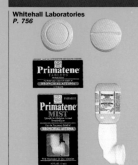

Available in 15 mL Inhaler Unit,
10 mL Suspension,
15 mL and 22.5 mL Refills
Tablets in 24's, 60's
Primatene®

Whitehall Laboratories
P. 756

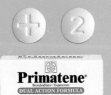

24's, 60's
**Primatene®
Dual Action Formula**

Whitehall Laboratories
P. 758

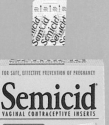

Vaginal Contraceptive Inserts
Semicid®

**Tamper-Resistant/
Evident Packaging**

Statements alerting con-
sumers to the specific type of
Tamper-Resistant/Evident
Packaging appear on the
bottle labels and cartons of
all over-the-counter products
of Wyeth-Ayerst. This includes
plastic cap seals on bottles,
individually wrapped tablets or
suppositories, and sealed
cartons. This packaging has
been developed to better
protect the consumer.

Wyeth-Ayerst Laboratories
P. 759

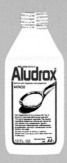

Suspension Antacid 12 Fl. oz.
Aludrox®

Wyeth-Ayerst Laboratories
P. 759

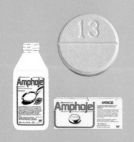

0.6 gram (10 gr.) Tablet shown above
12 Fl. oz. bottle and 100 tablets
Tablets and Suspension Antacid
Amphojel®

Wyeth-Ayerst Laboratories
P. 760

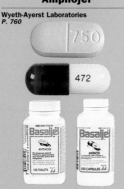

Antacid Tablets and Capsules
Basaljel®

Wyeth-Ayerst Laboratories
P. 760

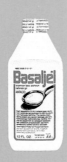

Antacid 12 Fl. oz.
Basaljel® Suspension

Wyeth-Ayerst Laboratories
P. 760

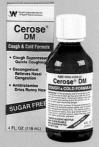

4 Fl. oz. Cough/Cold Formula
with Dextromethorphan
Also available in 1 pint bottles
Cerose® DM

Wyeth-Ayerst Laboratories
P. 761

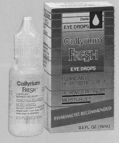

1/2 Fl. oz. (15 mL)
Eye drops with tetrahydrozoline HCl
plus glycerin
Collyrium Fresh™

Wyeth-Ayerst Laboratories
P. 761

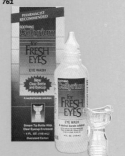

Eye Wash Lotion 4 Fl. oz. (118 mL)
with separate eyecup bottle cap
Collyrium for Fresh Eyes

Wyeth-Ayerst Laboratories
P. 761

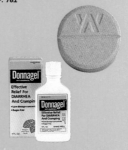

Available in bottles of 4, 8
and 16 Fl. oz. Chewable tablets
available in cartons of 18
Donnagel®

Wyeth-Ayerst Laboratories
P. 762

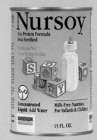

13 Fl. oz. Iron Fortified
Soy Protein Formula Concentrated Liquid
Also available in:
Ready-to-Feed Liquid and Powder
Nursoy®

Wyeth-Ayerst Laboratories
P. 762

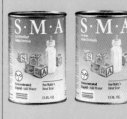

Iron Fortified Concentrated Liquid and
Lo-Iron Concentrated Liquid
Also available in Ready-to-Feed
Liquid and Powder
S.M.A.® Infant Formula

Wyeth-Ayerst Laboratories
P. 763

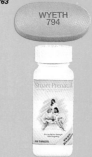

Multivitamin/Multimineral Supplement
for pregnant or lactating women
Stuart Prenatal®

Wyeth-Ayerst Laboratories
P. 764

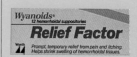

Box of 12 suppositories
Also available in boxes of 24
Wyanoids® Relief Factor

ZILA

Zila Pharmaceuticals, Inc.
P. 764

FAST RELIEF
From the pain, itching or burning of
CANKER SORES
FEVER BLISTERS &
COLD SORES
Long Lasting, Fast Acting
Zilactin®
Medicated Gel

Zilactin®
Medicated Gel

.25 oz. Medicated Gel

Also from Zila: Zilactin®-L Liquid
Treats cold sores and fever blisters
before they break out.

Zilactin®

PRODUCT INFORMATION

This section is made possible through the courtesy of the manufacturers whose products appear on the following pages. The information concerning each product has been prepared, edited, and approved by the medical department, medical director, and/or medical counsel of each manufacturer.

The product descriptions in this section comply with labeling regulations. They are designed to provide all information necessary for informed use, including, when applicable, active ingredients, indications, actions, warnings, cautions, drug interactions, symptoms and treatment of oral overdosage, dosage and directions for use, professional labeling, and how supplied. In some cases, additional information has been supplied to complement the standard labeling.

In compiling this section, the publisher has emphasized the necessity of describing products comprehensively. The descriptions seen here include all information made available by the manufacturer. The publisher does not warrant or guarantee any product described here, and does not perform any independent analysis of the information provided. Inclusion of a product in this book does not represent an endorsement, and the publisher does not necessarily advocate the use of any product listed.

AdvoCare International, L.L.C.
4100 ALPHA
SUITE 200
DALLAS, TX 75244

ACTOTHERM
Dietary Supplement

Ingredients: Each caplet contains: ThermoGen HC™ (Extracts of Gotu Kola, Cinnamon Ramulas, Peppermint, Lemon Verbena, Chamomile, Ginger, Chinese Licorice Root, Sweet Citrus Peel, Chicory); Guarana Extract; Potassium Phosphate; Magnesium Phosphate; Ascorbic Acid; Siberian Ginseng Extract; Mustard Seed; Niacin; Atlantic Kelp (standardized); Capsicum Extract (standardized); Green Tea Extract (standardized); Beta-Carotene.

Directions: Take 1–2 caplets two times a day, 30 minutes before meals, as a dietary supplement. Designed to be used in conjunction with AdvoCare's Weight Management Program.

Note: This product is not recommended for pregnant or lactating women. Keep out of reach of children.

LIPOTROL
Dietary Supplement

Ingredients: Each two caplets contain: [See table below.]
Garcinia Extract (standardized); Choline (Bitartrate); L-Carnitine; Zinc Monomethionine (**OPTIZINC®**); Inositol: Beta Sitosterol; Pullalan; Gymnema Sylvestre; Pantothenic Acid; Niacin; Pyridoxine (HCl); Vanadium (BMOV); Chromium (Polynicotinate-**CHROMEMATE® GTF**).
*% U.S. Recommended Daily Allowance for adults.

Directions: Take 1 caplet two times a day, 30 minutes before meals, as a dietary supplement. Designed to be used in conjunction with AdvoCare's Weight Management Program.

Note: This product is not recommended for pregnant or lactating women. Keep out of reach of children.

UNKNOWN DRUG?
Consult the
Product Identification Guide
(Gray Pages)
for full-color photos of
leading over-the-counter
medications

B.F. Ascher & Company, Inc.
15501 WEST 109th STREET
LENEXA, KS 66219
Mailing address:
P.O. BOX 717
SHAWNEE MISSION, KS
66201-0717

AYR® Saline Nasal Mist and Drops
[ār]

AYR Mist or Drops restores vital moisture to provide prompt relief for dry, crusted and inflamed nasal membranes due to chronic sinusitis, colds, low humidity, overuse of nasal decongestant drops and sprays, allergies, minor nose bleeds and other minor nasal irritations. AYR provides a soothing way to thin thick secretions and aid their removal from the nose and sinuses. AYR can be used as often as needed without the side effects associated with overuse of decongestant nose drops and sprays.

SAFE AND GENTLE ENOUGH FOR CHILDREN AND INFANTS
AYR Drops are particularly convenient for easy application with infants and children. AYR is formulated to prevent stinging, burning and irritation of delicate nasal tissue, even that of babies.

Directions For Use: SPRAY—Squeeze twice in each nostril as often as needed. Hold bottle upright. To spray, give the bottle short, firm squeezes. Take care not to aspirate nasal contents back into bottle. DROPS—Two to four drops in each nostril every two hours as needed, or as directed by your physician.

AYR is a specially formulated, buffered, isotonic saline solution containing sodium chloride 0.65% adjusted to the proper tonicity and pH with monobasic potassium phosphate/sodium hydroxide buffer to prevent nasal irritation. AYR also contains the non-irritating antibacterial and antifungal preservatives thimerosal and benzalkonium chloride and is formulated with deionized water.

How Supplied: AYR Mist in 50 ml spray bottles, AYR Drops in 50 ml dropper bottles.

Shown in Product Identification Guide, page 403

COUGH-X™

Active Ingredients: Each lozenge contains dextromethorphan hydrobromide 5 mg and benzocaine 2 mg. Also contains: Corn syrup, eucalyptus oil, menthol, propylene glycol and sucrose.

Indications: Temporarily suppresses cough due to minor throat and bronchial irritants. Also, for the temporary relief of occasional minor irritation and sore throat.

Warnings: A persistent cough may be a sign of a serious condition. If cough persists for more than 1 week, tends to recur or if sore throat is severe, persists for more than 2 days or if cough and/or sore throat is accompanied or followed by fever, persistent headache, rash, swelling, nausea or vomiting, consult a physician. Do not take this product for persistent or chronic cough such as occurs with smoking, asthma, emphysema or if cough is accompanied by excessive phlegm (mucus) unless directed by a physician. Do not exceed recommended dosage. Do not use this product if you have a history of allergy to local anesthetics such as procaine, butacaine, benzocaine or other "caine" anesthetics. As with any drug, if you are pregnant or nursing a baby, seek the advice of a health professional before using this product. KEEP THIS AND ALL DRUGS OUT OF REACH OF CHILDREN. In case of accidental overdose, seek professional assistance or contact a Poison Control Center immediately.

Drug Interaction Precaution: Do not use this product if you are now taking a prescription monoamine oxidase inhibitor (MAOI) (certain drugs for depression, psychiatric or emotional conditions, or Parkinson's disease), or for 2 weeks after stopping the MAOI drug. If you are uncertain whether your prescription drug contains an MAOI, consult a health professional before taking this product.

Directions: Allow lozenge to dissolve slowly in the mouth. Adults and children 6 years of age and older: One lozenge every 2 hours as needed not to exceed 12 lozenges in 24 hours or as directed by a physician. Children 2 to 6 years of age: One lozenge every 4 hours not to exceed 6 lozenges in 24 hours or as directed by a physician. Children under 2 years of age: Consult a physician.

How Supplied: Available in pleasant-tasting menthol eucalyptus flavor. 9 individually-wrapped lozenges come packaged in a carton.

Shown in Product Identification Guide, page 403

ITCH–X GEL®
Dual-acting, itch-relieving gel with aloe vera

Active Ingredients: Benzyl alcohol 10% and pramoxine HCl 1%.
Also contains: Aloe vera gel, carbomer 934, diazolidinyl urea, FD&C blue #1, methylparaben, propylene glycol, propylparaben, SD alcohol 40, styrene/acrylate copolymer, triethanolamine, and water.

Indications: For the temporary relief of pain and itching associated with minor skin irritations, allergic itches, rashes, hives, minor burns, insect bites, sunburns, poison ivy, poison oak, and poison sumac.

LIPOTROL		%USRDA*
Niacin	10 mg	50
Pantothenic Acid	10 mg	100
Pyridoxine (vitamin B6)	4 mg	200
Zinc (Monomethionine-**OPTIZINC®**)	5 mg	33

Warnings: For external use only. Avoid contact with the eyes. If condition worsens, or if symptoms persist for more than 7 days or clear up and occur again within a few days, discontinue use of this product and consult a physician. KEEP THIS AND ALL DRUGS OUT OF THE REACH OF CHILDREN. In case of accidental ingestion, seek professional assistance or contact a Poison Control Center immediately.

Directions: Adults and children 2 years of age and older: Apply to affected area not more than 3 to 4 times daily. Children under 2 years of age: consult a physician.

How Supplied: 35.4g (1.25 oz) tube
Shown in Product Identification Guide, page 403

MOBIGESIC® Analgesic Tablets
[mō'bǐ-jē'zǐk]
Breaks the cycle of pain. MOBIGESIC provides pain relief with a mild muscle relaxant effect.

Active Ingredients: Each tablet contains 325 mg of magnesium salicylate with 30 mg of phenyltoloxamine citrate.

Also Contains: Microcrystalline cellulose, magnesium stearate and colloidal silicon dioxide which aid in the formulation of the tablet and its dissolution in the gastrointestinal tract.

Indications: MOBIGESIC acts fast to provide relief from stress headache and other painful conditions by breaking the cycle of tension-stress pain. This formula relieves pain while relaxing tense, stiff muscles. Also effective in pain relief after dental procedures and minor surgery.

Caution: When used for the temporary symptomatic relief of colds, if relief does not occur within 7 days (3 days for fever), discontinue use and consult physician. This preparation may cause drowsiness. Do not drive or operate machinery while taking this medication. Do not administer to children under 6 years of age or exceed recommended dosage unless directed by physician.

Warnings: Keep this and all drugs out of the reach of children. In case of accidental overdose, call your doctor or poison control center immediately. As with any drug, if you are pregnant or nursing a baby, seek the advice of a health professional before using this product.

Usual Dosage: Adults—1 or 2 tablets every four hours, up to 10 tablets daily. Children (6 to 12 years)—1 tablet every 4 hours, up to 5 tablets daily. Do not use more than 10 days unless directed by physician.
Store at room temperature (59°–86°F).

How Supplied: Packages of 18's, 50's and 100's.
Shown in Product Identification Guide, page 403

MOBISYL® Analgesic Creme
[mō'bǐ-sǐl]
Penetrates to the site of pain to bring relief.

Active Ingredient: Trolamine salicylate 10%. Also Contains: Glycerin, methylparaben, mineral oil, polysorbate 60, propylparaben, sorbitan stearate, sorbitol, stearic acid, and water.

Description: MOBISYL is a greaseless, odorless, penetrating, non-burning, non-irritating analgesic creme.

Indications: For adults and children, 12 years of age and older, MOBISYL is indicated for the temporary relief of minor aches and pains of muscles and joints, such as simple backache, lumbago, arthritis, neuralgia, strains, bruises and sprains.

Actions: MOBISYL penetrates fast into sore, tender joints and muscles where pain originates. It works to reduce inflammation. Helps soothe stiff joints and muscles and gets you going again.

Warnings: For external use only. Avoid contact with the eyes. Discontinue use if condition worsens or if symptoms persist for more than 7 days, and consult a physician. Do not use on children under 12 years of age except under the advice and supervision of a physician. In case of accidental ingestion, seek professional assistance or contact a Poison Control Center immediately. Close cap tightly. Keep this and all drugs out of the reach of children. Store at room temperature.

Dosage and Administration: Place a liberal amount of MOBISYL Creme in your palm and massage into the area of pain and soreness three or four times a day, especially before retiring. MOBISYL may be worn under clothing or bandages.

How Supplied: MOBISYL is available in 35.4g (1.25 oz) tubes, 100g (3.5 oz) tubes, 226.8g (8 oz) jars.
Shown in Product Identification Guide, page 403

PEN•KERA® Creme with Keratin Binding Factor
A Therapeutic Moisturizing Creme for Chronic Dry Skin

Ingredients: Water, octyl palmitate, glycerin, mineral oil, polysorbate 60, sorbitan stearate, polyamino sugar condensate, urea, wheat germ glycerides, carbomer 940, triethanolamine, DMDMH, iodo propynyl butyl carbamate, diazolidinyl urea, and dehydroacetic acid.

Indications: PEN•KERA Therapeutic Creme for Chronic Dry Skin contains Keratin Binding Factor, a polyamino sugar condensate and urea, which is synthesized to match the same biological components as those found in skin. The Keratin Binding Factor in PEN•KERA Creme replaces the missing elements of dehydrated skin which absorb and retain moisture. The Keratin Binding Factor actually simulates the natural moisturizing mechanism of the skin, relieving itching, flaking, sensitive, dry skin symptoms.
PEN•KERA is fragrance-free, dye-free, paraben-free, lanolin-free, non-comedogenic and non-greasy for smooth, fast absorption.

Dosage and Administration: Apply in a thin layer. Because it penetrates quickly and is non-greasy, PEN•KERA may be used under make-up or sun screens. Regular use will reduce the frequency of application and quantity required to achieve moisturized skin.

Precautions: FOR EXTERNAL USE ONLY

How Supplied: PEN•KERA Therapeutic Creme is available in 8 oz. bottles.
Shown in Product Identification Guide, page 403

EDUCATIONAL MATERIAL

The following Patient Information Materials are available to physicians, pharmacists and consumers:
"How to Administer Nose Drops to an Infant" in English and Spanish
"Chronic Sinusitis" – Tips for alleviating sinus problems
"Dry, Irritated Nasal Passages"
"Decongestant Rebound" – Overuse of topical nasal decongestants
"Tension Headache: Break the Cycle of Stress-tension Headache"
"Chronic Dry Skin" – You don't have to live with it.
Write: Patient Information, B. F. Ascher & Co., Inc., P.O. Box 717, Shawnee Mission, KS 66201-0717

Astra USA, Inc.
50 OTIS ST.
WESTBORO, MA 01581-4500

XYLOCAINE® (lidocaine) 2.5%
[zī'lo-caine]
OINTMENT

For temporary relief of pain and itching due to minor burns, sunburn, minor cuts, abrasions, insect bites and minor skin irritations.

Composition: Lidocaine 2.5% in a water miscible ointment vehicle consisting of polyethylene glycols and propylene glycol.

Action and Uses: A topical anesthetic ointment for fast, temporary relief of pain and itching due to minor burns, sunburn, minor cuts, abrasions, insect bites and minor skin irritations. The ointment can be easily removed with water.

Administration and Dosage: Xylocaine 2.5% Ointment should be applied

Continued on next page

Astra—Cont.

liberally over the affected areas. Use enough to provide temporary relief and reapply Xylocaine 2.5% Ointment as needed for continued relief.

Important Warning: *Use only as directed by a physician in persistent, severe or extensive skin disorders. In case of accidental ingestion seek professional assistance or contact a poison control center immediately.* **KEEP OUT OF THE REACH OF CHILDREN.**

Caution: *Do not use in the eyes. Not for prolonged use. If the condition for which this preparation is used persists, or if a rash or irritation develops, discontinue use and consult a physician.*

How Supplied: 1.25 ounce tubes containing 2.5% lidocaine base.

Shown in Product Identification Guide, page 403

Au Pharmaceuticals, Inc.
P. O. BOX 131835
TYLER, TX 75713-1835

AURUM–Analgesic Lotion
Topical Analgesic
THERAGOLD–Analgesic Lotion
Topical Analgesic
THERAPEUTIC GOLD–
Analgesic Lotion
Topical Analgesic
PEDIGOLD
Analgesic Lotion
Topical Analgesic

Active Ingredients: The active ingredients are methyl salicylate 10%; menthol 3%; camphor 2.5%. These are combined in a rich, nonpetroleum base for easy and effective topical application.

Other Selected Ingredients: Special inactive ingredients include Deionized Water, C12–15 Alcohols, Propylene Glycol, Eucalyptus Oil, Stearic Acid, DEA Cetyl Phosphate, PEG 8-Distearate, Carboxy Polymethylene, Methyl Hydroxybenzoate, Ginseng, Imidazolidinyl Urea, Triethanolamine, Disodium EDTA, Urea, Jojoba Oil, Vitamins A & D$_3$, Vitamin E, FD&C Yellow No. 5, 24 Karat Gold, Aloe.

Indications: These lotions give fast, deep-penetrating, effective temporary relief from stiff, sore, aching muscles and joints associated with arthritis, bursitis, tendinitis and muscle disorders.

Actions: Methyl salicylate, menthol and camphor are classified as counterirritants which combine to provide both heat and cold stimulation to the pain receptors over and around the affected area. The lotions replace the perception of pain with the feeling of heat and/or cold to provide temporary relief of minor aches and pains.

Directions: Apply a liberal amount of lotion to painful area and allow to remain on skin for 30 seconds before rubbing lotion into the affected area. Apply product 3 or 4 times a day or as needed until pain is relieved, then reduce the frequency as needed.

Warnings: Use only as directed. For external use only. Avoid contact with eyes, mucous membranes, broken or irritated skin. Should contact occur, flush area with water. Do not use a heating pad with this lotion until one hour after application. Do not use on children under 12 years of age without advice of a physician. If condition worsens or persists for more than 7 days without relief, discontinue use of this product and consult a physician. Some individuals may experience sensitivity to some ingredients. If so, discontinue use immediately. Do not swallow. If swallowed, induce vomiting and call a physician.

Caution: contains 10% Methyl Salicylate and 24K GOLD. Persons who are allergic or hypersensitive to these ingredients should consult their physician before using this product.

How Supplied: These products are available in 128 ounce, 8 ounce, 2 ounce and 1.25 ounce bottles.
National Drug Code Registration #058796

FEMININE GOLD—
Analgesic Lotion
Topical Analgesic
MAXIMRELIEF
Analgesic Lotion
Topical Analgesic

Active Ingredients: The active ingredients are menthol 3%, camphor 2.5%. These are combined in a rich, nonpetroleum base for easy and effective topical application.

Other Selected Ingredients: Special inactive ingredients include Deionized Water, C12–15 Alcohols, Propylene Glycol, Eucalyptus Oil, Stearic Acid, DEA Cetyl Phosphate, PEG 8-Distearate, Carboxy Polymethylene, Methyl Hydroxybenzoate, Ginseng, Imidazolidinyl Urea, Triethanolamine, Disodium EDTA, Urea, Jojoba Oil, Vitamin A & D$_3$, Vitamin E, FD&C Yellow No. 5, 24 Karat Gold, Aloe.

Indications: This lotion gives fast, deep-penetrating, effective temporary relief from pain and discomfort of cramps and backache suffered during the menstrual cycle.

Actions: Menthol and camphor are classified as counterirritants which combine to provide both heat and cold stimulation to the pain receptors over and around the affected area. The lotion replaces the perception of pain with the feeling of heat and/or cold to provide temporary relief of minor aches and pains.

Directions: Apply a liberal amount of lotion to painful area and allow to remain on skin for 30 seconds before rubbing lotion into the affected area. Apply product 3 or 4 times a day or as needed until pain is relieved, then reduce the frequency to as needed.

Warnings: Use only as directed. For external use only. Avoid contact with eyes, mucous membranes, broken or irritated skin. Should contact occur, flush area with water. Do not use a heating pad with this lotion until one hour after application. Do not use on children under 12 years of age without advice of a physician. If condition worsens or persists for more than 7 days without relief, discontinue use of this product and consult a physician. Some individuals may experience sensitivity to some ingredients. If so discontinue use immediately. Do not swallow. If swallowed, induce vomiting and call a physician.

Caution: contains 24K GOLD. Persons who are allergic or hypersensitive to these ingredients should consult their physician before using this product.

How Supplied: These products are available in 8 ounce, 2 ounce and 1 ounce bottles.
National Drug Code Registration #058796

Ayerst Laboratories
Division of American Home
Products Corporation
685 THIRD AVE.
NEW YORK, NY 10017-4071

For information for Ayerst's consumer products, see product listings under Whitehall Laboratories.
Please turn to Whitehall Laboratories, page 753.

Baker Cummins Dermatologicals, Inc.
1950 SWARTHMORE AVENUE
LAKEWOOD, NJ 08701

AQUA-A® Cream

Description: Contains the vitamin A derivative, retinyl palmitate. Moisture-enriched smoothing concentrate.

Ingredients: Water, Caprylic/Capric Triglyceride, Methyl Gluceth-10, Glyceryl Stearate, Squalane, Mineral Oil, Dimethicone, Stearic Acid, PEG-50 Stearate, Retinyl Palmitate, Sodium Hyaluronate, Lecithin, Sodium Polyglutamate, Ascorbyl Palmitate, Carbomer 934, Dichlorobenzyl Alcohol, Cetyl Alcohol, BHT, Diazolidinyl Urea, Xanthan Gum, Menthol, Sodium Hydroxide, Tetrasodium EDTA.

Directions for Use: Use morning or night or both.

How Supplied: 2 oz. jars (58174-203-02)

AQUADERM® Sunscreen Moisturizer SPF 15

Description: Aquaderm® Sunscreen Moisturizer SPF 15 developed by leading dermatologists to deliver maximum moisturization. Regular daily use of Aquaderm's dual action moisturizer and sunscreen protects and preserves your youthful appearance. This specially developed formula contains sunscreens (SPF 15) that shield your skin from UVA and UVB rays, to protect it from wrinkles and reduce skin damage and possible skin cancer. Aquaderm® Sunscreen Moisturizer SPF 15 is safe and effective, hypo-allergenic, non-comedogenic, Paraben-free, and will not leave an artificial-feeling film. Aquaderm® Sunscreen Moisturizer SPF 15 is especially suited for patients undergoing Retin-A® therapy, who require maximum moisturization and sun protection. Retin-A® is a registered trademark of Johnson & Johnson.

Active Ingredients: Octyl Methoxycinnamate, 7.5%, Oxybenzone, 6%, in a moisturizing cream base.

Indications: Protects against harmful skin-aging rays of the sun.

Warnings: FOR EXTERNAL USE ONLY. Avoid contact with eyes. If irritation develops, discontinue use. Keep this and all drugs out of the reach of children. In case of accidental ingestion, seek professional assistance or contact a Poison Control Center immediately.

Directions for Use: Apply to face and neck as needed. Effective and compatible for daily use under make-up.

How Supplied: 3.5 oz. tube (58174-205-35)

Shown in Product Identification Guide, page 403

AQUADERM® Cream

Description: Ultrarich moisturizing cream concentrate. Softens, smooths, protects, absorbs quickly. Fragrance free—Ideal for use as a compounding base.

Ingredients: Water, Caprylic/Capric Triglyceride, Methyl Gluceth-10, Glyceryl Stearate, Mineral Oil, Squalane, Dimethicone, Stearic Acid, PEG-50 Stearate, Sodium Hyaluronate, Lecithin, Sodium Polyglutamate, Magnesium Aluminum Silicate, Carbomer 934, Dichlorobenzyl Alcohol, Cetyl Alcohol, BHT, Diazolidinyl Urea, Xanthan Gum, Menthol, Sodium Hydroxide, Tetrasodium EDTA.

Directions for Use: Apply to face or other dry areas morning or night or both.

How Supplied: 4 oz. jar (58174-202-04)
Shown in Product Identification Guide, page 403

AQUADERM® Lotion

Description: Ultrarich moisturizing lotion concentrate. Smooths, softens, protects, absorbs quickly. Ideal for use as a compounding base.

Ingredients: Water, Caprylic/Capric Triglyceride, Methyl Gluceth-10, Glyceryl Stearate, Dimethicone, Petrolatum, Mineral Oil, Squalane, PEG-50 Stearate, Stearic Acid, Sodium Hyaluronate, Lecithin, Sodium Polyglutamate, Magnesium Aluminum Silicate, Carbomer 934, Dichlorobenzyl Alcohol, Cetyl Alcohol, BHT, Diazolidinyl Urea, Xanthan Gum, Menthol, Tetrasodium EDTA, Sodium Hydroxide.

Directions for Use: Apply to hands and body morning or night or both.

How Supplied: 7.5 fl. oz. bottle (58174-201-75)
Shown in Product Identification Guide, page 403

P&S® Liquid

Ingredients: Mineral Oil, Water, Fragrance, Glycerin, Phenol, Sodium Chloride, D&C Yellow #11, D&C Red #17, D&C Green #6.

Indications: P&S® Liquid, used regularly, helps loosen and remove crusts and scales on the scalp.

Caution: FOR EXTERNAL USE ONLY. Do not apply to large portions of body surfaces. Discontinue use if excessive skin irritation develops. Avoid contact with eyes or mucous membranes. Keep out of the reach of children. In case of accidental ingestion, seek professional assistance or contact a Poison Control Center immediately.

Directions for Use: Apply liberally to scalp lesions each night before retiring. Massage gently to loosen scales and crusts. Leave on overnight and shampoo the next morning. Use daily as needed.

How Supplied: 8 fl. oz. bottle (58174-401-04); 4 fl. oz. bottle (58174-401-08)
Shown in Product Identification Guide, page 403

P&S® PLUS Tar Gel

Active Ingredient: 8% Coal Tar Solution (equivalent to 1.6% Crude Coal Tar).

Indications: For psoriasis and other scaling conditions. P&S® PLUS relieves the itching, irritation and skin flaking associated with seborrheic dermatitis, psoriasis and dandruff.

Warnings: FOR EXTERNAL USE ONLY. Avoid contact with the eyes; flush with water if product gets into eyes. If condition worsens or does not improve after regular use of this product as directed, consult a physician. Use caution in exposing skin to sunlight after applying this product; it may increase your tendency to sunburn for up to 24 hours after application. Do not use for prolonged periods without consulting a physician. Do not use this product in or around the rectum or in the genital area or groin except on the advice of a physician. Do not use this product with other forms of psoriasis therapy such as ultraviolet radiation or prescription drugs unless directed to do so by a physician. If condition covers a large area of the body, consult your physician before using this product.

Caution: Keep this and all drugs out of reach of children. In case of accidental ingestion, seek professional assistance or contact a Poison Control Center immediately.

Directions for Use: Apply to affected areas one to four times daily or as directed by physician.

How Supplied: 3.5 oz. tube (NDC 58174-409-35)

P&S® Shampoo

Active Ingredient: 2% Salicylic Acid.

Indications: P&S® Shampoo relieves the itching, irritation and skin flaking associated with seborrheic dermatitis of the scalp. It also relieves the itching, redness, and scaling associated with psoriasis of the scalp. P&S® Shampoo may be used alone as well as following treatment with P&S® Liquid. Its rich conditioning formula improves hair's manageability and helps prevent tangles.

Warnings: FOR EXTERNAL USE ONLY. Avoid contact with eyes or mucous membranes. If this occurs, rinse thoroughly with water. If condition worsens or does not improve after regular use of this product as directed, consult a physician. Do not use on children under 2 years of age except as directed by a physician. If condition covers a large area of the body, consult your doctor before using this product.

Caution: Keep this and all drugs out of reach of children. In case of accidental ingestion, seek professional assistance or contact a Poison Control Center immediately.

Directions for Use: For best results use twice weekly or as directed by a physician. Wet hair, apply to scalp and massage vigorously. Rinse and repeat.

How Supplied: 4 fl. oz. bottle (NDC 58174-407-04); 8 fl. oz. bottle (NDC 58174-407-08)
Shown in Product Identification Guide, page 403

ULTRA MIDE 25® Extra Strength Moisturizer

Ingredients: Water, Urea, Mineral Oil, Glycerin, Propylene Glycol, PEG-50 Stearate, Butyrolactone, Hydrogenated Lanolin, Sorbitan Laurate, Glyceryl Stearate, Magnesium Aluminum Silicate, Propylene Glycol Stearate SE, Ce-

Continued on next page

Baker Cummins Derm.—Cont.

tyl Alcohol, Fragrance, Diazolidinyl Urea, Tetrasodium EDTA.

Indications: Intensive moisturizer for extra dry, scaly or calloused skin. Contains ingredients to soften and moisturize areas of very dry, rough, cracked or calloused skin. This unique keratolytic patented formula contains a stabilized form of urea (25%) to help prevent the stinging and irritation often associated with moisturizers containing urea. ULTRA MIDE 25® Lotion contains no parabens.

Warnings: FOR EXTERNAL USE ONLY. Keep out of reach of children. Discontinue use if irritation occurs. Caution should be taken when used near the eyes. In case of accidental ingestion, seek professional assistance or contact a Poison Control Center immediately.

Directions for Use: Apply four times daily, or as directed by a physician. Each application should be rubbed in completely.

How Supplied: 8 fl. oz. bottle (58174-420-08)

Shown in Product Identification Guide, page 403

X–SEB® Shampoo

Active Ingredient: 1% Zinc Pyrithione.

Inactive Ingredients: Purified Water, Ammonium Lauryl Sulfate, Ammonium Laureth Sulfate, Ethylene Glycol Distearate, Lauramide DEA, Salicylic Acid, PEG 75 Lanolin, Ammonium Xylene Sulfate, Triethanolamine, Menthol, Methylchloroisothiazolinone and Methylisothiazolinone, Fragrance, FD&C Blue #1.

Indications: X-SEB® Shampoo provides effective relief of the itching and scalp flaking associated with dandruff. This unique formulation is gentle enough for daily use leaving hair healthy looking and manageable.

Warnings: FOR EXTERNAL USE ONLY. Avoid contact with the eyes; if this happens, rinse thoroughly with water. If condition worsens or does not improve after regular use of this product as directed, consult a physician. Do not use on children under 2 years of age except as directed by a physician.

Caution: Keep this and all drugs out of the reach of children. In case of accidental ingestion, seek professional assistance or contact a Poison Control Center immediately.

Directions for Use: For best results, use X-SEB® Shampoo twice a week or as directed by a physician. Wet hair, apply to scalp and massage vigorously. Rinse and repeat.

How Supplied: 4 fl. oz. bottle (NDC 58174-106-04); 8 fl. oz. bottle (NDC 58174-106-08)

Shown in Product Identification Guide, page 403

X–SEB® PLUS Conditioning Shampoo

Active Ingredient: 1% Zinc Pyrithione.

Inactive Ingredients: Purified Water, Ammonium Lauryl Sulfate, Ammonium Laureth Sulfate, Ethylene Glycol Distearate, Lauramide DEA, Salicylic Acid, PEG 75 Lanolin, Polyquaternium-7, Ammonium Xylene Sulfate, Triethanolamine, Menthol, Methylchloroisothiazolinone and Methylisothiazolinone, Fragrance, FD&C Blue #1.

Indications: X-SEB® PLUS conditioning shampoo provides effective relief of the itching and scalp flaking associated with dandruff. Ideal for dry, brittle hair. This unique formulation is gentle enough for daily use giving hair extra body, a healthy look and ease of manageability.

Warnings: FOR EXTERNAL USE ONLY. Avoid contact with the eyes; if this happens, rinse thoroughly with water. If condition worsens or does not improve after regular use of this product as directed, consult a physician. Do not use on children under 2 years of age except as directed by a physician.

Caution: Keep this and all drugs out of the reach of children. In case of accidental ingestion, seek professional assistance or contact a Poison Control Center immediately.

Directions for Use: For best results, use X-SEB® PLUS conditioning shampoo twice a week or as directed by a physician. Wet hair, apply to scalp and massage vigorously. Rinse and repeat.

How Supplied: 4 fl. oz. bottle (NDC 58174-116-04); 8 fl. oz. bottle (NDC 58174-116-08)

Shown in Product Identification Guide, page 403

X–SEB T® Pearl Shampoo

Active Ingredient: 10% Coal Tar Solution (2% Crude Coal Tar).

Inactive Ingredients: Purified water, TEA Lauryl Sulfate, Lauramide DEA, Ethylene Glycol Distearate, PEG-75 Lanolin, Salicylic Acid, Polyquaternium-7, Menthol, Hydroxypropyl Methylcellulose, Chloroxylenol, Disodium EDTA, Fragrance, FD&C Blue #1.

Indications: X-SEB T® Pearl shampoo relieves the itching, irritation and skin flaking associated with dandruff, seborrheic dermatitis, and psoriasis. This formulation is designed to effectively treat scaly conditions in a mild, gentle cleansing base leaving hair healthy looking and manageable. X-SEB T® Pearl will not discolor or damage hair that has been color treated or permed. Ideal for normal to oily hair type.

Warnings: FOR EXTERNAL USE ONLY. Avoid contact with the eyes; if this happens, rinse thoroughly with water. If irritation develops, discontinue use. If condition worsens or does not improve after regular use of this product as directed, consult a physician. Do not use on children under 2 years of age except as directed by a physician. Use caution in exposing skin to sunlight after applying this product; it may increase your tendency to sunburn for up to 24 hours after application. Do not use for prolonged periods without consulting a physician. Do not use this product with other forms of psoriasis therapy such as ultraviolet radiation or prescription drugs unless directed to do so by a physician. If condition covers a large area of the body, consult your physician before using this product.

Caution: Keep this and all drugs out of the reach of children. In case of accidental ingestion, seek professional assistance or contact a Poison Control Center immediately.

Directions for Use: For best results, use X-SEB T® Pearl shampoo at least twice a week or as directed by physician. Wet hair, apply to scalp and massage vigorously. Rinse and repeat or as directed by a physician.

How Supplied: 4 fl. oz. bottle (NDC 58174-104-04); 8 fl. oz. bottle (NDC 58174-104-08)

Shown in Product Identification Guide, page 403

X–SEB T® PLUS Conditioning Shampoo

Active Ingredient: 10% Coal Tar Solution (equivalent to 2% Crude Coal Tar).

Inactive Ingredients: Purified water, TEA Lauryl Sulfate, Lauramide DEA, Ethylene Glycol Distearate, PEG-75 Lanolin, Salicylic Acid, Polyquaternium-7, Menthol, Hydroxypropyl Methylcellulose, Chloroxylenol, Disodium EDTA, Fragrance, FD&C Blue #1.

Indications: X-SEB T® PLUS conditioning shampoo relieves the itching, irritation and skin flaking associated with dandruff, seborrheic dermatitis, and psoriasis. This formulation is designed to effectively treat scaly conditions in a mild, gentle cleansing base leaving hair healthy looking and manageable. X-SEB T® PLUS will not discolor or damage hair that has been color treated or permed. Ideal for normal to dry, brittle hair.

Warnings: FOR EXTERNAL USE ONLY. Avoid contact with the eyes; if this happens, rinse thoroughly with water. If irritation develops, discontinue use. If condition worsens or does not improve after regular use of this product as directed, consult a physician. Do not use on children under 2 years of age except as directed by a physician. Use caution in exposing skin to sunlight after applying this product; it may increase your tendency to sunburn for up to 24 hours after application. Do not use for prolonged periods without consulting a physician. Do not use this product with other forms of psoriasis therapy such as ultraviolet radiation or prescription drugs unless directed to do so by a physician. If condition covers a large area of the body, consult your physician before using this product.

Caution: Keep this and all drugs out of the reach of children. In case of accidental ingestion, seek professional assistance or contact a Poison Control Center immediately.

Directions for Use: For best results, use X-SEB T® PLUS at least twice a week or as directed by physician. Wet hair, apply to scalp and massage vigorously. Rinse and repeat or as directed by physician.

How Supplied: 4 fl. oz. bottle (NDC 58174-115-04); 8 fl. oz. bottle (NDC 58174-115-08)

Shown in Product Identification Guide, page 403

Beach Pharmaceuticals
Division of Beach Products, Inc.
5220 SOUTH MANHATTAN AVE. TAMPA, FL 33611

BEELITH Tablets
MAGNESIUM SUPPLEMENT WITH PYRIDOXINE HCl
Each tablet supplies 362 mg (30 mEq) of magnesium and 25 mg of pyridoxine HCL.

Description: Each tablet contains magnesium oxide 600 mg and pyridoxine hydrochloride (Vitamin B_6) 25 mg equivalent to B_6 20 mg. *Also, microcrystalline cellulose, sodium starch glycolate, D&C Yellow #10, FD&C Yellow #6 (Sunset Yellow), titanium dioxide, and other ingredients.* Each tablet yields 362 mg of magnesium and supplies 90% of the Adult U.S. Recommended Daily Allowance (RDA) for magnesium and 1000% of the Adult RDA for vitamin B_6.

Indications: As a dietary supplement for patients with magnesium and/or vitamin B_6 deficiencies resulting from malnutrition, alcoholism, magnesium depleting drugs and inadequate nutritional intake or absorption.

Dosage: One tablet daily or as directed by a physician.

Drug Interaction Precautions: Do not take this product if you are presently taking a prescription drug without consulting your physician or other health professional.

Warnings: If you have kidney disease, take only under the supervision of a physician. Excessive dosage may cause laxation. **KEEP OUT OF THE REACH OF CHILDREN.**

How Supplied: Golden yellow, film coated tablet with the name **BEACH** and the number **1132** printed on each tablet. Packaged in bottles of 100 (NDC 0486-1132-01) tablets.

Beiersdorf Inc.
360 Dr. Martin Luther King Dr. NORWALK, CT 06856-5529

AQUAPHOR®—Original Formula Ointment
NDC Numbers–10356-020-01
10356-020-02

Composition: Petrolatum, mineral oil, mineral wax and wool wax alcohol.

Actions and Uses: Aquaphor is a stable, neutral, odorless, anhydrous ointment base. Miscible with water or aqueous solutions, Aquaphor will absorb several times its own weight, forming smooth, creamy water-in-oil emulsions. In its pure form, Aquaphor is recommended for use as a topical preparation to help heal severely dry skin. Aquaphor contains no preservatives, fragrances or known irritants.

Administration and Dosages: Use Aquaphor alone or in compounding virtually any ointment using aqueous solutions or in combination with other oil-based substances and all common topical medications. Apply Aquaphor liberally to affected area.

Precautions: For external use only. Avoid contact with eyes. Not to be applied over third degree burns, deep or puncture wounds, infections or lacerations. If condition worsens or does not improve within 7 days, patient should consult a doctor.

How Supplied: 16 oz. jar—List No. 45585; 5 lb. jar—List. No. 45586
Shown in Product Identification Guide, page 403

AQUAPHOR® Antibiotic Ointment
NDC Number–10356-022-01

Composition: Polymyxin-B Sulfate/ Bacitracin Zinc, Petrolatum, Mineral Wax, Mineral Oil, Wool Wax Alcohol.

Actions and Uses: Aquaphor Antibiotic Formula is formulated to help reduce wound healing time and the risk of infection.[1] Recommended for prevention of infection in minor first-aid wounds and for use as a post-operative dressing. Aquaphor Antibiotic Formula is preservative-free, fragrance-free and hypoallergenic. It is recommended for patients with sensitive skin.

Administration and Dosage: Use Aquaphor Antibiotic Formula whenever a topical antibiotic ointment is needed to help prevent infection in minor cuts, scrapes and burns. Apply Aquaphor Antibiotic Formula liberally to affected area two to three times a day as needed.

Precautions: For external use only. Avoid contact with eyes, Not to be applied over third degree burns, deep or puncture wounds, infections or lacerations. If condition worsens or does not improve within seven days, patient should consult a physician.

How Supplied: .5 oz. tube.

1. Data on file, BDF Inc
Shown in Product Identification Guide, page 403

AQUAPHOR® Natural Healing Ointment
NDC Number–10356-021-01

Composition: Petrolatum, Mineral Oil, Mineral Wax, Wool Wax Alcohol, Panthenol, Bisabolol, Glycerin.

Actions and Uses: Aquaphor Natural Healing Formula is specially formulated for faster healing of severely dry skin, cracked skin and minor burns. It is recommended for patients suffering from severe skin chapping and from skin disorders that result in severely dry, damaged skin. This formula is also indicated as a follow-up skin treatment for patients undergoing radiation therapy or other drying/burning medical therapies. It is preservative-free, fragrance-free and hypoallergenic, and is clinically proven to reduce wound healing time.[1]

Administration and Dosage: Use Aquaphor Natural Healing Formula whenever a mild healing agent is needed. Apply liberally to affected areas two to three times a day. In the case of minor wounds, clean area prior to application.

Precautions: For external use only. Avoid contact with the eyes. Not to be applied over third degree burns, deep or puncture wounds, infections or lacerations. If condition worsens or does not improve within seven days, patient should consult a physician.

How Supplied: 1.75 oz. tube, List #45231

1. Data on file, BDF Inc
Shown in Product Identification Guide, page 403

EUCERIN®
[ū'sir-in]
Dry Skin Care Cleansing Bar

Actions and Uses: Eucerin® Cleansing Bar has been specially formulated for use on sensitive skin. The formulation contains Eucerite®, a special blend of ingredients that closely resemble the natural oils of the skin, thus providing excellent moisturizing properties. This

Continued on next page

Beiersdorf—Cont.

formulation is fragrance-free and non-comedogenic. Additionally, the pH value of Eucerin Cleansing Bar is neutral so as not to affect the skin's normal acid mantle.

Directions: Use during shower, bath, or regular cleansing, or as directed by physician.

How Supplied:
3 ounce bar
List Number 3852
Shown in Product Identification Guide, page 403

EUCERIN® Creme
[ū'sir-in]
Dry Skin Care
NDC Numbers—10356-090-01
10356-090-05
10356-090-04
10356-090-07

Composition: Water, petrolatum, mineral oil, wool wax alcohol, methylchloroisothiazolinone, methylisothiazolinone.

Actions and Uses: A gentle, non-comedogenic, fragrance-free water-in-oil emulsion. Eucerin can be used as a treatment for dry skin associated with eczema, psoriasis, chapped or chafed skin, sunburn, windburn and itching associated with dryness.

Administration and Dosages: Apply freely to affected areas of the skin as often as necessary or as directed by physician.

Precautions: For external use only.

How Supplied:
16 oz. jar—List Number 0090
8 oz. jar—List Number 3774
4 oz. jar—List Number 3797
2 oz. tube—List Number 3868
Shown in Product Identification Guide, page 403

EUCERIN® DAILY FACIAL LOTION
NDC Number–10356-972-01

Active Ingredients: Ethylhexyl p-methoxycinnamate, Titanium Dioxide, 2-Phenylbenzamidazole-5-Sulfonic Acid, 2-Ethylhexyl Salicylate. **Other Ingredients:** Triple Purified Water, Caprylic/Capric Triglyceride, Mineral Oil, Octyl Stearate, Cetearyl Alcohol, Glyceryl Stearate SE, Sodium Hydroxide, PEG-40 Castor Oil, Carbomer, Sodium Cetearyl Sulfate, Lanolin Alcohol, EDTA, Methylchloroisothiazolinone, Methylisothiazolinone.

Actions and Uses: Eucerin Daily Facial Lotion is fragrance-free, non-comedogenic and non-acnegenic. It has an SPF 20 and contains a non-sensitizing sunblock to protect skin from UVA and UVB light. It is specially formulated for dry, sensitive skin or for those undergoing therapies that irritate delicate facial skin such as Retin-A®* therapy, chemical peels and treatment with drying medications.[1] This light, oil-in-water formula is non-greasy and cosmetically elegant.

Administration and Dosage: Apply Eucerin Daily Facial Lotion twice a day (especially in the morning), or as directed by a physician. Can be used alone or under cosmetics.

Precautions: For external use only, not to be swallowed. Avoid contact with eyes. Discontinue use if signs of irritation or rash appear. Use on children under 6 months of age only with the advice of a physician.

How Supplied:
4-oz. bottle.
List #03972
1. Data on File, Beiersdorf Inc.
*Retin-A is a trademark of Ortho Pharmaceutical Corp.
Shown in Product Identification Guide, page 403

EUCERIN® Lotion
[ū'sir-in]
Dry Skin Care Lotion
NDC Numbers—10356-793-01
10356-793-04
10356-793-06

Composition: Water, Mineral Oil, Isopropyl Myristate, PEG-40 Sorbitan Peroleate, Lanolin Acid Glycerin Ester, Sorbitol, Propylene Glycol, Cetyl Palmitate, Magnesium Sulfate, Aluminum Stearate, Wool Wax Alcohol, BHT, Methylchloroisothiazolinone, Methylisothiazolinone.

Actions and Uses: Eucerin Lotion is a unique non-comedogenic, fragrance-free, water-in-oil formulation that will help to alleviate and soothe excessively dry skin, and provide long-lasting moisturization.

Administration and Dosage: Use daily as preventative care for skin exposed to sun, water, wind, cold or other drying elements.

Precautions: For external use only.

How Supplied:
8 fluid oz. plastic bottle—
List Number 3793
16 fluid oz. plastic bottle—
List number 3794
Shown in Product Identification Guide, page 403

**IF YOU SUSPECT
AN INTERACTION...**
The 1,400-page
*PDR Guide to Drug Interactions •
Side Effects • Indications*
can help.
Use the order form
in the front of this book.

Blaine Company, Inc.
1465 JAMIKE LANE
ERLANGER, KY 41018

MAG–OX 400

Description: Each tablet contains Magnesium Oxide 400 mg. U.S.P. (Heavy), or 241.3 mg. Elemental Magnesium (19.86 mEq.)

Indications and Usage: Hypomagnesemia, magnesium deficiencies and/or magnesium depletion during therapy with diuretics and/or digitalis, aminoglycosides, amphotericin B, cyclosporin, chemotherapy, and during pregnancy, PMS, menopause, diabetes, hyperoxaluria, malnutrition, weight/strength training, restricted diet, or alcoholism and as an antacid.

Warnings: Do not use this product except under the advice and supervision of a physician if you have a kidney disease. May have laxative effect.

Dosage: Adult dose 1 or 2 tablets daily with meals or as directed by a physician.

Professional Labeling: Serum magnesium levels do not accurately represent total body, tissue, or bone magnesium levels.

How Supplied: Bottles of 100, 1000, and hospital unit dose (U.D. 100s)

URO–MAG

Description: Each capsule contains Magnesium Oxide 140 mg. U.S.P. (Heavy), or 84.5 mg. Elemental Magnesium (6.93 mEq.)

Indications and Usage: Hypomagnesemia, magnesium deficiencies and/or magnesium depletion during therapy with diuretics and/or digitalis, aminoglycosides, amphotericin B, cyclosporin, chemotherapy, and during pregnancy, PMS, menopause, diabetes, hyperoxaluria, malnutrition, weight/strength training, restricted diet, or alcoholism and as an antacid.

Warnings: Do not use this product except under the advice and supervision of a physician if you have a kidney disease. May have laxative effect.

Dosage: Adult dose 3–4 capsules daily with meals or as directed by a physician.

Professional Labeling: Serum magnesium levels do not accurately represent total body, tissue, or bone magnesium levels.

How Supplied: Bottles of 100 and 1000.

EDUCATIONAL MATERIAL

Heart, female reproductive system and kidney stone charts, samples and literature available to physicians upon request.

Blairex Laboratories, Inc.
4810 TECUMSEH LANE
P.O. BOX 15190
EVANSVILLE, IN 47716-0190

BRONCHO SALINE®
0.9% Sodium Chloride Aerosol for the dilution of bronchodilator inhalation solutions. Sterile normal saline for diluting bronchodilator solutions for oral inhalation.

Description: Broncho Saline® is for patients using bronchodilator solutions for oral inhalation that require dilution with sterile normal saline solution. Broncho Saline is a sterile liquid solution consisting of 0.9% sodium chloride for oral inhalation with a pH of 4.5 to 7.5. Not to be used for injection.

Indications and Usage: Patients who use bronchodilator solutions for inhalation are instructed to dilute the medication with sterile normal saline solution. Bronchodilators that call for dilution with saline for administration by nebulization include:
  Alupent Inhalation Solution (Metaproterenol Sulfate, USP, 5%)
  Bronkosol (Isoetharine Hydrochloride, USP, 1%)
  Isuprel Hydrochloride (Isoproterenol Hydrochloride)
  Proventil Solution for Inhalation (Albuterol Sulfate, 0.5%)
  Ventolin Solution for Inhalation (Albuterol Sulfate, 0.5%)

Warnings: Use this product only with the approval of your physician, respiratory therapist or pharmacist. Contents under pressure. Do not puncture or incinerate. Keep out of reach of children. If you experience any complications, contact your physician immediately.

Directions for Use:
1. Add the prescribed dosage of bronchodilator medication to the nebulizer cup.
2. Pick up Broncho Saline® and look at the top parts. Line up parts so the half-circle under the valve cap fits over nozzle. This is necessary to press the valve cap down.
3. To dispense Broncho Saline®, aim nozzle, press, and release. Each time you press and release the valve, 1cc (mL) of saline is dispensed. If you need 2cc (mL), depress and release the valve twice. For 3cc (mL), depress and release the valve three times, and so on.
4. Dispense the recommended amount of saline into the nebulizer cup.
5. Proceed with the normal operation of your breathing apparatus.
6. When finished with your treatment, the reservoir should be rinsed clean with warm water. Please follow the cleaning instructions with your breathing apparatus.

How Supplied: Broncho Saline® comes in 90cc (mL) and 240cc (mL) Pressurized Containers.
Store between 15–25°C (59–77°F). Keep out of reach of children. See WARNINGS.

NASAL MOIST®
Sodium Chloride 0.65%

Description: Isotonic saline solution buffered with sodium bicarbonate. Preserved with Benzyl alcohol.

Actions and Uses: Use for dry nasal membranes caused by chronic sinusitis, allergy, asthma, dry air, oxygen therapy. May be used as often as needed.

Directions: Squeeze twice into each nostril as needed.

How Supplied: 45 mL (1.5 oz.) plastic squeeze bottle.

Block Drug Company, Inc.
257 CORNELISON AVENUE
JERSEY CITY, NJ 07302

BALMEX® OINTMENT
for diaper rash and minor skin irritations

Balmex® ointment helps treat and prevent diaper rash in four ways: 1. Soothes irritation. 2. Provides protection. 3. Promotes healing. 4. Reduces inflammation.

Directions: At the first sign of diaper rash or redness, apply Balmex® three or more times daily as needed. To help prevent diaper rash, apply Balmex® liberally as often as necessary, with each diaper change, especially at bedtime or anytime when exposure to wet diapers may be prolonged.

Warnings: Avoid contact with the eyes. For external use only. If condition worsens or does not improve within 7 days, contact a physician. Keep out of reach of children.

Active Ingredient: Zinc Oxide.

Inactive Ingredients: Balsam (Specially Purified Balsam Peru), Beeswax, Benzoic Acid, Bismuth Subnitrate, Mineral Oil, Purified Water, Silicone, Synthetic White Wax, and other ingredients.

How Supplied: 1, 2, 4 oz. tubes; 1 lb. plastic jars (½ oz. tubes for Hospitals only). Balmex Ointment-All Commercial Sizes-Safety Sealed.

BC® POWDER
ARTHRITIS STRENGTH BC® POWDER
BC® COLD POWDER

Description: BC® POWDER: Active Ingredients: Aspirin 650 mg per powder, Salicylamide 195 mg per powder and Caffeine 32 mg per powder. ARTHRITIS STRENGTH BC® POWDER: Active Ingredients: Aspirin 742 mg in combination with 222 mg Salicylamide and 36 mg Caffeine per powder.
BC® COLD POWDER
BC® COLD POWDER MULTI-SYMPTOM FORMULA (COLD-SINUS ALLERGY)
BC® COLD POWDER NON-DROWSY FORMULA (COLD-SINUS)
Active Ingredients: BC Cold Powder Multi-Symptom Formula (Cold-Sinus-Allergy)—Aspirin 650 mg, Phenylpropanolamine Hydrochloride 25 mg, and Chlorpheniramine Maleate 4 mg per powder. BC Cold Powder Non-Drowsy Formula (Cold-Sinus) Aspirin 650 mg and Phenylpropanolamine Hydrochloride 25 mg per powder.

Indications: BC Powder is for relief of simple headache; for temporary relief of minor arthritic pain, neuralgia, neuritis and sciatica; for relief of muscular aches, discomfort and fever of colds; and for relief of normal menstrual pain and pain of tooth extraction.
Arthritis Strength BC Powder is specially formulated to fight occasional minor pain and inflammation of arthritis. Like original formula BC, Arthritis Strength BC provides fast temporary relief of minor arthritis pain and inflammation, neuralgia, neuritis and sciatica; relief of muscular aches, discomfort and fever of colds; and pain of tooth extraction. BC Cold Powder Multi-Symptom (Cold-Sinus-Allergy) is for relief of cold symptoms such as body aches, fever, nasal congestion, sneezing, running nose, and watery itchy eyes. BC Cold Powder Non-Drowsy Formula (Cold-Sinus) is for relief of such symptoms as body aches, fever, and nasal congestions.

Warnings: Children and teenagers should not use this medicine for chicken pox or flu symptoms before a doctor is consulted about Reye Syndrome, a rare but serious illness reported to be associated with aspirin. Do not exceed recommended dosage or administer to children, including teenagers, with chicken pox or flu, unless directed by a physician. Do not take this product if you are allergic to aspirin, have asthma, gastric ulcer, or are taking a medication that affects the clotting of blood, except under the advice and supervision of a physician. If pain persists for more than 10 days or redness is present, discontinue use of this product and consult a physician immediately. Keep this and all medication out of children's reach. As with any drug, if you are pregnant or nursing a baby, consult your physician before using this product. IT IS ESPECIALLY IMPORTANT NOT TO USE ASPIRIN DURING THE LAST 3 MONTHS OF PREGNANCY UNLESS SPECIFICALLY DIRECTED TO DO SO BY A DOCTOR BECAUSE IT MAY CAUSE PROBLEMS IN THE UNBORN CHILD OR COMPLICATIONS DURING DELIVERY. Discontinue use if ringing

Continued on next page

Block Drug—Cont.

in the ears occurs. Do not exceed recommended dosage.

BC Cold Powder Family of Products: If symptoms do not improve within 7 days, or are accompanied by high fever, consult a physician before continuing use. Do not take this product if you have high blood pressure, heart disease, diabetes, or thyroid disease except under the advice and supervision of a physician. Do not take this product if you are presently taking a prescription antihypertensive or antidepressant drug containing a monoamine oxidase inhibitor except under the advice and supervision of a physician. This product contains aspirin and should not be taken by individuals who are sensitive to aspirin. BC Cold Powder Multi-Symptom with antihistamine may cause drowsiness. Avoid alcoholic beverages while taking this product. Use caution when driving a motor vehicle or operating machinery.

Overdosage: In case of accidental overdosage, contact a physician or poison control center immediately.

Dosage and Administration: BC Powder: Stir one powder into a glass of water or other liquid, or, place powder on tongue and follow with liquid. May be used every 3 or 4 hours up to 4 times a day. For children under 12 consult a physician.

Arthritis Strength BC Powder: Place one powder on tongue and follow with liquid. If you prefer, stir powder into glass of water or other liquid. May be used every three to four hours, up to 4 powders each 24 hours. For children under 12, consult a physician.

BC Cold Powder:

Adults—Stir one powder into a glass of water or other liquid, or place powder on tongue and following with liquid. May be used every 4 hours up to 4 times a day. For Children Under 12—consult a physician.

How Supplied: BC Powder: Available in tamper resistant over wrapped envelopes of 2 or 6 powders, as well as tamper resistant boxes of 24 and 50 powders.

Arthritis Strength BC Powder: Available in tamper resistant over wrapped envelopes of 6 powders, and tamper resistant over wrapped boxes of 24 and 50 powders.

BC Cold Powder: Available in tamper-resistant over wrapped envelopes of 6 powders, as well as tamper-resistant boxes of 24 powders.

NYTOL® TABLETS

Active Ingredient: Diphenhydramine Hydrochloride, 25 mg per tablet (NYTOL with DPH) and 50 mg per tablet (Maximum Strength NYTOL).

Indications: Diphenhydramine Hydrochloride is an antihistamine with anti-cholinergic and sedative effects which induces drowsiness and helps in falling asleep.

Warnings: Do not give children under 12 years of age. If sleeplessness persists continuously for more than 2 weeks, consult your doctor. Insomnia may be a symptom of serious underlying medical illness. Do not take this product if you have asthma, glaucoma, emphysema, chronic pulmonary disorders, shortness of breath, difficulty in breathing or difficulty in urination due to enlargement of the prostate gland unless directed by a doctor. Avoid alcoholic beverages while taking this product. Do not take this product if you are taking tranquilizers or sedatives, without first consulting your doctor. In case of accidental overdose seek professional assistance or contact a poison control center immediately. As with any drug, if your are pregnant or nursing a baby, seek the advice of a health professional before using this product. Keep this and all drugs out of the reach of children.

Drug Interaction: Alcohol and other drugs which cause CNS depression will heighten the depressant effect of this product. Monoamine oxidase (MAO) inhibitors will prolong and intensify the anticholinergic effects of antihistamines.

Symptoms and Treatment of Oral Overdosage: In adults overdose may cause CNS depression resulting in hypnosis and coma. In children CNS hyperexcitability may follow sedation; the stimulant phase may bring tremor, delirium and convulsions. Gastrointestinal reactions may include dry mouth, appetite loss, nausea and vomiting. Respiratory distress and cardiovascular complications (hypotension) may be evident. Treatment includes inducing emesis, and controlling symptoms.

Dosage and Administration: Adults and children 12 years of age and over, take 2 NYTOL with DPH or 1 Maximum Strength NYTOL tablet 20 minutes at bedtime if needed, or as directed by a physician.

How Supplied: Available in tamper resistant packages of 16, 32, and 72 tablets NYTOL with DPH; of 8 and 16 tablets Maximum Strength NYTOL.

PROMISE® SENSITIVE TOOTHPASTE
For Sensitive Teeth and Cavity Prevention

Active Ingredients: Potassium Nitrate and Sodium Monofluorophosphate in a pleasantly mint-flavored dentifrice.

Promise contains Potassium Nitrate for relief of dentinal hypersensitivity resulting from the exposure of tooth dentin due to periodontal surgery, cervical (gumline) erosion, abrasion or recession which causes pain on contact with hot, cold, or tactile stimuli. Promise also contains Sodium Monofluorophosphate for cavity prevention.

Indications: Promise builds increasing protection against painful sensitivity of the teeth to cold, heat, acids, sweets or contact and aids in the prevention of dental cavities.

Actions: Promise significantly reduces tooth hypersensitivity, with response to therapy evident after two weeks of use. Controlled double-blind clinical studies provide substantial evidence of the safety and effectiveness of Promise. The current theory on mechanism of action is that the potassium nitrate in Promise has an effect on neural transmission, interrupting the signal which would result in the sensation of pain. Sodium Monofluorophosphate protects the tooth surfaces to prevent cavities.

Warning: Sensitive teeth may indicate a serious problem that may need prompt care by a dentist. See your dentist if the problem persists or worsens. Do not use this product longer than 4 weeks unless recommended by a dentist or doctor. **Keep this and all drugs out of the reach of children.**

Directions: Adults and children 12 years of age and older:

Apply at least a 1-inch strip of the product onto a soft bristle toothbrush. Brush teeth thoroughly for at least 1 minute twice a day (morning and evening) or as recommended by a dentist or doctor.

How Supplied: Promise Sensitive is supplied in 1.6 oz. (46 g) and 3.0 oz. (85 g) tubes.

ORIGINAL FORMULA SENSODYNE® –SC
Toothpaste for Sensitive Teeth

Description: Each tube contains strontium chloride hexahydrate (10%) in a pleasantly flavored cleansing/polishing desensitizing dentifrice.

Actions/Indications: Tooth hypersensitivity is a condition in which individuals experience pain from exposure to hot, cold stimuli, from chewing fibrous foods, or from tactile stimuli (e.g. toothbrushing.) Hypersensitivity may also be caused by a reaction to sweet or acidic foods (OSMOTIC) stimuli. Hypersensitivity usually occurs when the protective enamel covering on teeth wears away (which happens most often at the gum line) or if gum tissue recedes and exposes the dentin underneath.

Running through the dentin are microscopic small "tubules" which, according to many authorities, carry the pain impulses to the nerve of the tooth.

Sensodyne–SC provides a unique ingredient—strontium chloride—which is believed to be deposited in the tubules where it blocks the pain. The longer Sensodyne–SC is used, the more of a barrier it helps build against pain.

The effect of Sensodyne–SC may not be manifested immediately and may require a few weeks or longer of use for relief to be obtained. A number of clinical studies in the U.S. and other countries have provided substantial evidence of the performance attributes of Sensodyne–SC. Complete relief of hypersensitivity has been reported in approximately 65% of users and measurable relief or reduction in hypersensitivity in approximately 90%. The Original Formula has been commercially available for over 30 years. The ADA Council on Dental Therapeutics has given Sensodyne–SC the Seal of Acceptance as an effective desensitizing dentifrice in otherwise normal teeth.

Contraindications: Subjects with severe dental erosion should brush properly and lightly with any dentifrice to avoid further removal of tooth structure.

Dosage and Administration: Apply at least a 1-inch strip of the product onto a soft bristle toothbrush. Brush teeth thoroughly for at least 1 minute twice a day (morning and evening) or as recommended by a dentist or doctor. Make sure to brush all sensitive areas of the teeth. Children under 12 years of age: consult a dentist or doctor.

Warnings: Sensitive teeth may indicate a serious problem that may need prompt care by a dentist. See your dentist if the problem persists or worsens. Do not use this product longer than 4 weeks unless recommended by a dentist or doctor.

How Supplied: SENSODYNE–SC Toothpaste is supplied in 2.1 oz. (60 g), 4.0 oz. (113 g), and 6.0 oz. (170 g).

FRESH MINT SENSODYNE®
COOL GEL SENSODYNE®
Toothpaste for Sensitive Teeth and Cavity Prevention
Desensitizing Dentifrice

Active Ingredients: 5% Potassium Nitrate and Sodium Monofluorophosphate (Fresh Mint) or Sodium Fluoride (Cool Gel) in a pleasantly mint-flavored dentifrice.
Fresh Mint Sensodyne and Cool Gel Sensodyne contain Potassium Nitrate for relief of dentinal hypersensitivity resulting from the exposure of tooth dentin due to periodontal surgery, cervical (gum line) erosion, abrasion or recession which causes pain on contact with hot, cold, or tactile stimuli and fluoride for cavity prevention. Fresh Mint Sensodyne has been given the Seal of Acceptance by the ADA Council on Dental Therapeutics as an effective desensitizing dentifrice for otherwise normal teeth.

Actions: Fresh Mint Sensodyne and Cool Gel Sensodyne significantly reduce tooth hypersensitivity, with response to therapy evident after two weeks of use. Controlled double-blind clinical studies provide substantial evidence of the safety and effectiveness of potassium nitrate. The current theory on mechanism

of action is that potassium nitrate has an effect on neural transmission, interrupting the signal which would result in the sensation of pain. Fluorides are anticariogenic, forming fluoroapatite in the outer surface of the dental enamel which is resistant to acids and caries.

Warnings: Sensitive teeth may indicate a serious problem that may need prompt care by a dentist. See your dentist if the problem persists or worsens. Do not use this product longer than 4 weeks unless recommended by a dentist or doctor.

Dosage and Administration: Apply at least a 1-inch strip of the product onto a soft bristle toothbrush. Brush teeth thoroughly for at least 1 minute twice a day (morning and evening) or as recommended by a dentist or doctor. Make sure to brush all sensitive areas of the teeth. Children under 12 years of age: consult a dentist or doctor.

How Supplied: Fresh Mint Sensodyne is supplied in 2.1 (60 g), 4.0 (113 g) and 6.0 oz. (170 g) tubes and in 4.0 oz. pumps. Cool Gel is available in 2.1 (60 g), 4.0 (113 g) and 6.0 oz. (170 g) tubes.

TEGRIN® DANDRUFF SHAMPOO
TEGRIN® FOR PSORIASIS LOTION, SKIN CREAM AND MEDICATED SOAP
TEGRIN®-HC WITH HYDROCORTISONE ANTI-ITCH OINTMENT

Description: Tegrin® Dandruff Shampoo contains 7% coal tar solution equivalent to 1.4% coal tar, in a pleasantly scented, high-foaming, cleansing shampoo base with emollients, conditioners and other formula components.
Tegrin® for Psoriasis Lotion, Skin Cream and Medicated Soap Tegrin Lotion, Skin Cream and Medicated Soap each contain 5% coal tar solution, equivalent to 0.8% coal tar. Both the Lotion and Cream also contain alcohol (4.9% and 4.7%, respectively). Tegrin®-HC is a special fragrance-free ointment which contains 1.0% hydrocortisone, an effective anti-itch ingredient in the maximum strength available without a prescription.

Actions/Indications: Coal Tar is obtained in the destructive distillation of bituminous coal and is a highly effective agent for controlling the flaking and itching of the scalp associated with dandruff, seborrheic dermatitis and psoriasis. The action of coal tar is believed to be keratolytic, antiseptic, antipruritic and astringent. The coal tar solution used in Tegrin Dandruff Shampoo is prepared in such a way as to reduce the pitch and other irritant components found in crude coal tar without reduction in therapeutic potency.
Coal tar solution has been used clincially for many years as a remedy for dandruff and for scaling associated with scalp disorders such as seborrhea and psoriasis.

Its mechanism of action has not been fully established, but it is believed to retard the rate of turnover of epidermal cells with regular use. A number of clinical studies have demonstrated the performance attributes of Tegrin Dandruff Shampoo against dandruff and seborrheic dermatitis. In addition to relieving the above symptoms, Tegrin shampoo, used regularly, maintains scalp and hair cleanliness and leaves the hair lustrous and manageable.
Tegrin-HC is for the temporary relief of itching associated with minor skin irritations, inflammation, rashes due to psoriasis, eczema and seborrheic dermatitis; other uses of this product should be only under the advice and supervision of a doctor.

Warnings: For external use only. Avoid contact with eyes. If contact occurs, rinse eyes thoroughly with water. If condition worsens or does not improve after regular use of this product as directed, consult a doctor. Use caution in exposing skin to sunlight after applying this product. It may increase tendency to sunburn for up to 24 hours after application. Do not use for prolonged periods without consulting a doctor. Do not use this product with other forms of psoriasis therapy, such as ultraviolet radiation or prescription drugs, unless directed by a doctor. Keep out of reach of children. In case of accidental ingestion, seek professional assistance or contact a Poison Control Center immediately.
Do not use any other hydrocortisone products with Tegrin-HC unless you have consulted a doctor. Do not use for the treatment of diaper rash; consult a doctor. KEEP OUT OF THE REACH OF CHILDREN.

Directions: Shake Tegrin Dandruff Shampoo well. Wet hair thoroughly. Rub Tegrin liberally into hair and scalp. Rinse thoroughly. Briskly massage a second application of the shampoo into a rich lather. Rinse thoroughly. For best results use at least twice a week or as directed by a doctor.
Apply Tegrin for Psoriasis lotion or cream to affected areas one to four times daily or as directed by a doctor. Use Tegrin Soap on affected areas in place of your regular soap.
Adults and children 2 years of age and older: apply Tegrin-HC to affected area not more than 3 to 4 times daily. Children under 2 years of age: Do not use, consult a doctor.

How Supplied: Tegrin Dandruff Shampoo is supplied in 7 fl. oz. (207 ml) plastic bottles.
Tegrin Lotion 7 fl. oz. (207 ml) bottle, Tegrin Cream 2 oz. (57 g) and 4.4 oz. (124 g) tubes, Tegrin Soap 4.5 oz. (127 g) bars.

Bock Pharmacal Company
P.O. BOX 419056
ST. LOUIS, MO 63141-9056

EMETROL®
(Phosphorated Carbohydrate Solution)
For the relief of nausea associated with upset stomach

Description: EMETROL is an oral solution containing balanced amounts of dextrose (glucose) and levulose (fructose) and phosphoric acid with controlled hydrogen ion concentration. Available in original lemon-mint or cherry flavor.

Ingredients: Each 5 mL teaspoonful contains dextrose (glucose), 1.87 g; levulose (fructose), 1.87 g; phosphoric acid, 21.5 mg; and the following inactive ingredients: glycerin, methylparaben, purified water; D&C yellow No. 10 and natural lemon-mint flavor in lemon-mint Emetrol; FD&C red No. 40 and artificial cherry flavor in cherry Emetrol.

Action: EMETROL quickly relieves nausea by local action on the wall of the hyperactive G.I. tract. There is no delay in therapeutic action such as that associated with systemic drugs.

Indications: For the relief of nausea due to upset stomach from intestinal flu, stomach flu, and food or drink indiscretions. For other conditions, take only as directed by your physician.

Advantages:
1. **Fast Action**—works quickly through local action relaxing hyperactive muscles of the G.I. tract.
2. **Effectiveness**—clinically proven to stop nausea.
3. **Safety**—all natural active ingredients won't mask symptoms of organic pathology. No salicylates makes Emetrol safe for children and teens with flu or fever. No known drug interactions.
4. **Convenience**—no ℞ required.
5. **Patient Acceptance**—pleasant tasting lemon-mint or cherry flavor.

Usual Adult Dose: One or two tablespoons. Repeat every 15 minutes until distress subsides.

Usual Children's Dose: One or two teaspoons. Repeat dose every 15 minutes until distress subsides.

Important: For maximum effectiveness never dilute EMETROL or drink fluids of any kind immediately before or after taking a dose.

Caution: Not to be taken for more than one hour (5 doses) without consulting a physician. If upset stomach continues or recurs frequently, consult a physician promptly as it may be a sign of a serious condition.
WARNING: KEEP THIS AND ALL MEDICATIONS OUT OF THE REACH OF CHILDREN. As with any drug, if you are pregnant or nursing a baby, seek the advice of a health professional before using this product.

This product contains fructose and should not be taken by persons with hereditary fructose intolerance (HFI).

> **This product contains sugar and should not be taken by diabetics except under the advice and supervision of a physician.**

In case of accidental overdose, contact a poison control center, emergency medical facility, or physician immediately for advice.

How Supplied: Each 5 mL teaspoonful of EMETROL contains dextrose (glucose), 1.87 g; levulose (fructose), 1.87 g; and phosphoric acid, 21.5 mg in a yellow, lemon-mint or red, cherry-flavored syrup.
Yellow, Lemon-Mint
NDC 0563-2113-04—Bottle of 4 fluid ounces (118 mL)
NDC 0563-2113-08—Bottle of 8 fluid ounces (236 mL)
NDC 0563-2113-16—Bottle of 1 pint (473 mL)
Red, Cherry
NDC 0563-2114-04—Bottle of 4 fluid ounces (118 mL)
NDC 0563-2114-08—Bottle of 8 fluid ounces (236 mL)
NDC 0563-2114-16—Bottle of 1 pint (473 mL)
Store at room temperature.
NOTICE: Each bottle is protected by a printed band around the cap. Do not use if band is damaged or missing.

Shown in Product Identification Guide, page 403

Boiron, The World Leader In Homeopathy
1208 AMOSLAND ROAD
NORWOOD, PA 19074

OSCILLOCOCCINUM®
[ah-sill 'o-cox-see 'num ']

Active Ingredient: Anas Barbariae Hepatis et Cordis Extractum HPUS 200C

Indications: For the relief of flu-like symptoms such as fever, chills, body aches and pains.

Actions: Like most Homeopathic remedies, Oscillococcinum® acts gently by stimulating the patient's natural defense mechanisms.

Warnings: If symptoms persist for more than three days or worsen, consult your physician. Keep all medication out of reach of children. As with any drug if you are pregnant or nursing a baby, seek professional advice before using this product.

Dosage and Administration: (Adults and Children over 2 years)
At the onset of symptoms, place the entire contents of one tube in your mouth and allow to dissolve under your tongue. Repeat every 6 hours as necessary. For maximum results, Oscillococcinum® should be taken early, at the onset of symptoms, and at least 15 minutes before or 1 hour after meals.

How Supplied: boxes of 3 unit doses or 6 unit doses of 0.04 oz. (1 gram) each (NDC #0220-9280-32 and NDC #0220-9288-33) Tamper resistant package. Manufactured by Boiron, France. Distributor: Boiron, Norwood, PA
Shown in Product Identification Guide, page 404

> **EDUCATIONAL MATERIAL**

Boiron Product Catalogue
General description of the most popular Boiron remedies and lines.
Oscillococcinum ® Brochure
Brochure on Oscillococcinum® describing clinical research on the product and its general use.
"What Is Homeopathy?"
Booklet free to physicians and pharmacists.
"An Introduction to Homeopathy for the Practicing Pharmacist"
A free continuing education booklet for pharmacists.

Bristol-Myers Products
(A Bristol-Myers Squibb Company)
345 PARK AVENUE
NEW YORK, NY 10154

ALPHA KERI®
Moisture Rich Body Oil

Composition: Contains mineral oil, Hydroloc™ brand of Westwood's PEG-4 dilaurate, lanolin oil, fragrance, benzophenone-3, D&C green 6.

Indications: ALPHA KERI is a water-dispersible oil for the care of dry skin. ALPHA KERI effectively deposits a thin, uniform, emulsified film of oil over the skin. This film lubricates and softens the skin. ALPHA KERI Moisture Rich Body Oil is an all-over skin moisturizer. Only Alpha Keri contains Hydroloc™—the unique emulsifier that provides a more uniform distribution of the therapeutic oils to moisturize dry skin. ALPHA KERI is valuable as an aid for dry skin and mild skin irritations.

Directions for Use: ALPHA KERI *should always be used with water, either added to water or rubbed on to wet skin.* Because of its inherent cleansing properties it is not necessary to use soap when ALPHA KERI is being used.
For external use only.
Label directions should be followed for use in shower, bath and cleansing.

Precaution: The patient should be warned to guard against slipping in tub or shower.

How Supplied: 4 fl. oz., 8 fl. oz., 12 fl. oz., and 16 fl. oz., plastic bottles. Also available in non-aerosol pump spray, 3.5 oz.

Shown in Product Identification Guide, page 404

ALPHA KERI®
Moisture Rich Cleansing Bar
Non-detergent Soap

Composition: Sodium tallowate, sodium cocoate, water, mineral oil, fragrance, PEG-75, glycerin, titanium dioxide, lanolin oil, sodium chloride. May contain: BHT, and/or Trisodium HEDTA, D&C Green 5, D&C Yellow 10.

Indications: ALPHA KERI Moisture Rich Cleansing Bar, rich in emollient oils, thoroughly cleanses as it soothes and softens the skin.

Indications: Adjunctive use in dry skin care.

Directions for Use: To be used as any other soap.

How Supplied: 4 oz. bar.

BACKACHE CAPLETS

Composition: Each caplet contains Magnesium Salicylate Tetrahydrate 580 mg (equivalent to 467 mg of anhydrous Magnesium Salicylate)
Other Ingredients: Carnauba Wax, Hydrogenated Vegetable Oil, Hydroxypropyl Methylcellulose, Magnesium Stearate, Microcrystalline Cellulose, Polyethylene Glycol, Polysorbate 80, Titanium Dioxide

Indications: For the temporary relief of minor aches and pains associated with backache and muscular aches (e.g., sprains and strains).

Directions: Adults: 2 caplets with water every 6 hours while symptoms persist, not to exceed 8 caplets in 24 hours or as directed by a doctor. Children under 12: Consult a doctor.

Warnings: Children and teenagers should not use this medicine for chicken pox or flu symptoms before a doctor is consulted about Reye syndrome, a rate but serious illness. **KEEP THIS AND ALL OTHER MEDICATIONS OUT OF THE REACH OF CHILDREN. IN CASE OF ACCIDENTAL OVERDOSE, SEEK PROFESSIONAL ASSISTANCE OR CONTACT A POISON CONTROL CENTER IMMEDIATELY.** As with any drug, if you are pregnant or nursing a baby, seek the advice of a health professional before using this product. Do not take this product for more than 10 days unless directed by a doctor. If pain persists or gets worse, if new symptoms occur, or if redness or swelling is present, consult a doctor because these could be

signs of a serious condition. Do not take this product if you are allergic to salicylates (including aspirin), have asthma, have stomach problems (such as heartburn, upset stomach or stomach pain) that persists or recur, or if you have ulcers or bleeding problems, unless directed by a doctor. If ringing in the ears or loss of hearing occurs, consult a doctor before taking any more of this product.

Drug Interaction Precaution: Do not take this product if you are taking a prescription drug for anticoagulation (thinning of blood), diabetes, gout or arthritis unless directed by a doctor.

How Supplied: BACKACHE is a white caplet with the logo "N-BACK" debossed on one side.
NDC 19810–0579–1 Blister cards of 24's
NDC 19810–0579–2 Bottles of 50's
The bottles of 50's are packaged in child resistant closures; the blister cards of 24's are recommended for households without young children and are packaged without a child resistant closure. Store at room temperature.

BUFFERIN®
[bŭf'fĕr-ĭn]
Analgesic

Composition:
Active Ingredient: Each coated tablet or caplet contains Aspirin 325 mg in a formulation buffered with Calcium Carbonate, Magnesium Oxide and Magnesium Carbonate.
Other Ingredients: Benzoic Acid, Citric Acid, Corn Starch, FD&C Blue No. 1, Hydroxypropyl Methylcellulose, Magnesium Stearate, Mineral Oil, Polysorbate 20, Povidone, Propylene Glycol, Simethicone Emulsion, Sodium Phosphate, Sorbitan Monolaurate, Titanium Dioxide. May also contain: Carnauba Wax, Zinc Stearate.

Indications: For temporary relief of headaches, pain and fever of colds, muscle aches, minor arthritis pain and inflammation, menstrual pain and toothaches.

Directions: Adults: 2 tablets or caplets with water every 4 hours while symptoms persist, not to exceed 12 tablets or caplets in 24 hours, or as directed by a doctor. Children 6 to under 12 years of age: One tablet or caplet with water every 4 hours, not to exceed 5 tablets or caplets in 24 hours or as directed by a doctor. Children under 6: Consult a doctor.

Warnings: Children and teenagers should not use this medicine for chicken pox or flu symptoms before a doctor is consulted about Reye syndrome, a rare but serious illness reported to be associated with aspirin. KEEP THIS AND ALL OTHER MEDICATIONS OUT OF THE REACH OF CHILDREN. IN CASE OF ACCIDENTAL OVERDOSE, SEEK PROFESSIONAL ASSISTANCE OR CONTACT A POISON CONTROL CENTER IMMEDIATELY. As with any drug,

if you are pregnant or nursing a baby, seek the advice of a health professional before using this product. **IT IS ESPECIALLY IMPORTANT NOT TO USE ASPIRIN DURING THE LAST 3 MONTHS OF PREGNANCY UNLESS SPECIFICALLY DIRECTED TO DO SO BY A DOCTOR BECAUSE IT MAY CAUSE PROBLEMS IN THE UNBORN CHILD OR COMPLICATIONS DURING DELIVERY.** Do not take this product for pain for more than 10 days (for adults) or 5 days (for children) or for fever for more than 3 days unless directed by a doctor. If pain or fever persists or gets worse, if new symptoms occur, or if redness or swelling is present, consult a doctor because these could be signs of a serious condition. Consult a dentist promptly for toothache. Do not give this product to children for the pain of arthritis unless directed by a doctor. Do not take this product if you are allergic to aspirin, have asthma, have stomach problems (such as heartburn, upset stomach or stomach pain) that persist or recur, or if you have ulcers or bleeding problems, unless directed by a doctor. If ringing in the ears or loss of hearing occurs, consult a doctor before taking or giving any more of this product.

Drug Interaction Precaution: This product should not be taken by any adult or child who is taking a prescription drug for anticoagulation (thinning of blood), diabetes, gout or arthritis unless directed by a doctor.

How Supplied: BUFFERIN is supplied as:
Coated circular white tablet with letter "B" debossed on one surface.
NDC 19810-0073-2 Bottle of 12's
NDC 19810-0093-3 Bottle of 30's
NDC 19810-0093-4 Bottle of 50's
NDC 19810-0073-5 Bottle of 100's
NDC 19810-0073-6 Bottle of 200's
NDC 19810-0073-9 Boxed 150 × 2 tablet foil pack for hospital and clinical use.
NDC 19810-0073-0 Vials of 10
Coated scored white caplet with letter "B" debossed on each side of scoring.
NDC 19810-0072-7 Bottle of 30's
NDC 19810-0072-8 Bottle of 50's
NDC 19810-0072-3 Bottle of 100's
All consumer sizes have child resistant closures except 100's for tablets and 50's for caplets which are sizes recommended for households without young children. Store at room temperature.
Also described in *PDR* for prescription drugs.

Professional Labeling

1. BUFFERIN® FOR RECURRENT TRANSIENT ISCHEMIC ATTACKS

Indication: For reducing the risk of recurrent transient ischemic attacks (TIA's) or stroke in men who have had transient ischemia of the brain due to fibrin platelet emboli. There is inadequate evidence that aspirin or buffered aspirin is effective in reducing TIA's in

Continued on next page

Bristol-Myers—Cont.

women at the recommended dosage. There is no evidence that aspirin or buffered aspirin is of benefit in the treatment of completed strokes in men or women.

Clinical Trials: The indication is supported by the results of a Canadian study (1) in which 585 patients with threatened stroke were followed in a randomized clinical trial for an average of 26 months to determine whether aspirin or sulfinpyrazone, singly or in combination, was superior to placebo in preventing transient ischemic attacks, stroke, or death. The study showed that, although sulfinpyrazone had no statistically significant effect, aspirin reduced the risk of continuing transient ischemic attacks, stroke, or death by 19 percent and reduced the risk of stroke or death by 31 percent. Another aspirin study carried out in the United States with 178 patients, showed a statistically significant number of "favorable outcomes," including reduced transient ischemic attacks, stroke, and death (2).

Precautions: Patients presenting with signs and symptoms of TIA's should have a complete medical and neurologic evaluation. Consideration should be given to other disorders that resemble TIA's. Attention should be given to risk factors: it is important to evaluate and treat, if appropriate, other diseases associated with TIA's and stroke, such as hypertension and diabetes.

Concurrent administration of absorbable antacids at therapeutic doses may increase the clearance of salicylates in some individuals. The concurrent administration of nonabsorbable antacids may alter the rate of absorption of aspirin, thereby resulting in a decreased acetylsalicylic acid/salicylate ratio in plasma. The clinical significance of these decreases in available aspirin is unknown. Aspirin at dosages of 1,000 milligrams per day has been associated with small increases in blood pressure, blood urea nitrogen, and serum uric acid levels. It is recommended that patients placed on long-term aspirin treatment be seen at regular intervals to assess changes in these measurements.

Adverse Reactions: At dosages of 1,000 milligrams or higher of aspirin per day, gastrointestinal side effects include stomach pain, heartburn, nausea and/or vomiting, as well as increased rates of gross gastrointestinal bleeding.

Dosage and Administration: Adult oral dosage for men is 1,300 milligrams a day, in divided doses of 650 milligrams twice a day or 325 milligrams four times a day.

References:
(1) The Canadian Cooperative Study Group. "A Randomized Trial of Aspirin and Sulfinpyrazone in Threatened Stroke," *New England Journal of Medicine*, 299:53–59, 1978.

(2) Fields, W.S., et al., "Controlled Trial of Aspirin in Cerebral Ischemia," *Stroke* 8:301–316, 1977.

2. BUFFERIN® FOR MYOCARDIAL INFARCTION

Indication: Aspirin is indicated to reduce the risk of death and/or nonfatal myocardial infarction in patients with a previous infarction or unstable angina pectoris.

Clinical Trials: The indication is supported by the results of six, large, randomized multicenter, placebo-controlled studies[1–7] involving 10,816, predominantly male, post-myocardial infarction (MI) patients and one randomized placebo-controlled study of 1,266 men with unstable angina. Therapy with aspirin was begun at intervals after the onset of acute MI varying from less than 3 days to more than 5 years and continued for periods of from less than one year to four years. In the unstable angina study, treatment was started within 1 month after the onset of unstable angina and continued for 12 weeks and complicating conditions such as congestive heart failure were not included in the study.

Aspirin therapy in MI patients was associated with about a 20 percent reduction in the risk of subsequent death and/or nonfatal reinfarction, a median absolute decrease of 3 percent from the 12 to 22 percent event rates in the placebo groups. In the aspirin-treated unstable angina patients the reduction in risk was about 50 percent, a reduction in the event rate of 5% from the 10% rate in the placebo group over the 12 weeks of the study.

Daily dosage of aspirin in the post-myocardial infarction studies was 300 mg. in one study and 900 and 1500 mg. in five studies. A dose of 325 mg. was used in the study of unstable angina.

Adverse Reactions: Gastrointestinal Reactions: Doses of 1000 mg. per day of aspirin caused gastrointestinal symptoms and bleeding that in some cases were clinically significant. In the largest post-infarction study (The Aspirin Myocardial Infaraction Study (AMIS) with 4,500 people), the percentage incidences of gastrointestinal symptoms for the aspirin (1000 mg. of a standard, solid-tablet formulation) and placebo-treated subjects, respectively, were: stomach pain (14.5%; 4.4%); heartburn (11.9%; 4.8%); nausea and/or vomiting (7.6%; 2.1%); hospitalization for gastrointestinal disorder (4.8%; 3.5%). In the AMIS and other trials, aspirin treated patients had increased rates of gross gastrointestinal bleeding. Symptoms and signs of gastrointestinal irritation were not significantly increased in subjects treated for unstable angina with buffered aspirin in solution.

Cardiovascular and Biochemical:
In the AMIS trial, the dosage of 1000 mg. per day of aspirin was associated with small increases in systolic blood pressure (BP) (average 1.5 to 2.1 mm) and diastolic BP (0.5 to 0.6 mm), depending upon whether maximal or last available readings were used. Blood urea nitrogen and uric acid levels were also increased, but by less than 1.0 mg%.

Subjects with marked hypertension or renal insufficiency had been excluded from the trial so that the clinical importance of these observations for such subjects or for any subjects treated over more prolonged periods is not known. It is recommended that patients placed on long-term aspirin treatment, even at doses of 300 mg. per day, be seen at regular intervals to assess changes in these measurements.

Administration and Dosage: Although most of the studies used dosages exceeding 300 mg., two trials used only 300 mg. and pharmacologic data indicate that this dose inhibits platelet function fully. Therefore, 300 mg. or a conventional 325 mg. aspirin dose is a reasonable, routine dose that would minimize gastrointestinal adverse reactions.

References: 1. Elwood P.C., et al., "A Randomized Controlled Trial of Acetylsalicylic Acid in the Secondary Prevention of Mortality from Myocardial Infarction," *British Medical Journal*, 1:436–440, 1974. 2. The Coronary Drug Project Research Group, "Aspirin in Coronary Heart Disease," *Journal of Chronic Disease*, 29:625–642, 1976. 3. Breddin K, et al., "Secondary Prevention of Myocardial Infarction; Comparison of Acetylsalicylic Acid Phenprocoumon and Placebo," *Thromb. Haemost.*, 41:225–236, 1979. 4. Aspirin Myocardial Infarction Study Research Group, "A Randomized, Controlled Trial of Aspirin in Persons Recovered from Myocardial Infarction," *Journal American Medical Association*, 243:661–669, 1980. 5. Elwood P.C., and Sweetnam, P.M., "Aspirin and Secondary Mortality after Myocardial Infarction," *Lancet*, pp. 1313–1315, December 22–29, 1979. 6. The Persantine-Aspirin Reinfarction Study Research Group. "Persantine and Aspirin in Coronary Heart Disease," *Circulation* 62;449–460, 1980. 7. Lewis H.D., et al., "Protective Effects of Aspirin Against Acute Myocardial Infarction and Death in Men with Unstable Angina, Results of a Veterans Administration Cooperative Study," *New England Journal of Medicine*, 309;396–403, 1983.

Shown in Product Identification Guide, page 404

BUFFERIN® AF Nite Time

Composition:
Active Ingredients: Each caplet contains Acetaminophen 500 mg. and Diphenhydramine Citrate 38 mg.
Other Ingredients: Benzoic Acid, Carnauba Wax, Corn Starch, D&C Yellow No. 10, D&C Yellow No. 10 Aluminum Lake, D&C Blue No. 1, FD&C Blue No. 1 Aluminum Lake, Hydroxypropyl Methylcellulose, Methylparaben, Magnesium Stearate, Propylene Glycol, Propylparaben, Simethicone Emulsion,

Stearic Acid, Titanium Dioxide. Remove cotton and recap bottle.

Indications: For temporary relief of occasional minor aches and pains accompanied by sleeplessness.

Warnings: KEEP THIS AND ALL OTHER MEDICATIONS OUT OF THE REACH OF CHILDREN. IN CASE OF ACCIDENTAL OVERDOSE, SEEK PROFESSIONAL ASSISTANCE OR CONTACT A POISON CONTROL CENTER IMMEDIATELY. PROMPT MEDICAL ATTENTION IS CRITICAL FOR ADULTS AS WELL AS FOR CHILDREN EVEN IF YOU DO NOT NOTICE ANY SIGNS OR SYMP-TOMS. As with any drug, if you are pregnant or nursing a baby, seek the advice of a health professional before using this product. Do not give this product to children under 12 years of age or use for more than 10 days unless directed by a doctor. Consult a doctor if symptoms persist or get worse or if new ones occur, or if sleeplessness persists continuously for more than 2 weeks because these may be symptoms of serious underlying medical illnesses. Do not take this product if you have asthma, glaucoma, emphysema, chronic pulmonary disease, shortness of breath, difficulty in breathing, or difficulty in urination due to enlargement of the prostate gland unless directed by a doctor. Avoid alcoholic beverages while taking this product. Do not take this product if you are taking sedatives or tranquilizers, without first consulting your doctor.

Directions: Adults: 2 caplets at bedtime if needed or as directed by a doctor.

Overdose: MUCOMYST (acetylcysteine) As An Antidote For Acetaminophen Overdose)
Acetaminophen is rapidly absorbed from the upper gastrointestinal tract with peak plasma levels occurring between 30 and 60 minutes after therapeutic doses and usually within 4 hours following an overdose. The parent compound, which is nontoxic, is extensively metabolized in the liver to form principally the sulfate and glucuronide conjugates which are also nontoxic and are rapidly excreted in the urine. A small fraction of an ingested dose is metabolized in the liver by the cytochrome P-450 mixed function oxidase enzyme system to form a reactive, potentially toxic, intermediate metabolite which preferentially conjugates with hepatic glutathione to form the nontoxic cysteine and mercapturic acid derivatives which are then excreted by the kidney. Therapeutic doses of acetaminophen do not saturate the glucuronide and sulfate conjugation pathways and do not result in the formation of sufficient reactive metabolite to deplete glutathione stores. However, following ingestion of a large overdose (150 mg/kg or greater) the glucuronide and sulfate conjugation pathways are saturated resulting in a larger fraction of the drug being metabolized via the P-450 pathway. The increased formation of reactive metabolite

may deplete the hepatic stores of glutathione with subsequent binding of the metabolite to protein molecules within the hepatocyte resulting in cellular necrosis. Acetylcysteine has been shown to reduce the extent of liver injury following acetaminophen overdose. Early symptoms following a potentially hepatotoxic overdose may include: nausea, vomiting, diaphoresis and general malaise. Clinical and laboratory evidence of hepatic toxicity may not be apparent until 48 to 72 hours postingestion. In adults and adolescents, regardless of the quantity of acetaminophen reported to have been ingested, administer MUCO-MYST® acetylcysteine immediately. MUCOMYST acetylcysteine therapy should be initiated and continued for a full course of therapy. Its effectiveness depends on early administration, with benefit seen principally in patients treated within 16 hours of the overdose. If acetaminophen plasma assay capability is not available, and the estimated acetaminophen ingestion exceeds 150 mg/kg, MUCOMYST acetylcysteine therapy should be initiated and continued for a full course of therapy.
For full prescribing information, refer to the MUCOMYST package insert. Do not await the results of assays for acetaminophen level before initiating treatment with MUCOMYST acetylcysteine. The following additional procedures are recommended: The stomach should be emptied promptly by lavage or by induction of emesis with syrup of ipecac. A serum acetaminophen assay should be obtained as early as possible, but no sooner than four hours following ingestion. Liver function studies should be obtained initially and repeated at 24-hour intervals.
For additional emergency information call your regional poison center or toll-free (1-800-525-6115) to the Rocky Mountain Poison Center for assistance in diagnosis and for directions in the use of MUCOMYST acetylcysteine as an antidote.

How Supplied: BUFFERIN® A/F Nite Time is supplied as: Light blue coated caplets with "BUFFERIN® Nite Time" imprinted in dark blue on one side.
NDC 19810-0084-1 Bottles of 24's
NDC 19810-0084-2 Bottles of 50's
The 50 caplet size does not have a child resistant closure and is recommended for households without young children.
Store at room temperature.

Arthritis Strength BUFFERIN®
[bŭf′fĕr-ĭn]
Analgesic

Composition:
Active Ingredient: Aspirin (500 mg) in a formulation buffered with Calcium Carbonate, Magnesium Oxide and Magnesium Carbonate.
Other Ingredients: Benzoic Acid, Citric Acid, Corn Starch, FD&C Blue No. 1, Hydroxypropyl Methylcellulose, Magne-

sium Stearate, Mineral Oil, Polysorbate 20, Povidone, Propylene Glycol, Simethicone Emulsion, Sodium Phosphate, Sorbitan Monolaurate, Titanium Dioxide. May also contain: Carnauba Wax, Zinc Stearate.

Indications: For temporary relief of the minor aches and pains, stiffness, swelling and inflammation of arthritis.

Directions: Adults: 2 caplets with water every 6 hours while symptoms persist, not to exceed 8 caplets in 24 hours, or as directed by a doctor. Children under 12 years of age: Consult a doctor.

Warnings: Children and teenagers should not use this medicine for chicken pox or flu symptoms before a doctor is consulted about Reye syndrome, a rare but serious illness reported to be associated with aspirin. KEEP THIS AND ALL OTHER MEDICATIONS OUT OF THE REACH OF CHILDREN. IN CASE OF ACCIDENTAL OVERDOSE, SEEK PROFESSIONAL ASSISTANCE OR CONTACT A POISON CONTROL CENTER IMMEDIATELY. As with any drug, if you are pregnant or nursing a baby, seek the advice of a health professional before using this product.
IT IS ESPECIALLY IMPORTANT NOT TO USE ASPIRIN DURING THE LAST 3 MONTHS OF PREGNANCY UNLESS SPECIFICALLY DIRECTED TO DO SO BY A DOCTOR BECAUSE IT MAY CAUSE PROBLEMS IN THE UNBORN CHILD OR COMPLICATIONS DURING DELIVERY. Do not take this product for pain for more than 10 days or for fever for more than 3 days unless directed by a doctor. If pain or fever persists or gets worse, if new symptoms occur, or if redness or swelling is present, consult a doctor because these could be signs of a serious condition. Do not take this product if you are allergic to aspirin, have asthma, have stomach problems (such as heartburn, upset stomach or stomach pain) that persist or recur, or if you have ulcers or bleeding problems, unless directed by a doctor. If ringing in the ears or loss of hearing occurs, consult a doctor before taking any more of this product.

Drug Interaction Precaution: Do not take this product if you are taking a prescription drug for anticoagulation (thinning of blood), diabetes, gout or arthritis unless directed by a doctor.

How Supplied: Arthritis Strength BUFFERIN® is supplied as:
Plain white coated caplet "ASB" debossed on one side.
NDC 19810-0051-1 Bottle of 40's
NDC 19810-0051-2 Bottle of 100's
The 40 caplet size does not have a child resistant closure and is recommended for households without young children.
Store at room temperature.
Shown in Product Identification Guide, page 404

Continued on next page

Bristol-Myers—Cont.

Extra Strength BUFFERIN®
[bŭf'fẽr-ĭn]
Analgesic

Composition:

Active Ingredient: Aspirin (500 mg) in a formulation buffered with Calcium Carbonate, Magnesium Oxide and Magnesium Carbonate.

Other Ingredients: Benzoic Acid, Citric Acid, Corn Starch, FD&C Blue No. 1, Hydroxypropyl Methylcellulose, Magnesium Stearate, Mineral Oil, Polysorbate 20, Povidone, Propylene Glycol, Simethicone Emulsion, Sodium Phosphate, Sorbitan Monolaurate, Titanium Dioxide. May also contain: Carnauba Wax, Zinc Stearate.

Indications: For temporary relief of headaches, pain and fever of colds, muscle aches, minor arthritis pain and inflammation, menstrual pain and toothaches.

Directions: Adults: 2 tablets with water every 6 hours while symptoms persist, not to exceed 8 tablets in 24 hours, or as directed by a doctor. Children under 12 years of age: Consult a doctor.

Warnings: Children and teenagers should not use this medicine for chicken pox or flu symptoms before a doctor is consulted about Reye syndrome, a rare but serious illness reported to be associated with aspirin. KEEP THIS AND ALL OTHER MEDICATIONS OUT OF THE REACH OF CHILDREN. IN CASE OF ACCIDENTAL OVERDOSE, SEEK PROFESSIONAL ASSISTANCE OR CONTACT A POISON CONTROL CENTER IMMEDIATELY. As with any drug, if your are pregnant or nursing a baby, seek the advice of a health professional before using this product. IT IS ESPECIALLY IMPORTANT NOT TO USE ASPIRIN DURING THE LAST 3 MONTHS OF PREGNANCY UNLESS SPECIFICALLY DIRECTED TO DO SO BY A DOCTOR BECAUSE IT MAY CAUSE PROBLEMS IN THE UNBORN CHILD OR COMPLICATIONS DURING DELIVERY. Do not take this product for more than 10 days or for fever for more than 3 days unless directed by a doctor. If pain or fever persists or gets worse, if new symptoms occur, or if redness or swelling is present, consult a doctor because these could be signs of a serious condition. Consult a dentist promptly for toothache. Do not take this product if you are allergic to aspirin, have asthma, have stomach problems (such as heartburn, upset stomach or stomach pain) that persist or recur, or if you have ulcers or bleeding problems, unless directed by a doctor. If ringing in the ears or loss of hearing occurs, consult a doctor before taking any more of this product.

Drug Interaction Precaution: Do not take this product if you are taking a prescription drug for anticoagulation (thinning of blood), diabetes, gout or arthritis unless directed by a doctor.

How Supplied: Extra Strength BUFFERIN® is supplied as:
White elongated coated tablet with "ESB" debossed on one side.
NDC 19810-0074-1 Bottle of 30's
NDC 19810-0074-4 Bottle of 50's
NDC 19810-0074-3 Bottle of 100's
All sizes have child resistant closures except 50's which is recommended for households without young children.
Store at room temperature.

Shown in Product Identification Guide, page 404

COMTREX®
[cŏm 'trĕx]
Multi-Symptom Cold Reliever

Composition: Each tablet, caplet, liquigel and fluidounce (30 ml.) contains:
[See table below.]

Indications: COMTREX® provides temporary relief of these major cold and flu symptoms: nasal and sinus congestion, runny nose, sneezing, coughing, minor sore throat pain, headache, fever, body aches and pain.

Directions:
Tablets or Caplets: Adults: 2 tablets or caplets every 4 hours while symptoms persist, not to exceed 8 tablets or caplets in 24 hours, or as directed by a doctor. Children 6 to under 12 years of age: One tablet or caplet every 4 hours while symptoms persist, not to exceed 4 tablets or caplets in 24 hours, or as directed by a doctor. Children under 6: Consult a doctor.
Liqui-Gel: Adults: 2 liqui-gels every 4 hours while symptoms persist, not to exceed 12 liqui-gels in 24 hours, or as directed by a doctor. Children 6 to under 12 years of age: 1 liqui-gel every 4 hours while symptoms persist, not to exceed 5 liqui-gels in 24 hours, or as directed by a doctor. Children under 6: Consult a doctor.
Liquid: Adults: One fluidounce (30 ml) in medicine cup provided or 2 tablespoons every 4 hours while symptoms persist, not to exceed 4 doses in 24 hours, or as directed by a doctor. Children 6 to under 12 years of age: ½ fluidounce (15 ml) or one tablespoon every 4 hours while symptoms persist, not to exceed 4 doses in 24 hours, or as directed by a doctor. Children under 6: Consult a doctor.

Warnings: KEEP THIS AND ALL OTHER MEDICATIONS OUT OF THE REACH OF CHILDREN. IN CASE OF ACCIDENTAL OVERDOSE, SEEK

	COMTREX Per Tablet or Caplet	COMTREX Liquid-Gel per Liqui-Gel	COMTREX Liquid Per Fl. Ounce
Acetaminophen:	325 mg.	325 mg.	650 mg.
Pseudoephedrine HCl:	30 mg.	—	60 mg.
Phenylpropanolamine HCl:	—	12.5 mg.	—
Chlorpheniramine Maleate:	2 mg.	2 mg.	4 mg.
Dextromethorphan HBr:	10 mg.	10 mg.	20 mg.

Other Ingredients:

Tablet	**Caplet**	**Liqui-Gels**	**Liquid**
Corn Starch	Benzoic Acid	D&C Yellow No. 10	Alcohol (20% by volume)
D&C Yellow No. 10 Lake	Carnauba Wax	FD&C Red No. 40	Citric Acid
FD&C Red No. 40 Lake	Corn Starch	Gelatin	D&C Yellow No. 10
Magnesium Stearate	D&C Yellow No. 10 Lake	Glycerin	FD&C Blue No. 1
Methylparaben	FD&C Red No. 40 Lake	Polyethylene Glycol	FD&C Red No. 40
Propylparaben	Hydroxypropyl Methylcellulose	Povidone	Flavors
Stearic Acid	Magnesium Stearate	Propylene Glycol	Polyethylene Glycol
May also contain:	Methylparaben	Silicon Dioxide	Povidone
Povidone	Mineral Oil	Sorbitol	Sodium Citrate
	Polysorbate 20	Titanium Dioxide	Sucrose
	Povidone	Water	Water
	Propylene Glycol		
	Propylparaben		
	Simethicone Emulsion		
	Sorbitan Monolaurate		
	Stearic Acid		
	Titanium Dioxide		

PROFESSIONAL ASSISTANCE OR CONTACT A POISON CONTROL CENTER IMMEDIATELY. PROMPT MEDICAL ATTENTION IS CRITICAL FOR ADULTS AS WELL AS FOR CHILDREN EVEN IF YOU DO NOT NOTICE ANY SIGNS OR SYMPTOMS. As with any drug, if you are pregnant or nursing a baby, seek the advice of a health professional before using this product. Do not take this product for more than 7 days (for adults) or 5 days (for children), unless directed by a doctor. If symptoms do not improve or are accompanied by a fever that lasts for more than 3 days, or if new symptoms occur, consult a doctor. Do not exceed recommended dosage because at higher doses nervousness, dizziness or sleeplessness may occur. May cause excitability especially in children. A persistent cough may be a sign of a serious condition. If cough persists for more than 7 days, tends to recur, or is accompanied by rash, persistent headache, fever that lasts for more than 3 days, or if new symptoms occur, consult a doctor. Do not take this product for persistent or chronic cough such as occurs with smoking, asthma or emphysema, or if cough is accompanied by excessive phlegm (mucus/sputum) unless directed by a doctor. If sore throat is severe, persists for more than 2 days, is accompanied or followed by a fever, headache, rash, nausea or vomiting, consult a doctor promptly. This product should not be taken by persons who have asthma, glaucoma, emphysema, chronic pulmonary disease, high blood pressure, heart disease, thyroid disease, diabetes, shortness of breath, difficulty in breathing or difficulty in urination due to enlargement of the prostate gland unless directed by a doctor. May cause marked drowsiness; alcohol may increase the drowsiness effect. Avoid alcoholic beverages, and do not take this product if you are taking sedatives or tranquilizers without first consulting your doctor. Use caution when driving a motor vehicle or operating machinery.

Drug Interaction Precaution: This product should not be taken by any adult or child who is taking a prescription medication for high blood pressure or depression without first consulting a doctor.

Overdose:
MUCOMYST (acetylcysteine) As An Antidote For Acetaminophen Overdose)
Acetaminophen is rapidly absorbed from the upper gastrointestinal tract with peak plasma levels occurring between 30 and 60 minutes after therapeutic doses and usually within 4 hours following an overdose. The parent compound, which is nontoxic, is extensively metabolized in the liver to form principally the sulfate and glucuronide conjugates which are also nontoxic and are rapidly excreted in the urine. A small fraction of an ingested dose is metabolized in the liver by the cytochrome P-450 mixed function oxidase enzyme system to form a reactive, potentially toxic, intermediate metabolite which preferentially conjugates with hepatic glutathione to form the nontoxic cysteine and mercapturic acid derivatives which are then excreted by the kidney. Therapeutic doses of acetaminophen do not saturate the glucuronide and sulfate conjugation pathways and do not result in the formation of sufficient reactive metabolite to deplete glutathione stores. However, following ingestion of a large overdose (150 mg/kg or greater) the glucuronide and sulfate conjugation pathways are saturated resulting in a larger fraction of the drug being metabolized via the P-450 pathway. The increased formation of reactive metabolite may deplete the hepatic stores of glutathione with subsequent binding of the metabolite to protein molecules within the hepatocyte resulting in cellular necrosis. Acetylcysteine has been shown to reduce the extent of liver injury following acetaminophen overdose. Early symptoms following a potentially hepatotoxic overdose may include: nausea, vomiting, diaphoresis and general malaise. Clinical and laboratory evidence of hepatic toxicity may not be apparent until 48 to 72 hours postingestion. In adults and adolescents, regardless of the quantity of acetaminophen reported to have been ingested, administer MUCOMYST® acetylcysteine immediately. MUCOMYST acetylcysteine therapy should be initiated and continued for a full course of therapy. Its effectiveness depends on early administration, with benefit seen principally in patients treated within 16 hours of the overdose. If acetaminophen plasma assay capability is not available, and the estimated acetaminophen ingestion exceeds 150 mg/kg, MUCOMYST acetylcysteine therapy should be initiated and continued for a full course of therapy.
For full prescribing information, refer to the MUCOMYST package insert. Do not await the results of assays for acetaminophen level before initiating treatment with MUCOMYST acetylcysteine. The following additional procedures are recommended: The stomach should be emptied promptly by lavage or by induction of emesis with syrup of ipecac. A serum acetaminophen assay should be obtained as early as possible, but no sooner than four hours following ingestion. Liver function studies should be obtained initially and repeated at 24-hour intervals.
For additional emergency information call your regional poison center or toll-free (1-800-525-6115) to the Rocky Mountain Poison Center for assistance in diagnosis and for directions in the use of MUCOMYST acetylcysteine as an antidote.

How Supplied:
COMTREX® is supplied as:
Yellow tablet with letter "C" debossed on one surface.
NDC 19810-0790-1 Blister packages of 24's

NDC 19810-0790-2 Bottles of 50's
NDC 19810-0790-3 Vials of 10's
Coated yellow caplet with "Comtrex" printed in red on one side.
NDC 19810-0792-3 Blister packages of 24's
NDC 19810-0792-4 Bottles of 50's
Yellow Liqui-Gel with "Comtrex" printed in red on one side.
NDC 19810-0561-1 Blister packages of 24's
NDC 19810-0561-2 Blister packages of 50's
Clear Red Cherry Flavored liquid:
NDC 19810-0791-1 6 oz. plastic bottles.
All sizes packaged in child resistant closures except for 24's for tablets, caplets and liqui-gels which are sizes recommended for households without young children. Store caplets, tablets and liquid at room temperature.
Store liqui-gels below 86° F. (30° C.). Keep from freezing.
Shown in Product Identification Guide, page 404

ALLERGY-SINUS COMTREX
[cŏm ′trĕx]
Multi-Symptom Allergy/Sinus Formula

Composition:
Active Ingredients: Each coated tablet or caplet contains 500 mg acetaminophen, 30 mg pseudoephedrine HCl, 2 mg chlorpheniramine maleate.
Other Ingredients: Benzoic acid, carnauba wax, corn starch, D&C yellow No. 10 lake, FD&C blue No. 1 lake, FD&C Red No. 40 lake, hydroxypropyl methylcellulose, mineral oil, polysorbate 20, povidone, propylene glycol, simethicone emulsion, sodium citrate, sorbitan monolaurate, stearic acid, titanium dioxide. May also contain: crospovidone, D&C yellow No. 10, erythorbic acid, FD&C blue No. 1, magnesium stearate, methylparaben, microcrystalline cellulose, polysorbate 80, propylparaben, silicon dioxide, wood cellulose.

Indications:
ALLERGY-SINUS COMTREX provides temporary relief of these upper respiratory allergy, hay fever, and sinusitis symptoms: sneezing, itchy watery eyes, runny nose, headache, nasal and sinus pressure and congestion.

Directions: Adults: 2 tablets or caplets every 6 hours while symptoms persist, not to exceed 8 tablets or caplets in 24 hours, or as directed by a doctor. Children under 12 years of age: Consult a doctor.

Warnings: KEEP THIS AND ALL OTHER MEDICATIONS OUT OF THE REACH OF CHILDREN. IN CASE OF ACCIDENTAL OVERDOSE, SEEK PROFESSIONAL ASSISTANCE OR CONTACT A POISON CONTROL CENTER IMMEDIATELY. PROMPT MEDICAL ATTENTION IS CRITICAL FOR ADULTS AS WELL AS FOR CHIL-

Continued on next page

Bristol-Myers—Cont.

DREN EVEN IF YOU DO NOT NOTICE ANY SIGNS OR SYMPTOMS. As with any drug, if you are pregnant or nursing a baby, seek the advice of a health professional before using this product. Do not take this product for more than 7 days unless directed by a doctor. If symptoms do not improve or are accompanied by a fever that lasts for more than 3 days, or if new symptoms occur, consult a doctor. Do not exceed recommended dosage because at higher doses nervousness, dizziness or sleeplessness may occur. May cause excitability especially in children. This product should not be taken by persons who have asthma, glaucoma, emphysema, chronic pulmonary disease, high blood pressure, heart disease, thyroid disease, diabetes, shortness of breath, difficulty in breathing or difficulty in urination due to enlargement of the prostate gland unless directed by a doctor. May cause drowsiness; alcohol, sedatives and tranquilizers may increase the drowsiness effect. Avoid alcoholic beverages, and do not take this product if you are taking sedatives or tranquilizers without first consulting your doctor. Use caution when driving a motor vehicle or operating machinery.

Drug Interaction Precaution: Do not take this product if you are presently taking a prescription drug for high blood pressure or depression, without first consulting your doctor.

Overdose:

MUCOMYST (acetylcysteine) As An Antidote For Acetaminophen Overdose)

Acetaminophen is rapidly absorbed from the upper gastrointestinal tract with peak plasma levels occurring between 30 and 60 minutes after therapeutic doses and usually within 4 hours following an overdose. The parent compound, which is nontoxic, is extensively metabolized in the liver to form principally the sulfate and glucuronide conjugates which are also nontoxic and are rapidly excreted in the urine. A small fraction of an ingested dose is metabolized in the liver by the cytochrome P-450 mixed function oxidase enzyme system to form a reactive, potentially toxic, intermediate metabolite which preferentially conjugates with hepatic glutathione to form the nontoxic cysteine and mercapturic acid derivatives which are then excreted by the kidney. Therapeutic doses of acetaminophen do not saturate the glucuronide and sulfate conjugation pathways and do not result in the formation of sufficient reactive metabolite to deplete glutathione stores. However, following ingestion of a large overdose (150 mg/kg or greater) the glucuronide and sulfate conjugation pathways are saturated resulting in a larger fraction of the drug being metabolized via the P-450 pathway. The increased formation of reactive metabolite may deplete the hepatic stores of glutathione with subsequent binding of the metabolite to protein molecules within the hepatocyte resulting in cellular necrosis. Acetylcysteine has been shown to reduce the extent of liver injury following acetaminophen overdose. Early symptoms following a potentially hepatotoxic overdose may include: nausea, vomiting, diaphoresis and general malaise. Clinical and laboratory evidence of hepatic toxicity may not be apparent until 48 to 72 hours postingestion. In adults and adolescents, regardless of the quantity of acetaminophen reported to have been ingested, administer MUCOMYST® acetylcysteine immediately. MUCOMYST acetylcysteine therapy should be initiated and continued for a full course of therapy. Its effectiveness depends on early administration, with benefit seen principally in patients treated within 16 hours of the overdose. If acetaminophen plasma assay capability is not available, and the estimated acetaminophen ingestion exceeds 150 mg/kg, MUCOMYST acetylcysteine therapy should be initiated and continued for a full course of therapy.

For full prescribing information, refer to the MUCOMYST package insert. Do not await the results of assays for acetaminophen level before initiating treatment with MUCOMYST acetylcysteine. The following additional procedures are recommended: The stomach should be emptied promptly by lavage or by induction of emesis with syrup of ipecac. A serum acetaminophen assay should be obtained as early as possible, but no sooner than four hours following ingestion. Liver function studies should be obtained initially and repeated at 24-hour intervals.

For additional emergency information call your regional poison center or toll-free (1-800-525-6115) to the Rocky Mountain Poison Center for assistance in diagnosis and for directions in the use of MUCOMYST acetylcysteine as an antidote.

How Supplied: Allergy-Sinus COMTREX® is supplied as:
Coated green tablets with "Comtrex A/S" printed in black on one side.
NDC 19810-0774-1 Blister packages of 24's
NDC 19810-0774-2 Bottles of 50's
Coated green caplets with "A/S" debossed on one surface.
NDC 19810-0081-4 Blister packages of 24's
NDC 19810-0081-5 Bottles of 50's
All sizes packaged in child resistant closures except 24's for tablets and caplets which are sizes recommended for households without young children.
Store at room temperature.
Shown in Product Identification Guide, page 404

DAY-NIGHT COMTREX®

Composition:
Active Ingredients: DAYTIME CAPLETS AND NIGHTTIME TABLETS BOTH CONTAIN: 325mg Acetaminophen; 30mg Pseudoephedrine HCl; 10mg Dextromethorphan HBr. NIGHTTIME TABLETS ALSO CONTAIN: 2mg Chlorpheniramine Maleate.
Other Ingredients: DAYTIME CAPLETS AND NIGHTTIME TABLETS BOTH CONTAIN: Benzoic Acid; Carnauba Wax; Corn Starch, Hydroxypropyl Methylcellulose; Magnesium Stearate; Methylparaben; Povidone; Propylparaben; Simethicone Emulsion; Stearic Acid; Titanium Dioxide. DAYTIME CAPLETS ALSO CONTAIN: D&C Yellow No. 10 Lake; FD&C Red No. 40 Lake; Mineral Oil, Polysorbate 20; Propylene Glycol; Sorbitan Monolaurate. NIGHTTIME TABLETS ALSO CONTAIN: FD&C Blue No. 1 Lake; Flavor; Polyethylene Glycol; Polysorbate 80; Saccharin Sodium.

Indications: Day/Night COMTREX provides you with two different formulas. COMTREX Daytime Caplets (orange) and COMTREX Nighttime Tablets (blue), for effective relief. COMTREX Daytime Caplets contain three ingredients for the temporary relief of these major cold and flu symptoms without causing drowsiness: a decongestant—to relieve stuffy nose and sinus congestion; a cough suppressant—to quiet cough; a non-aspirin analgesic—to relieve headache, fever, minor sore throat pain and body aches and pain. COMTREX Nighttime Tablets relieve all these symptoms plus they contain an antihistamine to temporarily relieve runny nose and sneezing.

Warnings for Daytime Caplets and Nighttime Tablets KEEP THESE AND ALL OTHER MEDICATIONS OUT OF THE REACH OF CHILDREN. IN CASE OF ACCIDENTAL OVERDOSE, SEEK PROFESSIONAL ASSISTANCE OR CONTACT A POISON CONTROL CENTER IMMEDIATELY. PROMPT MEDICAL ATTENTION IS CRITICAL FOR ADULTS AS WELL AS FOR CHILDREN EVEN IF YOU DO NOT NOTICE ANY SIGNS OR SYMPTOMS. As with any drug, if you are pregnant or nursing a baby, seek the advice of a health professional before using these products. Do not take these products for more than 7 days or for fever for more than 3 days unless directed by a doctor. If symptoms do not improve or are accompanied by a fever that lasts for more than 3 days, or if new symptoms occur, consult a doctor. Do not exceed recommended dosage because at higher doses nervousness, dizziness or sleeplessness may occur. A persistent cough may be a sign of a serious condition. If cough persists for more than 7 days, tends to recur or is accompanied by rash, persistent headache, fever that lasts for more than 3 days, or if new symptoms occur, consult a doctor. Do not take these products for persistent or chronic cough such as occurs with smoking, asthma or emphysema, or if cough is accompanied by excessive phlegm (mucus/sputum) unless directed by a doctor. If sore throat is severe, persists for more than 2 days, is accompanied or followed by a fever, headache, rash, nausea or vomiting, consult a doctor promptly. These products should not be taken by persons who have asthma, glaucoma, emphysema, chronic pulmonary disease, high blood pressure, heart disease, thyroid disease, diabetes, shortness of breath, difficulty in breathing, or difficulty in urination due to an enlargement of the prostate gland unless directed by a doctor.

Additional Warnings for Nighttime Tablets May cause marked drowsiness; alcohol may increase the drowsiness effect. Avoid alcoholic beverages, and do not take this product if you are taking sedatives or tranquilizers without first consulting your doctor. Use caution when driving a motor vehicle or operating machinery. May cause excitability especially in children.

DRUG INTERACTION PRECAUTION: Do not take these products if you are presently taking a prescription medication for high blood pressure or depression without first consulting your doctor.

Directions: Adults: 2 Daytime Caplets every 4 hours while symptoms persist, not to exceed 6 Daytime Caplets in 24 hours, or as directed by a doctor. 2 Nighttime Tablets at bedtime, if needed, to be taken no sooner than 4 hours after the last Daytime Caplets dose, or as directed by a doctor. **Children under 12:** Consult a doctor.

Overdose: MUCOMYST (acetylcysteine) As An Antidote For Acetaminophen Overdose)
Acetaminophen is rapidly absorbed from the upper gastrointestinal tract with peak plasma levels occurring between 30 and 60 minutes after therapeutic doses and usually within 4 hours following an overdose. The parent compound, which is nontoxic, is extensively metabolized in the liver to form principally the sulfate and glucuronide conjugates which are also nontoxic and are rapidly excreted in the urine. A small fraction of an ingested dose is metabolized in the liver by the cytochrome P-450 mixed function oxidase enzyme system to form a reactive, potentially toxic, intermediate metabolite which preferentially conjugates with hepatic glutathione to form the nontoxic cysteine and mercapturic acid derivatives which are then excreted by the kidney. Therapeutic doses of acetaminophen do not saturate the glucuronide and sulfate conjugation pathways and do not result in the formation of sufficient reactive metabolite to deplete glutathione stores. However, following ingestion of a large overdose (150 mg/kg or greater) the glucuronide and sulfate conjugation pathways are saturated resulting in a larger fraction of the drug being metabolized via the P-450 pathway. The increased formation of reactive metabolite may deplete the hepatic stores of glutathione with subsequent binding of the metabolite to protein molecules within the hepatocyte resulting in cellular necrosis. Acetylcysteine has been shown to reduce the extent of liver injury following acetaminophen overdose. Early symptoms following a potentially hepatotoxic overdose may include: nausea, vomiting, diaphoresis and general malaise. Clinical and laboratory evidence of hepatic toxicity may not be apparent until 48 to 72 hours postingestion. In adults and adolescents, regardless of the quantity of acetaminophen reported to have been ingested, administer MUCOMYST® acetylcysteine immediately. MUCOMYST acetylcysteine therapy should be initiated and continued for a full course of therapy. Its effectiveness depends on early administration, with benefit seen principally in patients treated within 16 hours of the overdose. If acetaminophen plasma assay capability is not available, and the estimated acetaminophen ingestion exceeds 150 mg/kg, MUCOMYST acetylcysteine therapy should be initiated and continued for a full course of therapy.

For full prescribing information, refer to the MUCOMYST package insert. Do not await the results of assays for acetaminophen level before initiating treatment with MUCOMYST acetylcysteine. The following additional procedures are recommended: The stomach should be emptied promptly by lavage or by induction of emesis with syrup of ipecac. A serum acetaminophen assay should be obtained as early as possible, but no sooner than four hours following ingestion. Liver function studies should be obtained initially and repeated at 24-hour intervals.

For additional emergency information call your regional poison center or toll-free (1-800-525-6115) to the Rocky Mountain Poison Center for assistance in diagnosis and for directions in the use of MUCOMYST acetylcysteine as an antidote.

How Supplied: DAY-NIGHT COMTREX® is supplied as:
Day-Coated orange caplet with letter "C" debossed on one surface.
Night-Coated blue tablet with letter "C" debossed on one surface.
NDC 19810-0078-1 Blister packages of 24's (18 caplets/6 tablets)
Store at room temperature.
Shown in Product Identification Guide, page 404

Non-Drowsy COMTREX®

Composition:
Active Ingredients: Each caplet contains 325mg Acetaminophen, 30 mg Pseudoephedrine HCl, 10mg Dextromethorphan HBr. Other Ingredients: Benzoic Acid, Carnauba Wax, Corn Starch, D&C Yellow No. 10 Lake, FD&C Red No. 40 Lake, Hydroxypropyl Methylcellulose, Magnesium Stearate, Methylparaben, Mineral Oil, Polysorbate 20, Povidone, Propylene Glycol, Propylparaben, Simethicone Emulsion, Sorbitan Monolaurate, Stearic Acid, Titanium Dioxide.

Indications: For temporary relief of nasal and sinus congestion, coughing, minor sore throat pain, headache, fever, body aches and pain.

Warnings: KEEP THIS AND ALL OTHER MEDICATIONS OUT OF THE REACH OF CHILDREN. IN CASE OF ACCIDENTAL OVERDOSE, SEEK PROFESSIONAL ASSISTANCE OR CONTACT A POISON CONTROL CENTER IMMEDIATELY. PROMPT MEDICAL ATTENTION IS CRITICAL FOR ADULTS AS WELL AS FOR CHILDREN EVEN IF YOU DO NOT NOTICE ANY SIGNS OR SYMPTOMS. As with any drug, if you are pregnant or nursing a baby, seek the advice of a health professional before using this product. Do not take this product for more than 7 days (for adults) or 5 days (for children) or for fever for more than 3 days unless directed by a doctor. Do not exceed recommended dosage because at higher doses nervousness, dizziness or sleeplessness may occur. A persistent cough may be a sign of a serious condition. If cough persists for more than 7 days, tends to recur or is accompanied by rash, persistent headache, fever that lasts for more than 3 days, or if new symptoms occur, consult a doctor. Do not take this product for persistent or chronic cough such as occurs with smoking, asthma or emphysema, or if cough is accompanied by excessive phlegm (mucus/sputum) unless directed by a doctor. If sore throat is severe, persists for more than 2 days, is accompanied or followed by a fever, headache, rash, nausea or vomiting, consult a doctor promptly. This product should not be taken by persons who have high blood pressure, heart disease, thyroid disease, diabetes or difficulty in urination due to enlargement of the prostate gland unless directed by a doctor.

DRUG INTERACTION PRECAUTION: This product should not be taken by any adult or child who is taking a prescription medication for high blood pressure or depression without first consulting a doctor.

Directions: Adults: 2 caplets every 4 hours while symptoms persist, not to exceed 8 caplets in 24 hours, or as directed by doctor. **Children 6 to under 12 years of age:** One caplet every 4 hours while symptoms persist, not to exceed 4 caplets in 24 hours, or as directed by a doctor. **Children under 6:** Consult a doctor.

Overdose: MUCOMYST (acetylcysteine) As An Antidote For Acetaminophen Overdose)
Acetaminophen is rapidly absorbed from the upper gastrointestinal tract with peak plasma levels occurring between 30 and 60 minutes after therapeutic doses and usually within 4 hours following an overdose. The parent compound, which is nontoxic, is extensively metabolized in the liver to form principally the sulfate and glucuronide conjugates which are

Continued on next page

Bristol-Myers—Cont.

also nontoxic and are rapidly excreted in the urine. A small fraction of an ingested dose is metabolized in the liver by the cytochrome P-450 mixed function oxidase enzyme system to form a reactive, potentially toxic, intermediate metabolite which preferentially conjugates with hepatic glutathione to form the nontoxic cysteine and mercapturic acid derivatives which are then excreted by the kidney. Therapeutic doses of acetaminophen do not saturate the glucuronide and sulfate conjugation pathways and do not result in the formation of sufficient reactive metabolite to deplete glutathione stores. However, following ingestion of a large overdose (150 mg/kg or greater) the glucuronide and sulfate conjugation pathways are saturated resulting in a larger fraction of the drug being metabolized via the P-450 pathway. The increased formation of reactive metabolite may deplete the hepatic stores of glutathione with subsequent binding of the metabolite to protein molecules within the hepatocyte resulting in cellular necrosis. Acetylcysteine has been shown to reduce the extent of liver injury following acetaminophen overdose. Early symptoms following a potentially hepatotoxic overdose may include: nausea, vomiting, diaphoresis and general malaise. Clinical and laboratory evidence of hepatic toxicity may not be apparent until 48 to 72 hours postingestion. In adults and adolescents, regardless of the quantity of acetaminophen reported to have been ingested, administer MUCOMYST® acetylcysteine immediately. MUCOMYST acetylcysteine therapy should be initiated and continued for a full course of therapy. Its effectiveness depends on early administration, with benefit seen principally in patients treated within 16 hours of the overdose. If acetaminophen plasma assay capability is not available, and the estimated acetaminophen ingestion exceeds 150 mg/kg, MUCOMYST acetylcysteine therapy should be initiated and continued for a full course of therapy. For full prescribing information, refer to the MUCOMYST package insert. Do not await the results of assays for acetaminophen level before initiating treatment with MUCOMYST acetylcysteine. The following additional procedures are recommended: The stomach should be emptied promptly by lavage or by induction of emesis with syrup of ipecac. A serum acetaminophen assay should be obtained as early as possible, but no sooner than four hours following ingestion. Liver function studies should be obtained initially and repeated at 24-hour intervals. For additional emergency information call your regional poison center or toll-free (1-800-525-6115) to the Rocky Mountain Poison Center for assistance in diagnosis and for directions in the use of MUCOMYST acetylcysteine as an antidote.

How Supplied: Non-Drowsy Comtrex® is supplied as:
Coated orange caplet with letter "C" debossed on one surface.
NDC 19810-0041-1 Blister packages of 24's
NDC 19810-0041-2 Bottles of 50's
The 24 size does not have a child resistant closure and is recommended for households without young children. Store at room temperature.
Shown in Product Identification Guide, page 404

CONGESPIRIN® for Children Aspirin Free Chewable Cold Tablets
[cŏn "gĕs 'pir-in]

Composition: Each tablet contains acetaminophen 81 mg. (1¼ grains), phenylephrine hydrochloride 1¼ mg. Also Contains: Calcium Stearate, D&C Red No. 30 Aluminum Lake, D&C Yellow No. 10 Aluminum Lake, Ethyl Cellulose, Flavor, Mannitol, Microcrystalline Cellulose, Polyethylene, Saccharin Calcium, Sucrose.

Indications: A non-aspirin analgesic/nasal decongestant that temporarily reduces fever and relieves aches, pains and nasal congestion associated with colds and "flu."

Warnings: KEEP THIS AND ALL MEDICINES OUT OF CHILDREN'S REACH. IN CASE OF ACCIDENTAL OVERDOSE, CONTACT A PHYSICIAN IMMEDIATELY.

Caution: If child is under medical care, do not administer without consulting physician. Do not exceed recommended dosage. Consult your physician if symptoms persist or if high blood pressure, heart disease, diabetes or thyroid disease is present. Do not administer for more than 10 days unless directed by physician.

Directions:
Under 2, consult your physician.
2–3 years ....2 tablets
4–5 years ....3 tablets
6–8 years ....4 tablets
9–10 years ....5 tablets
11–12 years ....6 tablets
over 12 years ....8 tablets
Repeat dose in four hours if necessary. Do not give more than four doses per day unless prescribed by your physician.

Overdose:
MUCOMYST (acetylcysteine) As An Antidote For Acetaminophen Overdose)
Acetaminophen is rapidly absorbed from the upper gastrointestinal tract with peak plasma levels occurring between 30 and 60 minutes after therapeutic doses and usually within 4 hours following an overdose. The parent compound, which is nontoxic, is extensively metabolized in the liver to form principally the sulfate and glucuronide conjugates which are also nontoxic and are rapidly excreted in

the urine. A small fraction of an ingested dose is metabolized in the liver by the cytochrome P-450 mixed function oxidase enzyme system to form a reactive, potentially toxic, intermediate metabolite which preferentially conjugates with hepatic glutathione to form the nontoxic cysteine and mercapturic acid derivatives which are then excreted by the kidney. Therapeutic doses of acetaminophen do not saturate the glucuronide and sulfate conjugation pathways and do not result in the formation of sufficient reactive metabolite to deplete glutathione stores. However, following ingestion of a large overdose (150 mg/kg or greater) the glucuronide and sulfate conjugation pathways are saturated resulting in a larger fraction of the drug being metabolized via the P-450 pathway. The increased formation of reactive metabolite may deplete the hepatic stores of glutathione with subsequent binding of the metabolite to protein molecules within the hepatocyte resulting in cellular necrosis. Acetylcysteine has been shown to reduce the extent of liver injury following acetaminophen overdose. Early symptoms following a potentially hepatotoxic overdose may include nausea, vomiting, diaphoresis and general malaise. Clinical and laboratory evidence of hepatic toxicity may not be apparent until 48 to 72 hours postingestion. In adults and adolescents, regardless of the quantity of acetaminophen reported to have been ingested, administer MUCOMYST® acetylcysteine immediately. MUCOMYST acetylcysteine therapy should be initiated and continued for a full course of therapy. Its effectiveness depends on early administration, with benefit seen principally in patients treated within 16 hours of the overdose. If acetaminophen plasma assay capability is not available, and the estimated acetaminophen ingestion exceeds 150 mg/kg, MUCOMYST acetylcysteine therapy should be initiated and continued for a full course of therapy. For full prescribing information, refer to the MUCOMYST package insert. Do not await the result of assays for acetaminophen level before initiating treatment with MUCOMYST acetylcysteine. The following additional procedures are recommended: The stomach should be emptied promptly by lavage or by induction of emesis with syrup of ipecac. A serum acetaminophen assay should be obtained as early as possible, but no sooner than four hours following ingestion. Liver function studies should be obtained initially and repeated at 24-hour intervals. For additional emergency information call your regional poison center or toll-free (1-800-525-6115) to the Rocky Mountain Poison Center for assistance in diagnosis and for directions in the use of MUCOMYST acetylcysteine as an antidote.

How Supplied: CONGESPIRIN Aspirin Free Chewable Cold Tablets are sup-

plied as scored orange tablets with "C" on one side.
NDC 19810-0748-1 Bottles of 24's.
Bottles are child resistant.
Store at room temperature.

Aspirin Free EXCEDRIN®

Composition: Each caplet contains Acetaminophen 500 mg. and Caffeine 65 mg. Other Ingredients: Benzoic Acid, Carnauba Wax, Corn Starch, Croscarmellose Sodium, D&C Red No. 27 Lake, D&C Yellow No. 10 Lake, FD&C Blue No. 1 Lake, Hydroxypropyl Methylcellulose, Magnesium Stearate, Methylparaben, Microcrystalline Cellulose, Propylparaben, Saccharin Sodium, Simethicone Emulsion, Stearic Acid, Titanium Dioxide. May also contain: Erythorbic Acid, Mineral Oil, Polyethylene Glycol, Polysorbate 20, Polysorbate 80, Povidone, Propylene Glycol, Sorbitan Monolaurate.

Indications: For temporary relief of the pain of headache, sinusitis, colds, muscular aches, menstrual discomfort, toothaches and minor arthritis pain.

Directions: Adults: 2 caplets every 6 hours while symptoms persist, not to exceed 8 caplets in 24 hours, or as directed by a doctor. Children under 12 years of age: Consult a doctor.

Warnings: KEEP THIS AND ALL OTHER MEDICATIONS OUT OF THE REACH OF CHILDREN. IN CASE OF ACCIDENTAL OVERDOSE, SEEK PROFESSIONAL ASSISTANCE OR CONTACT A POISON CONTROL CENTER IMMEDIATELY. PROMPT MEDICAL ATTENTION IS CRITICAL FOR ADULTS AS WELL AS FOR CHILDREN EVEN IF YOU DO NOT NOTICE ANY SIGNS OR SYMPTOMS. As with any drug, if you are pregnant or nursing a baby, seek the advice of a health professional before using this product. Do not take this product for pain for more than 10 days or for fever for more than 3 days unless directed by a doctor. If pain or fever persists or gets worse, if new symptoms occur, or if redness or swelling is present, consult a doctor because these could be signs of a serious condition. Consult a dentist promptly for toothache.

Overdose:
MUCOMYST (acetylcysteine) As An Antidote For Acetaminophen Overdose)
Acetaminophen is rapidly absorbed from the upper gastrointestinal tract with peak plasma levels occurring between 30 and 60 minutes after therapeutic doses and usually within 4 hours following an overdose. The parent compound, which is nontoxic, is extensively metabolized in the liver to form principally the sulfate and glucuronide conjugates which are also nontoxic and are rapidly excreted in the urine. A small fraction of an ingested dose is metabolized in the liver by the cytochrome P-450 mixed function oxidase enzyme system to form a reactive,

potentially toxic, intermediate metabolite which preferentially conjugates with hepatic glutathione to form the nontoxic cysteine and mercapturic acid derivatives which are then excreted by the kidney. Therapeutic doses of acetaminophen do not saturate the glucuronide and sulfate conjugation pathways and do not result in the formation of sufficient reactive metabolite to deplete glutathione stores. However, following ingestion of a large overdose (150 mg/kg or greater) the glucuronide and sulfate conjugation pathways are saturated resulting in a larger fraction of the drug being metabolized via the P-450 pathway. The increased formation of reactive metabolite may deplete the hepatic stores of glutathione with subsequent binding of the metabolite to protein molecules within the hepatocyte resulting in cellular necrosis. Acetylcysteine has been shown to reduce the extent of liver injury following acetaminophen overdose. Early symptoms following a potentially hepatotoxic overdose may include: nausea, vomiting, diaphoresis and general malaise. Clinical and laboratory evidence of hepatic toxicity may not be apparent until 48 to 72 hours postingestion. In adults and adolescents, regardless of the quantity of acetaminophen reported to have been ingested, administer MUCOMYST® acetylcysteine immediately. MUCOMYST acetylcysteine therapy should be initiated and continued for a full course of therapy. Its effectiveness depends on early administration, with benefit seen principally in patients treated within 16 hours of the overdose. If acetaminophen plasma assay capability is not available, and the estimated acetaminophen ingestion exceeds 150 mg/kg, MUCOMYST acetylcysteine therapy should be initiated and continued for a full course of therapy.
For full prescribing information, refer to the MUCOMYST package insert. Do not await the results of assays for acetaminophen level before initiating treatment with MUCOMYST acetylcysteine. The following additional procedures are recommended: The stomach should be emptied promptly by lavage or by induction of emesis with syrup of ipecac. A serum acetaminophen assay should be obtained as early as possible, but no sooner than four hours following ingestion. Liver function studies should be obtained initially and repeated at 24-hour intervals.
For additional emergency information call your regional poison center or toll-free (1-800-525-6115) to the Rocky Mountain Poison Center for assistance in diagnosis and for directions in the use of MUCOMYST acetylcysteine as an antidote.

How Supplied: Aspirin Free EXCEDRIN® is supplied as: Coated red caplets with "AF Excedrin" printed in white on one side.

NDC 19810-0089-1 Bottles of 24's
NDC 19810-0089-2 Bottles of 50's
NDC 19810-0089-3 Bottles of 100's
All sizes packaged in child resistant closures except 100's which is recommended for households without young children.
Store at room temperature.
*Shown in Product Identification
Guide, page 404*

Aspirin Free EXCEDRIN DUAL CAPLETS
[ĕx ″cĕd ′rĭn]

Composition: Each caplet contains Acetaminophen 500 mg; Calcium Carbonate 111 mg; Magnesium Carbonate 64 mg; Magnesium Oxide 30 mg.
Other Ingredients: Benzoic Acid, Carnauba Wax, Citric Acid, Corn Starch, Croscarmellose Sodium, D&C Red No. 27 Lake, Flavor, Hydroxypropyl Cellulose, Hydroxypropyl Methylcellulose, Magnesium Stearate, Methylparaben, Polyethylene Glycol, Povidone, Propylparaben, Saccharin Sodium, Simethicone Emulsion, Sodium Phosphate, Stearic Acid, Titanium Dioxide.

Indications: For the temporary relief of headache, minor aches and pains accompanied by heartburn, sour stomach, acid indigestion and upset stomach associated with these symptoms.

Directions: Adults: 2 caplets every 6 hours while symptoms persist, not to exceed 8 caplets in 24 hours, or as directed by a doctor. Children under 12: Consult a doctor.

Warnings: KEEP THIS AND ALL OTHER MEDICATIONS OUT OF THE REACH OF CHILDREN. IN CASE OF ACCIDENTAL OVERDOSE, SEEK PROFESSIONAL ASSISTANCE OR CONTACT A POISON CONTROL CENTER IMMEDIATELY. PROMPT MEDICAL ATTENTION IS CRITICAL FOR ADULTS AS WELL AS FOR CHILDREN EVEN IF YOU DO NOT NOTICE ANY SIGNS OR SYMPTOMS. As with any drug, if you are pregnant or nursing a baby, seek the advice of a health professional before using this product. Do not take this product for more than 10 days unless directed by a doctor. If pain persists or gets worse, if new symptoms occur, or if redness or swelling is present, consult a doctor because these could be signs of a serious condition. May have a laxative effect.

Overdose:
MUCOMYST (acetylcysteine As an Antidote for Acetaminophen Overdose)
Acetaminophen is rapidly absorbed from the upper gastrointestinal tract with peak plasma levels occurring between 30 and 60 minutes after therapeutic doses and usually within 4 hours following an overdose. The parent compound, which is nontoxic, is extensively metabolized in the liver to form principally the sulfate

Continued on next page

Bristol-Myers—Cont.

and glucuronide conjugates which are also nontoxic and are rapidly excreted in the urine. A small fraction of an ingested dose is metabolized in the liver by the cytochrome P-450 mixed function oxidase enzyme system to form a reactive, potentially toxic, intermediate metabolite which preferentially conjugates with hepatic glutathione to form the nontoxic cysteine and mercapturic acid derivatives which are then excreted by the kidney. Therapeutic doses of acetaminophen do not saturate the glucuronide and sulfate conjugation pathways and do not result in the formation of sufficient reactive metabolite to deplete glutathione stores. However, following ingestion of a larger overdose (150 mg/kg or greater) the glucuronide and sulfate conjugation pathways are saturated resulting in larger fraction of the drug being metabolized via the P-450 pathway. The increased formation of reactive metabolite may deplete the hepatic stores of glutathione with subsequent binding of the metabolite to protein molecules within the hepatocyte resulting in cellular necrosis. Acetylcysteine has been shown to reduce the extent of liver injury following acetaminophen overdose. Early symptoms following a potentially hepatotoxic overdose may include nausea, vomiting, diaphoresis and general malaise. Clinical and laboratory evidence of hepatic toxicity may not be apparent until 48 to 72 hours postingestion. In adults and adolescents, regardless of the quantity of acetaminophen reported to have been ingested, administer MUCOMYST® acetylcysteine immediately. MUCOMYST acetylcysteine therapy should be initiated and continued for a full course of therapy. Its effectiveness depends on early administration, with benefit seen principally in patients treated within 16 hours of the overdose. If acetaminophen plasma assay capability is not available, and the estimated acetaminophen ingestion exceeds 150 mg/kg, MUCOMYST acetylcysteine therapy should be initiated and continued for a full course of therapy.

For full prescribing information, refer to the MUCOMYST package insert. Do not await the results of assays for acetaminophen level before initiating treatment with MUCOMYST acetylcysteine. The following additional procedures are recommended. The stomach should be emptied promptly by lavage or by induction of emesis with syrup of ipecac. A serum acetaminophen assay should be obtained as early as possible, but no sooner than four hours following ingestion. Liver function studies should be obtained initially and repeated at 24-hour intervals.

For additional emergency information call your regional poison center or toll free (1-800-525-6115) to the Rocky Mountain Poison Center for assistance in diagnosis and for directions in the use of MUCOMYST acetylcysteine as an antidote.

How Supplied: Aspirin Free EXCEDRIN DUAL Caplets is a pink caplet with the logo "EX+" debossed on one side.
NDC 19810-0752-1 Bottles of 24's
NDC 19810-0752-2 Bottles of 50's
NDC 19810-0752-3 Bottles of 100's
The bottle of 24's and 100's are packaged in child resistant closures; the bottles of 50's are recommended for households without young children and are packaged without a child resistant closure. Store at room temperature.

EXCEDRIN® Extra-Strength Analgesic
[ĕx "cĕd 'rĭn]

Composition:
Each tablet or caplet contains Acetaminophen 250 mg.: Aspirin 250 mg.; and Caffeine 65 mg.
Other Ingredients: (Tablets or Caplets) Benzoic Acid, FD&C Blue No. 1, Hydroxypropyl Methylcellulose, Microcrystalline Cellulose, Mineral Oil, Polysorbate 20, Povidone, Propylene Glycol, Saccharin Sodium, Simethicone Emulsion, Sorbitan Monolaurate, Stearic Acid, Titanium Dioxide. May Also Contain: Carnauba Wax, Hydroxypropylcellulose.

Indications: For temporary relief of the pain of headache, sinusitis, colds, muscular aches, menstrual discomfort, toothaches and minor arthritis pain.

Directions: Adults: 2 tablets or caplets with water every 6 hours while symptoms persist, not to exceed 8 tablets or caplets in 24 hours, or as directed by a doctor. Children under 12 years of age: Consult a doctor.

Warnings: Children and teenagers should not use this medicine for chickenpox or flu symptoms before a doctor is consulted about Reye syndrome, a rare but serious illness reported to be associated with aspirin. KEEP THIS AND ALL OTHER MEDICATIONS OUT OF THE REACH OF CHILDREN. IN CASE OF ACCIDENTAL OVERDOSE, SEEK PROFESSIONAL ASSISTANCE OR CONTACT A POISON CONTROL CENTER IMMEDIATELY. PROMPT MEDICAL ATTENTION IS CRITICAL FOR ADULTS AS WELL AS FOR CHILDREN EVEN IF YOU DO NOT NOTICE ANY SIGNS OR SYMPTOMS. As with any drug, if you are pregnant or nursing a baby, seek the advice of a health professional before using this product. IT IS ESPECIALLY IMPORTANT NOT TO USE ASPIRIN DURING THE LAST 3 MONTHS OF PREGNANCY UNLESS SPECIFICALLY DIRECTED TO DO SO BY A DOCTOR BECAUSE IT MAY CAUSE PROBLEMS IN THE UNBORN CHILD OR COMPLICATIONS DURING DELIVERY. Do not take this product for pain for more than 10 days or for fever for more than 3 days unless directed by a doctor. If pain or fever persists or gets worse, if new symptoms occur, or if redness or swelling is present, consult a doctor because these could be signs of a serious condition. Consult a dentist promptly for toothache. Do not take this product if you are allergic to aspirin, have asthma, have stomach problems (such as heartburn, upset stomach or stomach pain) that persist or recur, or if you have ulcers or bleeding problems, unless directed by a doctor. If ringing in the ears or loss of hearing occurs, consult a doctor before taking any more of this product.

Drug Interaction Precaution: Do not take this product if you are taking a prescription drug for anticoagulation (thinning of blood), diabetes, gout or arthritis unless directed by a doctor.

Overdose:
MUCOMYST (acetylcysteine As An Antidote For Acetaminophen Overdose)
Acetaminophen is rapidly absorbed from the upper gastrointestinal tract with peak plasma levels occurring between 30 and 60 minutes after therapeutic doses and usually within 4 hours following an overdose. The parent compound, which is nontoxic, is extensively metabolized in the liver to form principally the sulfate and glucuronide conjugates which are also nontoxic and are rapidly excreted in the urine. A small fraction of an ingested dose is metabolized in the liver by the cytochrome P-450 mixed function oxidase enzyme system to form a reactive, potentially toxic, intermediate metabolite which preferentially conjugates with hepatic glutathione to form the nontoxic cysteine and mercapturic acid derivatives which are then excreted by the kidney. Therapeutic doses of acetaminophen do not saturate the glucuronide and sulfate conjugation pathways and do not result in the formation of sufficient reactive metabolite to deplete glutathione stores. However, following ingestion of a larger overdose (150 mg/kg or greater) the glucuronide and sulfate conjugation pathways are saturated resulting in larger fraction of the drug being metabolized via the P-450 pathway. The increased formation of reactive metabolite may deplete the hepatic stores of glutathione with subsequent binding of the metabolite to protein molecules within the hepatocyte resulting in cellular necrosis. Acetylcysteine has been shown to reduce the extent of liver injury following acetaminophen overdose. Early symptoms following a potentially hepatotoxic overdose may include nausea, vomiting, diaphoresis and general malaise. Clinical and laboratory evidence of hepatic toxicity may not be apparent until 48 to 72 hours postingestion. In adults and adolescents, regardless of the quantity of acetaminophen reported to have been ingested, administer MUCOMYST® acetylcysteine immediately. MUCOMYST acetylcysteine therapy should be initiated and continued for a full course of therapy. Its effectiveness depends on early administration, with

benefit seen principally in patients treated within 16 hours of the overdose. If acetaminophen plasma assay capability is not available, and the estimated acetaminophen ingestion exceeds 150 mg/kg, MUCOMYST acetylcysteine therapy should be initiated and continued for a full course of therapy.

For full prescribing information, refer to the MUCOMYST package insert. Do not await the results of assays for acetaminophen level before initiating treatment with MUCOMYST acetylcysteine. The following additional procedures are recommended. The stomach should be emptied promptly by lavage or by induction of emesis with syrup of ipecac. A serum acetaminophen assay should be obtained as early as possible, but no sooner than four hours following ingestion. Liver function studies should be obtained initially and repeated at 24-hour intervals.

For additional emergency information call your regional poison center or toll-free (1-800-525-6115) to the Rocky Mountain Poison Center for assistance in diagnosis and for directions in the use of MUCOMYST acetylcysteine as an antidote.

How Supplied: Extra Strength EXCEDRIN® is supplied as:
White circular tablet with letter "E" debossed on one side.
NDC 19810-0700-2 Bottles of 12's
NDC 19810-0782-3 Bottles of 24's
NDC 19810-0782-4 Bottles of 50's
NDC 19810-0700-5 Bottles of 100's
NDC 19810-0782-5 Bottles of 150's
NDC 19810-0061-9 Bottles of 175's
NDC 19810-0700-1 A metal tin of 12's
NDC 19810-0772-1 Vials of 10's
Coated white caplets with "Excedrin" printed in red on one side.
NDC 19810-0002-1 Bottles of 24's
NDC 19810-0002-2 Bottles of 50's
NDC 19810-0002-8 Bottles of 100's
NDC 19810-0091-1 Bottles of 175's
All sizes packaged in child resistant closures except 100's for tablets, 50's for caplets which are sizes recommended for households without young children.
Store at room temperature.

Shown in Product Identification Guide, page 404

EXCEDRIN P.M.®
[ĕx ″cĕd ′rĭn]
Analgesic Sleeping Aid

Composition: Each tablet, and caplet [See table above.]

Indications: For temporary relief of occasional headaches and minor aches and pains with accompanying sleeplessness.

Directions:
Tablets or Caplets:
Adults, 2 tablets or caplets at bedtime if needed or as directed by a doctor.

Warnings: KEEP THIS AND ALL OTHER MEDICATIONS OUT OF THE REACH OF CHILDREN. IN CASE OF

Acetaminophen
Diphenhydramine Citrate:
Other Ingredients:

	EXCEDRIN® PM
	Per Tablet or Caplet
Acetaminophen	500 mg.
Diphenhydramine Citrate:	38 mg.
	—

Tablet or Caplet
Benzoic Acid
Carnauba Wax
Corn Starch
D&C Yellow No. 10
D&C Yellow No. 10 Aluminum Lake
FD&C Blue No. 1
FD&C Blue No. 1 Aluminum Lake
Hydroxypropyl Methylcellulose
Methylparaben
Magnesium Stearate
Propylene Glycol
Propylparaben
Simethicone Emulsion
Stearic Acid
Titanium Dioxide

ACCIDENTAL OVERDOSE, SEEK PROFESSIONAL ASSISTANCE OR CONTACT A POISON CONTROL CENTER IMMEDIATELY. PROMPT MEDICAL ATTENTION IS CRITICAL FOR ADULTS AS WELL AS FOR CHILDREN EVEN IF YOU DO NOT NOTICE ANY SIGNS OR SYMPTOMS. As with any drug, if you are pregnant or nursing a baby, seek the advice of a health professional before using this product. Do not give this product to children under 12 years of age or use for more than 10 days unless directed by a doctor. Consult a doctor if symptoms persist or get worse or if new ones occur, or if sleeplessness persists continuously for more than 2 weeks because these may be symptoms of serious underlying medical illnesses. Do not take this product if you have asthma, glaucoma, emphysema, chronic pulmonary disease, shortness of breath, difficulty in breathing, or difficulty in urination due to enlargement of the prostate gland unless directed by a doctor. Avoid alcoholic beverages while taking this product. Do not take this product if you are taking sedatives or tranquilizers, without first consulting your doctor.

Overdose:
MUCOMYST (acetylcysteine) As An Antidote For Acetaminophen Overdose)
Acetaminophen is rapidly absorbed from the upper gastrointestinal tract with peak plasma levels occurring between 30 and 60 minutes after therapeutic doses and usually within 4 hours following an overdose. The parent compound, which is nontoxic, is extensively metabolized in the liver to form principally the sulfate and glucuronide conjugates which are also nontoxic and are rapidly excreted in the urine. A small fraction of an ingested dose is metabolized in the liver by the cytochrome P-450 mixed function oxidase enzyme system to form a reactive, potentially toxic, intermediate metabolite which preferentially conjugates with hepatic glutathione to form the nontoxic cysteine and mercapturic acid derivatives which are then excreted by the kid-

---

ney. Therapeutic doses of acetaminophen do not saturate the glucuronide and sulfate conjugation pathways and do not result in the formation of sufficient reactive metabolite to deplete glutathione stores. However, following ingestion of a large overdose (150 mg/kg or greater) the glucuronide and sulfate conjugation pathways are saturated resulting in a larger fraction of the drug being metabolized via the P-450 pathway. The increased formation of reactive metabolite may deplete the hepatic stores of glutathione with subsequent binding of the metabolite to protein molecules within the hepatocyte resulting in cellular necrosis. Acetylcysteine has been shown to reduce the extent of liver injury following acetaminophen overdose. Early symptoms following a potentially hepatotoxic overdose may include: nausea, vomiting, diaphoresis and general malaise. Clinical and laboratory evidence of hepatic toxicity may not be apparent until 48 to 72 hours postingestion. In adults and adolescents, regardless of the quantity of acetaminophen reported to have been ingested, administer MUCOMYST® acetylcysteine immediately. MUCOMYST acetylcysteine therapy should be initiated and continued for a full course of therapy. Its effectiveness depends on early administration, with benefit seen principally in patients treated within 16 hours of the overdose. If acetaminophen plasma assay capability is not available, and the estimated acetaminophen ingestion exceeds 150 mg/kg, MUCOMYST acetylcysteine therapy should be initiated and continued for a full course of therapy.

For full prescribing information, refer to the MUCOMYST package insert. Do not await the results of assays for acetaminophen level before initiating treatment with MUCOMYST acetylcysteine. The following additional procedures are recommended: The stomach should be emptied promptly by lavage or by induction of emesis with syrup of ipecac. A serum acetaminophen assay should be

Continued on next page

Bristol-Myers—Cont.

obtained as early as possible, but no sooner than four hours following ingestion. Liver function studies should be obtained initially and repeated at 24-hour intervals.

For additional emergency information call your regional poison center or toll-free (1-800-525-6115) to the Rocky Mountain Poison Center for assistance in diagnosis and for directions in the use of MUCOMYST acetylcysteine as an antidote.

How Supplied: EXCREDRIN P.M.® is supplied as:
Light blue circular coated tablets with "PM" debossed on one side.
NDC 19810-0763-6 Bottles of 10's
NDC 19810-0764-3 Bottles of 24's
NDC 19810-0763-4 Bottles of 50's
NDC 19810-0764-4 Bottles of 100's
Light blue coated caplet with "Excedrin P.M." imprinted on one side.
NDC 19810-0032-5 Bottles of 24's
NDC 19810-0032-3 Bottles of 50's
NDC 19810-0032-6 Bottles of 100's
All sizes packaged in child resistant closures except 50's tablets and caplets which are recommended for households without young children.
Store at room temperature
Shown in Product Identification Guide, page 404

Sinus EXCEDRIN®
[*ex "cĕd 'rĭn*]
Analgesic, Decongestant

Composition: Each coated tablet or caplet contains 500 mg Acetaminophen and 30 mg Pseudoephedrine HCl.

Other Ingredients: Corn Starch, D&C Yellow No. 10 Lake, FD&C Red No. 40 Lake, Hydroxypropyl Methylcellulose, Mineral Oil, Polysorbate 20, Povidone, Propylene Glycol, Simethicone Emulsion, Sorbitan Monolaurate, Stearic Acid, Titanium Dioxide. May also contain: Benzoic Acid, Carnauba Wax.

Indications: For temporary relief of headache, sinus pain and sinus pressure and congestion due to sinusitis or the common cold.

Directions: Adults: 2 tablets or caplets every 6 hours while symptoms persist, not to exceed 8 tablets or caplets in 24 hours, or as directed by a doctor. Children under 12 years of age: Consult a doctor.

Warnings: KEEP THIS AND ALL OTHER MEDICATIONS OUT OF THE REACH OF CHILDREN. IN CASE OF ACCIDENTAL OVERDOSE, SEEK PROFESSIONAL ASSISTANCE OR CONTACT A POISON CONTROL CENTER IMMEDIATELY. PROMPT MEDICAL ATTENTION IS CRITICAL FOR ADULTS AS WELL AS FOR CHILDREN EVEN IF YOU DO NOT NOTICE ANY SIGNS OR SYMPTOMS. As with any drug, if you are pregnant or nursing

a baby, seek the advice of a health professional before using this product. Do not take this product for more than 7 days unless directed by a doctor. If symptoms persist or get worse or are accompanied by a fever that lasts for more than 3 days, or if new symptoms occur, consult a doctor because these could be signs of a serious condition. Do not exceed recommended dosage because at higher doses nervousness, dizziness or sleeplessness may occur. Do not take this product if you have heart disease, high blood pressure, thyroid disease, diabetes, or difficulty in urination due to enlargement of the prostate gland unless directed by a doctor.

Drug Interaction Precaution: Do not take this product if you are taking a prescription medication for high blood pressure or depression without first consulting a doctor.

Overdose:
MUCOMYST (acetylcysteine) As An Antidote for Acetaminophen Overdose)
Acetaminophen is rapidly absorbed from the upper gastrointestinal tract with peak plasma levels occurring between 30 and 60 minutes after therapeutic doses and usually within 4 hours following an overdose. The parent compound, which is nontoxic, is extensively metabolized in the liver to form principally the sulfate and glucuronide conjugates which are also nontoxic and are rapidly excreted in the urine. A small fraction of an ingested dose is metabolized in the liver by the cytochrome P-450 mixed function oxidase enzyme system to form a reactive, potentially toxic, intermediate metabolite which preferentially conjugates with hepatic glutathione to form the nontoxic cysteine and mercapturic acid derivatives which are then excreted by the kidney. Therapeutic doses of acetaminophen do not saturate the glucuronide and sulfate conjugation pathways and do not result in the formation of sufficient reactive metabolite to deplete glutathione stores. However, following ingestion of a large overdose (150 mg/kg or greater) the glucuronide and sulfate conjugation pathways are saturated resulting in a larger fraction of the drug being metabolized via the P-450 pathway. The increased formation of reactive metabolite may deplete the hepatic stores of glutathione with subsequent binding of the metabolite to protein molecules within the hepatocyte resulting in cellular necrosis. Acetylcysteine has been shown to reduce the extent of liver injury following acetaminophen overdose. Early symptoms following a potentially hepatotoxic overdose may include: nausea, vomiting, diaphoresis and general malaise. Clinical and laboratory evidence of hepatic toxicity may not be apparent until 48 to 72 hours postingestion. In adults and adolescents, regardless of the quantity of acetaminophen reported to have been ingested, administer MUCO-MYST® acetylcysteine immediately. MUCOMYST acetylcysteine therapy

should be initiated and continued for a full course of therapy. Its effectiveness depends on early administration, with benefit seen principally in patients treated within 16 hours of the overdose. If acetaminophen plasma assay capability is not available, and the estimated acetaminophen ingestion exceeds 150 mg/kg, MUCOMYST acetylcysteine therapy should be initiated and continued for a full course of therapy.

For full prescribing information, refer to the MUCOMYST package insert. Do not await the results of assays for acetaminophen level before initiating treatment with MUCOMYST acetylcysteine. The following additional procedures are recommended: The stomach should be emptied promptly by lavage or by induction of emesis with syrup of ipecac. A serum acetaminophen assay should be obtained as early as possible, but no sooner than four hours following ingestion. Liver function studies should be obtained initially and repeated at 24-hour intervals.

For additional emergency information call your regional poison center or toll-free (1-800-525-6115) to the Rocky Mountain Poison Center for assistance in diagnosis and for directions in the use of MUCOMYST acetylcysteine as an antidote.

How Supplied: Sinus EXCEDRIN® is supplied as:
Coated circular orange tablets with "Sinus Excedrin" imprinted in green on one side.
NDC 19810-0080-1 Blister packages of 24's
NDC 19810-0080-2 Bottles of 50's
Coated orange caplets with "Sinus Excedrin" imprinted in green on one side.
NDC 19810-0077-1 Blister packages of 24's
NDC 19810-0077-2 Bottles of 50's
All sizes have child resistant closures except 24's for tablets and caplets which are recommended for households without young children.
Store at room temperature.
Shown in Product Identification Guide, page 405

4-WAY® Cold Tablets

Composition: Each tablet contains acetaminophen 325 mg., phenylpropanolamine HCl 12.5 mg., and chlorpheniramine maleate 2 mg. Other Ingredients: Corn Starch, Corn Starch Pregelatinized, Microcrystalline Cellulose, Sodium Starch Glycolate, Stearic Acid, Sucrose.

Indications: For temporary relief of nasal and sinus congestion, runny nose, sneezing, fever, minor sore throat pain, body aches and pain.

Directions:
Adults: 2 tablets every 4 hours while symptoms persist, not to exceed 12 tablets in 24 hours, or as directed by a doctor. Children 6 to under 12 years of age: One tablet every 4 hours while symptoms

persist, not to exceed 5 tablets in 24 hours, or as directed by a doctor. Children under 6: Consult a doctor.

Warnings: KEEP THIS AND ALL OTHER MEDICATIONS OUT OF THE REACH OF CHILDREN. IN CASE OF ACCIDENTAL OVERDOSE, SEEK PROFESSIONAL ASSISTANCE OR CONTACT A POISON CONTROL CENTER IMMEDIATELY. PROMPT MEDICAL ATTENTION IS CRITICAL FOR ADULTS AS WELL AS FOR CHILDREN EVEN IF YOU DO NOT NOTICE ANY SIGNS OR SYMPTOMS. As with any drug, if you are pregnant or nursing a baby, seek the advice of a health professional before using this product. Do not take this product for more than 10 days (for adults) or 5 days (for children) unless directed by a doctor. If symptoms do not improve or are accompanied by a fever that lasts for more than 3 days, or if new symptoms occur, consult a doctor. Do not exceed recommended dosage because at higher doses nervousness, dizziness or sleeplessness may occur. May cause excitability especially in children. If sore throat is severe, persists for more than 2 days, is accompanied or followed by a fever, headache, rash, nausea or vomiting, consult a doctor promptly. This product should not be taken by persons who have asthma, glaucoma, emphysema, chronic pulmonary disease, high blood pressure, heart disease, thyroid disease, diabetes, shortness of breath, difficulty in breathing or difficulty in urination due to enlargement of the prostate gland unless directed by a doctor. May cause drowsiness; alcohol may increase the drowsiness effect. Avoid alcoholic beverages, and do not take this product if you are taking sedatives or tranquilizers without first consulting your doctor. Use caution when driving a motor vehicle or operating machinery.

Drug Interaction Precaution: This product should not be taken by any adult or child who is taking a prescription medication for high blood pressure or depression without first consulting a doctor.

Overdose:
MUCOMYST (acetylcysteine) As An Antidote For Acetaminophen Overdose)
Acetaminophen is rapidly absorbed from the upper gastrointestinal tract with peak plasma levels occurring between 30 and 60 minutes after therapeutic doses and usually within 4 hours following an overdose. The parent compound, which is nontoxic, is extensively metabolized in the liver to form principally the sulfate and glucuronide conjugates which are also nontoxic and are rapidly excreted in the urine. A small fraction of an ingested dose is metabolized in the liver by the cytochrome P-450 mixed function oxidase enzyme system to form a reactive, potentially toxic, intermediate metabolite which preferentially conjugates with hepatic glutathione to form the nontoxic cysteine and mercapturic acid derivatives which are then excreted by the kidney. Therapeutic doses of acetaminophen do not saturate the glucuronide and sulfate conjugation pathways and do not result in the formation of sufficient reactive metabolite to deplete glutathione stores. However, following ingestion of a large overdose (150 mg/kg or greater) the glucuronide and sulfate conjugation pathways are saturated resulting in a larger fraction of the drug being metabolized via the P-450 pathway. The increased formation of reactive metabolite may deplete the hepatic stores of glutathione with subsequent binding of the metabolite to protein molecules within the hepatocyte resulting in cellular necrosis. Acetylcysteine has been shown to reduce the extent of liver injury following acetaminophen overdose. Early symptoms following a potentially hepatotoxic overdose may include: nausea, vomiting, diaphoresis and general malaise. Clinical and laboratory evidence of hepatic toxicity may not be apparent until 48 to 72 hours postingestion. In adults and adolescents, regardless of the quantity of acetaminophen reported to have been ingested, administer MUCOMYST® acetylcysteine immediately. MUCOMYST acetylcysteine therapy should be initiated and continued for a full course of therapy. Its effectiveness depends on early administration, with benefit seen principally in patients treated within 16 hours of the overdose. If acetaminophen plasma assay capability is not available, and the estimated acetaminophen ingestion exceeds 150 mg/kg, MUCOMYST acetylcysteine therapy should be initiated and continued for a full course of therapy.
For full prescribing information, refer to the MUCOMYST package insert. Do not await the results of assays for acetaminophen level before initiating treatment with MUCOMYST acetylcysteine. The following additional procedures are recommended: The stomach should be emptied promptly by lavage or by induction of emesis with syrup of ipecac. A serum acetaminophen assay should be obtained as early as possible, but no sooner than four hours following ingestion. Liver function studies should be obtained initially and repeated at 24-hour intervals.
For additional emergency information call your regional poison center or toll-free (1-800-525-6115) to the Rocky Mountain Poison Center for assistance in diagnosis and for directions in the use of MUCOMYST acetylcysteine as an antidote.

How Supplied: 4-WAY Cold Tablets are supplied as a white tablet with the number "4" debossed on one surface.
NDC 19810-0040-1 Bottle of 36's
All sizes packaged in child resistant bottle closures.
Store at room temperature.

4-WAY® Fast Acting Nasal Spray

Composition:
Phenylephrine hydrochloride 0.5%, naphazoline hydrochloride 0.05%, pyrilamine maleate 0.2%, in a buffered solution. Also Contains: Benzalkonium Chloride, Boric Acid, Sodium Borate, Water. Also available in a mentholated formula containing Phenylephrine hydrochloride 0.5%, naphazoline hydrochloride 0.05%, pyrilamine maleate 0.2%, in a buffered solution. Also Contains: Benzalkonium Chloride, Boric Acid, Camphor, Eucalyptol, Menthol, Poloxamer 188, Polysorbate 80, Sodium Borate, Water.

Indications: For prompt, temporary relief of nasal congestion due to the common cold, sinusitis, hay fever or other upper respiratory allergies.

Directions and Use Instructions:
Directions: Adults: Spray twice into each nostril not more often than every 4 hours. Do not give to children under 12 years of age unless directed by a doctor.
Use Instructions: For Metered Pump—Remove protective cap. Hold bottle with thumb at base and nozzle between first and second fingers. With head upright, insert metered pump spray nozzle into nostril. Depress pump all the way down, with a firm even stroke and sniff deeply. Repeat in other nostril. Do not tilt head backward while spraying. Wipe tip clean after each use. Note: This bottle is filled to correct level for proper pump action. Before using the first time, remove the protective cap from the tip and prime the metered pump by depressing pump firmly several times.
Use Instructions: For Atomizer—With head in a normal upright position, put atomizer tip into nostril. Squeeze bottle with firm, quick pressure while inhaling.

Warnings: KEEP THIS AND ALL OTHER MEDICATIONS OUT OF THE REACH OF CHILDREN. IN CASE OF ACCIDENTAL OVERDOSE OR INGESTION, SEEK PROFESSIONAL ASSISTANCE OR CONTACT A POISON CONTROL CENTER IMMEDIATELY. Do not exceed recommended dosage because burning, stinging, sneezing, or increase of nasal discharge may occur. The use of this container by more than one person may spread infection. Do not use this product for more than 3 days. If symptoms persist, consult a doctor. Adults and children who have heart disease, high blood pressure, thyroid disease, diabetes, or difficulty in urination due to enlargement of the prostate gland should not use this product unless directed by a doctor.

How Supplied:
Regular formula:
NDC 19810-0047-1 Atomizer of ½ fluid ounce.
NDC 19810-0047-2 Atomizer of 1 fluid ounce.

Continued on next page

Bristol-Myers—Cont.

NDC 19810-0047-3 Metered pump of ½ fluid ounce.
New Mentholated formula:
NDC 19810-0049-1 Atomizer of ½ fluid ounce.
Store at room temperature.
Shown in Product Identification Guide, page 404

4-WAY® Long Lasting Nasal Spray

Composition: Oxymetazoline Hydrochloride 0.05% in an isotonic aqueous solution. Phenylmercuric Acetate 0.002% added as a preservative. **Also Contains:** Benzalkonium Chloride, Glycine, Sorbitol, Water.

Indications: For prompt, temporary relief of nasal congestion due to the common cold, sinusitis, hay fever or other upper respiratory allergies.

Directions and Use Instructions:
Directions: Adults and children 6 to under 12 years of age (with adult supervision): 2 or 3 sprays in each nostril not more often than every 10 to 12 hours. Do not exceed 2 applications in any 24-hour period. Children under 6 years of age: Consult a doctor.
Use Instructions: For Metered Pump—Remove protective cap. Hold bottle with thumb at base and nozzle between first and second fingers. With head upright, insert metered pump spray nozzle into nostril. Depress pump all the way down, with a firm even stroke and sniff deeply. Repeat in other nostril. Do not tilt head backward while spraying. Wipe tip clean after each use. Note: This bottle is filled to correct level for proper pump action. Before using the first time, remove the protective cap from the tip and prime the metered pump by depressing pump firmly several times.
Use Instructions: For Atomizer—With head in a normal, upright position, put atomizer tip into nostril. Squeeze bottle with firm, quick pressure while inhaling.

Warnings: KEEP THIS AND ALL OTHER MEDICATIONS OUT OF THE REACH OF CHILDREN. IN CASE OF ACCIDENTAL OVERDOSE OR INGESTION, SEEK PROFESSIONAL ASSISTANCE OR CONTACT A POISON CONTROL CENTER IMMEDIATELY. Do not exceed recommended dosage because burning, stinging, sneezing, or increase of nasal discharge may occur. The use of this container by more than one person may spread infection. Do not use this product for more than 3 days. If symptoms persist, consult a doctor. Adults and children who have heart disease, high blood pressure, thyroid disease, diabetes, or difficulty in urination due to enlargement of the prostate gland should not use this product unless directed by a doctor.

How Supplied: 4-WAY Long Lasting Nasal Spray is supplied as:

NDC 19810-0048-1 Atomizer of ½ fluid ounce.
Store at room temperature.
Shown in Product Identification Guide, page 404

KERI LOTION
Skin Lubricant—Moisturizer

Available in three formulations:
KERI Original—recommended for dry skin.

Composition: Mineral oil in water, propylene glycol, glyceryl stearate/PEG-100 stearate, PEG-40 stearate, PEG-4 dilaurate, laureth-4, lanolin oil, methylparaben, propylparaben, fragrance, carbomer-934, triethanolamine, dioctyl sodium sulfosuccinate, quaternium-15.

KERI Silky Smooth with Vitamin E—recommended for daily use on dry skin.

Composition: Water, petrolatum, glycerin, dimethicone, steareth-2, cetyl alcohol, benzyl alcohol, laureth-23, magnesium aluminum silicate, tocopheryl linoleate, carbomer, BHT, fragrance, sodium hydroxide, disodium EDTA, quaternium-15.

KERI Silky Smooth Fragrance Free with Vitamin E—recommended for daily use on dry skin.

Composition: Water, petrolatum, glycerin, dimethicone, steareth-2, cetyl alcohol, benzyl alcohol, laureth-23, magnesium aluminum silicate, tocopheryl linoleate, carbomer, BHT, sodium hydroxide, disodium EDTA, quaternium-15.

Indications: KERI Lotion lubricates and helps hydrate the skin, making it soft and smooth. It relieves itching, helps maintain a normal moisture balance and supplements the protective action of skin lipids. Indicated for generalized dryness; detergent hands; chapped or chafed skin; "winter-itch," diaper rash; heat rash.

Directions for Use: Apply as often as needed. Use particularly after bathing and exposure to sun, water, soaps and detergents. For external use only.

How Supplied: KERI Lotion Original 6½ oz., 11 oz., 15 oz. and 20 oz. plastic bottles. KERI Silky Smooth 6½ oz., 11 oz. and 15 oz. plastic bottles. KERI Silky Smooth Fragrance Free 6½ oz., 11 oz. and 15 oz. plastic bottles.
Shown in Product Identification Guide, page 405

NO DOZ® Maximum Strength Caplets

Composition: Each caplet contains 200 mg. Caffeine. Other ingredients: Benzoic Acid, Corn Starch, FD&C Blue No. 1, Flavors, Hydroxypropyl Methylcellulose, Microcrystalline Cellulose, Propylene Glycol, Simethicone Emulsion, Stearic Acid, Sucrose, Titanium Dioxide. May also contain: Carnauba Wax, Mineral Oil, Polysorbate 20, Povidone, Sorbitan Monolaurate.

Indications: Helps restore mental alertness or wakefulness when experiencing fatigue or drowsiness.

Directions: Adults: one-half to one caplet not more often than every 3 to 4 hours.

Warnings: KEEP THIS AND ALL OTHER MEDICATIONS OUT OF THE REACH OF CHILDREN. IN CASE OF ACCIDENTAL OVERDOSE, SEEK PROFESSIONAL ASSISTANCE OR CONTACT A POISON CONTROL CENTER IMMEDIATELY. As with any drug, if you are pregnant or nursing a baby, seek the advice of a health professional before using this product. Do not give to children under 12 years of age. For occasional use only. Not intended for use as a substitute for sleep. If fatigue or drowsiness persists or continues to occur, consult a doctor. The recommended dose of this product contains about as much caffeine as a cup of coffee. Limit the use of caffeine-containing medications, foods, or beverages while taking this product because too much caffeine may cause nervousness, irritability, sleeplessness and, occasionally, rapid heart beat.

How Supplied: NO DOZ® Maximum Strength is supplied as: White coated caplets with "NO DOZ" debossed on one side. The opposite side is scored.
19810-0064-4 Bottles of 16's
19810-0064-5 Bottles of 36's
19810-0064-6 Bottles of 60's
Store at room temperature.
Shown in Product Identification Guide, page 405

NUPRIN®
(ibuprofen)
Analgesic

Warning: ASPIRIN SENSITIVE PATIENTS. Do not take this product if you have had a severe allergic reaction to aspirin, e.g.—asthma, swelling, shock or hives, because even though this product contains no aspirin or salicylates, cross-reactions may occur in patients allergic to aspirin. (See ADDITIONAL WARNINGS BELOW)

Composition: Each tablet or caplet contains ibuprofen USP, 200 mg. **Other Ingredients:** Carnauba wax, cornstarch, D&C Yellow No. 10, FD&C Yellow No. 6, hydroxypropyl methylcellulose, propylene glycol, silicon dioxide, stearic acid, titanium dioxide.

Indications: For the temporary relief of minor aches and pains associated with the common cold, headache, toothache, muscular aches, backache, for the minor pain of arthritis, for the pain of menstrual cramps and for reduction of fever.

Additional Warnings: The following warnings are stated on the Nuprin label: Do not take for pain for more than 10 days or for fever for more than 3 days unless directed by a doctor. If pain or fever persists or gets worse, if new symptoms occur, or if the painful area is red or swollen, consult a doctor. These could be signs of serious illness. If you are under a doctor's care for any serious condition, consult a doctor before taking this product. As with aspirin and acetaminophen, if you have any condition which requires you to take prescription drugs or if you have had any problems or serious side effects from taking any non-prescription pain reliever, do not take NUPRIN without first discussing it with your doctor. If you experience any symptoms which are unusual or seem unrelated to the condition for which you took ibuprofen, consult a doctor before taking any more of it. Although ibuprofen is indicated for the same conditions as aspirin and acetaminophen, it should not be taken with them except under a doctor's direction. Do not combine this product with any other ibuprofen-containing product. As with any drug, if you are pregnant or nursing a baby, seek the advice of a health professional before using this product. IT IS ESPECIALLY IMPORTANT NOT TO USE IBUPROFEN DURING THE LAST 3 MONTHS OF PREGNANCY UNLESS SPECIFICALLY DIRECTED TO DO SO BY A DOCTOR BECAUSE IT MAY CAUSE PROBLEMS IN THE UNBORN CHILD OR COMPLICATIONS DURING DELIVERY. Keep this and all drugs out of the reach of children. In case of accidental overdose, seek professional assistance or contact a poison control center immediately.

Caution: Store at room temperature. Avoid excessive heat 40°C (104°F).

Directions: Adults: Take 1 tablet or caplet every 4 to 6 hours while symptoms persist. If pain or fever does not respond to 1 tablet or caplet, 2 tablets or caplets may be used but do not exceed 6 tablets or caplets in 24 hours, unless directed by a doctor. The smallest effective dose should be used. Take with food or milk if occasional and mild heartburn, upset stomach, or stomach pain occurs with use. Consult a doctor if these symptoms are more than mild or if they persist. Children: Do not give this product to children under 12 except under the advice and supervision of a doctor.

How Supplied:
NUPRIN® is supplied as:
Golden yellow round tablets with "NU-PRIN" printed in black on one side.
NDC 19810-0767-2 Bottles of 24's
NDC 19810-0767-3 Bottles of 50's
NDC 19810-0767-4 Bottles of 100's
NDC 19810-0767-7 Bottles of 150's
NDC 19810-0767-9 Vials of 10's
Golden yellow caplets with "NUPRIN" printed in black on one side.
NDC 19810-0796-1 Bottles of 24's
NDC 19810-0796-2 Bottles of 50's
NDC 19810-0796-3 Bottles of 100's
All sizes packaged in child resistant closures except 24's for tablets and 24's for caplets, which are sizes recommended for households without young children.
Store at room temperature. Avoid excessive heat 40°C. (104°F.).

Distributed by Bristol-Myers Company
Shown in Product Identification Guide, page 405

PAZO® Hemorrhoid Ointment/Suppositories

Composition:
Ointment: Active Ingredients: Camphor, 2%; Ephedrine Sulfate, 0.2%; Zinc Oxide, 5%. Other Ingredients: Lanolin, Petrolatum.
Suppositories (per suppository): Active Ingredients: Ephedrine Sulfate, 3.86 mg; Zinc Oxide, 96.5 mg. Other Ingredients: Hydrogenated Vegetable Oil.

Indications:
Ointment: For the temporary relief of local pain, itching, and discomfort associated with inflamed hemorrhoidal tissues. Temporarily shrinks hemorrhoidal tissue.
Suppositories: For the temporary relief of local itching and discomfort associated with inflamed hemorrhoidal tissues. Temporarily shrinks hemorrhoidal tissue.

Directions:
Ointment — Adults: When practical, cleanse the affected area with soap and warm water and rinse thoroughly. Gently dry by patting or blotting with toilet tissue or a soft cloth before application of this product. Apply externally to the affected area up to 4 times daily. Do not put this product into the rectum by using fingers or any mechanical device or applicator. Children under 12 years of age: consult a doctor.
Suppositories—Adults: When practical, cleanse the affected area with mild soap and warm water and rinse thoroughly. Gently dry by patting or blotting with toilet tissue or a soft cloth before application of this product. Remove foil wrapper and insert suppository into the rectum. Use rectally up to 4 times daily. Children under 12 years of age: consult a doctor.

Warnings: KEEP THIS AND ALL OTHER MEDICATIONS OUT OF THE REACH OF CHILDREN. IN CASE OF ACCIDENTAL INGESTION OR OVERDOSE, SEEK PROFESSIONAL ASSISTANCE OR CONTACT A POISON CONTROL CENTER IMMEDIATELY. As with any drug, if you are pregnant or nursing a baby, seek the advice of a health professional before using this product. If condition worsens or does not improve within 7 days, consult a doctor. Do not exceed the recommended daily dosage unless directed by a doctor. In case of bleeding consult a doctor promptly. Do not use this product if you have heart disease, high blood pressure, thyroid disease, diabetes, or difficulty in urination due to enlargement of the prostate gland unless directed by a doctor. Some users of this product may experience nervousness, tremor, sleeplessness, nausea, and loss of appetite. If these

symptoms persist or become worse consult your doctor.
DRUG INTERACTION PRECAUTION: Do not use this product if you are taking a prescription drug for high blood pressure or depression without first consulting your doctor. Store at room temperature.

How Supplied: PAZO® ointment is supplied as:
NDC 19810-0768-1 One ounce tubes
PAZO® suppositories are silver foil wrapped and supplied as:
NDC 19810-0703-1 Box of 12's

PRESUN® ACTIVE 15 AND 30
Clear Gel Sunscreens

Active Ingredients: Oxybenzone. Octyl Methoxycinnamate. Octyl Salicylate.
PRESUN® 15 Also contains: S.D. Alcohol 40, 71.5% PPG-15 Stearyl Ether, Acrylates/t-Ocylpropenamide Copolymer, Hydroxypropylcellulose.
PRESUN® 30 Also contains: S.D. Alcohol 40, 69% PPG-15 Stearyl Ether, Acrylates/t-Ocylpropenamide Copolymer, Hydroxypropylcellulose.

Indications: 15 OR 30 TIMES NATURAL UVB PROTECTION: Used liberally and regularly PreSun® 15 or 30 Active Clear Gel Sunscreens provide 15 or 30 times your natural UVB sunburn protection and may help reduce the chance of premature wrinkling of the skin caused by repeated and prolonged overexposure to the sun.
UVA/UVB PROTECTION: PreSun® 15 or 30 Active Clear Gel Sunscreens are formulated to provide protection from sunburn caused by both UVA and UVB rays.
CLEAR GEL FORMULA: PreSun® Active Sunscreens are cool refreshing Clear Gels that feel non-greasy. They are fragrance and PABA free, which fits your Active lifestyle.
WATERPROOF: PreSun® 15 or 30 Active Clear Gel Sunscreens maintain their degree of protection even after 80 minutes in the water.

Directions: Smooth evenly and liberally onto dry skin before sun exposure. Massage in gently. Reapply to dry skin after swimming, excessive perspiration or towel drying.

Warnings: For external use only. As with all sunscreens, avoid contact with eyes. Discontinue use if irritation or rash appears. Consult a physician before using on children under six months of age.

How Supplied: 4 oz. plastic bottles

PRESUN® FOR KIDS
Children's Sunscreen

Active Ingredients: Octyl methoxycinnamate, oxybenzone, octyl salicylate.
Also contains: Water, isopropyl myristate, PG dioctanoate, isodecyl neopen-

Continued on next page

Bristol-Myers—Cont.

tanoate, DEA cetyl phosphate, PVP/ Eicosene copolymer, stearic acid, cetyl alcohol, dimethicone, diazolidinyl urea, Carbomer-940, triethanolamine, methyl-chloroisothiazolinone, and methyliso-thiazolinone.

Indications: 29 TIMES NATURAL PROTECTION: Used as directed, PRE-SUN For Kids provides 29 times your child's natural sunburn protection and may help reduce the chance of prema-ture aging and wrinkling of the skin.
NONSTINGING: A non-PABA, fra-grance-free formula that is designed not to sting sensitive skin. (Avoid contact with eyes since all sunscreens can cause irritation and stinging of the eye.)
HYPOALLERGENIC: PRESUN For Kids is hypoallergenic and, because the known sensitizers common to most sun-screens have been removed, is suitable for your child's sensitive skin.
WATERPROOF 29: PRESUN For Kids maintains its degree of protection (SPF 29) even after 80 minutes in the water.

Warnings: For external use only. Pro-tect from freezing. *As with all sunscreens:* Apply to a small area; check after 24 hours. Discontinue use if irritation or rash appears. Avoid contact with eyes. In case of contact, flush eyes with water. Keep out of the reach of children. Use on children under six months of age only with the advice of a physician.

Directions for Use: For maximum protection, smooth evenly and liberally onto dry skin before sun exposure. Mas-sage in gently. Reapplication to dry skin after prolonged swimming, excessive per-spiration or towel drying is recom-mended for all-day protection.

How Supplied: 4 oz. plastic bottle.

PRESUN® 15 AND 25 MOISTURIZING SUNSCREENS WITH KERI

PreSun® 15 Moisturizing Sunscreen

Active Ingredient: Oxybenzone, octyl dimethyl PABA. Also contains: Water, petrolatum, isopropyl myristate, PG di-octanoate, isodecyl neopentanoate, DEA cetyl phosphate, PVP/Eicosene copo-lymer, stearic acid, cetyl alcohol, dimeth-icone, diazolidinyl urea, Carbomer-940, triethanolamine, methylchloroisothi-azolinone and methylisothiazolinone. May also contain fragrance.

PreSun® 25 Moisturizing Sunscreen

Active Ingredient: Octyl methoxycin-namate, oxybenzone, octyl salicylate. Also contains: Water, isopropyl myris-tate, isodecyl neopentanoate, propylene glycol dioctanoate, petrolatum, DEA-cetyl phosphate, PVP-Eicosene copo-lymer, stearic acid, cetyl alcohol, dimeth-icone, diazolidinyl urea, Carbomer-940,

triethanolamince, methylchloroiso-thiazolinone and methylisothiazolinone.

Indications: 15 or 25 TIMES NATU-RAL UVB PROTECTION: Used liber-ally and regularly, PreSun® Moisturiz-ing Sunscreens provide 15 or 25 times your natural UVB sunburn protection and may help reduce the chance of pre-mature wrinkling of the skin caused by repeated and prolonged exposure to the sun. **UVA/UVB Protection:** PreSun® Moisturizing Sunscreens are formulated to provide protection from sunburn caused by both UVA and UVB rays.
Moisturizing: PreSun® Moisturizing Sunscreen with Keri moisturizing is a moisture-rich formula that is absorbed in quickly to provide a high degree of UVB sunburn protection while helping to re-lieve the drying effects of the sun.
Waterproof: PreSun® Moisturizing Sunscreen maintains its degree of protec-tion even after 80 minutes in the water.

Directions: Smooth evenly and liber-ally onto dry skin before sun exposure. Massage in gently. Reapply to dry skin after swimming, excessive perspiration or towel drying.

Warning: For external use only. As with all sunscreens, avoid contact with eyes. Discontinue use if irritation or rash appears. Consult a physician before us-ing on children under six months of age.

How Supplied: 4 oz. plastic bottles

PRESUN® 23 and PRESUN® FOR KIDS Spray Mist Sunscreens

Active Ingredients: Octyl dimethyl PABA, octyl methoxycinnamate, oxy-benzone, octyl salicylate. Also contains: C_{12-15} alcohols benzoate, cyclomethi-cone, PG dioctanoate, PVP hexadecene, copolymer, and 19% (w/w) SD alcohol 40.

Indications: 23 TIMES NATURAL PROTECTION: Used as directed, PRESUN 23 and PRESUN For Kids Spray Mist Sunscreens provide 23 times your natural sunburn protection and may help reduce the chance of prema-ture aging and wrinkling of the skin.
WATERPROOF 23: PRESUN 23 and PRESUN For Kids Spray Mist Sun-screens maintain their degree of protec-tion (SPF 23) even after 80 minutes in the water.
Convenience Spray: This revolutionary new spray bottle design is non-aerosol.

Directions for Use: For best results, hold bottle about ten inches away from body while spraying. Massage in gently. Reapplication to dry skin after prolonged swimming, excessive perspiration or towel drying is recommended for all-day protection.

Warnings: For external use only. Do not use if sensitive to *p*-aminobenzoic acid (PABA) or related compounds. Avoid flame. Do not expose to heat or store above 86°F. As with all sunscreens: Apply to a small area; check after

24 hours. Discontinue use if irritation or rash appears. Avoid spraying in the eyes. In case of contact, flush eyes with water. Keep out of reach of children. Use on children under six months of age only with the advice of a physician.

How Supplied: 23 Spray Mist Sun-screen: 3.5 oz. plastic bottle with non-aerosol spray. For Kids Spray Mist Sun-screen: 3.5 oz. plastic bottle with non-aerosol spray.

PRESUN® 15 and 29 SENSITIVE SKIN SUNSCREENS PABA-FREE Sunscreen Protection

Active Ingredients: Octyl methoxy-cinnamate, oxybenzone, octyl salicylate. Also contains: Water, isopropyl myris-tate, PG dioctanoate, isodecyl neopen-tanoate, DEA cetyl phosphate, PVP/ Eicosene copolymer, stearic acid, cetyl alcohol, dimethicone, diazolidinyl urea, Carbomer-940, triethanolamine, methyl-chloroisothiazolinone, and methyliso-thiazolinone.

Indications:
15 or 29 TIMES NATURAL PROTEC-TION: Used as directed, PRESUN 15 or 29 Sensitive Skin Sunscreen provides 15 or 29 times your natural *sunburn* protec-tion and may help reduce the chance of premature aging and wrinkling of the skin as well as skin cancer caused by overexposure to the sun.
PABA-FREE FORMULAS: PABA- and fragrance-free formulas that provide a very high degree of sunburn protection and, because the known sensitizers com-mon to most sunscreens have been re-moved, is suitable for sensitive skin.
WATERPROOF: PRESUN Sensitive Skin Sunscreen maintains its degree of protection even after 80 minutes in the water.

Directions for Use: For maximum protection, smooth evenly and liberally onto dry skin before sun exposure. Mas-sage in gently. Reapplication to dry skin after prolonged swimming, excessive per-spiration or towel drying is recom-mended for all-day protection.

Warnings: For external use only. Pro-tect from freezing. *As with all sunscreens:* Apply to a small area; check after 24 hours. Discontinue use if irritation or rash appears. Avoid contact with eyes. In case of contact, flush eyes with water. Keep out of the reach of children. Use on children under six months of age only with the advice of a physician.

How Supplied: 29 Sensitive Skin: 4 oz. (NSN 6505-01-267-1483) plastic bottle. 15 Sensitive Skin: 4 oz. plastic bottle.

PRESUN® 46 MOISTURIZING SUNSCREEN

Active Ingredient: Octyl dimethyl PABA, oxybenzone. Also contains: wa-ter, isopropyl myristate, PG dioctanoate, isodecyl neopentanoate, DEA cetyl phosphate, PVP/Eicosene copolymer, stearic acid, cetyl alcohol, dimethicone, diazolidinyl urea, carbomer-940, triethanolamine, methylchloroisothiazolinone and methylisothiazolinone. May also contain fragrance.

Indications: 46 TIMES NATURAL UVB PROTECTION: Used liberally and regularly, PreSun® 46 Moisturizing Sunscreen provides 46 times your natural UVB sunburn protection and may help reduce the chance of premature wrinkling of the skin caused by repeated and prolonged exposure to the sun. UVA/UVB: PreSun 46 Moisturizing Sunscreen is formulated to provide protection from sunburn caused by both UVA nd UVB rays.

Moisturizing: A moisture-rich formula that is absorbed in quickly to provide a high degree of UVB sunburn protection while helping to relieve the drying effects of the sun.

Waterproof: PreSun® 46 Moisturizing Sunscreen maintains its degree of protection even after 80 minutes in the water.

Directions: Smooth evenly and liberally onto dry skin before sun exposure. Massage in gently. Reapply to dry skin after swimming, excessive perspiration or towel drying.

Warnings: For external use only. As with all sunscreens, avoid contact with eyes. Discontinue use if irritation or rash appears. Consult a physician before using on children under six months of age.

How Supplied: 4 oz. plastic bottle

THERAGRAN® LIQUID with Niacin & Vitamin C
High Potency Vitamin Supplement

Each 5 ml. teaspoonful contains:

		Percent US RDA*
Vitamin A	5,000 IU	100
Vitamin D	400 IU	100
Vitamin C	200 mg	333
Thiamine	10 mg	667
Riboflavin	10 mg	588
Niacin	100 mg	500
Vitamin B6	4.1 mg	205
Vitamin B12	5 mcg	83
Pantothenic Acid	21.4 mg	214

*US Recommended Daily Allowance

Ingredients: purified water, sucrose, glycerine, propylene glycol, sodium ascorbate, niacinamide, polysorbate 80, ascorbic acid, thiamine hydrochloride, d-panthenol, carboxymethylcellulose sodium, riboflavin-5-phosphate sodium, artificial and natural flavors, (sodium benzoate and methylparaben as preservatives), pyridoxine hydrochloride, vitamin A palmitate, cholecalciferol, ferric ammonium citrate, cyanocobalamin Take 1 teaspoonful daily or as directed by physician.

How Supplied: In bottles of 4 fl. oz. NO REFRIGERATION REQUIRED

Storage: Store at room temperature; avoid excessive heat.
(P9163-00)

ADVANCED FORMULA THERAGRAN® TABLETS
(High Potency Multivitamin Formula)

FOR ADULTS—PERCENTAGE OF U.S. RECOMMENDED DAILY ALLOWANCE

Vitamins	Quantity	US RDA
Vitamin A	5000 IU	100%
(as Acetate and Beta Carotene)		
Vitamin B1	3 mg	200%
Vitamin B2	3.4 mg	200%
Vitamin B6	3 mg	150%
Vitamin B12	9 mcg	150%
Vitamin C	90 mg	150%
Vitamin D	400 I.U.	100%
Vitamin E	30 I.U.	100%
Niacin	20 mg	100%
Folic Acid	400 mcg	100%
Pantothenic Acid	10.0 mg	100%
Biotin	30 mcg	10%

Ingredients: Lactose, ascorbic acid, microcrystalline cellulose, gelatin, dl-alpha-tocopheryl acetate, niacinamide, starch, calcium pantothenate, sodium caseinate, hydroxypropyl methylcellulose, sucrose, povidone, pyridoxine hydrochloride, riboflavin, silicon dioxide, magnesium stearate, thiamine mononitrate, vitamin A acetate, polyethylene glycol, triacetin, stearic acid, titanium dioxide, annatto, beta carotene, FD&C Red 40, folic acid, biotin, ergocalciferol, cyanocobalamin.

Warning: KEEP OUT OF REACH OF CHILDREN.

Recommended Adult Intake—1 tablet daily or as directed by physician.

How Supplied: Packs of 130; and Unimatic® cartons of 100.

Storage: Store at room temperature; avoid excessive heat; keep tightly closed. UNIMATIC® is a trademark of E.R. Squibb & Sons, Inc.
Shown in Product Identification Guide, page 405

COMPLETE FORMULA with Beta Carotene
THERAGRAN-M® TABLETS
(High Potency Multivitamin Formula with Minerals)
[See table at top of next column]

Ingredients: Magnesium oxide, dibasic calcium phosphate, lactose, ascorbic acid, ferrous fumarate, gelatin, dl-alpha tocopheryl, acetate, crospovidone, niacinamide, hydroxypropyl methylcellulose, zinc oxide, povidone, manganese sulfate, potassium chloride, starch, calcium pantothenate, sodium caseinate, pyridoxine hydrochloride, cupric sulfate, magnesium stearate, sucrose, silicon dioxide, riboflavin, thiamine mononitrate, stearic acid, polyethylene glycol, triacetin, Vitamin A acetate, FD&C Red 40, potassium citrate, beta carotene, tita-

TABLET CONTENTS:
FOR ADULTS—PERCENTAGE OF U.S. RECOMMENDED DAILY ALLOWANCE

Vitamins	Quantity	US RDA
Vitamin A	5000 IU	100%
(as Acetate and Beta Carotene)		
Vitamin B1	3 mg	200%
Vitamin B2	3.4 mg	200%
Vitamin B6	3 mg	150%
Vitamin B12	9 mcg	150%
Vitamin C	90 mg	150%
Vitamin D	400 IU	100%
Vitamin E	30 IU	100%
Niacin	20 mg	100%
Folic Acid	400 mcg	100%
Pantothenic Acid	10.0 mg	100%
Biotin	30 mcg	10%
Minerals		
Iron	27 mg	150%
Copper	2 mg	100%
Iodine	150 mcg	100%
Zinc	15 mg	100%
Magnesium	100 mg	25%
Calcium	40 mg	4%
Phosphorus	31 mg	3%
Chromium	15 mcg	*
Molybdenum	15 mcg	*
Selenium	10 mcg	*
Manganese	5 mg	*
ELECTROLYTES		
Chloride	7.5 mg	*
Potassium	7.5 mg	*

*US RDA not established.

nium dioxide, folic acid, potassium iodide, FD&C Blue No. 2, chromic chloride, sodium molybdate, biotin, sodium selenate, ergocalciferol, cyanocobalamin

Warning: KEEP OUT OF REACH OF CHILDREN.

Usage: For adults—1 tablet daily

How Supplied: Packs of 90, 130 and 240; and Unimatic® cartons of 100.

Storage: Store at room temperature; avoid excessive heat; keep tightly closed. UNIMATIC® is a trademark of E.R. Squibb & Sons, Inc.
Shown in Product Identification Guide, page 405

THERAGRAN® STRESS FORMULA
High Potency Multivitamin Stress Formula with Iron and Vitamin C

TABLET CONTENTS: For Adults—Percentage of US Recommended Daily Allowance

Ingredients	Quantity	US RDA
Vitamin B1	15 mg	1000%
Vitamin B2	15 mg	882%
Vitamin B6	25 mg	1250%
Vitamin B12	12 mcg	200%
Vitamin C	600 mg	1000%
Vitamin E	30 IU	100%
Niacin	100 mg	500%
Pantothenic Acid	20 mg	200%
Iron	27 mg	150%
Folic Acid	400 mcg	100%
Biotin	45 mcg	15%

Continued on next page

Bristol-Myers—Cont.

Ingredients: Ascorbic acid, niacinamide, ferrous fumarate, starch, lactose, pyridoxine hydrochloride, crospovidone, dl-alpha tocopheryl acetate, gelatin, calcium pantothenate, riboflavin, povidone, thiamine mononitrate, hydroxypropyl methylcellulose, sodium caseinate, magnesium stearate, silicon dioxide, stearic acid, polyethylene glycol, triacetin, titanium dioxide, FD&C Red No. 40, FD&C Yellow No. 6, folic acid, biotin, cyanocobalamin

Warning: KEEP OUT OF REACH OF CHILDREN.

Recommended Adult Intake—1 tablet daily or as directed by physician.

How Supplied: Bottles of 75.

Storage: Store at room temperature; avoid excessive heat.
(P893-01)
Shown in Product Identification Guide, page 405

THERAPEUTIC MINERAL ICE®

Composition:
Active Ingredient: Menthol 2%
Other Ingredients: Ammonium Hydroxide, Carbomer 934, Cupric Sulfate, FD&C Blue No. 1, Isopropyl Alcohol, Magnesium Sulfate, Sodium Hydroxide, Thymol, Water.

Indications: For the temporary relief of minor aches and pains of muscles and joints associated with arthritis, simple backache, strains, bruises, sprains and sports injuries. **USE ONLY AS DIRECTED. Read all warnings before use.**

Warnings: KEEP OUT OF THE REACH OF CHILDREN. For external use only. Not for internal use. Avoid contact with eyes and mucous membranes. Do not use with other ointments, creams, sprays, or liniments. **Do not use with Heating Pads or Heating Devices.** If condition worsens, or if symptoms persist for more than 7 days, or clear up and occur again within a few days, discontinue use of this product and consult your doctor. Do not apply to wounds or damaged skin. Do not bandage tightly. If you have sensitive skin, consult doctor before use. If skin irritation develops, discontinue use and consult your doctor. As with any drug, if you are pregnant or nursing a baby, seek the advice of a health professional before using this product. Keep cap tightly closed. Do not use, pour, spill or store near heat or open flame. **Note:** You can always use Mineral Ice as directed, but its use is never intended to replace your doctor's advice.

Directions: Adults and children 2 years of age and older: Clean skin of all other ointments, creams, sprays, or liniments. Apply to affected areas not more than 3 to 4 times daily. May be used with wet or dry bandages or with ice packs. No protective cover needed. Children under 2 years of age: Consult a doctor.

How Supplied:
NDC 19810-0034-4 3.5 oz.
NDC 19810-0034-2 8 oz.
NDC 19810-0034-3 16 oz.
Store at room temperature.
Shown in Product Identification Guide, page 405

THERAPEUTIC MINERAL ICE®
Exercise Formula, Pain Relieving Gel

Composition:
Active Ingredient: Menthol 4%.
Other Ingredients: Ammonium Hydroxide, Carbomer 934P or Carbomer 934, Cupric Sulfate, FD&C Blue No. 1, Fragrance, Isopropyl Alcohol, Magnesium Sulfate, Sodium Hydroxide, Thymol, Water.

Indications: For the temporary relief of minor aches and pains of muscles and joints associated with strains, sprains, bruises, sports injuries and simple backache. **USE ONLY AS DIRECTED. Read all warnings before use.**

Warnings: KEEP OUT OF REACH OF CHILDREN. For external use only. Not for internal use. Avoid contact with eyes and mucous membranes. Do not use with other ointments, creams, sprays, or liniments. **Do not use with heating pad or heating devices.** If condition worsens, or if symptoms persist for more than 7 days, or clear up and occur again within a few days, discontinue use of this product and consult your doctor. Do not apply to wounds or damaged skin. Do not bandage tightly. If you have sensitive skin, consult doctor BEFORE use. If skin irritation develops, discontinue use and consult your doctor. As with any drug, if you are pregnant or nursing a baby, seek the advice of a health professional before using this product. Do not use, pour, spill, or store near heat or open flame. NOTE: You can always use MINERAL ICE® EXERCISE FORMULA as directed, but its use is never intended to replace your doctor's advice.

Directions: Adults and children 2 years of age and older: Clean skin of all other ointments, creams, sprays, or liniments. Apply to affected areas not more than 3 to 4 times daily. May be used with wet or dry bandages or with ice packs. Not greasy. No protective cover needed. Children: Do not use on children under 2 years of age, except under the advice and supervision of a doctor.

How Supplied: Available in 3 oz. tubes.
STORE AT ROOM TEMPERATURE.
KEEP CAP TIGHTLY CLOSED.
Shown in Product Identification Guide, page 405

THERAPEUTIC MINERAL ICE PLUS MOISTURIZERS

Composition: THERAPEUTIC MINERAL ICE PLUS MOISTURIZERS CONTAINS Menthol 4% in a base of ammonium hydroxide, carbomer, cupric sulfate, FD&C Blue No. 1, fragrance, isopropyl alcohol, magnesium sulfate, petrolatum, polysorbate 20, sodium hydroxide, thymol and water.

For the temporary relief of minor aches and pains of msucles and joints associated with:
● Arthritis
● Simple backache
● Strains, sprains, and bruises
● Sports injuries

Directions: Adults and children 2 years of age and older: Clean skin of all other ointments, creams, sprays, or liniments. Apply to affected areas not more often than 3 to 4 times daily. May be used with wet or dry bandages or with ice packs. No protective cover needed. Children under 2 years of age: Consult a doctor. **USE ONLY AS DIRECTED. Read all warnings before use.**

Warnings: KEEP OUT OF REACH OF CHILDREN. For external use only. Not for interal use. Avoid contact with eyes and mucous membranes. Do not use with other ointments, creams, sprays, or liniments. **DO NOT USE WITH HEATING PADS OR HEATING DEVICES.** If condition worsens, or if sypmtoms persist for more than 7 days, or clear up and occur again within a few days, discontinue use of this product and consult a doctor **before** use. If skin irritation develops, discontinue use and consult your doctor. As with any drug, if you are pregnant or nursing a baby, seek the advice of a health professional before using this product. Keep cap tightly closed. Do not use, pour, spill or store near heat or open flame. **NOTE:** You can always use **MINERAL ICE® PLUS MOISTURIZER** as directed, but its use is never intended to replace your doctor's advice.

How Supplied: THERAPEUTIC MINERAL ICE PLUS MOISTURIZERS is a light blue gel with a pleasant fragrance.
NDC 19810-0569-1 2 oz. Tube
NDC 19810-0569-2 4 oz. Tube
Store at room temperature.

W.K. Buckley, Inc.
P.O. BOX 5022
WESTPORT, CT 06881-5022

BUCKLEY'S MIXTURE

Each teaspoonful (5mL) contains 12.5 mg dextromethorphan hydrobromide in a sugar-free base. Also contains: ammonium carbonate, camphor, Canada balsam, carrageenan, glycerine, menthol, pine needle oil, sodium butylparaben and sodium propylparaben (as preservatives), sodium saccharin, tincture of calcium, water.

Indications: Temporarily relieves coughs due to minor throat and bronchial irritation as may occur with a cold.

Dosage and Administration: ADULT: One and a half teaspoonsful every four hours. CHILDREN: 6 to 12 years—Three quarters of a teaspoonful every four hours. Do not exceed recommended dosage or give to children under 6 years of age unless directed by a physician.

Warnings: A persistent cough may be a sign of a serious condition. If a cough persists for more than 1 week, tends to recur, or is accompanied by fever, rash, or persistent headache, consult a doctor. Do not take this product for persistent or chronic cough such as occurs with smoking, asthma, emphysema, or if a cough is accompanied by excessive phlegm (mucus) unless directed by a doctor. As with any drug, if you are pregnant or nursing a baby, seek professional advice before using this product.

Drug Interaction Precaution: Do not take this product if you are presently taking a prescription monoamine oxidase inhibitor without first consulting your doctor.
Keep this and all drugs out of reach of children: In case of accidental overdose, seek professional assistance or contact a poison control center immediately. Store at controlled room temperature between 15°C and 30°C (59°F and 86°F).

How Supplied: Bottles of 4 fl oz and 8 fl oz.

Shown in Product Identification Guide, page 405

UNKNOWN DRUG?
Consult the
Product Identification Guide
(Gray Pages)
for full-color photos of
leading over-the-counter
medications

Burroughs Wellcome Co.
3030 CORNWALLIS ROAD
RESEARCH TRIANGLE PARK,
NC 27709

ACTIFED® ALLERGY DAYTIME/NIGHTTIME CAPLETS
[ăk 'tuh-fĕd]

Actifed® Allergy DAYTIME (white caplets) is a no-drowsiness product. Actifed® Allergy NIGHTTIME (blue caplets) may cause marked drowsiness. Read directions carefully for both products.
ACTIFED® ALLERGY DAYTIME (white caplets)
ANTIHISTAMINE-FREE. CONTAINS NO INGREDIENTS THAT MAY CAUSE DROWSINESS.

Product Benefits: The **DAYTIME** no-drowsiness product (white caplets) contains a nasal decongestant (pseudoephedrine) that provides temporary relief of nasal congestion due to hay fever or other upper respiratory allergies. Helps decongest sinus openings and passages; relieves sinus pressure; reduces swollen nasal passages.

Directions: Adults and children 12 years and over, **2 caplets every 4 to 6 hours** during waking hours. Do not exceed a total of 8 caplets (Daytime or Nighttime) in 24 hours. **Do not take Actifed Allergy Daytime within 4 hours of Actifed Allergy Nighttime.** Not recommended for children under 12.

Each Actifed Allergy Daytime Caplet Contains: pseudoephedrine hydrochloride 30 mg. Also contains: carnauba wax, crospovidone, hydroxypropyl methylcellulose, lactose, magnesium stearate, microcrystalline cellulose, polyethylene glycol, and titanium dioxide.

ACTIFED® ALLERGY NIGHTTIME (blue caplest) **MAY CAUSE MARKED DROWSINESS.**

Product Benefits: The **NIGHTTIME** product (blue caplets) contains a nasal decongestant (pseudoephedrine) and an antihistamine (diphenhydramine) that provide temporary relief of nasal congestion, sinus pressure, swollen nasal passages, runny nose, and sneezing due to hay fever or other upper respiratory allergies. Also relieves itching of the nose or throat and itchy, watery eyes due to hay fever.

Directions: Adults and children 12 years and over, **2 caplets at bedtime.** Due to potential marked drowsiness, do not take during waking hours unless confined to bed or resting at home; 2 caplets then may be taken every 4 to 6 hours. Do not exceed a total of 8 caplets (Daytime and/or Nighttime) in 24 hours. **Do not take Actifed Allergy Nighttime within 4 hours of Actifed Daytime.** Not recommended for children under 12.

Warning: May cause marked drowsiness; alcohol, sedatives and tranquilizers may increase the drowsiness effect. Avoid alcoholic beverages while taking Actifed Allergy Nighttime. Do not take

this product if you are taking sedatives or tranquilizers, without first consulting your doctor. Use caution when driving a motor vehicle or operating machinery.

Each Actifed Allergy Nighttime Caplet Contains: diphenhydramine hydrochloride 25 mg and pseudoephedrine hydrochloride 30 mg. Also contains: carnauba wax, crospovidone, FD&C Blue No. 1 Lake, hydroxypropyl methylcellulose, lactose, magnesium stearate, microcrystalline cellulose, polyethylene glycol, polysorbate 80, and titanium dioxide.
ACTIFED® DAYTIME/NIGHTTIME products do not contain triprolidine hydrochloride, the antihistamine found in other ACTIFED products.

Warnings: Do not exceed a combined total of 8 caplets (Actifed Allergy Daytime *plus* Actifed Allergy Nighttime) in 24 hours. These products may cause excitability, especially in children. Do not exceed recommended dosage for these products because at higher doses nervousness, dizziness, or sleeplessness may occur. If symptoms do not improve within 7 days or are accompanied by high fever, consult a doctor before continuing use. Do not take these products, unless directed by a doctor, if you have high blood pressure, heart disease, thyroid disease, glaucoma, a breathing problem such as emphysema or chronic bronchitis, or difficulty in urination due to enlargement of the prostate gland. As with any drug, if you are pregnant or nursing a baby, seek the advice of a health professional before using these products.

Drug Interaction Precaution: Do not take these products if you are presently taking a prescription antihypertensive or antidepressant drug containing a monoamine oxidase inhibitor except under the advice and supervision of a doctor.
KEEP THESE AND ALL DRUGS OUT OF THE REACH OF CHILDREN. In case of accidental overdose, seek professional assistance or contact a Poison Control Center immediately. Store at 15° to 25°C (59° to 77°F) in a dry place and protect from light.

How Supplied: Package contains 24 Daytime caplets and 8 Nighttime Caplets.
Shown in Product Identification Guide, page 405

ACTIFED® PLUS Caplets
[ăk 'tuh-fĕd]

Product Benefits: Each ACTIFED® PLUS Coated Caplet contains three maximum strength ingredients for temporary relief from symptoms of the common cold, seasonal allergies (hay fever) and sinus congestion.
The **ANTIHISTAMINE** (triprolidine) temporarily dries runny nose and relieves sneezing associated with the common cold, hay fever or other upper respi-

Continued on next page

Burroughs Wellcome—Cont.

ratory allergies. Also relieves itching of the nose or throat, and itchy, watery eyes due to hay fever.

The **DECONGESTANT** (pseudoephedrine) temporarily relieves nasal congestion due to the common cold, hay fever or other upper respiratory allergies, or associated with sinusitis. Temporarily relieves nasal stuffiness. Reduces the swelling of nasal passages; shrinks swollen membranes; and temporarily restores freer breathing through the nose. Also, helps to decongest sinus openings and passages; relieves sinus pressure.

The non-aspirin **ANALGESIC** (acetaminophen) temporarily relieves occasional minor aches, pains and headache, and reduces fever due to the common cold.

Each ACTIFED PLUS Coated Caplet Contains: acetaminophen 500 mg, pseudoephedrine hydrochloride 30 mg and triprolidine hydrochloride 1.25 mg. Also contains: carnauba wax, crospovidone, FD&C Blue No. 1 Lake, D&C Yellow No. 10 Lake, hydroxypropyl methylcellulose, magnesium stearate, microcrystalline cellulose, polyethylene glycol, polysorbate 80, povidone, pregelatinized corn starch, stearic acid, and titanium dioxide.

Directions: Adults and children 12 years of age and over, 2 caplets every 6 hours. Do not exceed 8 caplets in 24 hours. Not recommended for children under 12 years of age.

Warnings: May cause drowsiness; alcohol, sedatives, and tranquilizers may increase the drowsiness effect. Avoid alcoholic beverages while taking this product. Do not take this product if you are taking sedatives or tranquilizers, without first consulting your doctor. Use caution when driving a motor vehicle or operating machinery. May cause excitability, especially in children. Do not exceed recommended dosage because at higher doses nervousness, dizziness, or sleeplessness may occur. Do not take this product for more than 7 days. If symptoms do not improve or are accompanied by fever that lasts for more than 3 days, or if new symptoms occur, consult a doctor. Do not take this product, unless directed by a doctor, if you have high blood pressure, heart disease, diabetes, thyroid disease, glaucoma, a breathing problem such as emphysema or chronic bronchitis, or difficulty in urination due to enlargement of the prostate gland. As with any drug, if you are pregnant or nursing a baby, seek the advice of a health professional before using this product.

Drug Interaction Precaution: Do not take this product if you are presently taking a prescription antihypertensive or antidepressant drug containing a monoamine oxidase inhibitor except under the advice and supervision of a doctor.

KEEP THIS AND ALL DRUGS OUT OF THE REACH OF CHILDREN. In case of accidental overdose, seek professional assistance or contact a Poison Control Center immediately. Prompt medical attention is critical for adults as well as for children even if you do not notice any signs or symptoms.

Store at 15° to 25°C (59° to 77°F) in a dry place and protect from light.   402907

How Supplied: Boxes of 20, 40.
Shown in Product Identification Guide, page 405

ACTIFED® SINUS DAYTIME/ NIGHTTIME Caplets
[ak 'tuh-fĕd]

> This package contains 2 separate products: Actifed Sinus DAYTIME (white caplets) is a no-drowsiness product; Actifed Sinus NIGHTTIME (blue caplets) may cause marked drowsiness. Read directions carefully for both products.

ACTIFED® SINUS DAYTIME (white caplets)
CONTAINS NO INGREDIENTS THAT MAY CAUSE DROWSINESS.

Product Benefits: The **DAYTIME** no-drowsiness product (white caplets) contains a non-aspirin pain reliever (acetaminophen) and nasal decongestant (pseudoephedrine) that provide temporary relief of sinus headache pain, sinus pressure and nasal congestion due to the common cold, hay fever, or other allergies.

Directions: Adults and children 12 years and over, **2 caplets** every 4 to 6 hours during waking hours. Do not exceed a total of 8 caplets (Daytime or Nighttime) in 24 hours. **Do not take Actifed Sinus Daytime within 6 hours of Actifed Sinus Nighttime.** Not recommended for children under 12.

Each Actifed Sinus Daytime Caplet Contains: acetaminophen 325 mg and pseudoephedrine hydrochloride 30 mg. Also contains: carnauba wax, crospovidone, hydroxypropyl methylcellulose, magnesium stearate, microcrystalline cellulose, polyethylene glycol, povidone, pregelatinized corn starch, sodium starch glycolate, stearic acid, and titanium dioxide.

ACTIFED® SINUS NIGHTTIME (blue caplets)
MAY CAUSE MARKED DROWSINESS.

Product Benefits: The **NIGHTTIME** product (blue caplets) contains a non-aspirin pain reliever (acetaminophen), a nasal decongestant (pseudoephedrine), and an antihistamine (diphenhydramine) that provide temporary relief of sinus headache pain, sinus pressure, nasal congestion, runny nose, and sneezing due to the common cold, hay fever, or

other allergies. Also relieves itching of the nose or throat and itchy, watery eyes due to hay fever.

Directions: Adults and children 12 years and over, **2 caplets** at bedtime. Due to potential marked drowsiness, do not take during waking hours unless confined to bed or resting at home; 2 caplets then may be taken every 6 hours. Do not exceed a total of 8 caplets (Daytime or Nighttime) in 24 hours. **Do not take Actifed Sinus Nighttime within 6 hours of Actifed Sinus Daytime.** Not recommended for children under 12.

Warning: May cause marked drowsiness; alcohol, sedatives, and tranquilizers may increase the drowsiness effect. Avoid alcoholic beverages while taking Actifed Sinus Nighttime. Do not take this product if you are taking sedatives or tranquilizers, without first consulting your doctor. Use caution when driving a motor vehicle or operating machinery.

Each Actifed Sinus Nighttime Caplet Contains: acetaminophen 500 mg, diphenhydramine hydrochloride 25 mg and pseudoephedrine hydrochloride 30 mg. Also contains: carnauba wax, crospovidone, FD&C Blue No. 1 Lake, hydroxypropyl methylcellulose, magnesium stearate, microcrystalline cellulose, polyethylene glycol, polysorbate 80, povidone, pregelatinized corn starch, sodium starch glycolate, stearic acid, and titanium dioxide.

ACTIFED DAYTIME/NIGHTTIME products do not contain triprolidine hydrochloride, the antihistamine found in other ACTIFED products.

Warnings: Do not exceed a combined total of 8 caplets (Actifed Sinus Daytime *plus* Actifed Sinus Nighttime) in 24 hours. These products may cause excitability, especially in children. Do not exceed recommended dosage for these products because at higher doses nervousness, dizziness, or sleeplessness may occur. Do not take these products for more than 7 days. If symptoms do not improve or are accompanied by fever that lasts for more than 3 days, or if new symptoms occur, consult a doctor. Do not take these products, unless directed by a doctor, if you have high blood pressure, heart disease, diabetes, thyroid disease, glaucoma, a breathing problem such as emphysema or chronic bronchitis, or difficulty in urination due to enlargement of the prostate gland. As with any drug, if you are pregnant or nursing a baby, seek the advice of a health professional before using these products.

Drug Interaction: Do not take these products if you are presently taking a prescription antihypertensive or antidepressant drug containing a monoamine oxidase inhibitor except under the advice and supervision of a doctor.

KEEP THESE AND ALL DRUGS OUT OF THE REACH OF CHILDREN. In case of accidental overdose, seek professional assistance or contact a Poison Control Center immediately. Prompt medical attention is critical for adults as well as for children even if you do not notice any signs or symptoms.

Store at 15° to 25°C (59° to 77°F) in a dry place and protect from light.

How Supplied: Package contains 18 Daytime Caplets and 6 Nighttime Caplets. 402136

Shown in Product Identification Guide, page 405

ACTIFED® SINUS DAYTIME/ NIGHTTIME Tablets
[ak'tuh-fĕd]

This package contains 2 separate products: Actifed Sinus DAYTIME (white tablets) is a no-drowsiness product; Actifed Sinus NIGHTTIME (blue tablets) may cause marked drowsiness. Read directions carefully for both products.

ACTIFED® SINUS DAYTIME (white tablets)
CONTAINS NO INGREDIENTS THAT MAY CAUSE DROWSINESS.

Product Benefits: The **DAYTIME** no-drowsiness product (white tablets) contains a non-aspirin pain reliever (acetaminophen) and nasal decongestant (pseudoephedrine) that provide temporary relief of sinus headache pain, sinus pressure and nasal congestion due to the common cold, hay fever, or other allergies.

Directions: Adults and children 12 years and over, **2 tablets** every 4 to 6 hours during waking hours. Do not exceed a total of 8 tablets (Daytime and/or Nighttime) in 24 hours. **Do not take Actifed Sinus Daytime within 6 hours of Actifed Sinus Nighttime.** Not recommended for children under 12.

Each Actifed Sinus Daytime Tablet Contains: acetaminophen 325 mg and pseudoephedrine hydrochloride 30 mg. Also contains: carnauba wax, crospovidone, hydroxypropyl methylcellulose, magnesium stearate, microcrystalline cellulose, polyethylene glycol, povidone, pregelatinized corn starch, sodium starch glycolate, stearic acid, and titanium dioxide.

ACTIFED® SINUS NIGHTTIME (blue tablets)
MAY CAUSE MARKED DROWSINESS.

Product Benefits: The **NIGHTTIME** product (blue tablets) contains a non-aspirin pain reliever (acetaminophen), a nasal decongestant (pseudoephedrine), and an antihistamine (diphenhydramine) that provide temporary relief of sinus headache pain, sinus pressure, nasal congestion, runny nose, and sneezing due to the common cold, hay fever, or other allergies. Also relieves itching of the nose or throat and itchy, watery eyes due to hay fever.

Directions: Adults and children 12 years and over, **2 tablets** at bedtime. Due to potential marked drowsiness, do not take during waking hours unless confined to bed or resting at home; 2 tablets then may be taken every 6 hours. Do not exceed a total of 8 tablets (Daytime and/ or Nighttime) in 24 hours. **Do not take Actifed Sinus Nighttime within 6 hours of Actifed Sinus Daytime.** Not recommended for children under 12.

Warning: May cause marked drowsiness; alcohol, sedatives, and tranquilizers may increase the drowsiness effect. Avoid alcoholic beverages while taking Actifed Sinus Nighttime. Do not take this product if you are taking sedatives or tranquilizers, without first consulting your doctor. Use caution when driving a motor vehicle or operating machinery.

Each Actifed Sinus Nighttime Tablet Contains: acetaminophen 500 mg, diphenhydramine hydrochloride 25 mg and pseudoephedrine hydrochloride 30 mg. Also contains: carnauba wax, crospovidone, FD&C Blue No. 1 Lake, hydroxypropyl methylcellulose, magnesium stearate, microcrystalline cellulose, polyethylene glycol, polysorbate 80, povidone, pregelatinized corn starch, sodium starch glycolate, stearic acid, and titanium dioxide.

ACTIFED DAYTIME/NIGHTTIME products do not contain triprolidine hydrochloride, the antihistamine found in other ACTIFED products.

Warnings: Do not exceed a combined total of 8 tablets (Actifed Sinus Daytime *plus* Actifed Sinus Nighttime) in 24 hours. These products may cause excitability, especially in children. Do not exceed recommended dosage for these products because at higher doses nervousness, dizziness, or sleeplessness may occur. Do not take these products for more than 7 days. If symptoms do not improve or are accompanied by fever that lasts for more than 3 days, or if new symptoms occur, consult a doctor. Do not take these products, unless directed by a doctor, if you have high blood pressure, heart disease, diabetes, thyroid disease, glaucoma, a breathing problem such as emphysema or chronic bronchitis, or difficulty in urination due to enlargement of the prostate gland. As with any drug, if you are pregnant or nursing a baby, seek the advice of a health professional before using these products.

Drug Interaction: Do not take these products if you are presently taking a prescription antihypertensive or antidepressant drug containing a monoamine oxidase inhibitor except under the advice and supervision of a doctor.
KEEP THESE AND ALL DRUGS OUT OF THE REACH OF CHILDREN. In case of accidental overdose, seek professional assistance or contact a Poison Control Center immediately. Prompt medical attention is critical for adults as well as for children even if you do not notice any signs or symptoms.

Store at 15° to 25°C (59° to 77°F) in a dry place and protect from light.

How Supplied: Package contains 18 Daytime Tablets and 6 Nighttime Tablets. 402063
Shown in Product Identification Guide, page 405

ACTIFED® Syrup
[ăk'tuh-fĕd]

Product Benefits: ACTIFED Syrup contains two maximum strength ingredients for temporary relief from symptoms of the common cold, seasonal allergies (hay fever) and sinus congestion.
The **ANTIHISTAMINE** (triprolidine) temporarily dries runny nose and relieves sneezing associated with the common cold, hay fever, or other upper respiratory allergies. Also relieves itching of the nose or throat, and itchy, watery eyes due to hay fever.
The **DECONGESTANT** (pseudoephedrine) temporarily relieves nasal congestion due to the common cold, hay fever or other upper respiratory allergies, or associated with sinusitis. Temporarily relieves nasal stuffiness. Reduces the swelling of nasal passages; shrinks swollen membranes; and temporarily restores freer breathing through the nose. Also, helps to decongest sinus openings and passages; relieves sinus pressure.

Each 5 mL (1 teaspoonful) Actifed Syrup Contains: pseudoephedrine hydrochloride 30 mg and triprolidine hydrochloride 1.25 mg. Also contains: methylparaben 0.1% and sodium benzoate 0.1% (added as preservatives), D&C Yellow No. 10, glycerin, purified water, and sorbitol.

Directions: Adults and children 12 years and over, 2 teaspoonfuls every 4 to 6 hours. Children 6 to under 12 years of age, 1 teaspoonful every 4 to 6 hours. Do not exceed 4 doses in 24 hours. Children under 6, consult a doctor.

Warnings: May cause drowsiness; alcohol, sedatives, and tranquilizers may increase the drowsiness effect. Avoid alcoholic beverages while taking this product. Do not take this product if you are taking sedatives or tranquilizers, without first consulting your doctor. Use caution when driving a motor vehicle or operating machinery. May cause excitability, especially in children. Do not exceed recommended dosage because at higher doses nervousness, dizziness or sleeplessness may occur. If symptoms do not improve within 7 days or are accompanied by high fever, consult a doctor before continuing use. Do not take this product, unless directed by a doctor, if you have high blood pressure, heart disease, diabetes, thyroid disease, asthma, glaucoma, a breathing problem such as emphysema or chronic bronchitis, or difficulty in urination due to enlargement of the prostate gland. As with any drug, if you are

Continued on next page

Burroughs Wellcome—Cont.

pregnant or nursing a baby, seek the advice of a health professional before using this product.

Drug Interaction Precaution: Do not take this product if you are presently taking a prescription antihypertensive or antidepressant drug containing a monoamine oxidase inhibitor except under the advice and supervision of a physician.

KEEP THIS AND ALL DRUGS OUT OF THE REACH OF CHILDREN. In case of accidental overdose, seek professional assistance or contact a Poison Control Center immediately.

Store at 15° to 25°C (59° to 77°F) and protect from light.

How Supplied: Bottles of 4 fl oz (118 mL) and 1 pint. (473 mL)   402360

Shown in Product Identification Guide, page 405

ACTIFED® Tablets
[ăk 'tuh-fĕd]

Product Benefits: Each ACTIFED Tablet contains two maximum strength ingredients for temporary relief from symptoms of the common cold, seasonal allergies (hay fever) and sinus congestion.

The **ANTIHISTAMINE** (triprolidine) temporarily dries runny nose and relieves sneezing associated with the common cold, hay fever or other upper respiratory allergies. Also relieves itching of the nose or throat, and itchy, watery eyes due to hay fever.

The **DECONGESTANT** (pseudoephedrine) temporarily relieves nasal congestion due to the common cold, hay fever or other upper respiratory allergies, or associated with sinusitis. Temporarily relieves nasal stuffiness. Reduces the swelling of nasal passages; shrinks swollen membranes; and temporarily restores freer breathing through the nose. Also, helps to decongest sinus openings and passages; relieves sinus pressure.

Each Actifed Tablet Contains: pseudoephedrine hydrochloride 60 mg and triprolidine hydrochloride 2.5 mg. Also contains: flavor, hydroxypropyl methylcellulose, lactose, magnesium stearate, polyethylene glycol, potato starch, povidone, sucrose, and titanium dioxide.

Directions: Adults and children 12 years of age and over, 1 tablet every 4 to 6 hours. Children 6 to under 12 years of age, ½ tablet every 4 to 6 hours. Do not exceed 4 doses in 24 hours. Children under 6 years of age, consult a doctor.

Warnings: May cause drowsiness; alcohol, sedatives, and tranquilizers may increase the drowsiness effect. Avoid alcoholic beverages while taking this product. Do not take this product if you are taking sedatives or tranquilizers, without first consulting your doctor. Use caution when driving a motor vehicle or operating machinery. May cause excitability, especially in children. Do not exceed recommended dosage because at higher doses nervousness, dizziness or sleeplessness may occur. If symptoms do not improve within 7 days or are accompanied by high fever, consult a doctor before continuing use. Do not take this product, unless directed by a doctor, if you have high blood pressure, heart disease, diabetes, thyroid disease, glaucoma, a breathing problem such as emphysema or chronic bronchitis, or difficulty in urination due to enlargement of the prostate gland. As with any drug, if you are pregnant or nursing a baby, seek the advice of a health professional before using this product.

Drug Interaction Precaution: Do not take this product if you are presently taking a prescription antihypertensive or antidepressant drug containing a monoamine oxidase inhibitor except under the advice and supervision of a doctor.

KEEP THIS AND ALL DRUGS OUT OF THE REACH OF CHILDREN. In case of accidental overdose, seek professional assistance or contact a Poison Control Center immediately.

Store at 15° to 25°C (59° to 77°F) in a dry place and protect from light.

How Supplied: Boxes of 12, 24, 48 and bottles of 100 and 1000; unit dose pack box of 100.   402304

Shown in Product Identification Guide, page 405

ACTIFED® PLUS Tablets
[ăk 'tuh-fĕd]

Product Benefits: Each ACTIFED PLUS Coated Tablet contains three maximum strength ingredients for temporary relief from symptoms of the common cold, seasonal allergies (hay fever) and sinus congestion.

The **ANTIHISTAMINE** (triprolidine) temporarily dries runny nose and relieves sneezing associated with the common cold, hay fever or other upper respiratory allergies. Also relieves itching of the nose or throat, and itchy, watery eyes due to hay fever.

The **DECONGESTANT** (pseudoephedrine) temporarily relieves nasal congestion due to the common cold, hay fever or other upper respiratory allergies, or associated with sinusitis. Temporarily relieves nasal stuffiness. Reduces the swelling of nasal passages; shrinks swollen membranes; and temporarily restores freer breathing through the nose. Also, helps to decongest sinus openings and passages; relieves sinus pressure.

The non-aspirin **ANALGESIC** (acetaminophen) temporarily relieves occasional minor aches, pains and headache, and reduces fever due to the common cold.

Each ACTIFED PLUS Coated Tablet Contains: acetaminophen 500 mg, pseudoephedrine hydrochloride 30 mg and triprolidine hydrochloride 1.25 mg. Also

contains: carnauba wax, crospovidone, FD&C Blue No. 1 Lake, D&C Yellow No. 10 Lake, hydroxypropyl methylcellulose, magnesium stearate, microcrystalline cellulose, polyethylene glycol, polysorbate 80, povidone, pregelatinized corn starch, stearic acid, and titanium dioxide.

Directions: Adults and children 12 years of age and over, 2 tablets every 6 hours. Do not exceed 8 tablets in 24 hours. Not recommended for children under 12 years of age.

Warnings: May cause drowsiness: alcohol, sedatives, and tranquilizers may increase the drowsiness effect. Avoid alcoholic beverages while taking this product. Do not take this product if you are taking sedatives or tranquilizers, without first consulting your doctor. Use caution when driving a motor vehicle or operating machinery. May cause excitability, especially in children. Do not exceed recommended dosage because at higher doses nervousness, dizziness, or sleeplessness may occur. Do not take this product for more than 7 days. If symptoms do not improve, or are accompanied by fever that lasts for more than 3 days, or if new symptoms occur, consult a doctor. Do not take this product, unless directed by a doctor, if you have high blood pressure, heart disease, diabetes, thyroid disease, glaucoma, a breathing problem such as emphysema or chronic bronchitis, or difficulty in urination due to enlargement of the prostate gland. As with any drug, if you are pregnant or nursing a baby, seek the advice of a health professional before using this product.

Drug Interaction Precaution: Do not take this product if you are presently taking a prescription antihypertensive or antidepressant drug containing a monoamine oxidase inhibitor except under the advice and supervision of a doctor.

KEEP THIS AND ALL DRUGS OUT OF THE REACH OF CHILDREN. In case of accidental overdose, seek professional assistance or contact a Poison Control Center immediately. Prompt medical attention is critical for adults as well as for children even if you do not notice any signs or symptoms.

Store at 15° to 25°C (59° to 77°F) in a dry place and protect from light.

How Supplied: Boxes of 20, 40.
      402717

BOROFAX® Skin Protectant
[bôr 'uh-făks]

Indications: Helps treat and prevent diaper rash. Protects chafed skin due to diaper rash and helps seal out wetness.

Directions: Change wet and soiled diapers promptly, cleanse the diaper area, and allow to dry. Apply ointment liberally as often as necessary, with each diaper change, especially at bedtime or anytime when exposure to wet diapers may be prolonged.

Warnings: For external use only. Avoid contact with the eyes. If condition worsens or does not improve within 7 days, consult a doctor. Keep this and all drugs out of the reach of children. In case of accidental ingestion, seek professional assistance or contact a Poison Control Center immediately.

Active Ingredients: Zinc oxide 15% and white petrolatum 68.6%.
Also contains: Lanolin, mineral oil, and fragrance.
Store at 15° to 25°C (59° to 77°F).

How Supplied: Tube, 1.8 oz (50 g)
433191
Shown in Product Identification Guide, page 406

EMPIRIN® ASPIRIN
[ĕm 'puh-rŭn]

For relief of headache, minor muscular aches and pains, toothache, discomfort and fever of colds and flu, pain of the premenstrual and menstrual periods, and temporary relief of minor arthritis pain (see CAUTION below).

Directions: Adults: 1 or 2 tablets with a full glass of water. Repeat every 4 hours as needed, up to 12 tablets a day. **Children:** Consult a physician (see WARNINGS).

Caution: In arthritic conditions, if pain persists for more than 10 days or redness is present, consult a physician immediately.

Warnings: Children and teenagers should not use this medicine for chicken pox or flu symptoms before a doctor is consulted about Reye syndrome, a rare but serious illness reported to be associated with aspirin. Keep this and all medicines out of children's reach. In case of accidental overdose, contact a physician immediately.
High or continued fever, severe or persistent sore throat especially when accompanied by high fever, headache, nausea or vomiting, may be serious. Consult your physician. Do not exceed dose unless directed by a physician. Do not take this product if you are allergic to aspirin, have asthma, a gastric ulcer or its symptoms, or are taking a medication that affects the clotting of blood, except under the advice of a physician. As with any drug, if you are pregnant or nursing a baby, seek the advice of a health professional before using this product.
IT IS ESPECIALLY IMPORTANT NOT TO USE ASPIRIN DURING THE LAST 3 MONTHS OF PREGNANCY UNLESS SPECIFICALLY DIRECTED TO DO SO BY A DOCTOR BECAUSE IT MAY CAUSE PROBLEMS IN THE UNBORN CHILD OR COMPLICATIONS DURING DELIVERY.

Active Ingredients: Each tablet contains aspirin 325 mg (5 gr).

Inactive Ingredients: microcrystalline cellulose and potato starch.
Store at 15° to 25°C (59° to 77°F) in a dry place.

How Supplied: Bottles of 50, 100.
488151
Shown in Product Identification Guide, page 406

NEOSPORIN® Ointment
[nē 'uh-spō 'rŭn]

Indications: First aid to help prevent infection in minor cuts, scrapes, and burns.

Directions: Clean the affected area. Apply a small amount of this product (an amount equal to the surface area of the tip of a finger) on the area 1 to 3 times daily. May be covered with a sterile bandage.

Warnings: For external use only. Stop use and consult a physician if the condition persists or gets worse, or if a rash or other allergic reaction develops. Do not use this product if you are allergic to any of the listed ingredients. Do not use in the eyes or apply over large areas of the body. In case of deep or puncture wounds, animal bites, or serious burns, consult a physician. Do not use longer than 1 week unless directed by a physician. Keep this and all drugs out of the reach of children. In case of accidental ingestion, seek professional assistance or contact a Poison Control Center immediately.

Each Gram Contains: polymyxin B sulfate 5,000 units, bacitracin zinc 400 units and neomycin 3.5 mg in a special white petrolatum base.
Store at 15° to 25°C (59° to 77°F).

How Supplied: Tubes, ½ oz (14.2 g) (with applicator tip), 1 oz (28.4 g); 1/32 oz (0.9 g) (approx.) foil packets packed 144 per carton.

Professional Labeling: Consult *1994 Physicians' Desk Reference®.* 561595
Shown in Product Identification Guide, page 406

NEOSPORIN® PLUS MAXIMUM STRENGTH Cream
[nē "uh-spō 'rŭn]

Indications: First aid to help prevent infection and provide temporary relief of pain or discomfort in minor cuts, scrapes, and burns.

Directions: Adults and children 2 years of age and older: Clean the affected area. Apply a small amount of this product (an amount equal to the surface area of the tip of a finger) on the area 1 to 3 times daily. May be covered with a sterile bandage. **Children under 2 years of age: Consult a physician.**

Warnings: For external use only. If condition worsens, or if symptoms persist for more than 1 week or clear up and oc-

cur again within a few days, or if a rash or other allergic reaction develops, discontinue use of this product and consult a physician. Do not use this product if you are allergic to any of the listed ingredients. Do not use in the eyes or apply over large areas of the body. Do not use in large quantities, particularly over raw surfaces or blistered areas. In case of deep or puncture wounds, animal bites, or serious burns, consult a physician. Do not use longer than 1 week unless directed by a physician. Keep this and all drugs out of the reach of children. In case of accidental ingestion, seek professional assistance or contact a Poison Control Center immediately.

Each Gram Contains: polymyxin B sulfate 10,000 units, neomycin 3.5 mg, and lidocaine 40 mg. Also contains: methylparaben 0.25% (added as a preservative), emulsifying wax, mineral oil, poloxamer 188, propylene glycol, purified water, and white petrolatum.
Store at 15° to 25°C (59° to 77°F).

How Supplied: ½ oz (14.2 g) tubes.
561208
Shown in Product Identification Guide, page 406

NEOSPORIN® PLUS MAXIMUM STRENGTH Ointment
[nē "uh-spō 'rŭn]

Indications: First aid to help prevent infection and provide temporary relief of pain or discomfort in minor cuts, scrapes, and burns.

Directions: Adults and children 2 years of age and older: Clean the affected area. Apply a small amount of this product (an amount equal to the surface area of the tip of a finger) on the area 1 to 3 times daily. May be covered with a sterile bandage. **Children under 2 years of age: Consult a physician.**

Warnings: For external use only. If condition worsens, or if symptoms persist for more than 1 week or clear up and occur again within a few days, or if a rash or other allergic reaction develops, discontinue use of this product and consult a physician. Do not use this product if you are allergic to any of the listed ingredients. Do not use in the eyes or apply over large areas of the body. Do not use in large quantities, particularly over raw surfaces or blistered areas. In case of deep or puncture wounds, animal bites, or serious burns, consult a physician. Do not use longer than 1 week unless directed by a physician. Keep this and all drugs out of the reach of children. In case of accidental ingestion, seek professional assistance or contact a Poison Control Center immediately.

Each Gram Contains: polymyxin B sulfate 10,000 units, bacitracin zinc 500 units, neomycin 3.5 mg, and lidocaine 40 mg in a special white petrolatum base.

Continued on next page

Burroughs Wellcome—Cont.

Store at 15° to 25°C (59° to 77°F).

How Supplied: ½ oz (14.2 g) and 1 oz (28.4 g) tubes.

561204

Shown in Product Identification Guide, page 406

NIX®
Permethrin
Lice Treatment

Product Benefits: Nix Creme Rinse kills lice and their unhatched eggs with only one application. Nix protects against head lice reinfestation for a full 14 days. The unique creme rinse formula leaves hair manageable and easy to comb.

Indications: For the treatment of head lice.

Directions for Use: Nix Creme Rinse should be used after hair has been washed with your regular shampoo, rinsed with water and towel dried. A sufficient amount should be applied to saturate hair and scalp (especially behind the ears and on nape of the neck). Leave on hair for 10 minutes but no longer. Rinse with water. A single application is sufficient. Retreatment is required in less than 1% of patients. If live lice are observed seven days or more after the first application of this product, a second treatment should be given. For proper head lice management, remove nits with the nit comb provided.

Head lice live on the scalp and lay small white eggs (nits) on the hair shaft close to the scalp. The nits are most easily found on the nape of the neck or behind the ears. All personal headgear, scarfs, coats, and bed linen should be disinfected by machine washing in hot water and drying, using the hot cycle of a dryer for at least 20 minutes. Personal articles of clothing or bedding that cannot be washed may be dry-cleaned, sealed in a plastic bag for a period of about 2 weeks, or sprayed with a product specifically designed for this purpose. Personal combs and brushes may be disinfected by soaking in hot water (above 130°F) for 5 to 10 minutes. Thorough vacuuming of rooms inhabited by infected patients is recommended.

Warnings: For external use only. Itching, redness, or swelling of the scalp may occur. If skin irritation persists or infection is present or develops, discontinue use and consult a doctor. Do not use near the eyes or permit contact with mucous membranes. If product gets into the eyes, immediately flush with water. Consult a doctor if infestation of eyebrows or eyelashes occurs. This product may cause breathing difficulty or an asthmatic episode in susceptible persons. This product should not be used on children less than 2 months of age. As with any drug, if you are pregnant or nursing a baby, seek the advice of a health professional before using this product. Keep this and all drugs out of the reach of children. In case of accidental ingestion, seek professional assistance or contact a Poison Control Center immediately.

Each Fluid Ounce Contains: permethrin 280 mg (1%). Inactive ingredients are: balsam canada, cetyl alcohol, citric acid, FD&C Yellow No. 6, fragrance, hydrolyzed animal protein, hydroxyethylcellulose, polyoxyethylene 10 cetyl ether, propylene glycol, and stearalkonium chloride. Also contains: isopropyl alcohol 5.6 g (20%) and added as preservatives, methylparaben 56 mg (0.2%) and propylparaben 22 mg (0.08%). Store at 15° to 25°C (59° to 77°F).

How Supplied: Bottles of 2 fl oz (50 mL) with special comb and Family Pack of 2 bottles, 2 fl oz (50 mL) each, with special comb.

585095

Shown in Product Identification Guide, page 406

POLYSPORIN® Ointment
[pŏl 'ē-spō 'rŭn]

Indications: First aid to help prevent infection in minor cuts, scrapes, and burns.

Directions: Clean the affected area. Apply a small amount of this product (an amount equal to the surface area of the tip of a finger) on the area 1 to 3 times daily. May be covered with a sterile bandage.

Warnings: For external use only. Stop use and consult a physician if the condition persists or gets worse, or if a rash or other allergic reaction develops. Do not use this product if you are allergic to any of the listed ingredients. Do not use in the eyes or apply over large areas of the body. In case of deep or puncture wounds, animal bites, or serious burns, consult a physician. Do not use longer than 1 week unless directed by a physician. Keep this and all drugs out of the reach of children. In case of accidental ingestion, seek professional assistance or contact a Poison Control Center immediately.

Each Gram Contains: polymyxin B sulfate 10,000 units and bacitracin zinc 500 units in a special white petrolatum base. Store at 15° to 25°C (59° to 77°F).

How Supplied: Tubes, ½ oz (14.2 g) with applicator tip, 1 oz (28.4 g); ¹⁄₃₂ oz (0.9 g) (approx.) foil packets packed in cartons of 144.

576087

Shown in Product Identification Guide, page 406

POLYSPORIN® Powder
[pŏl 'ē-spō 'rŭn]

Indications: First aid to help prevent infection in minor cuts, scrapes, and burns.

Directions: Clean the affected area. Apply a light dusting of the powder on the area 1 to 3 times daily. May be covered with a sterile bandage.

Warnings: For external use only. Stop use and consult a physician if the condition persists or gets worse, or if a rash or other allergic reaction develops. Do not use this product if you are allergic to any of the listed ingredients. Do not use in the eyes or apply over large areas of the body. In case of deep or puncture wounds, animal bites, or serious burns, consult a physician. Do not use longer than 1 week unless directed by a physician. Keep this and all drugs out of the reach of children. In case of accidental ingestion, seek professional assistance or contact a Poison Control Center immediately.

Each Gram Contains: polymyxin B sulfate 10,000 units and bacitracin zinc 500 units in a lactose base. Store at 15° to 25°C (59° to 77°F). Do not store under refrigeration.

How Supplied: 0.35 oz (10 g) shaker-vial. 575975

Shown in Product Identification Guide, page 406

Children's
SUDAFED® Liquid
[sū 'duh-fěd]

Each 5 mL (1 teaspoonful) contains pseudoephedrine hydrochloride 30 mg. Also contains: methylparaben 0.1% and sodium benzoate 0.1% (added as preservatives), citric acid, FD&C Red No. 40, flavor, glycerin, purified water, sorbitol and sucrose.

Indications: For temporary relief of nasal congestion due to the common cold, hay fever or other upper respiratory allergies and nasal congestion associated with sinusitis; promotes nasal and/or sinus drainage.

Directions: To be given every 4 to 6 hours. Do not exceed 4 doses in 24 hours. Children 6 to under 12 years of age, 1 teaspoonful. Children 2 to under 6 years of age, ½ teaspoonful. For children under 2 years of age, consult a physician.

Warnings: Do not exceed recommended dosage because at higher doses nervousness, dizziness or sleeplessness may occur. Do not give this product to children for more than 7 days. If symptoms do not improve or are accompanied by high fever, consult a physician. Do not give this product to children who have heart disease, high blood pressure, thyroid disease, or diabetes unless directed by a physician.

Drug Interaction Precaution: Do not give this product to a child who is taking a prescription drug for high blood pressure or depression, without first consulting the child's physician.

KEEP THIS AND ALL MEDICINES OUT OF CHILDREN'S REACH. In case of accidental overdose, seek professional assistance or contact a Poison Control Center immediately.

Store at 15° to 25°C (59° to 77°F) and protect from light.

How Supplied: Bottles of 4 fl oz. (118 mL)

605225

Shown in Product Identification Guide, page 406

SUDAFED® COLD AND COUGH LIQUIDCAPS
[sū duh 'fĕd]

Indications: The COUGH SUPPRESSANT (dextromethorphan) temporarily relieves cough due to the common cold. The DECONGESTANT (pseudoephedrine) temporarily relieves stuffy nose and sinus congestion due to the common cold. The non-aspirin PAIN RELIEVER/FEVER REDUCER (acetaminophen) temporarily relieves minor sore throat pain, headache, fever, and body aches due to the common cold or flu. The EXPECTORANT (guaifenesin) helps loosen phlegm (mucus) to drain bronchial tubes and make coughs more productive.

Directions: Adults and children 12 years of age and over, 2 liquid caps every 4 hours, not to exceed 8 liquid caps in 24 hours. Not recommended for children under 12 years of age.

Each Liquid Cap Contains: acetaminophen 250 mg, dextromethorphan hydrobromide 10 mg, guaifenesin 100 mg, and pseudoephedrine hydrochloride 30 mg. Also contains D&C Yellow No. 10, FD&C Red No. 40, gelatin, glycerin, polyethylene glycol, povidone, propylene glycol, purified water, and sorbitol.

Warnings: Do not exceed recommended dosage because at higher doses nervousness, dizziness, or sleeplessness may occur. Do not take this product for more than 7 days. A persistent cough may be a sign of a serious condition. If cough or other symptoms persist for more than 7 days, tend to recur, or are accompanied by rash, persistent headache, fever that lasts for more than 3 days, or if new symptoms occur, consult a physician. Do not take this product for persistent or chronic cough such as occurs with smoking, asthma, chronic bronchitis, emphysema, or where cough is accompanied by excessive phlegm (mucus) unless directed by a physician. If sore throat is severe, persists for more than 2 days, is accompanied or followed by fever, headache, rash, nausea, or vomiting, consult a physician promptly. Do not take this product if you have high blood pressure, heart disease, diabetes, thyroid disease, or difficulty in urination due to enlargement of the prostate gland except under the advice and supervision of a physician. As with any drug, if you are pregnant or nursing a baby, seek the advice of a health professional before using this product.

Drug Interaction Precaution: Do not take this product if you are presently taking a prescription antihypertensive or antidepressant drug containing a monoamine oxidase inhibitor except under the advice and supervision of a physician.

KEEP THIS AND ALL DRUGS OUT OF THE REACH OF CHILDREN. In case of accidental overdose, seek professional assistance or contact a Poison Control Center immediately. Prompt medical attention is critical for adults as well as children even if you do not notice any signs or symptoms.

Store at 15° to 25°C (59° to 77°F) in a dry place and protect from light.

How Supplied: Box of 10 and 20.

Shown in Product Identification Guide, page 406

SUDAFED® Cough Syrup
[sū 'duh-fĕd]

Each 5 mL (1 teaspoonful) contains pseudoephedrine hydrochloride 15 mg, dextromethorphan hydrobromide 5 mg and guaifenesin 100 mg. Also contains: alcohol 2.4%, methylparaben 0.1% and sodium benzoate 0.1% (added as preservatives), citric acid, D&C Yellow No. 10, FD&C Blue No. 1, flavor, glycerin, purified water, sodium chloride and sucrose.

Indications: For temporary relief of cough due to minor throat and bronchial irritation as may occur with the common cold or inhaled irritants. For temporary relief of nasal congestion due to the common cold. Helps loosen phlegm (mucus) and thin bronchial secretions to rid the bronchial passageways of bothersome mucus.

Directions: To be given every 4 hours. Do not exceed 4 doses in 24 hours. Adults and children 12 years of age and over, 4 teaspoonfuls. Children 6 to under 12 years of age, 2 teaspoonfuls. Children 2 to under 6 years of age, 1 teaspoonful. For children under 2 years of age, consult a physician.

Warnings: Do not give this product to children under 2 years of age unless directed by a physician. Do not exceed recommended dosage because at higher doses nervousness, dizziness or sleeplessness may occur. Do not take this product for persistent or chronic cough such as occurs with smoking, asthma, chronic bronchitis, or emphysema, or where cough is accompanied by excessive phlegm (mucus) unless directed by a physician. A persistent cough may be a sign of a serious condition. If cough persists for more than 1 week, tends to recur, or is accompanied by fever, rash, or persistent headache, consult a physician. Do not take this preparation if you have high blood pressure, heart disease, diabetes, thyroid disease, or difficulty in urination due to enlargement of the prostate gland, except under the advice and supervision of a physician. As with any drug, if you are pregnant or nursing a baby, seek the advice of a health professional before using this product.

Drug Interaction Precaution: Do not take this product if you are presently taking a prescription antihypertensive or antidepressant drug containing a monoamine oxidase inhibitor except under the advice and supervision of a physician.

KEEP THIS AND ALL DRUGS OUT OF THE REACH OF CHILDREN. In case of accidental overdose, seek professional assistance or contact a Poison Control Center immediately.

Store at 15° to 25°C (59° to 77°F).
DO NOT REFRIGERATE.

How Supplied: Bottles of 4 fl oz (118 mL).

604043

Shown in Product Identification Guide, page 406

SUDAFED® Tablets 30 mg
[sū 'duh-fĕd]

Each tablet contains pseudoephedrine hydrochloride 30 mg. Also contains: acacia, carnauba wax, dibasic calcium phosphate, FD&C Red No. 40 Lake and Yellow No. 6 Lake, magnesium stearate, pharmaceutical glaze, polysorbate 60, potato starch, povidone, sodium benzoate, stearic acid, talc, and titanium dioxide. Printed with edible black ink.

Indications: For temporary relief of nasal congestion due to the common cold, hay fever or other upper respiratory allergies, and nasal congestion associated with sinusitis; promotes nasal and/or sinus drainage.

Directions: To be given every 4 to 6 hours. Do not exceed 4 doses in 24 hours. Adults and children 12 years of age and over, 2 tablets. Children 6 to under 12 years of age, 1 tablet. Children 2 to under 6 years of age, use Children's Sudafed Liquid. For children under 2 years of age, consult a physician.

Warnings: Do not exceed recommended dosage because at higher doses nervousness, dizziness or sleeplessness may occur. If symptoms do not improve within 7 days, or are accompanied by a high fever, consult a physician before continuing use. Do not take this preparation if you have high blood pressure, heart disease, diabetes, thyroid disease, or difficulty in urination due to enlargement of the prostate gland, except under the advice and supervision of a physician. As with any drug, if you are pregnant or nursing a baby, seek the advice of a health professional before using this product.

Drug Interaction Precaution: Do not take this product if you are presently taking a prescription antihypertensive or antidepressant drug containing a monoamine oxidase inhibitor, except under the advice and supervision of a physician.

Continued on next page

Burroughs Wellcome—Cont.

KEEP THIS AND ALL MEDICINES OUT OF CHILDREN'S REACH. In case of accidental overdose, seek professional assistance or contact a Poison Control Center immediately.

Store at 15° to 25°C (59° to 77°F) in a dry place and protect from light.

How Supplied: Boxes of 24, 48. Bottles of 100. Institutional Pack, Carton of 500 x 2. 604270

Shown in Product Identification Guide, page 406

SUDAFED® Tablets 60 mg (Adult Strength)
[sū 'duh-fĕd]

Each tablet contains pseudoephedrine hydrochloride 60 mg. Also contains: acacia, carnauba wax, corn starch, dibasic calcium phosphate, hydroxypropyl methylcellulose, magnesium stearate, pharmaceutical glaze, polysorbate 60, sodium starch glycolate, stearic acid, sucrose, talc, and titanium dioxide. Printed with edible red ink.

Indications: For temporary relief of nasal congestion due to the common cold, hay fever or other upper respiratory allergies, and nasal congestion associated with sinusitis; promotes nasal and/or sinus drainage.

Directions: To be given every 4 to 6 hours. Do not exceed 4 doses in 24 hours. Adults and children 12 years of age and over, 1 tablet. Children 6 to under 12 years of age, use Sudafed 30 mg Tablets. Children 2 to under 6 years of age, use Children's Sudafed Liquid. For children under 2 years of age, consult a physician.

Warnings: Do not exceed recommended dosage because at higher doses nervousness, dizziness or sleeplessness may occur. If symptoms do not improve within 7 days, or are accompanied by a high fever, consult a physician before continuing use. Do not take this preparation if you have high blood pressure, heart disease, diabetes, thyroid disease, or difficulty in urination due to enlargement of the prostate gland, except under the advice and supervision of a physician. As with any drug, if you are pregnant or nursing a baby, seek the advice of a health professional before using this product.

Drug Interaction Precaution: Do not take this product if you are presently taking a prescription antihypertensive or antidepressant drug containing a monoamine oxidase inhibitor, except under the advice and supervision of a physician.

KEEP THIS AND ALL MEDICINES OUT OF CHILDREN'S REACH. In case of accidental overdose, seek professional assistance or contact a Poison Control Center immediately.

Store at 15° to 25°C (59° to 77°F) in a dry place and protect from light.

How Supplied: Bottles of 100. 605656

Shown in Product Identification Guide, page 406

SUDAFED PLUS® Liquid
[sū 'duh-fĕd]

Product Benefits: For the temporary relief of nasal or sinus congestion, sneezing, runny nose, and itchy, watery eyes associated with the common cold, hay fever, or other upper respiratory allergies.

EACH 5 mL (1 TEASPOONFUL) SUDAFED PLUS LIQUID CONTAINS: pseudoephedrine hydrochloride 30 mg and chlorpheniramine maleate 2 mg. Also contains: methylparaben 0.1% and sodium benzoate 0.1% (added as preservatives), citric acid, D&C Yellow No. 10, FD&C Yellow No. 6, flavor, glycerin, purified water and sucrose.

Directions: Adults and children 12 years and over, 2 teaspoonfuls every 4 to 6 hours. Children 6 to under 12 years, 1 teaspoonful every 4 to 6 hours. Do not exceed 4 doses in 24 hours. Children under 6, consult a doctor.

Warnings: May cause drowsiness; alcohol, sedatives, and tranquilizers may increase the drowsiness effect. Avoid alcoholic beverages while taking this product. Do not take this product if you are taking sedatives or tranquilizers, without first consulting your doctor. Use caution when driving a motor vehicle or operating machinery. May cause excitability, especially in children. Do not exceed recommended dosage because at higher doses nervousness, dizziness or sleeplessness may occur. If symptoms do not improve within 7 days, or are accompanied by a high fever, consult a doctor before continuing use. Do not take this product, unless directed by a doctor, if you have high blood pressure, heart disease, diabetes, thyroid disease, glaucoma, a breathing problem such as emphysema or chronic bronchitis, or difficulty in urination due to enlargement of the prostate gland. As with any drug, if you are pregnant or nursing a baby, seek the advice of a health professional before using this product.

Drug Interaction Precaution: Do not take this product if you are presently taking a prescription antihypertensive or antidepressant drug containing a monoamine oxidase inhibitor except under the advice and supervision of a doctor.

KEEP THIS AND ALL DRUGS OUT OF THE REACH OF CHILDREN. In case of accidental overdose, seek professional assistance or contact a Poison Control Center immediately.

Store at 15° to 25°C (59° to 77°F) and protect from light.

Store at 15° to 25°C (59° to 77°F) in a dry place and protect from light.

How Supplied: Bottles of 4 fl oz (118 mL). 605290

Shown in Product Identification Guide, page 406

SUDAFED PLUS® Tablets
[sū 'duh-fĕd]

Product Benefits: For the temporary relief of nasal or sinus congestion, sneezing, runny nose, and itchy, watery eyes associated with the common cold, hay fever, or other upper respiratory allergies.

EACH SUDAFED PLUS TABLET CONTAINS: pseudoephedrine hydrochloride 60 mg and chlorpheniramine maleate 4 mg. Also contains: lactose, magnesium stearate, potato starch and povidone.

Directions: Adults and children 12 years and over, 1 tablet every 4 to 6 hours. Children 6 to under 12 years, ½ tablet every 4 to 6 hours. Do not exceed 4 doses in 24 hours. Children under 6, consult a doctor.

Warnings: May cause drowsiness; alcohol, sedatives, and tranquilizers may increase the drowsiness effect. Avoid alcoholic beverages while taking this product. Do not take this product if you are taking sedatives or tranquilizers, without first consulting your doctor. Use caution when driving a motor vehicle or operating machinery. May cause excitability, especially in children. Do not exceed recommended dosage because at higher doses nervousness, dizziness or sleeplessness may occur. If symptoms do not improve within 7 days, or are accompanied by a high fever, consult a doctor before continuing use. Do not take this product, unless directed by a doctor, if you have high blood pressure, heart disease, diabetes, thyroid disease, glaucoma, a breathing problem such as emphysema or chronic bronchitis, or difficulty in urination due to enlargement of the prostate gland. As with any drug, if you are pregnant or nursing a baby, seek the advice of a health professional before using this product.

Drug Interaction Precaution: Do not take this product if you are presently taking a prescription antihypertensive or antidepressant drug containing a monoamine oxidase inhibitor except under the advice and supervision of a physician.

KEEP THIS AND ALL DRUGS OUT OF THE REACH OF CHILDREN. In case of accidental overdose, seek professional assistance or contact a Poison Control Center immediately.

Store at 15° to 25°C (59° to 77°F) in a dry place and protect from light.

How Supplied: Boxes of 24, 48. 605390

Shown in Product Identification Guide, page 406

SUDAFED® Severe Cold Formula Caplets
[sū' duh-fĕd]

Product Benefits: Maximum allowable levels of nasal decongestant, cough suppressant, and non-aspirin pain reliever/fever reducer provide temporary relief from symptoms of the common cold and flu. This product contains no ingredients that may cause drowsiness. The **DECONGESTANT** (pseudoephedrine) temporarily relieves nasal and sinus congestion due to the common cold. It temporarily relieves nasal stuffiness; reduces the swelling of nasal passages; shrinks swollen membranes; and temporarily restores freer breathing through the nose. The **COUGH SUPPRESSANT** (dextromethorphan) temporarily relieves cough due to the common cold. The non-aspirin **PAIN RELIEVER/FEVER REDUCER** (acetaminophen) temporarily relieves headache, body aches and pains, minor sore throat pain, and reduces fever due to the common cold.

Directions: Adults and children 12 years of age and over, 2 caplets every 6 hours, not to exceed 8 caplets in 24 hours. Not recommended for children under 12 years of age.

Each Coated Caplet Contains: acetaminophen 500 mg, dextromethorphan hydrobromide 15 mg, and pseudoephedrine hydrochloride 30 mg. Also contains: carnauba wax, crospovidone, hydroxypropyl methylcellulose, magnesium stearate, microcrystalline cellulose, polyethylene glycol, povidone, pregelatinized corn starch, stearic acid, and titanium dioxide.

Warnings: Do not exceed recommended dosage because at higher doses nervousness, dizziness or sleeplessness may occur. Do not take this product for more than 10 days. A persistent cough may be a sign of a serious condition. If cough persists for more than 7 days, tends to recur, or is accompanied by rash, persistent headache, fever that lasts for more than 3 days, or if new symptoms occur, consult a physician. Do not take this product for persistent or chronic cough such as occurs with smoking, asthma, emphysema, or if cough is accompanied by excessive phlegm (mucus) unless directed by a physician. If sore throat is severe, persists for more than 2 days, is accompanied or followed by fever, headache, rash, nausea, or vomiting, consult a physician promptly. Do not take this product if you have high blood pressure, heart disease, diabetes, thyroid disease, or difficulty in urination due to enlargement of the prostate gland except under the advice and supervision of a physician. As with any drug, if you are pregnant or nursing a baby, seek the advice of a health professional before using this product.

Drug Interaction Precaution: Do not take this product if you are presently taking a prescription antihypertensive or antidepressant drug containing a monoamine oxidase inhibitor except under the advice and supervision of a physician.

KEEP THIS AND ALL DRUGS OUT OF THE REACH OF CHILDREN. In case of accidental overdose, seek professional assistance or contact a Poison Control Center immediately. Prompt medical attention is critical for adults as well as for children even if you do not notice any signs or symptoms.

Store at 15° to 25°C (59° to 77°F) in a dry place.

How Supplied: Boxes of 10, 20.

604119

Shown in Product Identification Guide, page 406

SUDAFED® Severe Cold Formula Tablets
[sū' duh-fĕd]

Product Benefits: Maximum allowable levels of nasal decongestant, cough suppressant, and non-aspirin pain reliever/fever reducer provide temporary relief from symptoms of the common cold and flu. This product contains no ingredients that may cause drowsiness. The **DECONGESTANT** (pseudoephedrine) temporarily relieves nasal and sinus congestion due to the common cold. It temporarily relieves nasal stuffiness; reduces the swelling of nasal passages; shrinks swollen membranes; and temporarily restores freer breathing through the nose. The **COUGH SUPPRESSANT** (dextromethorphan) temporarily relieves cough due to the common cold. The non-aspirin **PAIN RELIEVER/FEVER REDUCER** (acetaminophen) temporarily relieves headache, body aches and pains, minor sore throat pain, and reduces fever due to the common cold.

Directions: Adults and children 12 years of age and over, 2 tablets every 6 hours, not to exceed 8 tablets in 24 hours. Not recommended for children under 12 years of age.

Each Coated Tablet Contains: acetaminophen 500 mg, dextromethorphan hydrobromide 15 mg, and pseudoephedrine hydrochloride 30 mg. Also contains: carnauba wax, crospovidone, hydroxypropyl methylcellulose, magnesium stearate, microcrystalline cellulose, polyethylene glycol, povidone, pregelatinized corn starch, stearic acid, and titanium dioxide.

Warnings: Do not exceed recommended dosage because at higher doses nervousness, dizziness or sleeplessness may occur. Do not take this product for more than 10 days. A persistent cough may be a sign of a serious condition. If cough persists for more than 7 days, tends to recur, or is accompanied by rash, persistent headache, fever that lasts for more than 3 days, or if new symptoms occur, consult a physician. Do not take this product for persistent or chronic cough such as occurs with smoking, asthma, emphysema, or if cough is accompanied by excessive phlegm (mucus) unless directed by a physician. If sore throat is severe, persists for more than 2 days, is accompanied or followed by fever, headache, rash, nausea, or vomiting, consult a physician promptly. Do not take this product if you have high blood pressure, heart disease, diabetes, thyroid disease, or difficulty in urination due to enlargement of the prostate gland except under the advice and supervision of a physician. As with any drug, if you are pregnant or nursing a baby, seek the advice of a health professional before using this product.

Drug Interaction Precaution: Do not take this product if you are presently taking a prescription antihypertensive or antidepressant drug containing a monoamine oxidase inhibitor except under the advice and supervision of a physician.

KEEP THIS AND ALL DRUGS OUT OF THE REACH OF CHILDREN. In case of accidental overdose, seek professional assistance or contact a Poison Control Center immediately. Prompt medical attention is critical for adults as well as for children even if you do not notice any signs or symptoms.

Store at 15° to 25°C (59° to 77°F) in a dry place.

How Supplied: Boxes of 10, 20.

604117

Shown in Product Identification Guide, page 406

SUDAFED® SINUS Caplets
[sū' duh-fĕd sī' nəs]

Product Benefits:
- Maximum allowable levels of non-aspirin pain reliever and nasal decongestant provide temporary relief of sinus headache pain, pressure and nasal congestion due to colds and flu or hay fever and other allergies.
- Contains no ingredients which may cause drowsiness.

Directions: Adults and children 12 years and over, 2 caplets every 6 hours, not to exceed 8 caplets in a 24-hour period. Not recommended for children under 12 years of age.

Each Coated Caplet Contains: acetaminophen 500 mg and pseudoephedrine hydrochloride 30 mg. Also contains: carnauba wax, crospovidone, FD&C Yellow No. 6 Lake, hydroxypropyl methylcellulose, magnesium stearate, microcrystalline cellulose, polyethylene glycol, polysorbate 80, povidone, pregelatinized corn starch, stearic acid, and titanium dioxide.

Warnings: Do not exceed recommended dosage because at higher doses nervousness, dizziness, or sleeplessness may occur. Do not take this product for more than 10 days. If symptoms do not improve or are accompanied by fever that lasts for more than 3 days, or if new symptoms occur, consult a physician. Do not take this product if you have high

Continued on next page

Burroughs Wellcome—Cont.

blood pressure, heart disease, diabetes, thyroid disease, or difficulty in urination due to enlargement of the prostate gland except under the advice and supervision of a physician. As with any drug, if you are pregnant or nursing a baby, seek the advice of a health professional before using this product.

Drug Interaction Precaution: Do not take this product if you are presently taking a prescription antihypertensive or antidepressant drug containing a monoamine oxidase inhibitor except under the advice and supervision of a physician.

KEEP THIS AND ALL DRUGS OUT OF THE REACH OF CHILDREN. In case of accidental overdose, seek professional assistance or contact a Poison Control Center immediately. Prompt medical attention is critical for adults as well as children even if you do not notice any signs or symptoms.

Store at 15° to 25°C (59° to 77°F) in a dry place and protect from light.

How Supplied: Boxes of 24 and 48.
605834

Shown in Product Identification Guide, page 406

SUDAFED® SINUS Tablets
[sū' duh-fĕd sī' nəs]

Product Benefits:

• Maximum allowable levels of non-aspirin pain reliever and nasal decongestant provide temporary relief of sinus headache pain, pressure and nasal congestion due to colds and flu or hay fever and other allergies.

• Contains no ingredients which may cause drowsiness.

Directions: Adults and children 12 years and over, 2 tablets every 6 hours, not to exceed 8 tablets in a 24-hour period. Not recommended for children under 12 years of age.

Each Coated Tablet Contains: Acetaminophen 500 mg and pseudoephedrine hydrochloride 30 mg. Also contains: carnauba wax, crospovidone, FD&C Yellow No. 6 Lake, hydroxypropyl methylcellulose, magnesium stearate, microcrystalline cellulose, polyethylene glycol, polysorbate 80, povidone, pregelatinized corn starch, stearic acid, and titanium dioxide.

Warnings: Do not exceed recommended dosage because at higher doses nervousness, dizziness, or sleeplessness may occur. Do not take this product for more than 10 days. If symptoms do not improve or are accompanied by fever that lasts for more than 3 days, or if new symptoms occur, consult a physician. Do not take this product if you have high blood pressure, heart disease, diabetes, thyroid disease, or difficulty in urination due to enlargement of the prostate gland

except under the advice and supervision of a physician. As with any drug, if you are pregnant or nursing a baby, seek the advice of a health professional before using this product.

Drug Interaction Precaution: Do not take this product if you are presently taking a prescription antihypertensive or antidepressant drug containing a monoamine oxidase inhibitor except under the advice and supervision of a physician.

KEEP THIS AND ALL DRUGS OUT OF THE REACH OF CHILDREN. In case of accidental overdose, seek professional assistance or contact a Poison Control Center immediately. Prompt medical attention is critical for adults as well as children even if you do not notice any signs or symptoms.

Store at 15° to 25°C (59° to 77°F) in a dry place and protect from light.

How Supplied: Boxes of 24 and 48.
605836

Shown in Product Identification Guide, page 406

SUDAFED® 12 Hour Caplets
[sū 'duh-fĕd]

Each coated extended-release caplet contains pseudoephedrine hydrochloride 120 mg in a capsule-shaped tablet. Also contains: hydroxypropyl methylcellulose, magnesium stearate, microcrystalline cellulose, polyethylene glycol, povidone, and titanium dioxide. Printed with edible blue ink.

Indications: For temporary relief of nasal congestion due to the common cold, hay fever, or other upper respiratory allergies, and nasal congestion associated with sinusitis; promotes nasal and/or sinus drainage.

Directions: Adults and children 12 years and over—One caplet every 12 hours, not to exceed two caplets in 24 hours. Sudafed 12 Hour is not recommended for children under 12 years of age.

Warnings: Do not exceed recommended dosage because at higher doses, nervousness, dizziness, or sleeplessness may occur. Do not take this product if you have heart disease, high blood pressure, thyroid disease, diabetes, or difficulty in urination due to enlargement of the prostate gland unless directed by a doctor. If symptoms do not improve within 7 days or are accompanied by fever, consult your doctor before continuing use. As with any drug, if you are pregnant or nursing a baby, seek the advice of a health professional before using this product.

Drug Interaction Precaution: Do not take this product if you are presently taking a prescription drug for high blood pressure or depression, without first consulting your doctor.

KEEP THIS AND ALL DRUGS OUT OF THE REACH OF CHILDREN. In case of accidental overdose, seek profes-

sional assistance or contact a Poison Control Center immediately.

Store at 15° to 25°C (59° to 77°F) in a dry place and protect from light.

How Supplied: Boxes of 10 and 20.
605571

Shown in Product Indentification Guide, page 406

Campbell Laboratories Inc.
300 EAST 51st STREET
P.O. BOX 812, FDR STATION
NEW YORK, NY 10150

HERPECIN–L® Cold Sore Lip Balm
[her "puh-sin-el "]

PRODUCT OVERVIEW

Key Facts: HERPECIN-L Lip Balm is a convenient, easy-to-use treatment for perioral herpes simplex infections. Sunscreens provide an SPF of 15.

Major Uses: HERPECIN-L not only treats cold sores, sun and fever blisters, but with prophylactic use, its sunscreens also protect to help prevent them. Users report early use at the prodromal stages of an attack will often abort the lesions and prevent scabbing. Prescribe: Apply "early, often and liberally."

Safety Information: For topical use only. A rare sensitivity may occur.

PRESCRIBING INFORMATION
HERPECIN–L® Cold Sore Lip Balm

Composition: A soothing, emollient, lip balm incorporating allantoin, the sunscreen, Padimate O, in a balanced, slightly acidic lipid base that includes petrolatum and titanium dioxide at a cosmetically acceptable level. (Does not contain any caines, antibiotics, phenol or camphor.) (NDC 38083-777-31)

Actions and Uses: HERPECIN-L® relieves dryness and chapping by providing a lipid barrier to help restore normal moisture balance to the lips. Skin protectants help to soften the crusts and scabs of "cold sores." The sunscreen is effective in 2900-3200 AU range while titanium dioxide, though at low levels, helps to block, scatter and reflect the sun's rays. Applied as a lip balm, SPF is 15. Reapply often during sun exposure.

Administration: (1) *Recurrent "cold sores, sun and fever blisters":* Simply put, use *soon* and *often.* Frequent sufferers report that with *prophylactic* use (BID/PRN), attacks are fewer and less severe. Most recurrent herpes labialis patients are aware of the prodromal symptoms: tingling, itching, burning. At this stage, or if the lesion has already developed, HERPECIN-L should be applied liberally as often as convenient—at least *every hour.* (2) *Outdoor protection:* Apply before and during sun exposure, after swimming and again at bedtime (h.s.). (3) *Dry, chapped lips:* Apply as needed.

Adverse Reactions: If sensitive to any of the ingredients, discontinue use.

Contraindications: None.

How Supplied: 2.8 gm. swivel tubes.

Samples Available: Yes. (Request on professional letterhead or Rx pad.)

Care-Tech Laboratories
Div. of Consolidated Chemical, Inc.
**3224 SOUTH KINGSHIGHWAY BOULEVARD
ST. LOUIS, MO 63139**

BARRI–CARE®

Composition: Active Ingredient: Chloroxylenol
Inactive Ingredients: Petrolatum, Water, Paraffin, Propylene Glycol, Milk Protein, Cod Liver Oil, Aloe Vera Gel, Fragrance, Potassium Hydroxide, Methyl Paraben, Propyl Paraben, Vitamin A & D₃, (E) dl Alpha-Tocopheryl Acetate, (E) dl-Alpha-Tocopherol, D&C Yellow #11 and D&C Red #17.

Actions and Uses: Barri-Care is an antimicrobial ointment formulated to provide a moisture proof barrier against urine, detergent irritants, feces and drainage from wounds or skin lesions. Proven antimicrobial action against E. coli, MRSA, S. aureus and Pseudomonas aeruginosa. Protects perineal area of the incontinent patient from painful skin rashes and relieves irritation around stoma sites. Utilize on Grades I–IV pressure ulcers to halt skin breakdown. Can be used also on minor burns. Will not melt under feverish conditions.

Precautions: External Use Only. Non-Toxic. Avoid eye contact.

Directions: Cleanse affected area with Satin thoroughly. Apply ointment topically to affected area. Reapply 2–3 times daily or as directed by physician.

How Supplied: 2 oz. jar, 4 oz. tubes, 8 oz. jar. NDC #46706-206

CARE CREME®

Composition: Active Ingredient: Chloroxylenol
Inactive Ingredients: Water, Cetyl Alcohol, Lanolin Oil, Cod Liver Oil, Sodium Laureth Sulfate, Triethanolamine, Propylene Glycol, Petrolatum, Lanolin Alcohol, Methyl Gluceth 20 Distearate, Beeswax, Citric Acid, Methyl Paraben, Fragrance, Propyl Paraben, Vitamins A, D₃ and E-dl Alpha-Tocopherol.

Actions and Uses: Care Creme is an antimicrobial skin care creme specially formulated for use on severely dry skin such as Sjogren's Syndrome, atopic dermatitis, psoriasis, minor burns, urine or fecal exposure, scaling and inter-tissue ammonia related rash. Extremely effective on oncology radiation burns. Use at first sign of reddened skin or initial breakdown. Vitamin and oil enriched to promote skin integrity. Contains no metallic ions.

Precautions: Non-toxic, External Use Only. Avoid use around eye area.

Directions: Cleanse affected area with Satin and gently massage Care Creme into skin until completely absorbed or as directed by physician.

How Supplied: 2 oz., 4 oz. tubes, 9 oz. jar. NDC #46706-205

CLINICAL CARE® WOUND CLEANSER

Composition: Active Ingredient: Benzethonium Chloride
Inactive Ingredients: Water, Amphoteric 2, Aloe Vera Gel, DMDM Hydantoin, Citric Acid.

Actions and Uses: Clinical Care is an antimicrobial, emulsifying solution which aids in removing debris and particulate matter from open, dermal wounds. Clinical Care inhibits the growth of pathogenic organisms. Proven effective at eliminating S. aureus, P. aeruginosa, S. typhimurium, Aspergillus, E. coli, MRSA, S. pyogenes and K. pneumonia. Will not produce dermal irritation.

Precautions: External Use Only. Non-Toxic. No contra-indicators.

Directions: Spray affected area as necessary to debride. Use sterile gauze to gently remove debris and necrotic tissue at dermal surface.

How Supplied: 4 oz. spray, 8 oz. spray

CONCEPT®

Composition: Active Ingredient: Chloroxylenol
Inactive Ingredients: Water, Amphoteric 9, Polysorbate 20, PEG-150 Distearate, Cocamide DEA, Cocoyl Sarcosine, Fragrance, D&C Green #5.

Actions and Uses: Concept is a geriatric shampoo and body wash for patients whose skin is irritated by soaps and harsh detergents. Concept is non-eye irritating and reduces bacteria on the skin. Excellent for replenishing moisture in dry, flaky dermal tissues and eliminating body odors. Utilize on children over 6 months of age to address rashing or atopic dermatitis.

Precautions: External Use Only. Non-Toxic.

Directions: Use in normal manner of bathing and shampooing. Rinse thoroughly.

How Supplied: 8 oz., Gallons

FORMULA MAGIC®

Composition: Active Ingredient: Benzethonium Chloride
Inactive Ingredients: Talc, Mineral Oil, Magnesium Carbonate, Fragrance, DMDM Hydantoin.

Actions and Uses: Formula Magic is primarily a geriatric care powder and nursing lubricant. Aids in preventing excoriation, friction chafing and eliminating odor. Antibacterial action proven effective at 99.9% inhibition where Formula Magic is applied. Excellent for use on diabetic patients, feet and under breasts to relieve redness and skin irritation.

Precautions: Non-irritating to skin, non-toxic, slightly irritating to eyes.

Directions: Apply liberally to body and rub gently into skin.

How Supplied: 4 oz. and 12 oz. NDC #46706-202

ORCHID FRESH II®
Perineal/Ostomy Cleanser

Composition: Active Ingredient: Benzethonium Chloride
Inactive Ingredients: Water, Amphoteric 2, DMDM Hydantoin, Fragrance, Citric Acid.

Actions and Uses: Orchid Fresh II is an amphoteric, topical antimicrobial cleansing solution which gently cleans and emulsifies feces and urine on the incontinent patient. Use also on stoma sites and ostomy bags to deodorize and eliminate odor. Outstanding antimicrobial action on Pseudomonas, E. coli, Staphylococcus aureus, MRSA, etc. Orchid Fresh II will aid in reducing skin breakdown.

Precautions: External Use Only, Non-Toxic—Non-Dermal Irritating

Directions: Spray topically and remove feces and urine with warm, moist washcloth. Spray directly on peristomal skin areas, clean gently and pat dry. Utilize Care Creme on reddened skin areas.

How Supplied: 4 oz., 8 oz. and Gallons NDC #46706-115

SATIN® ANTIMICROBIAL SKIN CLEANSER

Composition: Active Ingredient: Chloroxylenol
Inactive Ingredients: Water, Sodium Laureth Sulfate, Cocamidopropyl Betaine, PEG-8, Cocamide DEA, Glycol Stearate, Lanolin Oil, Tetrasodium EDTA, D&C Yellow #10.

Actions and Uses: Satin has been specially formulated for use on sensitive or aging dermal tissue, atopic dermatitis and psoriasis. Effective in eliminating gram-positive and gram-negative pathogens such as E. coli, S. aureus, Pseudomonas, etc. Contains emollients to replenish natural oils and proteins. Satin also eliminates skin odor and dry, itchy skin.

Continued on next page

Care-Tech—Cont.

Precautions: No contra-indicators. External use only. Non-Toxic.

Directions: Use during shower, bath or regular cleansing or as directed by physician.

How Supplied: 4 oz., 8 oz., 12 oz. 16 oz., 1 Gallon NDC #46706-101

TECHNI–CARE® SURGICAL SCRUB

Composition: Active Ingredient: Chloroxylenol 3%
Inactive Ingredients: Water, Sodium Lauryl Sulfate, Cocamide DEA, Propylene Glycol, Cocamidopropyl Betaine, Cocamidopropyl PG-Dimonium Chloride Phosphate, Citric Acid, Tetrasodium EDTA, Aloe Vera Gel, Hydrolyzed Animal Protein, D&C Yellow #10.

Actions and Uses: Techni-Care represents entirerly new technology in a broad-spectrum, topical, antiseptic microbicide for skin degerming. 99.99% Bacterial reduction in 30 second contact usage. Techni-Care may be used for disinfection of wounds, for pre-op and post-op along with surgical scrub applications. Non-staining and non-irritating to dermal tissue. Techni-Care conditions dermal tissue and promotes more rapid rate of healing.

Precautions: Non-Toxic, Non-Irritating, External Use Only. Can be used safely around ears and eyes or as directed by a physician.

Directions: Apply, lather and rinse well. For pre-op, apply and let dry, no rinsing required.

How Supplied: 20 mL packets, 8 oz., 16 oz., 32 oz., Gallons and peel paks

---

Chesebrough-Pond's USA Co.
**33 BENEDICT PLACE
GREENWICH, CT 06830**

DERMASIL™ DRY SKIN TREATMENT
Concentrated Treatment

Active Ingredients: Glycerin, dimethicone

Other Ingredients: Cyclomethicone, water, sunflower seed oil, petrolatum, oleth-10, soya sterol, borage seed oil, lecithin, tocopheryl acetate (Vitamin E acetate), retinyl palmitate (Vitamin A palmitate), cholecalciferol (Vitamin D3), ascorbyl palmitate, stearic acid, TEA, carbomer, corn oil, disodium EDTA, methylparaben, DMDM hydantoin, iodopropynyl butylcarbamate.

Indications/Actions: Suitable for severe dry skin, and the control of symptoms such as chapping, cracking, flaking, roughness, redness, soreness, and the itching associated with dry skin. This concentrated treatment contains four systems to control and provide long-lasting relief from severe dry skin:
Occlusives to block moisture loss from the skin's surface
Humectant to bind water in the skin's outermost layers
Skin lipids to enhance the skin's natural ability to retain moisture
EFA's an important component of the skin's moisture barrier
Hypoallergenic and fragrance free.

Directions: Apply sparingly. Use in combination with Dermasil Lotion or Cream on patches of extreme dryness, such as fingertips and knuckles.

Warnings: Keep out of reach of children. For externl use only. Avoid contact with eyes. If condition worsens or does not improve within seven days, consult a doctor or pharmacist. Not to be applied over deep or puncture wounds, infections or lacerations.

How Supplied: 1 oz. (28 g.)

DERMASIL™ DRY SKIN TREATMENT CREAM

Active Ingredient: Dimethicone

Other Ingredients: Water, petrolatum, myreth-3 myristate, glycerin, sunflower seed oil, cetearyl alcohol, TEA, lecithin, borage seed oil, cholesterol, stearic acid, carbomer, ceteareth-20, palmarosa oil, rose extract, sweet almond oil, sandalwood oil, vanilla, ethylene brassylate, methylparaben, propylparaben, DMDM hydantoin.

Indications/Actions: Suitable for severe dry skin, and control of symptoms such as chapping, cracking, flaking, roughness, soreness, and the itching associated with dry skin. This cream contains four systems to control, and provide long-lasting relief from severe dry skin:
— occlusives to block moisture loss from the skin's surface
— humectant to bind water in the skin's outermost layers
— skin lipids to enhance the skin's natural ability to retain moisture
— EFA's an important compound of the skin's moisture barrier
Hypoallergenic and fragrance free.

Directions: Apply as needed to areas of dry skin. Use in combination with Dermasil Treatment on patches of extreme dryness, such as fingertips and knuckles.

Warning: Keep out of reach of children. For external use only. Avoid contact with eyes. If condition worsens or does not improve within seven days, consult a doctor or pharmacist. Not to be applied over deep or puncture wounds, infections and lacerations.

How Supplied: 4 oz (113 g)
2 oz (56 g)

DERMASIL™ DRY SKIN TREATMENT LOTION

Active Ingredient: dimethicone

Other Ingredients: water, petrolatum, glycerin, mineral oil, stearic acid, sunflower seed oil, glycol stearate, cetyl acetate, glyceryl stearate, TEA, lecithin, borage seed oil, cholesterol, ascorbyl, palmitate, carbomer, PEG-40 stearate, cetyl alcohol, acetylated lanolin alcohol, magnesium aluminum silicate, palmarosa oil, rose extract, sweet almond oil, sandalwood oil, vanilla, ethylene brassylate, stearamide amp, disodium EDTA, methylparaben, propylparaben, DMDM hydantoin.

Indications/Actions: Suitable for severe dry skin, and control of symptoms such as chapping, cracking, flaking, roughness, redness, soreness, and the itch associated with dry skin. This lotion contains four systems to control, and provide long-lasting relief from severe dry skin:
Occlusives to block moisture loss from the skin's surface
Humectant to bind water in the skins outermost layers
Skin lipids to enhance the skin's natural ability to retain moisture EFA's an important component of the skin's moisture barrier
Hypoallergenic and fragrance free.

Directions: Apply as needed to areas of dry skin. Use in combination with Dermasil concentrated Treatment on patches of extreme dryness, such as fingertips and knuckles.

Warnings: Keep out of reach of children. For external use only. Avoid contact with eyes. If condition worsens or does not improve within seven days, consult a doctor or pharmacist. Not to be applied over deep or puncture wounds, infections or lacerations.

How Supplied: 8 oz (236 ml)
4 oz (118 ml)

VASELINE®
100% Pure Petroleum Jelly Skin Protectant

Composition: White Petrolatum U.S.P.

Indication: A soothing protectant for minor skin irritations such as burns, scrapes, abrasions, chafing, detergent hands, dry or chapped skin, and sunburn. Helps prevent diaper rash, soothes chapped skin and temporarily soothes minor sunburn due to its emollient and lubricant properties. Helps prevent and heal dry, chapped sun- and windburned skin. Vaseline products are non-comedogenic.

Directions: Cleanse affected areas with soap and water prior to application, then apply generously to provide a continuous protective film. Apply as needed, before, during and following exposure to sun, wind, water, and cold weather.

Drug Interaction: No known drug interactions. Product is innocuous, physiologically inert with no known sensitization potential.

Warning: Keep out of reach of children. For external use only. Not to be applied over deep or puncture wounds, infections or lacerations.

How Supplied: 1 oz. and 2.5 oz. plastic tubes. (NDC 0521-8120-01, -31). 1.75 oz., 3.75 oz., 7.5 oz., and 13 oz. plastic jars (NDC 0521-8120-24, -28, -29, -32).

VASELINE® INTENSIVE CARE® MOISTURIZING SUNBLOCK LOTION

Active Ingredients: Ethylhexyl *p*-methoxycinnamate, oxybenzone, 2-ethylhexyl salicylate.*

Inactive Ingredients: Water, glycerin, stearic acid, aloe vera gel, PVP/Eicosene copolymer, dimethicone, TEA, DEA-cetylphosphate, cetyl alcohol, petrolatum, tocopheryl acetate, magnesium aluminum silicate, carbomer 934, fragrance, methylparaben, propylparaben, disodium EDTA, DMDM hydantin.

Indications/Actions: Vaseline Intensive Care Moisturizing Sunblock Lotion provides broad-spectrum protection from the sun's harmful rays. Good for all skin types, especially those that burn easily. It combines sunscreens with moisturizers that are hypo-allergenic and will penetrate into the skin quickly to help replenish moisture loss due to sun and wind exposure. Vaseline Intensive Care Moisturizing Sunblock Lotion is also PABA-free,† gentle, and waterproof for up to eight hours in water.

Directions: Apply generously and evenly to exposed areas. Apply product liberally prior to exposure to sun. Re-apply after prolonged swimming or excessive perspiration.

---

*SPF 25, only.
†Not SPF 40.

Warnings: Keep out of reach of children. For external use only. Avoid contact with eyes.

How Supplied: 4 oz. and 6 oz. SPF 4 through SPF 40.

VASELINE® INTENSIVE CARE®
Extra Strength LOTION

Active Ingredient: Dimethicone

Other Ingredients: Water, glycerin, stearic acid, C11–13 isoparaffin, glycol stearate, petrolatum, glyceryl stearate, TEA, zinc oxide, cetyl alcohol, potassium cetyl phosphate, carbomer, cetyl acetate, acetylated lanolin alcohol, stearamide AMP, fragrance, magnesium aluminum silicate, methylparaben, propylparaben, disodium EDTA, DMDM hydantoin

Indications: Vaseline® Intensive Care® Extra Strength Lotion is specially formulated to help treat and prevent severe dry skin. Its clinically tested formula contains a proven ingredient —Dimethicone—to treat extremely dry, red, sore skin. The Vaseline Intensive Care Extra Strength Lotion is hypo-allergenic and non-comedogenic.

Directions: Apply liberally to severely dry skin, particularly hands, elbows and feet. Use to moisturize and treat skin after bathing/showering; under shaving cream; after shaving; overnight.

Warnings: Keep out of reach of children. For external use only. Avoid contact with eyes. If condition worsens or does not improve within 7 days, consult a doctor. Not to be applied over deep or puncture wounds, infections or lacerations.

How Supplied: 6 oz., 10 oz. and 15 oz.

VASELINE PETROLEUM JELLY CREAM
CREAMY FORMULA

Active Ingredient: Petrolatum

Other Ingredients: Water, aluminum starch octenylsuccinate, C12–15 alkyllactate, myreth-3 myristate, cetosearyl alcohol, glycerin, diglycerol, microcrystalline wax, tocopheryl acetate (Vitamin E acetate), ceteareth-20, carbomer, TEA, ethylene brassylate, methylparaben, DMDM hydantoin, disodium EDTA, iodopropynyl butyl-carbamate.

Indications/Actions: Moisturizes, protects and restores severely dry skin to its natural suppleness. Use on hands, elbows, knees, heels and face. This rich, smooth cream penetrates deeply, absorbs completely and is proven to be as effective as Vaseline 100% Pure Petroleum Jelly in moisturizing and protection. Hypo-allergenic. Fragrance Free. Non-comedeogenic.

Directions: Apply liberally as often as needed for long-lasting protection of dry, irritated skin.

Warnings: For external use only. Avoid contact with eyes. Not for eye makeup removal. If condition worsens or does not improve within seven days, consult a doctor. Not to be applied over diaper rash, deep or puncture wounds, infections or lacerations. Keep out of reach of children.

How Supplied: 4.75 oz (134 g)
4.5 oz (127 g)
2 oz (57 g)
.85 oz (24 g)

Church & Dwight Co., Inc.
469 N. HARRISON STREET
PRINCETON, NJ 08540

ARM & HAMMER®
Pure Baking Soda

Active Ingredient: Sodium Bicarbonate U.S.P.

Indications: For alleviation of acid indigestion, also known as heartburn or sour stomach. Not a remedy for other types of stomach complaints such as nausea, stomachache, abdominal cramps, gas pains, or stomach distention caused by overeating and/or overdrinking. In the latter case, one should not ingest solids, liquids or antacid but rather refrain from all physical activity and—if uncomfortable—call a physician.

Actions: ARM & HAMMER® Pure Baking Soda provides fast-acting, effective neutralization of stomach acids. Each level ½ teaspoon dose will neutralize 20.9 mEq of acid.

Warnings: Except under the advice and supervision of a physician: (1) do not administer to children under five years of age, (2) do not take more than eight level ½ teaspoons per person up to 60 years old or four level ½ teaspoons per person 60 years or older in a 24-hour period, (3) do not use this product if you are on a sodium restricted diet, (4) do not use the maximum dose for more than two weeks, (5) do not ingest food, liquid or any antacid when stomach is overly full to avoid possible injury to the stomach.

Dosage and Administration: Level ½ teaspoon in ½ glass (4 fl. oz.) of water every two hours up to maximum dosage or as directed by a physician. Accurately measure level ½ teaspoon. Each level ½ teaspoon contains 20.9 mEq (.476 gm) sodium.

How Supplied: Available in 8 oz., 16 oz., 32 oz., and 64 oz. boxes.

CIBA Consumer Pharmaceuticals
Division of CIBA-GEIGY Corporation
MACK WOODBRIDGE II
581 MAIN STREET
WOODBRIDGE, NJ 07095

ALLEREST® MAXIMUM STRENGTH TABLETS, NO DROWSINESS TABLETS, HEADACHE STRENGTH TABLETS, SINUS PAIN FORMULA TABLETS, CHILDREN'S CHEWABLE TABLETS AND 12 HOUR CAPLETS

Active Ingredients:
Maximum Strength Tablets —Chlorpheniramine maleate 2 mg, pseudoephedrine HCl 30 mg.
No Drowsiness Tablets —Acetaminophen 325 mg, pseudoephedrine HCl 30 mg.
Headache Strength Tablets —Acetaminophen 325 mg, chlorpheniramine maleate 2 mg, pseudoephedrine HCl 30 mg.
Sinus Pain Formula Tablets —Acetaminophen 500 mg, chlorpheniramine maleate 2 mg, pseudoephedrine HCl 30 mg.
Children's Chewable Tablets —Chlorpheniramine maleate 1 mg, phenylpropanolamine HCl 9.4 mg.
12 Hour Caplets —Chlorpheniramine maleate 12 mg, phenylpropanolamine HCl 75 mg.

Other Ingredients:
Maximum Strength Tablets —Blue 1 lake, dibasic calcium phosphate, magnesium stearate, microcrystalline cellulose, povidone, pregelatinized starch, sodium starch glycolate. *No Drowsiness and Headache Strength Tablets* —Magnesium stearate, microcrystalline cellulose, povidone, pregelatinized starch.
Sinus Pain Formula Tablets —Magnesium stearate, microcrystalline cellulose, povidone, pregelatinized starch, sodium starch glycolate.
Children's Chewable Tablets —Calcium stearate, citric acid, flavor, magnesium trisilicate, mannitol, saccharin sodium, sorbitol.
12 Hour Caplets —Carnauba wax, colloidal silicon dioxide, lactose, methylcellulose, polyethylene glycol, povidone, Red 30, stearic acid, titanium dioxide, Yellow 6.

Indications:
Maximum Strength, Headache Strength, Sinus Pain Formula, Children's Chewable Tablets and 12 Hour Caplets —Temporarily relieves nasal congestion, runny nose, sneezing, itching of the nose or throat, and itchy, watery eyes due to hay fever or other upper respiratory allergies; also *Headache Strength and Sinus Pain Formula Tablets* —For the temporary relief of minor aches, pains, and headache; also *12 Hour Caplets* —For temporary relief of nasal congestion due to the common cold, hay fever or other upper respiratory allergies, or associated with sinusitis.
No Drowsiness Tablets —Temporarily relieves nasal congestion due to hay fever, other upper respiratory allergies, or the common cold, or associated with sinusitis. For the temporary relief of minor aches, pains, and headache.

Warnings: *All Products* —Do not exceed recommended dosage because at higher doses, nervousness, dizziness, or sleeplessness may occur. Do not take this product if you have heart disease, high blood pressure, thyroid disease, diabetes, or difficulty in urination due to enlargement of the prostate gland, unless directed by a physician. As with any drug, if you are pregnant or nursing a baby, seek the advice of a health professional before using this product. **Keep this and all drugs out of the reach of children.** In case of accidental overdose, seek professional assistance or contact a Poison Control Center immediately. Prompt medical attention (for products containing acetaminophen) is critical for adults as well as children even if you do not notice any signs or symptoms. And, *All Products Except No Drowsiness Tablets* —Do not take this product if you have a breathing problem such as emphysema or chronic bronchitis, or if you have glaucoma, unless directed by a physician. May cause excitability, especially in children. May cause drowsiness; alcohol, sedatives, and tranquilizers may increase the drowsiness effect. Avoid alcoholic beverages while taking this product. Do not take this product if you are taking sedatives or tranquilizers, without first consulting your physician. Use caution when driving a motor vehicle or operating machinery.
Maximum Strength Tablets, Children's Chewable Tablets and 12 Hour Caplets —Do not take this product for more than 7 days. If symptoms do not improve or are accompanied by fever, consult a physician.
Headache Strength, Sinus Pain Formula, and No Drowsiness Tablets —Do not take this product for more than 10 days (for adults) or 5 days (for children). If symptoms do not improve or are accompanied by fever that lasts more than 3 days, or if new symptoms occur, consult a physician.

Drug Interaction Precaution: *All Products* —Do not take this product if you are presently taking a prescription drug for high blood pressure or depression, without first consulting your physician; and *Children's Chewable Tablets*—Do not take this product if you are presently taking another medication containing phenylpropanolamine.

Directions: Dose as follows while symptoms persist, or as directed by a physician.
Maximum Strength, No Drowsiness and Headache Strength Tablets —Adults and children 12 years of age and over: 2 tablets every 4 to 6 hours, not to exceed 8 tablets in 24 hours. Children 6 to under 12 years of age: 1 tablet every 4 to 6 hours, not to exceed 4 tablets in 24 hours. Children under 6 years of age: Consult a physician.
Sinus Pain Formula Tablets —Adults and children 12 years of age and over: 2 tablets every 6 hours, not to exceed 8 tablets in 24 hours. Children under 12 years of age: Consult a physician.
Children's Chewable Tablets —Children 6 to under 12 years of age: 2 tablets every 4 to 6 hours, not to exceed 8 tablets in 24 hours. Children under 6 years of age: Consult a physician.
12 Hour Caplets —Adults and children 12 years of age and over: 1 caplet swallowed whole every 12 hours, not to exceed 2 caplets in 24 hours.

How Supplied:
Maximum Strength Tablets —Boxes of 24, 48, and 72.
No Drowsiness Tablets —Boxes of 20.
Headache Strength Tablets —Boxes of 24.
Sinus Pain Formula Tablets —Boxes of 20.
Children's Chewable Tablets —Boxes of 24.
12 Hour Caplets —Boxes of 10.
ALLEREST is a registered trademark of Ciba-Geigy Corporation

ACUTRIM® 16 HOUR* STEADY CONTROL APPETITE SUPPRESSANT TABLETS
Caffeine Free

ACUTRIM® —MAXIMUM STRENGTH APPETITE SUPPRESSANT TABLETS
Caffeine Free

ACUTRIM LATE DAY® STRENGTH* APPETITE SUPPRESSANT TABLETS
Caffeine Free

Description: ACUTRIM® tablets are an aid to appetite control in conjunction with a sensible weight loss program. ACUTRIM® tablets deliver their maximum strength dosage of appetite suppressant at a precisely controlled rate. This timed release is scientifically targeted to effectively distribute the appetite suppressant all day.*
ACUTRIM makes it easier to follow the kind of reduced calorie diet needed for best weight control results.
A diet plan developed by an expert dietician is included in the package for your personal use as a further aid.

Formula: Each ACUTRIM® tablet contains: Active Ingredient—phenylpropanolamine HCl 75 mg (appetite suppressant time release).
Inactive Ingredients—ACUTRIM® 16 HOUR Steady Control: Cellulose Acetate, Hydroxypropyl Methylcellulose, Stearic Acid—ACUTRIM® MAXIMUM STRENGTH: Cellulose Acetate, D&C Yellow #10, FD&C Blue #1, FD&C Yellow #6, Hydroxypropyl Methylcellulose, Povidone, Propylene Glycol, Stearic Acid, Titanium Dioxide—ACUTRIM LATE DAY® Strength: Cellulose Acetate, FD&C Yellow #6, Hydroxypropyl

Methylcellulose, Isopropyl Alcohol, Propylene Glycol, Riboflavin, Stearic Acid, Titanium Dioxide.

Directions: Adult oral dosage is **one tablet** at mid-morning with a full glass of water. Swallow each tablet whole; do not divide, crush, chew, or dissolve the tablet. Exceeding the recommended dose has not been shown to result in greater weight loss. This product's effectiveness is directly related to the degree to which you reduce your usual daily food intake. Attempts at weight reduction which involve the use of this product should be limited to periods not exceeding 3 months, because this should be enough time to establish new eating habits. Read and follow important Diet Plan enclosed.
WARNINGS: FOR ADULT USE ONLY. Do not take more than one tablet per day (24 hours). Exceeding the recommended dose may cause serious health problems. Do not give this product to children under 12 years of age. Persons between 12 and 18 are advised to consult their physician before using this product. If nervousness, dizziness, sleeplessness, palpitations or headache occurs, stop taking this medication and consult your physician. If you are being treated for high blood pressure, depression, or an eating disorder or have heart disease, diabetes, or thyroid disease, do not take this product except under the supervision of a physician. As with any drug, if you are pregnant or nursing a baby, seek the advice of a health professional before using this product.

Drug Interaction Precaution: If you are taking a cough/cold or allergy medication containing any form of phenylpropanolamine, or any type of nasal decongestant, do not take this product. Do not take this product if you are taking any prescription drug, except under the advice and supervision of a physician. Do not use this product if you are presently taking a prescription monoamine oxidase inhibitor (MAOI) for depression or for two weeks after stopping use of a MAOI without first consulting a physician.
KEEP THIS AND ALL MEDICATION OUT OF THE REACH OF CHILDREN. In case of accidental overdose, seek professional assistance or contact a poison control center immediately.

How Supplied: Tamper-evident blister packages of 20 and 40 tablets. Do not use if individual seals are broken.
DO NOT STORE ABOVE 30°C (86°F). PROTECT FROM MOISTURE
*Peak Strength and extent of duration relate solely to blood levels.
Shown in Product Identification Guide, page 407

AMERICAINE® HEMORRHOIDAL OINTMENT
[a-mer 'i-kān]

Active Ingredient: Benzocaine 20%.

Other Ingredients: Benzethonium chloride, polyethylene glycol 300, polyethylene glycol 3350.

Indications: For the temporary relief of local pain, itching and soreness associated with hemorrhoids and anorectal inflammation.

Warnings: If condition worsens, or does not improve within 7 days, consult a physician. Do not exceed the recommended daily dosage unless directed by a physician. In case of bleeding, consult a physician promptly. Do not put this product into the rectum by using fingers or any mechanical device or applicator. Certain persons can develop allergic reactions to ingredients in this product. If the symptom being treated does not subside or if redness, irritation, swelling, pain, or other symptoms develop or increase, discontinue use and consult a physician. **Keep this and all drugs out of the reach of children.** In case of accidental ingestion, seek professional assistance or contact a Poison Control Center immediately.

Directions: *Adults:* When practical, cleanse the affected area with mild soap and warm water and rinse thoroughly. Gently dry by patting or blotting with toilet tissue or a soft cloth before application of this product. Apply externally to the affected area up to 6 times daily. *Children under 12 years of age:* Consult a physician.

How Supplied: *Hemorrhoidal Ointment* —1 oz. tube.
AMERICAINE is a registered trademark of Ciba-Geigy Corporation.
Shown in Product Identification Guide, page 407

AMERICAINE® TOPICAL ANESTHETIC SPRAY AND FIRST AID OINTMENT
[a-mer 'i-kān]

Active Ingredient: Benzocaine 20%.

Other Ingredients: *Spray* —Butane (propellant), isobutane (propellant), polyethylene glycol 200, propane (propellant). *Ointment* —Benzethonium chloride, polyethylene glycol 300, polyethylene glycol 3350.

Indications: For the temporary relief of pain and itching associated with minor cuts, scrapes, burns, sunburn, insect bites, or minor skin irritations.

Warnings: For external use only. Avoid contact with the eyes. If condition worsens, or if symptoms persist for more than 7 days or clear up and occur again within a few days, discontinue use of this product and consult a physician. **Keep this and all drugs out of the reach of children.** In case of accidental ingestion,

seek professional assistance or contact a Poison Control Center immediately. *For Spray only* —Contents under pressure. Do not puncture or incinerate. Flammable mixture; do not use near fire or flame. Do not store at temperature above 120°F. Use only as directed. Intentional misuse by deliberately concentrating and inhaling the contents can be harmful or fatal.

Directions: Adults and children 2 years of age and older: Apply liberally to affected area not more than 3 to 4 times daily. Children under 2 years of age: Consult a physician.

How Supplied: *Topical Anesthetic Spray* —⅔ oz., 2 oz. and 4 oz. aerosol containers. *First Aid Ointment* —¾ oz. tube, which is a clear, fragrance-free gel formula that is nonstaining, easy to apply, and is easily removed with soap and water.
AMERICAINE is a registered trademark of Ciba-Geigy Corporation.
Shown in Product Identification Guide, page 407

CALDECORT® ANTI-ITCH CREAM AND SPRAY; CALDECORT LIGHT® CREAM
[kal 'de-kort]

Active Ingredient: *Cream* —Hydrocortisone acetate (equivalent to hydrocortisone 1%). *Light Cream* —Hydrocortisone acetate (equivalent to hydrocortisone ½%). *Spray* —Hydrocortisone 1%.

Other Ingredients: *Cream* —Isopropyl myristate, methylparaben, polysorbate 60, propylparaben, purified water, sorbitan monostearate, sorbitol solution, stearic acid. *Light Cream* —Aloe vera gel, isopropyl myristate, methylparaben, polysorbate 60, propylparaben, purified water, sorbitan monostearate, sorbitol solution, stearic acid. *Spray* —Isobutane (propellant), isopropyl myristate, SD alcohol 40-B 62.7% (w/w).

Indications: For the temporary relief of itching associated with minor skin irritations, inflammation, and rashes due to eczema, insect bites, poison ivy, poison oak, poison sumac, soaps, detergents, cosmetics, jewelry, seborrheic dermatitis, psoriasis, and for external feminine itching. Other uses of this product should be only under the advice and supervision of a doctor.

Warnings: **For external use only.** Avoid contact with the eyes. If condition worsens, or if symptoms persist for more than 7 days or clear up and occur again within a few days, stop use of this product and do not begin use of any other hy-

Continued on next page

The full prescribing information for each CIBA Consumer Pharmaceuticals product is contained herein and is that in effect as of December 15, 1993

CIBA Consumer—Cont.

drocortisone product unless you have consulted a doctor. Do not use for the treatment of diaper rash. Consult a doctor. Do not use if you have a vaginal discharge. Consult a doctor. **Keep this and all drugs out of the reach of children.** In case of accidental ingestion, seek professional assistance or contact a Poison Control Center immediately. *For Spray only*—Avoid contact with the eyes or on other mucous membranes. Contents under pressure. Do not puncture or incinerate. Flammable mixture, do not use near fire or flame. Do not store at temperature above 120°F. Use only as directed. Intentional misuse by deliberately concentrating and inhaling the contents can be harmful or fatal.

Directions: *Cream and Light Cream:* Adults and children 2 years of age and older: Apply to affected area not more than 3 or 4 times daily. Children under 2 years of age: Do not use, consult a doctor.

Spray: Shake well, hold 4" to 6" from affected area. Apply to affected area not more than 3 to 4 times daily. Children under 2 years of age: Do not use, consult a doctor.

How Supplied: *Cream* —½ oz. and 1 oz. tubes. *Light Cream* —½ oz. tubes. *Spray*—1.5 oz. aerosol container. CALDECORT and CALDECORT LIGHT are registered trademarks of Ciba-Geigy Corporation.

Shown in Product Identification Guide, page 407

CALDESENE® MEDICATED POWDER AND OINTMENT
[kal 'de-sēn]

Active Ingredients: *Powder* —Calcium undecylenate 10%. *Ointment* —White petrolatum 53.9%; zinc oxide 15%.

Other Ingredients: *Powder* — Fragrance, talc. *Ointment* —Cod liver oil, fragrance, lanolin, methylparaben, propylparaben, talc.

Indications: Caldesene Medicated Powder is indicated to help relieve, treat and prevent diaper rash, prickly heat and chafing. Caldesene Ointment helps relieve, treat and prevent diaper rash, protects sensitive skin against wetness, and soothes chafed skin.

Actions: Only Caldesene Medicated Powder contains calcium undecylenate, an antimicrobial that inhibits growth of the organisms frequently associated with diaper rash. Also forms a protective coating to repel moisture, and helps treat and prevent chafing and prickly heat. Caldesene Ointment is specially formulated to soothe and treat diaper rash while protecting sensitive skin against wetness. Unlike other ointments containing zinc oxide, Caldesene Ointment has a mild fragrance and is easily removed from the diaper area with soap and water.

Warnings: For external use only. Avoid contact with eyes. If condition worsens or does not improve within 7 days, consult a physician. **Keep this and all drugs out of the reach of children.** In case of accidental ingestion, seek professional assistance or contact a Poison Control Center immediately. Powder only: Keep powder away from child's face to avoid inhalation, which can cause breathing problems. Do not use on broken skin. Ointment only: Do not apply over deep or puncture wounds, infections and lacerations.

Directions: Use on baby after every bath or diaper change as directed by a pediatrician. Cleanse and thoroughly dry baby's skin, then smooth on Caldesene. Powder only: Apply powder close to the body away from child's face. (Shake bottle—don't squeeze—to apply powder to your hand or directly into the diaper.)

How Supplied: *Medicated Powder*—2 oz (57 g) and 4 oz (113 g) shaker containers. *Medicated Powder* —1.25 oz (35 g). CALDESENE is a registered trademark of Ciba-Geigy Corporation.

Shown in Product Identification Guide, page 407

CRUEX® ANTIFUNGAL POWDER, SPRAY POWDER AND CREAM
[kru 'ex]

Active Ingredients: *Powder* —Calcium undecylenate 10%. *Spray Powder* —Total undecylenate 19%, as undecylenic acid and zinc undecylenate. *Cream* —Total undecylenate 20%, as undecylenic acid and zinc undecylenate.

Other Ingredients: *Powder* —Colloidal silicon dioxide, fragrance, isopropyl myristate, talc. *Spray Powder* —Fragrance, isobutane (propellant), isopropyl myristate, menthol, talc, trolamine. *Cream* —Fragrance, glycol stearate SE, lanolin, methylparaben, PEG-8 laurate, PEG-6 stearate, propylparaben, sorbitol solution, stearic acid, trolamine, purified water, white petrolatum.

Indications: Cures jock itch, relieves itching, chafing, and burning. Soothes irritation. Cruex powders also absorb perspiration.

Warnings: Do not use on children under 2 years of age except under the advice and supervision of a doctor. For external use only. If irritation occurs, or if there is no improvement within 2 weeks, discontinue use and consult a doctor. **Keep this and all drugs out of the reach of children.** In case of accidental ingestion, seek professional assistance or contact a Poison Control Center immediately. *For Spray Powder only*—Avoid inhaling. Avoid spraying in eyes or on other mucous membranes. Contents under pressure. Do not puncture or incinerate. Flammable mixture, do not use near fire or flame. Do not expose to heat or temperatures above 49°C (120°F.) Use

only as directed. Intentional misuse by deliberately concentrating and inhaling the contents can be harmful or fatal.

Directions: Cleanse skin with soap and water and dry thoroughly. Apply Cruex to affected area morning and night, before and after athletic activity, or as directed by a doctor. Best results are usually obtained with 2 weeks' use of this product. If satisfactory results have not occurred within this time, consult a doctor. Children under 12 years of age should be supervised in the use of this product. This product is not effective on the scalp or nails.

How Supplied: *Powder* —1.5 oz (43 g) plastic squeeze bottle. *Spray Powder* —1.8 oz (51 g), 3.5 oz (99 g) and 5.5 oz (156 g) aerosol containers. *Cream* —½ oz (14 g) tube. CRUEX is a registered trademark of Ciba-Geigy Corporation.

Shown in Product Identification Guide, page 407

DESENEX® ANTIFUNGAL POWDER, SPRAY POWDER, CREAM, OINTMENT, AND SPRAY LIQUID
[dess 'i-nex]

Active Ingredients: *Cream, Ointment, Powder, and Spray Powder,* —Total undecylenate 25%, as undecylenic acid and zinc undecylenate. *Spray Liquid* —Tolnaftate 1%.

Other Ingredients: *Cream, Ointment* —Fragrance, glycol stearate SE, lanolin, methylparaben, PEG-8 laurate, PEG-6 stearate, propylparaben, purified water, sorbitol solution, stearic acid, trolamine, white petrolatum. *Powder* —Fragrance, talc. *Spray Powder* —Fragrance, isobutane (propellant), isopropyl myristate, menthol, talc, trolamine. *Spray Liquid* —BHT, fragrance, isobutane (propellant), polyethylene glycol 400, SD alcohol 40-B (41% w/w).

Indications: Proven clinically effective in the treatment of athlete's foot (tinea pedis). Relieves the painful itching, cracking and discomfort associated with athlete's foot. Desenex Spray Liquid prevents the recurrence of athlete's foot with daily use.

Warnings: Do not use on children under 2 years of age except under the advice and supervision of a doctor. For external use only. Avoid contact with the eyes. If irritation occurs, or if there is no improvement within 4 weeks, discontinue use and consult a doctor. **Keep this and all drugs out of the reach of children.** In case of accidental ingestion, seek professional assistance or contact a Poison Control Center immediately. *For Spray Powder* and *Spray Liquid*—Avoid inhaling. Avoid contact with the eyes or other mucous membranes. Contents under pressure. Do not puncture or incinerate. Flammable mixture, do not use near fire or flame. Do not expose to heat or temperatures above 49°C (120°F). Use only as directed. Intentional misuse by deliberately concentrating and inhaling the contents can be harmful or fatal.

Directions: Cleanse skin with soap and water and dry thoroughly. Apply over affected area morning and night or as directed by a doctor, paying special attention to the spaces between the toes. It is also helpful to wear well-fitting, ventilated shoes and to change shoes and socks at least once daily. Best results are usually obtained with 4 weeks' use of this product. If satisfactory results have not occurred within this time, consult a doctor. Children under 12 years of age should be supervised in the use of this product. This product is not effective on the scalp or nails. For persistent cases of athlete's foot, use Desenex Ointment or Cream at night and Desenex Powder or Spray Powder during the day. To prevent recurrence of athlete's foot, apply Desenex Spray Liquid to feet once or twice daily following the above directions.

How Supplied: *Cream* —½ oz (14 g) tube. *Ointment* —½ oz (14 g) and 1 oz (28 g) tubes. *Powder* —1.5 oz (43 g) and 3 oz (85 g) shaker containers. *Spray Powder* —2.7 oz (77 g) and 5.5 oz (156 g) aerosol containers. *Spray Liquid* —3 oz (85 g) aerosol container. DESENEX is a registered trademark of Ciba-Geigy Corporation.
Shown in Product Identification Guide, page 407

DESENEX® FOOT & SNEAKER DEODORANT SPRAY

[dess 'i-nex]

Ingredients: Isobutane (propellant), SD alcohol 40-B, talc, aluminum chlorohydrex, silica, diisopropyl adipate, fragrance, menthol, tartaric acid.

Description: Foot & Sneaker Deodorant Spray cools and comforts feet, helping them feel clean and refreshed. Helps foster good foot hygiene with regular use. Specially formulated to absorb wetness, deodorize and relieve the discomfort of hot, perspiring, active feet. Sprays on like a liquid—dries quickly to a fine powder.

Directions: **Shake well,** hold 6 inches from area and spray onto soles of your feet and between your toes daily. Also, spray liberally over entire area of shoes or sneakers before wearing.

Warnings: Avoid spraying in eyes or on other mucous membranes. Contents under pressure. Do not puncture or incinerate. Flammable mixture, do not use near fire or flame. Do not expose to heat or temperatures above 49°C (120°F). Use only as directed. Intentional misuse by deliberately concentrating and inhaling the contents can be harmful or fatal. **Keep out of reach of children.**

How Supplied: *Desenex Foot & Sneaker Deodorant Spray Powder* —3 oz (85 g) aerosol container. Also available, Desenex Foot & Sneaker Deodorant Powder Plus with an antifungal—2 oz (57 g) shaker container.
DESENEX is a registered trademark of Ciba-Geigy Corporation.
Shown in Product Identification Guide, page 407

EXTRA STRENGTH DOAN'S®
Analgesic Caplets

Indications: For temporary relief of minor backache pain.

Directions: Adults—Two caplets with water every 6 hours while symptoms persist, not to exceed 8 caplets during a 24-hour period or as directed by a doctor. Children under 12: consult a doctor.

Warnings: Children and teenagers should not use this medicine for chicken pox or flu symptoms before a doctor is consulted about Reye syndrome, a rare but serious illness. As with any drug, if you are pregnant or nursing a baby, seek the advice of a health professional before using this product. Do not take this product for pain for more than 10 days unless directed by a doctor. If pain or fever persists or gets worse, if new symptoms occur, or if redness or swelling is present, consult a doctor because these could be signs of a serious condition. Do not take this product if you are allergic to salicylates (including aspirin), have stomach problems (such as heartburn, upset stomach, or stomach pain) that persist or recur, or if you have ulcers or bleeding problems, unless directed by a doctor. If ringing in the ears or a loss of hearing occurs, consult a doctor before taking any more of this product.
KEEP THIS AND ALL MEDICINES OUT OF THE REACH OF CHILDREN. In case of accidental overdose, seek professional assistance or contact a Poison Control Center immediately.

Drug Interaction Precaution: Do not take this product if you are taking a prescription drug for anticoagulation (thinning of the blood), diabetes, gout, or arthritis unless directed by a doctor.

Active Ingredient: Each caplet contains Magnesium Salicylate Tetrahydrate 580 mg. (equivalent to 467.2 mg. of anhydrous Magnesium Salicylate).

Also Contains: Magnesium Stearate, Microcrystalline Cellulose, Opadry White, Polyethylene Glycol, Stearic Acid.
Shown in Product Identification Guide, page 407

Extra Strength
DOAN'S® P.M.
Magnesium Salicylate/
Diphenhydramine
Analgesic/Sleep Aid Caplets

Indications: For temporary relief of minor back pain accompanied by sleeplessness.

Directions: Adults and children 12 years of age or older: Take 2 caplets with water at bedtime if needed, or as directed by a doctor.

Warnings: Children and teenagers should not use this medicine for chicken pox or flu symptoms before a doctor is consulted about Reye syndrome, a rare but serious illness. **KEEP THIS AND ALL OTHER MEDICATIONS OUT OF THE REACH OF CHILDREN.** IN CASE OF ACCIDENTAL OVERDOSE, SEEK PROFESSIONAL ASSISTANCE OR CONTACT A POISON CONTROL CENTER IMMEDIATELY. DO NOT GIVE THIS PRODUCT TO CHILDREN UNDER 12 YEARS OF AGE. As with any drug, if you are pregnant or nursing a baby, seek the advice of a health professional before using this product. Do not take this product for pain for more than 10 days unless directed by a doctor. If pain or fever persists or gets worse, if new symptoms occur, or if redness or swelling is present, consult a doctor because these could be signs of a serious condition. If sleeplessness persists continuously for more than 2 weeks, consult your doctor. Insomnia may be a symptom of serious underlying medical illness. Do not take this product if you have asthma, glaucoma, emphysema, chronic pulmonary disease, shortness of breath, difficulty in breathing, or difficulty in urination due to enlargement of the prostate gland, stomach problems (such as heartburn, upset stomach, or stomach pain) that persist or recur, ulcers or bleeding problems, or if you are allergic to aspirin or salicylates unless directed by a doctor. If ringing in the ears or a loss of hearing occurs, consult a doctor before taking any more of this product. Avoid alcoholic beverages while taking this product. Do not take this product if you are taking sedatives or tranquilizers without first consulting your doctor.

Drug Interaction Precaution: Do not take this product if you are taking a prescription drug for anticoagulation (thinning of the blood), diabetes, gout, or arthritis unless directed by a doctor.

Active Ingredients: Each caplet contains Magnesium Salicylate Tetrahydrate 580mg. (equivalent to 467.2mg. of anhydrous Magnesium Salicylate) and Diphenydramine HCl 25mg.

Also Contains: Carnauba Wax, Colloidal Silicon Dioxide, Croscarmellose Sodium, Microcrystalline Cellulose, Magnesium Stearate, Opadry Blue, Stearic Acid, Talc.
Shown in Product Identification Guide, page 407

Continued on next page

The full prescribing information for each CIBA Consumer Pharmaceuticals product is contained herein and is that in effect as of December 15, 1993

CIBA Consumer—Cont.

REGULAR STRENGTH DOAN'S®
Analgesic Caplets

Indications: For temporary relief of occasional minor backache pain.

Directions: Adults—Two caplets every 4 hours as needed, not to exceed 12 caplets during a 24-hour period or as directed by a physician. Not intended for use by children or teenagers except under the advice of a physician. If pain persists for more than 10 days, discontinue use and consult your physician.

Warning: Children and teenagers should not use this medicine for chicken pox or flu symptoms before a doctor is consulted about Reye syndrome, a rare but serious illness. As with any drug, if you are pregnant or nursing a baby, seek the advice of a health professional before using this product. Do not use this product if you are under medical care or are allergic to aspirin or salicylates, except under the advice and supervision of your physician. **KEEP THIS AND ALL MEDICINES OUT OF THE REACH OF CHILDREN.** In case of accidental overdose, seek professional assistance or consult a Poison Control Center immediately.

Active Ingredient: Each caplet contains Magnesium Salicylate 325 mg.

Also Contains: Magnesium Stearate, Microcrystalline Cellulose, Opadry Light Green, Polyethylene Glycol, Stearic Acid.
Store at 15°–30°C (59°–86°F). PROTECT FROM MOISTURE.
Shown in Product Identification Guide, page 407

DULCOLAX®
[dul'co-lax]
brand of bisacodyl USP
Tablets of 5 mg
Suppositories of 10 mg
Laxative

Ingredients: Each enteric coated tablet contains: Active: Bisacodyl USP 5 mg. Also contains: Acacia, acetylated monoglyceride, carnauba wax, cellulose acetate phthalate, corn starch, D&C Red No. 30 aluminum lake, D&C Yellow No. 10 aluminum lake, dibutyl phthalate, docusate sodium, gelatin, glycerin, iron oxides, kaolin, lactose, magnesium stearate, methylparaben, pharmaceutical glaze, polyethylene glycol, povidone, propylparaben, sodium benzoate, sorbitan monooleate, sucrose, talc, titanium dioxide, white wax.
Each suppository contains: Active: Bisacodyl USP 10 mg. Also contains: Hydrogenated vegetable oil.
SODIUM CONTENT: Tablets and suppositories contain less than 0.2 mg per dosage unit and are thus dietetically sodium free.

Indications: For the relief of occasional constipation and irregularity. Physicians should refer to the "Professional Labeling" section for additional indications and information.

Directions:
Tablets
Adults and children 12 years of age and over: Take 2 or 3 tablets (usually 2) in a single dose once daily.
Children 6 to under 12 years of age: Take 1 tablet once daily.
Children under 6 years of age: Consult a physician.
Expect results in 8–12 hours if taken at bedtime or within 6 hours if taken before breakfast.
Suppositories
Adults and children 12 years of age and over: 1 suppository once daily. Remove foil wrapper. Lie on your side and, with pointed end first, push suppository high into the rectum so it will not slip out. Retain it for 15 to 20 minutes. If you feel the suppository must come out immediately, it was not inserted high enough and should be pushed higher.
Children 6 to under 12 years of age: ½ suppository once daily.
Children under 6 years of age: Consult a physician.
If the suppository seems soft, hold in foil wrapper under cold water for one or two minutes. In the presence of anal fissures or hemorrhoids, suppository may be coated at the tip with petroleum jelly before insertion.

Warnings: Do not use laxative products when abdominal pain, nausea, or vomiting are present unless directed by a physician. The process of restoring normal bowel function by use of a laxative may result in some abdominal discomfort. Laxative products should not be used for a period longer than 1 week unless directed by a physician. Rectal bleeding or failure to have a bowel movement after use of a laxative may indicate a serious condition. If this occurs, discontinue use and consult your physician. As with any drug, if you are pregnant or nursing a baby, seek the advice of a health care professional before using this product. KEEP THIS AND ALL MEDICATION OUT OF THE REACH OF CHILDREN. In case of accidental overdose or ingestion, seek professional assistance or contact a poison control center immediately. For tablets: Do not chew or crush. Do not give to children under 6 years of age unless directed by a physician. Do not take this product within 1 hour after taking an antacid or milk.

How Supplied: Dulcolax, brand of bisacodyl: Yellow, enteric-coated tablets of 5 mg in boxes of 10, 25, 50 and 100; suppositories of 10 mg in boxes of 4, 8, 16 and 50.

NDC 0083-6200 (tablets)
NDC 0083-6100 (suppositories)

Note: Store Dulcolax suppositories and tablets at temperatures below 77°F (25°C). Avoid excessive humidity.

Also Available: Dulcolax® Bowel Prep Kit. Each kit contains:
1 Dulcolax suppository of 10 mg bisacodyl;
4 Dulcolax tablets of 5 mg bisacodyl;
Complete patient instructions.

PROFESSIONAL LABELING:

Description and Clinical Pharmacology: Dulcolax is a contact stimulant laxative, administered either orally or rectally, which acts directly on the colonic mucosa to produce normal peristalsis throughout the large intestine. The active ingredient in Dulcolax, bisacodyl, is a colorless, tasteless compound that is practically insoluble in water or alkaline solution. Its chemical name is: bis(p-acetoxyphenyl)-2-pyridylmethane. Bisacodyl is very poorly absorbed, if at all, in the small intestine following oral administration, nor in the large intestine following rectal administration. On contact with the mucosa or submucosal plexi of the large intestine, bisacodyl stimulates sensory nerve endings to produce parasympathetic reflexes resulting in increased peristaltic contractions of the colon. It has also been shown to promote fluid and ion accumulation in the colon, which increases the laxative effect. A bowel movement is usually produced approximately 6 hours after oral administration (8–12 hours if taken at bedtime), and approximately 15 minutes to 1 hour after rectal administration, providing satisfactory cleansing of the bowel which may, under certain circumstances, obviate the need for colonic irrigation.

Indications and Usage: For use as part of a bowel cleansing regimen in preparing the patient for surgery or for preparing the colon for x-ray endoscopic examination. Dulcolax will not replace the colonic irrigations usually given patients before intracolonic surgery, but is useful in the preliminary emptying of the colon prior to these procedures.
Also for use as a laxative in postoperative care (i.e., restoration of normal bowel hygiene), antepartum care, postpartum care, and in preparation for delivery.

Contraindications: Stimulant laxatives, such as Dulcolax, are contraindicated for patients with acute surgical abdomen, appendicitis, rectal bleeding, or intestinal obstruction.

Precautions: Long-term administration of Dulcolax is not recommended in the treatment of chronic constipation.

Dosage and Administration:
Preparation for x-ray endoscopy: For barium enemas, no food should be given following oral administration to prevent reaccumulation of material in the cecum, and a suppository should be administered one to two hours prior to examination.
Children under 6 years of age: Oral administration is not recommended due to the requirement to swallow tablets

whole. For rectal administration, the suppository dosage is 5 mg (½ of 10 mg suppository) in a single daily dose.
Shown in Product Identification Guide, page 407

EFIDAC/24
Nasal decongestant

Indications: Provides temporary relief of nasal congestion due to the common cold, hay fever, or other upper respiratory allergies, and nasal congestion associated with sinusitis; reduces swelling of nasal passages; shrinks swollen membranes; relieves sinus pressure; and temporarily restores freer breathing through the nose.

Directions: Adults and children 12 years and over: Take just one tablet with fluid every 24 hours. DO NOT EXCEED ONE TABLET IN 24 HOURS. SWALLOW EACH TABLET WHOLE; DO NOT DIVIDE, CRUSH, CHEW, OR DISSOLVE THE TABLET. The tablet does not completely dissolve and may be seen in the stool (this is normal). Not for use in children under 12 years of age.

Warnings: DO NOT EXCEED RECOMMENDED DOSAGE because at higher doses nervousness, dizziness, or sleeplessness may occur. Do not take this product for more than 7 days. If symptoms do not improve or are accompanied by fever, consult a physician. Do not take this product if you have heart disease, high blood pressure, thyroid disease, diabetes, or difficulty in urination due to enlargement of the prostate gland, unless directed by a physician.
Rarely, tablets of this kind may cause bowel obstruction (blockage), usually in people with severe narrowing of the bowel (esophagus, stomach or intestine). If you have had obstruction or narrowing of the bowel, do not take this product without consulting your physician. Contact your physician if you experience persistent abdominal pain or vomiting. As with any drug, if you are pregnant or nursing a baby, seek the advice of a health professional before using this product.
KEEP THIS AND ALL DRUGS OUT OF THE REACH OF CHILDREN. In case of accidental overdose, seek professional assistance or contact a Poison Control Center immediately.

Drug Interaction Precaution: Do not take this product if you are presently taking a prescription drug for high blood pressure or depression, or any product containing a decongestant, without first consulting your physician.
Store in a dry place between 4°–30°C (39°–86°F).
QUESTIONS? Please write Consumer Affairs at the address below.

Distributed by: Ciba Consumer Pharmaceuticals, 581 Main Street, Woodbridge, NJ 07095

Inactive Ingredients: Cellulose, cellulose acetate, FD&C Blue #1, hydroxypropl cellulose, hydroxypropl methylcellulose, magnesium stearate, polyethylene glycol, polysorbate 80, povidone, sodium chloride, and titanium dioxide.
Shown in Product Identification Guide, page 407

EUCALYPTAMINT®
Arthritis Pain Reliever
Maximum Strength
External Analgesic

Description: Maximum Strength topical analgesic that provides hours of effective relief.

Active Ingredient: Natural Menthol (16%)

Inactive Ingredients: Lanolin and Eucalyptus Oil

Indications: For the temporary relief of minor aches and pains of muscles and joints associated with arthritis.

Directions: Adults and children 2 years of age and older: Gently massage a conservative amount into affected area not more than 3 to 4 times daily. Children under 2 years of age: Consult a physician.

Warning: FOR EXTERNAL USE ONLY. Avoid contact with eyes. Do not apply to wounds or damaged skin. Do not bandage tightly. Do not use with heating pads or heating devices. If condition worsens, or if symptoms persist for more than 7 days, discontinue use of this product and consult a physician. Keep this and all drugs out of the reach of children. In case of accidental ingestion, seek professional assistance or contact a Poison Control Center immediately. Store at room temperature 15°–30°C (59°–86°F). Do not freeze. It is normal for the consistency of Eucalyptamint to vary with temperature changes. If thickening does occur, warm the tube in the palms of your hands or run under warm water.

How Supplied: Eucalyptamint Ointment is supplied in a 2 oz. easy to squeeze tube.
Shown in Product Identification Guide, page 407

EUCALYPTAMINT®
Muscle Pain Relief Formula
External Analgesic

Description: A uniquely scented gel creme formulation providing hours of effective pain relief for overworked muscles.

Active Ingredient: Menthol 8%

Other Ingredients: Carbomer 980, Eucalyptus Oil, Fragrance, Propylene Glycol, SD 3A Alcohol, Triethanolamine, TWEEN 80, Water.

Indications: For the temporary relief of minor aches and pains of muscles associated with simple backache, strains, sprains and sports injuries.

Directions: Adults and children 2 years of age and older. Shake tube with cap facing downward. Gently massage a conservative amount into affected area not more than 3 to 4 times daily. Children under 2 years of age: Consult a physician.

Warning: FOR EXTERNAL USE ONLY. Avoid contact with eyes. Do not apply to wounds or damaged skin. Do not bandage tightly. Do not use with heating pads or heating devices. If condition worsens, or if symptoms persist for more than 7 days, discontinue use of this product and consult a physician. Keep this and all drugs out of the reach of children. In case of accidental ingestion, seek professional assistance or contact a Poison Control Center immediately. Store at room temperature 15°–30°C (59°–86°F). DO NOT FREEZE.

How Supplied: Eucalyptamint Muscle Pain Relief Formula is supplied in 2.25 oz. bottles and is available in two scents: Alpine Breeze and Powder Fresh. *Eucalyptamint is a registered trademark of Ciba-Geigy.*
Shown in Product Identification Guide, page 407

FIBERALL® Chewable Tablets
[fi'ber-all]
Lemon Creme Flavor

Description: Fiberall Chewable Tablets are a bulk-forming, nonirritant laxative which contain less than 1.5 grams of sugar per tablet. The active ingredient is calcium polycarbophil, a bulk-forming man-made fiber. The smooth gelatinous bulk formed by Fiberall Chewable Tablets encourages peristaltic activity and a more normal elimination of the bowel contents.
The recommended dose of one tablet contains the equivalent to 1 gram of polycarbophil.

Inactive Ingredients: Crospovidone, dextrose, flavors, magnesium stearate and yellow No. 10 aluminum lake. Each dose contains less than 1 mg of sodium, 225 mg of calcium and less than 6 calories.

Indications: Fiberall Chewable Tablets are indicated for the management of chronic constipation, temporary constipation caused by illness or pregnancy, irritable bowel syndrome, and for constipation related to duodenal ulcer or diverticulosis. Fiberall Chewable Tablets are

Continued on next page

The full prescribing information for each CIBA Consumer Pharmaceuticals product is contained herein and is that in effect as of December 15, 1993

CIBA Consumer—Cont.

also indicated for stool softening in patients with hemorrhoids or after anorectal surgery.

Actions: After the tablet is chewed it readily disperses and acts without irritants or stimulants. Polycarbophil absorbs water in the gastrointestinal tract to form a gelatinous bulk which encourages a more normal bowel movement.

Directions: Take this product (child or adult dose) with at least 8 ounces (a full glass) of water or other fluid. Taking this product without enough liquid may cause choking. See Warnings.

Dosage and Administration: *Adults and children 12 years and older:* chew and swallow 1 tablet, 1–4 times a day. *Children 6 to under 12 years:* one-half the usual adult dose or as recommended by a physician. *Children under 6:* consult a physician. **Drink a full glass (8 fl oz) of liquid with each dose.** Drinking additional liquid helps Fiberall work even more effectively. Continued use for 2 to 3 days may be desired for maximum laxative benefits.

Warnings: Taking this product without adequate fluid may cause it to swell and block your throat or esophagus and may cause choking. Do not take this product if you have difficulty in swallowing. If you experience chest pain, vomiting or difficulty in swallowing or breathing after taking this product, seek immediate medical attention.

Contraindications: Fecal impaction or intestinal obstruction. Any disease state in which consumption of extra calcium is contraindicated.

Drug Interactions: This product contains calcium, which may interact with some forms of TETRACYCLINE if taken concomitantly. The tetracycline product should be taken 1 hour before or 2–3 hours after taking a Fiberall Chewable Tablet.

How Supplied: Boxes containing 18 tablets.

FIBERALL® Fiber Wafers
[fi'ber-all]
Fruit & Nut, Oatmeal Raisin

Description: Fiberall Fiber Wafers are a bulk-forming, nonirritant laxative. The active ingredient is psyllium hydrophilic mucilloid, a dietary fiber extracted from the seed husk of blond psyllium seed *(Plantago ovata)*. The smooth gelatinous bulk formed by Fiberall Wafers encourages peristaltic activity and a more normal elimination of the bowel contents.
One (1) Fiberall Fiber Wafer contains 3.4 g of psyllium hydrophilic mucilloid in a good-tasting wafer form, of which approximately 2.2 g is soluble fiber. One wafer is equivalent to one teaspoonful of Fiberall Powder.

Inactive Ingredients: Fruit & Nut Flavor: Baking powder, brown sugar, butter flavor, cinnamon, corn syrup, crisp rice, dried ground apricots, flour, glycerin, granulated sugar, granulated walnuts, lecithin, margarine, molasses, oats, salt, vegetable oil shortening (soybean and cottonseed oil), water and wheat bran. Fiberall Fruit & Nut Fiber Wafers contain approximately 79 calories and 110 mg of sodium per wafer.
Oatmeal Raisin Flavor: Baking powder, cinnamon, cinnamon flavor, cloves, corn syrup, flour, glycerin, granulated sugar, lecithin, molasses, oats, raisins, vegetable oil shortening (soybean and cottonseed oil), water and wheat bran. Fiberall Oatmeal Raisin Fiber Wafers contain approximately 78 calories and 30 mg of sodium per wafer.

Indications: Fiberall Fiber Wafers are indicated for the management of chronic constipation, temporary constipation caused by illness or pregnancy, irritable bowel syndrome, and for constipation related to duodenal ulcer or diverticulosis. Fiberall Wafers are also indicated for stool softening in patients with hemorrhoids or after anorectal surgery.

Actions: The homogenous high-fiber formula of Fiberall Fiber Wafers, eaten with 8 oz of a beverage of the patient's choice, acts without irritants or stimulants in the gastrointestinal tract.

Directions: Take this product (child or adult dose) with at least 8 ounces (a full glass) of water or other fluid. Taking this product without enough liquid may cause choking. See Warnings.

Dosage and Administration: The recommended dosage for adults is one to two Fiberall Fiber Wafers 1 to 3 times daily, with a full 8 oz glass of water or other liquid with each wafer. The recommended daily dose for children 6 to under 12 years old is one-half the usual adult dose (with liquid), or as recommended by a physician. For children under 6, consult a physician. Drinking additional liquid is recommended and helps Fiberall work even more effectively. Two to three days' usage may be required for optimal laxative benefits.

Warnings: Taking this product without adequate fluid may cause it to swell and block your throat or esophagus and may cause choking. Do not take this product if you have difficulty in swallowing. If you experience chest pain, vomiting or difficulty in swallowing or breathing after taking this product, seek immediate medical attention.

Contraindications: Fecal impaction or intestinal obstruction.

Precaution: As with any grain product, inhaled or ingested psyllium powder may cause an allergic reaction in individuals sensitive to it.

How Supplied: Boxes containing 14 wafers.

Shown in Product Identification Guide, page 407

FIBERALL® Powder, Orange or Natural Flavor
[fi'ber-all]

Description: Fiberall is a bulk-forming, nonirritant laxative which contains no sugar. The active ingredient is psyllium hydrophilic mucilloid, a dietary fiber extracted from the seed husk of blond psyllium seed *(Plantago ovata)*. The smooth gelatinous bulk formed by Fiberall encourages peristaltic activity and a more normal elimination of the bowel contents.
The recommended dose contains 3.4 g psyllium hydrophilic mucilloid, of which approximately 2.2 g is soluble fiber.

Inactive Ingredients: Natural Flavor: Citric acid, flavor, polysorbate 60 and wheat bran. Orange Flavor: Beta-carotene, citric acid, flavor, polysorbate 60, saccharin, wheat bran and yellow No. 6 lake. Each dose contains less than 10 mg of sodium, less than 60 mg of potassium, and provides less than 6 calories (10 calories for Orange).

Indications: Fiberall is indicated for the management of chronic constipation, temporary constipation caused by illness or pregnancy, irritable bowel syndrome, and for constipation related to duodenal ulcer or diverticulosis. Fiberall is also indicated for stool softening in patients with hemorrhoids or after anorectal surgery.

Actions: The homogenous, high-fiber formula of Fiberall is readily dispersed in liquids and acts without irritants or stimulants in the gastro-intestinal tract.

Directions: Take this product (child or adult dose) with at least 8 ounces (a full glass) of water or other fluid. Taking this product without enough liquid may cause choking. See Warnings.

Dosage and Administration:
Adults: Natural: Place one scoopful filled to the line (5 g) or one slightly rounded teaspoonful in a glass and add 8 oz. of cool water or other liquid. Stir to mix. Orange: Place one level scoopful (5.9 g) or one rounded teaspoonful in glass and add liquid as above. Take orally one to three times daily according to individual response.
Children 6 to under 12 years old: One-half the usual adult dose (with liquid) or as recommended by a physician. Drinking additional liquid is recommended and helps Fiberall work even more effectively. Two to three days' usage may be required for maximum laxative benefits.
New Users: Start by taking 1 dose each day. Gradually increase to 3 doses per day if needed or recommended by doctor. If minor gas or bloating occurs, reduce the amount taken until system adjusts.

Warnings: Taking this product without adequate fluid may cause it to swell and block your throat or esophagus and may cause choking. Do not take this product if you have difficulty in swallowing. If you experience chest pain, vomiting or difficulty in swallowing or breathing after taking this product, seek immediate medical attention.

Contraindications: Fecal impaction or intestinal obstruction.

Precaution: As with any grain product, inhaled or ingested psyllium powder may cause an allergic reaction in individuals sensitive to it.

How Supplied: Powder, in 10 or 15 oz containers.

Shown in Product Identification Guide, page 407

ISOCLOR® TIMESULE® Capsules
[*īs 'ŏ-klŏr*]

Active Ingredients: Chlorpheniramine maleate 8 mg and phenylpropanolamine hydrochloride 75 mg.

Inactive Ingredients: Benzyl alcohol, butyl paraben, edetate calcium disodium, gelatin, methyl paraben, pharmaceutical glaze, propyl paraben, sodium lauryl sulfate, sodium propiomate, starch, sucrose and other ingredients.

Indications: For the temporary relief of nasal congestion due to the common cold, hay fever, or other upper respiratory allergies and associated with sinusitis. Helps decongest sinus openings, sinus passages and promotes nasal and/or sinus drainage; temporarily restores freer breathing through the nose. For the temporary relief of running nose, sneezing, itching of the nose or throat, and itchy and watery eyes as may occur in allergic rhinitis (such as hay fever).

Warnings: Do not give this product to children under 12 years except under the advice and supervision of a physician. Do not exceed the recommended dosage because at higher doses, nervousness, dizziness, or sleeplessness may occur. If symptoms do not improve within seven days or are accompanied by high fever, consult a physician before continuing use. Do not take this product if you have high blood pressure, heart disease, diabetes, thyroid disease, asthma, glaucoma or difficulty in urination due to enlargement of the prostate gland except under the advice and supervision of a physician. Do not take this product if you are taking another medication containing phenylpropanolamine. Avoid alcoholic beverages while taking this product. Avoid driving a motor vehicle or operating heavy machinery. This preparation may cause drowsiness; this preparation may cause excitability, especially in children. As with any drug, if you are pregnant or nursing a baby, seek the advice of a health professional before using this product.
Keep this and all drugs out of the reach of children. In case of accidental overdose, seek professional assistance or contact a Poison Control Center immediately.

Drug Interaction Precaution: Do not take this product if you are presently taking a prescription antihypertensive or antidepressant drug containing a monoamine oxidase inhibitor except under the advice and supervision of a physician.

Directions: Adults and children over 12 years of age: one capsule every 12 hours. Do not exceed two capsules in 24 hours.

How Supplied: Packaged on blister cards in cartons of 10's and 20's, and bottles of 100.
ISOCLOR® and TIMESULE® are registered trademarks of Ciba-Geigy Corporation.
Distributed by:
Ciba Consumer Pharmaceuticals

MYOFLEX® EXTERNAL ANALGESIC CREME
[*mī 'ō-flex*]

Description: Odorless, stainless and non-burning topical pain reliever.

Active Ingredient: Trolamine salicylate 10%.

Other Ingredients: Cetyl alcohol, disodium EDTA, fragrance, propylene glycol, purified water, sodium lauryl sulfate, stearyl alcohol, white wax.

Indications: For the temporary relief of minor aches and pains of muscles and joints associated with simple backache, arthritis, strains and sprains.

Warning: FOR EXTERNAL USE ONLY. Do not apply to irritated skin or if excessive irritation develops. Avoid contact with eyes. If condition worsens, or if symptoms persist for more than 7 days or clear up and occur again within a few days, discontinue use of this product and consult a physician. Keep this and all other medication out of the reach of children. In case of accidental ingestion, seek professional assistance or contact a Poison Control Center immediately. As with any drug, if you are pregnant or nursing a baby, seek the advice of a health professional before using this product. Protect from freezing or excessive heat. Store at controlled room temperature 15°–30°C (59°–86°F).

Directions: Use only as directed. **Adults and children 2 years of age and older:** Apply to affected area not more than three to four times daily. Affected areas may be wrapped loosely with two- or three-inch elastic bandage. **Children under 2 years of age:** Consult a physician.

How Supplied: Myoflex Creme is supplied in 2 oz. and 4 oz. easy-squeeze tubes, and 8 oz. and 16 oz. jars.
MYOFLEX is a registered trademark of Ciba-Geigy Corporation.

Shown in Product Identification Guide, page 407

NŌSTRIL® Nasal Decongestant
[*nō 'stril*]
phenylephrine HCl, USP

Active Ingredient: phenylephrine HCl 0.25% (¼% Mild strength) or phenylephrine HCl 0.5% (½% Regular strength). Also contains benzalkonium chloride 0.004% as a preservative, boric acid, sodium borate, water.

Indications: For temporary relief of nasal congestion due to the common cold, hay fever, other upper respiratory allergies, or associated with sinusitis.

Actions: NŌSTRIL metered pump spray for nasal decongestion delivers measured, uniform doses. The medication constricts the smaller arterioles of the nasal passages, producing a gentle, predictable, decongestant effect. Nōstril penetrates and shrinks swollen membranes, restoring freer breathing and unclogs sinus passages, bringing the effective medication in contact with inflamed, swollen tissues. It will not hurt tender membranes since it is formulated to match the pH of normal nasal secretions. The one-way pump helps prevent draw-back contamination of the medication.

Warnings: Do not exceed recommended dosage because burning, stinging, sneezing, or increased nasal discharge may occur. Do not use for more than 3 days. If symptoms persist, consult a physician. Use of the dispenser by more than one person may spread infection. Do not use this product if you have heart disease, high blood pressure, thyroid disease, diabetes or difficulty in urination due to enlargement of the prostate gland, unless directed by a physician. Keep this and all drugs out of reach of children.

Symptoms and Treatment of Oral Overdosage: In case of accidental ingestion, seek professional assistance or consult a poison control center immediately.

Dosage and Administration:
¼% Mild—Adults and children 6 to under 12 years of age (with adult supervision): 2 or 3 sprays in each nostril not more often than every 4 hours. Children under 6 years of age: consult a doctor.
½% Regular—Adults: 2 or 3 sprays in each nostril not more often than every 4 hours. Do not give to children under 12 years of age unless directed by a doctor. Remove protective cap. Hold bottle with thumb at base and nozzle between first and second fingers. With head upright, insert nozzle into nostril. Depress pump 2 or 3 times, all the way down, and sniff deeply. Repeat in other nostril. Before

Continued on next page

The full prescribing information for each CIBA Consumer Pharmaceuticals product is contained herein and is that in effect as of December 15, 1993

CIBA Consumer—Cont.

using the first time, prime pump by depressing it firmly several times.

How Supplied: Metered nasal pump spray in white plastic bottles of ½ fl. oz. (15 ml) packaged in tamper-resistant outer cartons.

0.25% (¼% Mild strength) for children 6 years and over and adults who prefer a milder decongestant.

0.5% (½% Regular strength) for adults and children 12 years or older.

Shown in Product Identification Guide, page 407

NŌSTRILLA® Long Acting
[*nō-stril 'a*]
Nasal Decongestant
oxymetazoline HCl, USP

Active Ingredient: oxymetazoline HCl 0.05%. Also contains benzalkonium chloride 0.02% as a preservative, glycine, sorbitol solution, water. (Mercury preservatives are not used in this product.)

Indications: For temporary relief of nasal congestion due to the common cold, hay fever, other upper respiratory allergies, or associated with sinusitis.

Actions: NŌSTRILLA metered pump spray for nasal decongestion delivers measured, uniform doses. The medication constricts the smaller arterioles of the nasal passages, producing a prolonged (up to 12 hours), gentle, predictable, decongestant effect. Nōstrilla penetrates and shrinks swollen membranes, restoring freer breathing and unclogs sinus passages, bringing the effective medication in contact with inflamed, swollen tissues. It will not hurt tender membranes since it is formulated to match the pH of normal nasal secretions. Use at bedtime restores freer nasal breathing through the night. The one-way pump helps prevent draw-back contamination of the medication.

Warnings: Do not exceed recommended dosage because burning, stinging, sneezing or increased nasal discharge may occur. Do not use for more than 3 days. If symptoms persist, consult a physician. Use of the dispenser by more than one person may spread infection. Do not use this product if you have heart disease, high blood pressure, thyroid disease, diabetes or difficulty in urination due to enlargement of the prostate gland unless directed by a doctor. Keep this and all drugs out of reach of children.

Symptoms and Treatment of Oral Overdosage: In case of accidental ingestion, seek professional assistance or contact a poison control center immediately.

Dosage and Administration: Adults and children 6 to under 12 years of age (with adult supervision): 2 or 3 sprays in each nostril not more often than every

10 to 12 hours. Do not exceed 2 applications in any 24-hour period. Children under 6 years of age: consult a doctor. Remove protective cap. Hold bottle with thumb at base and nozzle between first and second fingers. With head upright, insert nozzle into nostril. Depress pump 2 or 3 times, all the way down, and sniff deeply. Repeat in other nostril. Before using the first time, prime pump by depressing it firmly several times.

How Supplied: Metered nasal pump spray in white plastic bottles of ½ fl. oz. (15 ml) packaged in tamper-resistant outer cartons.

NUPERCAINAL®
Dibucaine
Hemorrhoidal and Anesthetic
Ointment

Active Ingredient: 1% dibucaine USP. Also contains: acetone sodium bisulfite, lanolin, light mineral oil, purified water, and white petrolatum.

Indications: For prompt, temporary relief of pain, itching and burning due to hemorrhoids or other anorectal disorders. May also be used topically for temporary relief of pain and itching associated with sunburn, minor burns, cuts, scrapes, insect bites, or minor skin irritation.

Directions: Adults: When practical, cleanse the affected area with mild soap and water and rinse thoroughly. Gently dry by patting or blotting with toilet tissue or a soft cloth before application of this product. Puncture tube seal with cap or sharp object. Apply externally to the affected area up to 3 or 4 times daily. Children 2–12: Do not use except under the advice and supervision of a physician. DO NOT USE IN INFANTS UNDER 2 YEARS OF AGE OR LESS THAN 35 LBS. WEIGHT.

Warnings: IF SWALLOWED, CONSULT A PHYSICIAN OR POISON CONTROL CENTER IMMEDIATELY. **Do not use in or near the eyes.** If condition worsens or does not improve within 7 days, consult a physician. Do not put this product into the rectum by using fingers or any mechanical device. Do not exceed recommended daily dosage unless directed by a physician. Certain persons can develop allergic reactions to ingredients in this product. If the symptom being treated does not subside or if redness, irritation, swelling, pain, bleeding or other symptoms develop or increase, discontinue use and consult a physician promptly. As with any drug, if you are pregnant or nursing a baby, seek the advice of a health care professional before using this product. KEEP THIS AND ALL MEDICATION OUT OF REACH OF CHILDREN.

How Supplied: Nupercainal Hemorrhoidal and Anesthetic Ointment is available in tamper-evident packaged tubes of 1 and 2 ounces. See crimp of tube

for lot number and expiration date. Store between 15°–30°C (59°–86°F).
NDC 0083-5812.

Shown in Product Identification Guide, page 408

NUPERCAINAL
HYDROCORTISONE 1% CREAM
Anti-Itch Cream

Indications: For the temporary relief of external anal itching. May also be used for the temporary relief of itching associated with minor skin irritations and rashes due to eczema, insect bites, poison ivy, poison oak, poison sumac, soaps, detergents, cosmetics, jewelry, seborrheic dermatitis, or psoriarsis. Other uses of this product should be only under the advice and supervision of a physician.

Directions: Adults: When practical, cleanse the affected area with mild soap and warm water and rinse thoroughly. Gently dry by patting or blotting with toilet tissue or a soft cloth before application of this product. Apply to affected area not more than 3 to 4 times daily. Children under 12 years of age: Consult a physician.

Warnings: For external use only. Avoid contact with the eyes. If condition worsens, or if symptoms persist for more than 7 days or clear up and occur again within a few days, stop use of this product and do not begin use of any other hydrocortisone product unless you consulted a physician. Do not use for the treatment of diaper rash; consult a physician. Do not exceed the recommended daily dosage unless directed by a physician. In case of bleeding, consult a physician promptly. Do not put this product into the rectum by using fingers or any mechanical device or applicator. KEEP THIS AND ALL MEDICATION OUT OF REACH OF CHILDREN. In case of accidental ingestion, seek professional assistance or contact a poison control center immediately.

Inactive Ingredients: Cetostearyl Alcohol, Sodium Lauryl Sulfate, White Petrolatum, Propylene Glycol, Purified Water.

Store at room temperature 15–30°C (59°–86°F).

Questions? Write to Consumer Affairs at the address below.

Distributed by: Ciba Consumer Pharmaceuticals, 581 Main Street, Woodbridge, NJ 07095
Made in Canada

Shown in Product Identification Guide, page 407

NUPERCAINAL®
Pain Relief Cream

Active Ingredient: 0.5% dibucaine USP.

Also contains: acetone sodium bisulfite, fragrance, glycerin, potassium hydroxide, purified water, stearic acid, and trolamine.

Indications: For prompt, temporary relief of pain and itching due to sunburn, minor burns, cuts, scrapes, scratches, and nonpoisonous insect bites.

Directions: Puncture tube seal with cap or sharp object. Apply to affected area, rub in gently. **Do not use in or near eyes.**

Caution: IF SWALLOWED, CONSULT A PHYSICIAN OR POISON CONTROL CENTER IMMEDIATELY. Not for prolonged use. Not more than $\frac{2}{3}$ tube should be applied in 24 hours for adults or $\frac{1}{6}$ tube to a child. If the symptom being treated does not subside or rash, irritation, swelling, pain, or other symptoms develop or increase, discontinue use and consult a physician.

How Supplied: Nupercainal Pain-Relief Cream is available in tamper-evident packaged tubes of $1\frac{1}{2}$ ounces. See crimp of tube for lot number and expiration date. NDC 0083-5830-91.

Shown in Product Identification Guide, page 407

NUPERCAINAL®
Suppositories

Indications: Nupercainal Rectal Suppositories give temporary relief of itching, burning, and discomfort associated with hemorrhoids or other anorectal disorders.

Each suppository contains 2.1 grams cocoa butter, NF and .25 gram zinc oxide. Also contains acetone sodium bisulfite and bismuth subgallate.

Directions: ADULTS—When practical, cleanse the affected area. Tear one suppository at the "V" cut, peel foil downward and remove foil wrapper before inserting into the rectum. Gently insert the suppository rectally, rounded end first. Use one suppository up to 6 times daily or after each bowel movement. CHILDREN UNDER 12 YEARS OF AGE—Consult a physician.

WARNING: IF ACCIDENTALLY SWALLOWED, CONSULT A PHYSICIAN OR POISON CONTROL CENTER IMMEDIATELY.
If condition worsens or does not improve within 7 days, consult a physician. Do not exceed the recommended daily dosage unless directed by a physician. In case of bleeding consult a physician promptly. As with any drug, if you are pregnant or nursing a baby, seek the advice of a health professional before using this product.
Keep this and all medications out of reach of children.
Nupercainal Suppositories are available in tamper-evident packages of 12 and 24. Do not store above 30°C (86°F).
C86-42 (Rev. 9/86)

OTRIVIN®
xylometazoline hydrochloride USP
Nasal Spray and Nasal Drops 0.1%
Pediatric Nasal Drops 0.05%
Nasal Decongestant

One application provides rapid and long-lasting relief of nasal congestion for up to 10 hours.
Quickly clears stuffy noses due to common cold, sinusitis, hay fever.
Nasal congestion can make life miserable—you can't breathe, smell, taste, or sleep comfortably. That is why Otrivin is so helpful. It clears away that stuffy feeling.
Otrivin has been prescribed by doctors for many years. Here is how you use it:
Nasal Spray 0.1%—for adults and children 12 years and older. Spray 2 or 3 times into each nostril every 8–10 hours. With head upright, squeeze sharply and firmly while inhaling (sniffing) through the nose. For adult use only.
Nasal Drops 0.1%—for adults and children 12 years and older. Put 2 or 3 drops into each nostril every 8 to 10 hours. Tilt head as far back as possible. Immediately bend head forward toward knees, hold for a few seconds, then return to upright position.
Do not give Nasal Spray 0.1% or Nasal Drops 0.1% to children under 12 years except under the advice and supervision of a physician.
Pediatric Nasal Drops 0.05%—for children 2 to 12 years of age. Put 2 or 3 drops into each nostril every 8 to 10 hours. Tilt head as far back as possible. Immediately bend head forward toward knees, hold a few seconds, then return to upright position.
Do not give this product to children under 2 years except under the advice and supervision of a physician.
Otrivin Nasal Spray/Nasal Drops contain 0.1% xylometazoline hydrochloride, USP. Also contains benzalkonium chloride, dibasic sodium phosphate, disodium edetate, monobasic sodium phosphate, purified water and sodium chloride. They are available in an unbreakable plastic spray package of 0.66 fl oz (20 ml) and in a plastic dropper bottle of 0.83 fl oz (25 ml).
Otrivin Pediatric Nasal Drops contain 0.05% xylometazoline hydrochloride, USP. Also contains benzalkonium chloride, dibasic sodium phosphate, disodium edetate, monobasic sodium phosphate, purified water and sodium chloride. It is available in a plastic dropper bottle of 0.83 fl oz (25 ml).

Warnings: Do not exceed recommended dosage, because symptoms such as burning, stinging, sneezing, or increase of nasal discharge may occur. Do not use this product for more than 3 days. If symptoms persist, consult a physician. The use of this dispenser by more than one person may cause infection.
Keep this and all medicines out of the reach of children. Overdosage in young children may cause marked sedation. In case of accidental ingestion, seek profes-

sional assistance or contact a Poison Control Center immediately.

Caution: Do not use if the clear overwrap with the name Otrivin® or the printed band on the bottle is missing or damaged.
Shown in Product Identification Guide, page 408

PRIVINE®
naphazoline hydrochloride, USP
0.05% Nasal Solution
0.05% Nasal Spray
Nasal Decongestant

Privine is a nasal decongestant that comes in three forms: Nasal Drops (in a bottle with a dropper), Nasal Spray (in a plastic squeeze bottle) and Nasal Solution (in a 16 fl oz bottle). All are for prompt, and prolonged relief of nasal congestion due to common colds, sinusitis, hay fever, etc.
Privine is an effective nasal decongestant **when you use it in the recommended dosage.** If you use too much, too long, or too often, Privine may be harmful to your nasal mucous membranes and cause burning, stinging, sneezing or an increased runny nose.
Do not use Privine by mouth.
IF NASAL STUFFINESS PERSISTS AFTER 3 DAYS OF TREATMENT, DISCONTINUE USE AND CONSULT A DOCTOR.
Keep this and all medications out of the reach of children. Do not use Privine in children under 12 years of age, except with the advice and supervision of a doctor.

Caution: Do not use Privine if you have glaucoma.
OVERDOSAGE IN YOUNG CHILDREN MAY CAUSE MARKED SEDATION AND IF SEVERE, EMERGENCY TREATMENT MAY BE NECESSARY. IN CASE OF ACCIDENTAL INGESTION, SEEK PROFESSIONAL ASSISTANCE OR CONTACT A POISON CONTROL CENTER IMMEDIATELY.
How to use Nasal Drops.
Use only 1 to 2 drops in each nostril. Do not repeat this dosage more than every 6 hours. Squeeze rubber bulb to fill dropper with proper amount of medication. For best results, tilt head as far back as possible and put 1 to 2 drops of solution into your right nostril. Then lean head forward, inhaling and turning your head to the left. Refill dropper by squeezing bulb. Now tilt head as far back as possible and put 1 to 2 drops of solution into your left nostril. Then lean head forward, inhaling, and turning your head to the right.

Continued on next page

The full prescribing information for each CIBA Consumer Pharmaceuticals product is contained herein and is that in effect as of December 15, 1993

CIBA Consumer—Cont.

The Privine dropper bottle is designed to make administration of the proper dosage easy. Privine will not cause sleeplessness, so you may use it before going to bed.

Important: After use, be sure to rinse the dropper with very hot water. This helps prevent contamination of the bottle with bacteria from nasal secretions. Use of the dispenser by more than one person may spread infection.

Note: Privine Nasal Solution may be used with glass, plastic, stainless steel and specially treated metals used in atomizers. Do not let the solution come in contact with reactive metals, especially aluminum. If solution becomes discolored, it should be discarded.

How to use Nasal Spray.

Spray 1 or 2 times in each nostril, not more often than every 6 hours. Avoid overdosage. Follow directions for use carefully. For best results do **not** shake the plastic squeeze bottle.

Remove cap. With head held upright, spray twice into each nostril. Squeeze the bottle sharply and firmly while sniffing through the nose.

Privine Nasal Drops contain 0.05% naphazoline HCl, USP. It also contains benzalkonium chloride, dibasic sodium phosphate, disodium edetate, monobasic sodium phosphate, purified water and sodium chloride.

Privine Nasal Solution contains 0.05% naphazoline hydrochloride, USP. It also contains benzalkonium chloride, disodium edetate dihydrate, hydrochloric acid, purified water, sodium chloride, and trolamine. It is available in bottles of 16 fl. oz. (473 ml).

Privine Nasal Spray contains 0.05% naphazoline hydrochloride USP. It also contains benzalkonium chloride, dibasic sodium phosphate, disodium edetate, monobasic sodium phosphate, purified water, and sodium chloride. It is available in plastic squeeze bottles of 0.66 fl oz (20 ml).

Caution: Do not use if the clear overwrap on the box with the name Privine® or the printed band on the bottle is missing or damaged.

Shown in Product Identification Guide, page 408

Q–VEL®
Muscle Relaxant/Pain Reliever

Active Ingredient: Quinine Sulfate 1 gr. (64.8 mg).

Contains: Vitamin E (400 I.U. *dl* -alpha tocopheryl acetate) in a lecithin base.

Indications: For prevention and temporary relief of night leg cramps.

Warnings: Do not take if pregnant or nursing a baby. Q-Vel is also not indicated for those sensitive to quinine or

under 12 years of age. Discontinue use and consult your physician if ringing in the ears, deafness, diarrhea, nausea, skin rash, bruising or visual disturbances occur. In case of accidental overdose, seek medical assistance or contact Poison Control Center at once. Keep this and all medicine out of reach of children.

Dosage: To prevent night leg cramps take 2 soft caplets after the evening meal plus 2 at bedtime. For relief in case of sudden attack, take 2 soft caplets at once plus 2 after ½ hour if needed. Do not exceed 4 soft caplets daily.

How Supplied: Bottles of 16, 30, 50 and 100 softgels.
Store at 15°–30°C (59°–86°F) and protect from moisture.

Shown in Product Identification Guide, page 408

SINAREST® TABLETS, EXTRA STRENGTH TABLETS AND NO DROWSINESS TABLETS
[*sīn 'a-rest*]

Active Ingredients:
Tablets —Acetaminophen 325 mg, chlorpheniramine maleate 2 mg, pseudoephedrine HCl 30 mg.
Extra Strength Tablets —Acetaminophen 500 mg, chlorpheniramine maleate 2 mg, pseudoephedrine HCl 30 mg.
No Drowsiness Tablets —Acetaminophen 500 mg, pseudoephedrine HCl 30 mg.

Other Ingredients:
All Products —Magnesium stearate, microcrystalline cellulose, povidone, pregelatinized starch.
Extra Strength and No Drowsiness Tablets also contain—Sodium starch glycolate. *Tablets and Extra Strength Tablets* also contain—Yellow 6 lake, Yellow 10 lake.

Indications:
Tablets and Extra Strength Tablets —Temporarily relieves nasal congestion, runny nose, sneezing, itching of the nose and throat, and itchy, watery eyes due to hay fever or other upper respiratory allergies, or associated with sinusitis. For temporary relief of minor aches, pains, and headache.
No Drowsiness Tablets —Temporarily relieves nasal congestion due to hay fever or other upper respiratory allergies, or associated with sinusitis. For temporary relief of minor aches, pains, and headache.

Warnings: *Tablets* —Do not take this product for more than 10 days (for adults) or 5 days (for children). *Extra Strength and No Drowsiness Tablets* —Do not take this product for more than 10 days. *All Products* —Do not exceed recommended dosage because at higher doses, nervousness, dizziness, or sleeplessness may occur. If symptoms do not improve or are accompanied by fever that lasts more than 3 days, or if new symptoms occur, consult a physician. Do not take this product if you have heart

disease, high blood pressure, thyroid disease, diabetes, or difficulty in urination due to enlargement of the prostate gland, unless directed by a physician. As with any drug, if you are pregnant or nursing a baby, seek the advice of a health professional before using this product. **Keep this and all drugs out of the reach of children.** In case of accidental overdose, seek professional assistance or contact a Poison Control Center immediately. Prompt medical attention is critical for adults as well as children even if you do not notice any signs or symptoms. Also, *Tablets and Extra Strength Tablets* —Do not take this product, unless directed by a physician, if you have a breathing problem such as emphysema or chronic bronchitis, or if you have glaucoma. May cause excitability, especially in children. May cause drowsiness; alcohol, sedatives, and tranquilizers may increase the drowsiness effect. Avoid alcoholic beverages while taking this product. Do not take this product if you are taking sedatives or tranquilizers, without first consulting your physician. Use caution when driving a motor vehicle or operating machinery.

Drug Interaction Precautions: *All Products* —Do not take this product if you are presently taking a prescription drug for high blood pressure or depression, without first consulting your physician.

Directions: Dose as follows while symptoms persist, or as directed by a physician.
Tablets —Adults and children 12 years of age and older: 2 tablets every 4–6 hours, not to exceed 8 tablets in 24 hours. Children 6 to under 12 years of age: 1 tablet every 4–6 hours, not to exceed 4 tablets in 24 hours. Children under 6 years of age: Consult a physician.
Extra Strength and No Drowsiness Tablets —Adults and children 12 years of age and older: 2 tablets every 6 hours, not to exceed 8 tablets in 24 hours. Children under 12 years of age: Consult a physician.

How Supplied:
Tablets —Boxes of 20, 40, and 80.
Extra Strength Tablets —Boxes of 24.
No Drowsiness Tablets —Boxes of 20.
SINAREST is a registered trademark of Ciba-Geigy Corporation

SLOW FE®
Slow Release Iron Tablets

Description: SLOW FE supplies ferrous sulfate for the treatment of iron deficiency and iron deficiency anemia with a significant reduction in the incidence of the common side effects of oral iron preparations. The wax matrix delivery system of SLOW FE is designed to maximize the release of ferrous sulfate in the duodenum and the jejunum where it is best tolerated and absorbed. SLOW FE has been clinically shown to be associated with a lower incidence of constipation, diarrhea and abdominal discomfort when compared to regular iron tablets and the leading capsule.

Formula: Each tablet contains 160 mg. dried ferrous sulfate USP, equivalent to 50 mg. elemental iron. Also contains cetostearyl alcohol, colloidal silicon dioxide, hydroxypropyl methylcellulose, shellac, lactose, magnesium stearate, polyethylene glycol.

Dosage: ADULTS—one or two tablets daily or as recommended by a physician. A maximum of four tablets daily may be taken. CHILDREN—one tablet daily. Tablets must be swallowed whole.

Warning: Close tightly and keep out of reach of children. Contains iron, which can be harmful or fatal to children in large doses. In case of accidental overdose, seek professional assistance or contact a Poison Control Center immediately. The treatment of any anemic condition should be on the advice and under the supervision of a physician. As oral iron products interfere with absorption of oral tetracycline antibiotics, these products should not be taken within two hours of each other. As with any drug, if you are pregnant or nursing a baby, seek the advice of a health professional before using this product.
Keep this and all medicines out of reach of children.
Tamper-Evident Packaging.

How Supplied: Blister packages of 30, 60, and child-resistant bottles of 100. Do Not Store Above 86°F. Protect From Moisture.
Shown in Product Identification Guide, page 408

SUNKIST® CHILDREN'S CHEWABLE MULTIVITAMINS— REGULAR

Vitamin Ingredients: Each tablet contains:
[See table above.]

Indication: Dietary supplementation.

Dosage and Administration: One chewable tablet daily for adults and children two years and older.

Warning: Phenylketonurics: Contains Phenylalanine

How Supplied: SUNKIST Children's Multivitamins-Regular are supplied in bottles of 60 chewable tablets with child resistant safety caps.
SUNKIST® is a registered trademark of SUNKIST Growers, Inc., Sherman Oaks, CA 91423. ©
Shown in Product Identification Guide, page 408

SUNKIST® CHILDREN'S CHEWABLE MULTIVITAMINS—PLUS EXTRA C

Vitamin Ingredients: Each tablet contains the ingredients of the Regular

VITAMINS	QUANTITY PER TABLET	PERCENT U.S. RDA	
		FOR CHILD. 2 TO 4 YRS OF AGE (1 TABLET)	FOR ADULTS & CHILD. OVER 4 YRS OF AGE (1 TABLET)
Vitamin A (as Palmitate + Beta Carotene)	2500 IU	100	50
Vitamin D-3	400 IU	100	100
Vitamin E	15 IU	150	50
Vitamin C	60 mg	150	100
Folic Acid	0.3 mg	150	75
Niacinamide	13.5 mg	150	68
Vitamin B-6	1.05 mg	150	53
Vitamin B-12	4.5 mcg	150	75
Vitamin B-1	1.05 mg	150	70
Vitamin B-2	1.20 mg	150	71
Vitamin K-1	5 mcg	*	*

*Recognized as essential in human nutrition, but no U.S. RDA established.

multivitamin product plus extra Vitamin C (a total of 250 mg).

Indication: Dietary supplementation.

Dosage and Administration: One chewable tablet daily for adults and children two years and older.

Warning: Phenylketonurics: Contains Phenylalanine.

How Supplied: SUNKIST Children's Multivitamins Plus Extra C are supplied in bottles of 60 chewable tablets with child resistant caps.
Sunkist® is a registered trademark of Sunkist Growers, Inc., Sherman Oaks, CA 91423.©
Shown in Product Identification Guide, page 408

SUNKIST® CHILDREN'S CHEWABLE MULTIVITAMINS— PLUS IRON

Vitamin Ingredients: Each tablet contains the vitamins of the Regular multivitamin product plus 15 mg of Iron.

Indication: Dietary supplementation.

Dosage and Administration: One chewable tablet daily for adults and children two years and older.

Warning: Close tightly and keep out of reach of children. Contains iron, which can be harmful or fatal to children in large doses. In case of accidental overdose, seek professional assistance or contact a Poison Control Center immediately.
Phenylketonurics: Contains phenylalanine.

How Supplied: SUNKIST Children's Multivitamins Plus Iron are supplied in bottles of 60 chewable tablets with child resistant safety caps.
Sunkist® is a registered trademark of Sunkist Growers, Inc., Sherman Oaks, CA 91423.©
Shown in Product Identification Guide, page 408

SUNKIST® CHILDREN'S CHEWABLE MULTIVITAMINS— COMPLETE

Vitamin Ingredients: Each tablet contains the following ingredients:
[See table on next page.]

Indication: Dietary supplementation.

Dosage and Administration: Children ages 2 to 4: one-half chewable tablet daily; One chewable tablet daily for adults and children four years and older.

Warning: Close tightly and keep out of reach of children. Contains iron, which can be harmful or fatal to children in large doses. In case of accidental overdose, seek professional assistance or contact a Poison Control Center immediately.
Phenylketonurics: Contains phenylalanine.

How Supplied: SUNKIST Children's Multivitamins Complete are supplied in bottles of 60 chewable tablets with child resistant safety caps.
Sunkist® is a registered trademark of Sunkist Growers, Inc., Sherman Oaks, CA 91423.©
Shown in Product Identification Guide, page 408

SUNKIST® VITAMIN C
**Citrus Complex
Chewable Tablets
Easy to Swallow Caplets**

Description: All Sunkist Vitamin C chewable tablets have a delicious orange flavor unlike any other Vitamin C tablet. Each 60 mg chewable tablet contains 100% of the U.S. RDA* of Vitamin C. Each 250 mg chewable tablet contains 417% of the U.S. RDA* of Vitamin C.

Continued on next page

The full prescribing information for each CIBA Consumer Pharmaceuticals product is contained herein and is that in effect as of December 15, 1993

CIBA Consumer—Cont.

Each 500 mg chewable tablet contains 833% of the U.S. RDA* of Vitamin C.

Each 500 mg easy to swallow caplet contains 833% of the U.S. RDA* of Vitamin C.

Sunkist Vitamin C chewable tablets and easy to swallow caplets do not contain artificial flavors or colors.

*U.S. Recommended Daily Allowance for adults and children over 4 years of age.

Indication: Dietary supplementation.

How Supplied: 60 mg Chewable Tablets—Rolls of 11.
250 mg and 500 mg Chewable Tablets—Bottles of 60.
500 mg Easy to Swallow Caplets—Bottles of 60.

Sunkist® is a registered trademark of Sunkist Growers, Inc., Sherman Oaks, CA 91423.©

Shown in Product Identification Guide, page 408

TING® ANTIFUNGAL CREAM, POWDER, SPRAY LIQUID, and SPRAY POWDER

Active Ingredient: Tolnaftate, 1%.

Other Ingredients: *Cream* —BHT, fragrance, polyethylene glycol 400, polyethylene glycol 3350, titanium dioxide. *Powder* —Corn starch, fragrance, talc. *Spray Liquid* —BHT, fragrance, isobutane (propellant), polyethylene glycol 400, SD alcohol 40-B (41% w/w). *Spray Powder* —BHT, fragrance, isobutane (propellant), PPG-12-buteth-16, SD alcohol 40-B (14% w/w), talc.

Indications: Cures athlete's foot and jock itch with a clinically proven ingredient. Relieves itching and burning. Prevents the recurrence of athlete's foot with daily use.

Warnings: Do not use on children under 2 years of age except under the advice and supervision of a doctor. For external use only. Avoid contact with the eyes. If irritation occurs, or if there is no improvement within 4 weeks for athlete's foot, or within 2 weeks for jock itch, discontinue use and consult a doctor. **Keep this and all drugs out of the reach of children.** In case of accidental ingestion, seek professional assistance or contact a Poison Control Center immediately. *For Spray Liquid and Spray Powder only* —Avoid inhaling. Avoid contact with the eyes or other mucous membranes. Contents under pressure; do not puncture or incinerate. Flammable mixture, do not use near fire or flame. Do not expose to heat or temperatures above 49°C (120°F). Use only as directed. Intentional misuse by deliberately concentrating and inhaling contents can be harmful or fatal.

Directions: Cleanse skin with soap and water and dry thoroughly. Apply over affected area morning and night or as directed by a doctor. For athlete's foot pay special attention to the spaces between the toes. It is also helpful to wear well-fitting, ventilated shoes and to change shoes and socks at least once daily. Best results in athlete's foot are usually obtained with 4 weeks' use of this product, and in jock itch, with two weeks' use. If satisfactory results have not occurred within these times, consult a doctor. Children under 12 years of age should be supervised in the use of this product. This product is not effective on the scalp or nails. To prevent recurrence of athlete's foot, apply Ting to feet once or twice daily following the above directions.

How Supplied: *Cream* —½ oz (14 g) tube, *Powder* —1.5 oz (43 g) shaker container, *Spray Liquid and Spray Powder* —3 oz (85 g) aerosol containers.
TING is a registered trademark of Ciba-Geigy Corporation.

Shown in Product Identification Guide, page 408

VITRON-C® TABLETS
[vī'tron c]

Active Ingredients: Each tablet contains
Ferrous fumarate, USP .... 200 mg equivalent to 66 mg elemental iron (365% U.S. RDA)
Ascorbic acid .... 125 mg (200% U.S. RDA)
Present in part as sodium ascorbate, USP

Other Ingredients: Colloidal silicon dioxide, flavor, glycine, hydroxypropyl methylcellulose, iron oxides, magnesium stearate, microcrystalline cellulose, polyethylene glycol, polysorbate 80, povidone, saccharin sodium, talc, titanium dioxide.

Indications: For iron deficiency anemia.

Actions: Vitron-C contains ferrous fumarate with ascorbic acid to enhance iron absorption. Vitron-C, a well-tolerated formula, is especially useful when pregnancy, menstruation, or chronic blood loss increases iron needs.

Warning: Close tightly and keep out of reach of children. Contains iron, which can be harmful or fatal to children in large doses. In case of accidental overdose, seek professional assistance or contact a Poison Control Center immediately.
The treatment of any anemic condition should be under the advice and supervision of a physician. As oral iron products interfere with absorption of oral tetracycline antibiotics, these products should not be taken within two hours of each other. As with any drug, if you are pregnant or nursing a baby, seek the advice of a health professional before using this product.

Directions: Adults—one or two tablets daily or as directed by a physician. Tablet may be swallowed whole, chewed or sucked like a lozenge.

How Supplied: Bottles of 100 and 1000 tablets with child-resistant safety closures.

SUNKIST CHILDREN'S CHEWABLE MULTIVITAMINS—COMPLETE

VITAMINS	QUANTITY PER TABLET	PERCENT U.S. RDA FOR CHILD. 2 TO 4 YRS OF AGE (½ TABLET)	FOR ADULTS & CHILD. OVER 4 YRS OF AGE (1 TABLET)
Vitamin A (as Palmitate + Beta Carotene)	5000 IU	100	100
Vitamin D-3	400 IU	50	100
Vitamin E	30 IU	150	100
Vitamin C	60 mg	75	100
Folic Acid	0.4 mg	100	100
Biotin	40 mcg	13	13
Pantothenic Acid	10 mg	100	100
Niacinamide	20 mg	111	100
Vitamin B-6	2 mg	143	100
Vitamin B-12	6 mcg	100	100
Vitamin B-1	1.5 mg	107	100
Vitamin B-2	1.7 mg	106	100
Vitamin K-1	10 mcg	*	*
MINERALS			
Iron	18 mg	90	100
Magnesium	20 mg	5	5
Iodine	150 mcg	107	100
Zinc	10 mg	63	67
Manganese	1 mg	*	*
Calcium	100 mg	6	10
Phosphorus	78 mg	5	8
Copper	2 mg	100	100

*Recognized as essential in human nutrition, but no U.S. RDA established.

Columbia Laboratories, Inc.
2665 SOUTH BAYSHORE DRIVE
MIAMI, FL 33133

DIASORB®
[dī 'ă-zorb]
Activated Nonfibrous Attapulgite Liquid and Tablets

Description: Diasorb relieves cramps and pain associated with diarrhea. It is available as a pleasant-tasting cola-flavored liquid and as easy-to-swallow tablets. Diasorb is safe for children.

Active Ingredient: Each liquid teaspoonful and tablet contains 750 mg activated nonfibrous attapulgite.

Inactive Ingredients: *Liquid*—Benzoic acid, citric acid, flavor, glycerin, magnesium aluminum silicate, methylparaben, polysorbate, propylene glycol, propylparaben, saccharin, sodium hypochlorite solution, sorbitol, xanthan gum, and water. *Tablet*—D&C Red No. 30 Al Lake, Gelatin, Hydroxypropyl Cellulose, Hydroxypropyl Methylcellulose, Magnesium Stearate, Pharmaceutical Shellac, Polyethylene Glycol, Povidone, Propylene Glycol, Sorbitol, Titanium Dioxide, and Water.

Directions for Use: Take the full recommended starting dose at the first sign of diarrhea, and repeat after each subsequent bowel movement. Do not exceed maximum recommended dose per day. Shake liquid well before using.
Swallow tablets with water. Do not chew.

Caution: Do not use if foil seal around tablet is broken.

Warning: Do not use for more than 2 days or in the presence of fever or in infants or children under 3, unless directed by a physician. In case of accidental overdose, seek professional assistance or contact a poison control center immediately.
Store at room temperature (59° to 86° F) in a dry place.
KEEP THIS AND ALL MEDICATIONS OUT OF THE REACH OF CHILDREN.

Dosage: See Table for recommended dosage for acute diarrhea.
[See table above.]

How Supplied: *Liquid*—In plastic bottles of 4 fl oz (120 mL).
Tablets—Packaged in blister packs of 24.
Shown in Product Identification Guide, page 408

LEGATRIN®
[leg 'a-trin]

Active Ingredient: Quinine Sulfate, 162.5 mg per tablet.

Other Ingredients: Calcium phosphate dibasic, cellulose, croscarmellose sodium, FD&C blue No. 2 aluminum lake, FD&C red No. 40 aluminum lake, gelatin, hydroxypropyl cellulose, hydroxypropyl methylcellulose, magnesium stearate, polyethylene glycol 400, silica, starch, stearic acid, titanium dioxide.

Age	Initial Dose	Maximum Dose per 24 hours
Adults and children over 12 years	4 tsp or 4 Tablets	12 tsp or 12 Tablets
Children 6–12 years	2 tsp or 2 Tablets	6 tsp or 6 Tablets
Children 3–6 years	1 tsp or 1 Tablet	3 tsp or 3 Tablets
Infants and children under 3 years	Only as directed by a physician	

Indications: For relief of night leg cramps, muscle spasms, restless legs.

Warnings: Discontinue use and consult a physician immediately if swelling, bruising, skin rash, skin discoloration or bleeding occurs. These symptoms may indicate a serious condition. Discontinue use if ringing in the ears, deafness, diarrhea, nausea or visual disturbances occur. In case of accidental overdose, seek medical assistance or contact Poison Control Center immediately. Do not take if pregnant, nursing a baby, allergic or sensitive to quinine or under 12 years of age. Keep this and all medication out of reach of children.

Caution: Do not use if Legatrin printed foil seal is damaged or missing.

Dosage: When a leg cramp occurs, take two tablets at once. To help prevent future night leg cramp attacks, take two tablets two hours before bedtime. Do not exceed two tablets daily. Consult a physician if symptoms persist longer than ten days.

How Supplied: Blister packages of 30 and 50 tablets.
Shown in Product Identification Guide, page 408

Copley Pharmaceutical Inc.
25 JOHN RD
CANTON, MA 02021

MICONAZOLE NITRATE VAGINAL CREAM 2%
7-DAY VAGINAL CREAM
CURES MOST VAGINAL YEAST INFECTIONS
FULL PRESCRIPTION STRENGTH

Indication: For the treatment of vaginal yeast infections (candidiasis).
If you have any or all of the symptoms of a yeast infection (vaginal itching, burning, discharge) and if some time in the past your doctor has told you that these symptoms are due to a yeast infection, then MICONAZOLE vaginal cream should work for you. If, however, you never have had these symptoms before, you should see your doctor before using MICONAZOLE vaginal cream.
MICONAZOLE NITRATE VAGINAL CREAM IS FOR THE TREATMENT OF VAGINAL YEAST INFECTIONS ONLY. IT DOES NOT TREAT OTHER INFECTIONS AND DOES NOT PREVENT PREGNANCY.
WHAT ARE VAGINAL YEAST INFECTIONS (CANDIDIASIS)?
A yeast infection is a common type of vaginal infection. Your doctor may call it candidiasis. This condition is caused by an organism called Candida, which is a type of yeast. Even healthy women usually have this yeast on the skin, in the mouth, in the digestive tract, and in the vagina. At times, the yeast can grow very quickly. In fact, the infection is sometimes called yeast (Candida) "overgrowth."
A yeast infection can occur at almost any time of life. It is most common during the childbearing years. The infection tends to develop most often in some women who are pregnant, diabetic, taking antibiotics, taking birth control pills, or have a damaged immune system.
Various medical conditions can damage the body's normal defenses against infection. One of the most serious of these conditions is infection with the human immunodeficiency virus (HIV—the virus that causes AIDS). Infection with HIV causes the body to be more susceptible to infections, including vaginal yeast infections. Women with HIV infection may have frequent vaginal yeast infections or, especially, vaginal yeast infections that do not clear up easily with proper treatment. If you may have been exposed to HIV and are experiencing either frequently recurring vaginal yeast infections or, especially, vaginal yeast infections that do not clear up easily with proper treatment, you should see your doctor promptly. If you wish further information on risk factors for HIV infection or on the relationship between recurrent or persistent vaginal yeast infections and HIV infection, please contact your doctor or the CDC National AIDS HOTLINE at 1-800-342-AIDS (English), 1-800-344-7432 (Spanish), or 1-800-243-7889 (hearing impaired, TDD).
IF YOU EXPERIENCE VAGINAL YEAST INFECTIONS FREQUENTLY (THEY RECUR WITHIN A TWO MONTH PERIOD) OR IF YOU HAVE

Continued on next page

Copley—Cont.

VAGINAL YEAST INFECTIONS THAT DO NOT CLEAR UP EASILY WITH PROPER TREATMENT, YOU SHOULD SEE YOUR DOCTOR PROMPTLY TO DETERMINE THE CAUSE AND TO RECEIVE PROPER MEDICAL CARE.

Symptoms of Vaginal Yeast Infections: There are many signs and symptoms of a yeast infection. They can include:

- Vaginal itching (ranging from mild to intense);
- A clumpy, white vaginal discharge that may look like cottage cheese;
- Vaginal soreness, irritation or burning, especially during intercourse;
- Rash or redness around the vagina.
Note: Vaginal discharge that is different from above, for example, a yellow/green discharge or a discharge that smells "fishy," may indicate that you have something other than a yeast infection. If this is the case, you should consult your doctor before using MICONAZOLE vaginal cream.

Warnings: • This product is only effective in treating vaginal infection caused by yeast. Do not use in eyes or take by mouth.

- **Do not use MICONAZOLE vaginal cream if you have any of the following signs and symptoms. Also, if they occur while using MICONAZOLE vaginal cream, STOP using the product and contact your doctor right away. You may have a more serious illness.**
  - **Fever (above 100°F orally).**
  - **Pain in the lower abdomen, back or either shoulder.**
  - **A vaginal discharge that smells bad.**
- If there is no improvement or if the infection worsens within 3 days, or complete relief is not felt within 7 days, or your symptoms return within two months, then you may have something other than a yeast infection. You should consult your doctor.
If you may have been exposed to the human immunodeficiency virus (HIV, the virus that causes AIDS) and are now having recurrent vaginal infections, especially infections that don't clear up easily with proper treatment, see your doctor promptly to determine the cause of your symptoms and to receive proper medical care.
- This cream contains mineral oil. Mineral oil may weaken latex in condoms or in diaphragms. Do not rely on condoms or diaphragms to prevent sexually transmitted diseases or pregnancy while using MICONAZOLE vaginal cream.
- Do not use tampons while using this medication.

- Do not use in girls less than 12 years of age.
- If you are pregnant or think you may be, do not use this product except under the advice and supervision of a doctor.
- Keep this and all drugs out of the reach of children.
- In case of accidental ingestion, seek professional assistance or contact a poison control center immediately.

Contents: One tube of vaginal cream containing miconazole nitrate 2%. One plastic applicator.
IMPORTANT: THE TUBE OPENING IS SEALED FOR YOUR PROTECTION. DO NOT USE IF THE TUBE SEAL HAS A HOLE IN IT OR IF THE SEAL CANNOT BE SEEN. RETURN THE PRODUCT TO THE STORE WHERE YOU BOUGHT IT.

Directions for Use: To begin treatment, wait until bedtime.
Before going to bed:

1 To open the tube, unscrew the cap. Turn the cap upside down and place the cap on the end of the tube. Push down firmly until the seal is broken (as shown).

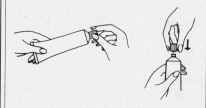

2 Attach the applicator to the tube by turning applicator clockwise (as shown).

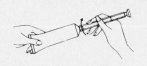

3 Squeeze the tube from the bottom. This will force the cream into the applicator. Do this until the inside piece of the applicator is pushed out as far as it will go and the applicator is completely filled. Separate applicator from tube.

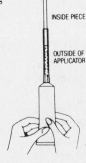

INSIDE PIECE

OUTSIDE OF APPLICATOR

4 Hold the applicator containing the cream by the opposite end from where the cream is. Gently insert the applicator

into the vagina as far as it will go comfortably.

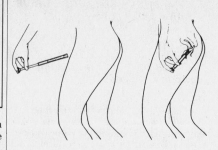

As shown in the pictures, this can be done while standing with your feet spread a few inches apart and your knees bent. Or, you can lie on your back with your knees bent. Once you are ready, push the inside piece of the applicator in and place the cream as far back in the vagina as possible. Then remove the applicator from the vagina. You should go to bed as soon as possible after inserting the cream. This will reduce leakage.
You may want to use deodorant-free minipads or pantyshields during the time that you are using MICONAZOLE vaginal cream. This is because the cream can leak and/or you may see some discharge. <u>DO NOT USE TAMPONS</u>.

5 After each use, replace the cap and roll tube from bottom (as shown).

6 Be sure to clean the applicator after each use. Pull the two pieces apart. Wash them with soap and warm water. To rejoin, gently push the inside piece into the outside piece as far as it will go.

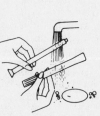

7 Repeat steps 1 through 6 before going to bed on each of the next six evenings.

Adverse Reactions (Side Effects): The following side effects have been reported with the use of MICONAZOLE vaginal cream: a temporary increase in burning, itching, and/or irritation when the cream is inserted. Abdominal cramping, headaches, hives, and skin rash, have also been reported. If any of these occur, stop using MICONAZOLE vaginal cream and consult your doctor.

For Best Results:

1. Be sure to use for seven days in a row even if your symptoms go away before then.

2. Use one applicatorful of cream at bedtime for seven nights in a row, even during your menstrual period.
3. Wear cotton underwear.
4. If your partner has any penile itching, redness, or discomfort, he should consult his doctor and mention that you are treating a yeast infection.
5. Dry the outside vaginal area thoroughly after a shower, bath, or swim. Change out of a wet bathing suit or damp workout clothes as soon as possible. A dry area is less likely to encourage the growth of yeast.
6. Wipe from front to rear (away from the vagina) after a bowel movement.
7. Don't douche unless your doctor tells you to do so. Douching may disturb the vaginal bacterial balance.
8. Do not scratch if you can help it. Scratching can cause more irritation and can spread the infection.
9. Discuss with your doctor any medication you are now taking. Certain types of medication can make your vagina more prone to infection.

If You Have a Question: Questions of a medical nature should be taken up with your doctor.

Active Ingredient: miconazole nitrate 2% (100 mg per dose)

Storage: Store at room temperature, 15°–30°C (59°–86°F). Avoid heat (over 30°C or 86°F).
COPLEY PHARMACEUTICAL, INC
CANTON, MA 02021
Revised: December 1992
RM #5850
MG #8397
Shown in Product Identification Guide, page 408

Del Pharmaceuticals, Inc.
A Subsidiary of Del Laboratories, Inc.
163 E. BETHPAGE ROAD
PLAINVIEW, NY 11803

DERMAREST® DriCort™
Anti-Itch Creme
(Hydrocortisone 1.0%)

Description: Dermarest DriCort contains the maximum strength of hydrocortisone available without a prescription. Plus, through a unique patented base, DriCort goes on feeling powder dry immediately. As a result, it gives dry, scaly skin a soft silky feeling.

Active Ingredients: Hydrocortisone Acetate (equivalent to Hydrocortisone, 1.0%).

Other Ingredients: Caprylic/Capric Triglyceride, Colloidal Silicon Dioxide, Polyethylene, White Petrolatum.

Indications: For the temporary relief of itching associated with minor skin irritations, inflammation, and rashes due to eczema, insect bites, psoriasis, seborrheic dermatitis, poison ivy, poison oak, or poi-

son sumac, soaps, detergents, cosmetics, jewelry, and for external genital, feminine, and anal itching. Other uses of this product should be only under the advice and supervision of a physician.

Warnings: For external use only. Avoid contact with the eyes. If condition worsens, or if symptoms persist for more than 7 days or clear up and occur again within a few days, stop use of this product and do not begin use of any other hydrocortisone product unless you have consulted a physician. Do not use for the treatment of diaper rash. Consult a physician. Do not use if you have a vaginal discharge. Consult a physician. For external anal itching use: Do not exceed the recommended daily dosage unless directed by a physician. In case of bleeding, consult a physician promptly. Do not put this product into the rectum by using fingers or any mechanical device or applicator. Keep this and all drugs out of the reach of children. In case of accidental ingestion, seek professional assistance or contact a Poison Control Center immediately.

Dosage and Administration: Adults and children 2 years of age and older: Apply to affected area not more than 3 to 4 times daily. Children under 2 years of age: Do not use, consult a physician. For external anal itching use: Adults: When practical, cleanse the affected area with mild soap and warm water and rinse thoroughly. Gently dry by patting or blotting with toilet tissue or a soft cloth before application of this product. Children under 12 years of age: Consult a physician.

How Supplied: 0.5 oz (14 g) and 1 oz (28 g) tubes
Shown in Product Identification Guide, page 408

DERMAREST® Plus Gel
Cooling, Anti-itch Gel

Description: Dermarest Plus is a cooling, anti-itch gel that contains maximum strength antihistamine plus a cooling anesthetic to stop the itch and fight its cause.

Active Ingredients: Diphenhydramine Hydrochloride 2.0%, Menthol 1.0%.

Inactive Ingredients: Aloe Vera Gel, Benzalkonium Chloride, Fragrance, Hydroxypropylcellulose, Isopropyl Alcohol, Methylparaben, Propylene Glycol, Purified Water.

Indications: For fast temporary relief of intense itching and pain associated with minor skin irritation, skin allergies, insect bites, poison ivy, rashes and sunburn.
Warnings: For external use only. Avoid contact with the eyes. Do not apply over large areas of the body. Do not apply to blistered, raw or oozing areas of the skin. If condition worsens, or if symptoms persist for more than 7 days, or clear up and occur again within a few

days, discontinue use of this product and consult a physician. Keep this and all drugs out of the reach of children. In case of accidental ingestions, seek professional assistance or contact a Poison Control Center immediately.

Dosage and Administration: For adults and children two years of age or older: Apply liberally to the affected area not more than three or four times daily, or as directed by your physician. For children under two years of age: Consult a physician.

How Supplied: Available in 0.5 oz. (14g) and 1.0 oz. (21g) tube(s).
Shown in Product Identification Guide, page 408

BABY ORAJEL®

Description: Baby Orajel with fast-acting benzocaine (7.5%) relieves teething pain within one minute. It's pleasant tasting and contains no alcohol.

Active Ingredient: Benzocaine 7.5%.

Inactive Ingredients: FD&C Red No. 40, Flavor, Glycerin, Polyethylene Glycols, Purified Water, Sodium Saccharin, Sorbic Acid, Sorbitol.

Indications: For the temporary relief of sore gums due to teething in infants and children 4 months of age and older. Baby Orajel is a safe, soothing, pleasantly flavored product which helps to immediately relieve teething pain by its topical anesthetic effect on the gums.

Actions: Benzocaine is a topical, local anesthetic commonly used for pain, discomfort, or pruritis associated with wounds, mucous membranes and skin irritations.

Warnings: Do not use this product for more than 7 days unless directed by a dentist or physician. If sore mouth symptoms do not improve in 7 days; if irritation, pain or redness persists or worsens; or if swelling, rash or fever develops, see your dentist or physician promptly. Do not exceed recommended dosage. Do not use this product if you have a history of allergy to local anesthetics such as procaine, butacaine, benzocaine, or other "caine" anesthetics. Fever and nasal congestion are not symptoms of teething and may indicate the presence of infection. If these symptoms persist, consult your physician. Keep this and all drugs out of the reach of children. In case of accidental overdose, seek professional assistance or contact a Poison Control Center immediately. Do not use if tube tip is cut prior to opening.

Precaution: For persistent or excessive teething pain, consult your physician.

Directions: Wash hands. Cut open tip of tube on score mark. Use your fingertip or cotton applicator to apply a small pea-size amount of Baby Orajel. Apply to affected area not more than four times

Continued on next page

Del—Cont.

daily or as directed by a dentist or physician. For infants under 4 months of age.

How Supplied: Baby Orajel: Gel in ⅓ oz (9.45 g) tube.

Shown in Product Identification Guide, page 408

BABY ORAJEL® TOOTH & GUM CLEANSER

Description: Baby Orajel Tooth & Gum Cleanser is specifically designed for children under four. Safe to swallow, non-foaming, fluoride- and abrasive-free, it contains Microdent™, which helps remove plaque and fight its build-up. Available in fruit and vanilla flavors.

Active Ingredients: Microdent™ (Poloxamer 407 2.0%, Simethicone 0.12%).

Inactive Ingredients: Carboxymethylcellulose Sodium, Citric Acid, Flavor, Glycerin, Methylparaben, Potassium Sorbate, Propylene Glycol, Propylparaben, Purified Water, Sodium Saccharin, Sorbitol.

Indications and Actions: Baby Orajel Tooth & Gum Cleanser is the first and only oral cleanser specially formulated to remove the plaque-like film on babies' teeth and gums. It's fluoride-Free, non-abrasive and does not foam so it's safe to use every day. It's sugar-free and has a flavor babies love. Only Baby Orajel Tooth & Gum Cleanser contains patented Microdent™—shown in clinical testing to help remove plaque and fight its buildup.

Warnings: Keep out of the reach of children. Do not use if tube tip is cut prior to opening.

Dosage and Administration: Wash hands. Cut open tip of tube on score mark. Apply a small amount to baby's gums and teeth with your finger or a gauze pad or a toothbrush. Gently rub the gums and teeth to remove food and plaque-like film. For best results, use in the morning and at bedtime.

How Supplied: Gel in ½ oz. (14.2g) tube and 1 oz. (28.3g) tube. Available in Vanilla or Fruit flavor.

Shown in Product Identification Guide, page 408

Maximum Strength ORAJEL®
[ōr ′ah-jel]

Description: Maximum Strength Orajel with 20% benzocaine provides immediate, long lasting toothache pain relief.

Active Ingredient: Benzocaine 20%.

Inactive Ingredients: Clove Oil, Flavor, Polyethylene Glycols, Sodium Saccharin, Sorbic Acid. May contain Citric Acid.

Indications: Maximum Strength Orajel is formulated to provide fast, long

lasting relief from toothache pain for hours.

Actions: Benzocaine is a topical, local anesthetic commonly used for pain, discomfort, or pruritis associated with wounds, mucous membranes and skin irritation.

Warning: Keep this and all drugs out of the reach of children. Do not use if tube tip is cut prior to opening. Do not use this product if you have a history of allergy to local anesthetics such as procaine, butacaine, benzocaine or other "caine" anesthetics. In case of accidental overdose, seek professional assistance or contact a Poison Control Center immediately.

Precaution: This preparation is intended for use in cases of toothache only as a temporary expedient until a dentist can be consulted. Do not use continuously.

Directions: Remove cap. Cut open tip of tube on score mark. Squeeze a small quantity of Maximum Strength Orajel directly into cavity and around gum surrounding the teeth.

How Supplied: Gel in two sizes—³⁄₁₆ oz (5.3 g) and ⅓ oz (9.45 g) tubes.

Shown in Product Identification Guide, page 408

ORAJEL® Mouth-Aid®
[ōr ′ah-jel]

Description: Orajel Mouth-Aid is a unique triple-acting medication which provides fast relief from painful minor mouth and lip sores. It stays on the sore for added protection.

Active Ingredients: Benzocaine 20%, Benzalkonium Chloride 0.02%, Zinc Chloride 0.1%.

Inactive Ingredients: Allantoin, Carbomer, Edetate Disodium, Peppermint Oil, Polyethylene Glycol, Polysorbate 60, Propyl Gallate, Propylene Glycol, Purified Water, Povidone, Sodium Saccharin, Sorbic Acid, Stearyl Alcohol.

Indications: For the temporary relief of pain associated with canker sores, cold sores, fever blisters and minor irritation or injury of the mouth and gums.

Actions: Benzocaine is a topical, local anesthetic commonly used for pain, discomfort, or pruritis associated with wounds, mucous membranes and skin irritations. Benzalkonium chloride is a rapidly acting surface disinfectant and detergent. Zinc chloride provides an astringent effect.

Warnings: Do not use this product for more than 7 days unless directed by a dentist or physician. If sore mouth symptoms do not improve in 7 days; if irritation, pain, or redness persists or worsens; or if swelling, rash or fever develops, see your dentist or physician promptly. Do not exceed recommended dosage. Do not use this product if you have a history of

allergy to local anesthetics such as procaine, butacaine, benzocaine or other "caine" anesthetics. Keep this and all drugs out of the reach of children. In case of accidental overdose, seek professional assistance or contact a Poison Control Center immediately. Do not use if tube tip is cut prior to opening.

Precaution: If condition persists, discontinue use and consult your physician or dentist. Not for prolonged use.

Directions: Cut open tip of tube on score mark. Adults and children 2 years and older: Apply to the affected area. Use up to 4 times daily or as directed by a dentist or physician. Children under 12 years of age should be supervised in the use of the product. Children under 2 years of age: Consult a dentist or physician.

How Supplied: Gel in 2 sizes—a ⅓ oz (9.45 g) tube and a ³⁄₁₆ oz (5.3 g) tube.

Shown in Product Identification Guide, page 408

PRONTO® Lice Killing Shampoo & Conditioner in One Kit

Description: Pronto Concentrate Lice Killing Shampoo & Conditioner in One contains the maximum strength of pyrethrins and piperonyl butoxide. In addition, a conditioner is included in the formulation to reduce tangles, for easy, effective comb-out of lice and eggs.

Active Ingredients: Pyrethrins 0.33%, piperonyl butoxide technical 4.00% [equivalent to 3.2% (butylcarbityl), (6-propylpiperonyl) ether and 0.80% related compounds].

Indications: One treatment of pediculicide shampoo kills head, body and pubic lice on contact.

Actions: Pronto Lice Killing Shampoo & Conditioner in One contains the maximum strength of pyrethrins and piperonyl butoxide. Pyrethrins act directly on the nervous system of insects and piperonyl butoxide enhances the neurotoxic effect of pyrethrins by inhibiting the oxidative breakdown of the pyrethrins by the insect's detoxification system. This results in a longer amount of time which the pyrethrins may exert their toxic effect on the insect.

Caution: Causes moderate eye irritation. Avoid contact with eyes or clothing. May cause skin irritation. Wash thoroughly with soap and water after handling. If product should get into eyes, immediately flush with water. Follow directions carefully.
Not to be used by persons allergic to ragweed. Harmful if swallowed. In case of infection or skin irritation, discontinue use and consult a physician. In order to prevent reinfestation with lice, all clothing and bedding must be sterilized or treated concurrent with the application of this preparation. Do not exceed two consecutive applications within 24 hours.

Precautionary Statements: Hazards to Humans and Domestic Animals.

Directions for Use: It is a violation of Federal Law to use this product in a manner inconsistent with its labeling. Shake well.

Instruct child to close eyes and cover eyes with clean wet towel. Apply Pronto Shampoo Concentrate cautiously to dry hair, scalp or any affected areas. Add a generous amount of water to work Pronto Shampoo Concentrate into a rich lather. Allow the shampoo to remain on area for 10 minutes, but no longer. Rinse treated areas thoroughly with warm water. Rinse eyes out with water following use. A fine-toothed metal or plastic comb (included) may be used to help remove dead lice and their eggs (nits) from hair. Handy applicator gloves are provided for your convenience in applying the shampoo to avoid contact with lice. Reapply follow-up treatment within 7–10 days to prevent self reinfestation from hatching eggs not killed by first application.
Storage and Disposal: Do not reuse empty container. Rinse thoroughly. Securely wrap original container in several layers of newspaper and discard in waste container.

How Supplied: 2 fl oz (59 ml) and 4 fl oz (118 ml) plastic bottles.
Shown in Product Identification Guide, page 408

TANAC® Medicated Gel
Fever Blister/Cold Sore Treatment

Description: Tanac Medicated Gel treats cold sores with a unique, long lasting maximum strength pain reliever with Dyclonine Hydrochloride (1.0%). It also protects lip sores while it treats them.

Active Ingredients: Dyclonine Hydrochloride 1.0%, Allantoin 0.5%.

Inactive Ingredients: Citric Acid, Flavor, Hydroxylated Lanolin, Petrolatum, Propylene Glycol, Purified Water, PVP/Hexadecene Copolymer, Yellow Wax.

Indications: For the temporary relief of pain and itching associated with fever blisters and cold sores. Relieves dryness and softens cold sores and fever blisters.

Warnings: DO NOT USE IF TIP IS CUT PRIOR TO OPENING. For external use only. Avoid contact with the eyes. If conditions worsens, or if symptoms persist for more than 7 days or clear up and occur again within a few days, discontinue use of this product and consult a physician. Keep this and all other drugs out of reach of children. In case of accidental ingestion, seek professional assistance, or contact a Poison Control Center immediately.

Dosage and Administration: Cut open tip of tube on score mark. Adults and children 2 years of age and older: Apply to fever blisters/cold sores not

more than 3 to 4 times daily. Children under 2 years of age: consult a physician.

How Supplied: Available in ⅓ oz. (9.45g) plastic tube.
Shown in Product Identification Guide, page 408

TANAC® No Sting Liquid

Description: Tanac Liquid provides fast, soothing relief from painful canker sores and other gum irritations because it contains an effective anesthetic plus an antiseptic. It's alcohol-free so it doesn't sting.

Active Ingredients: Benzocaine 10%, Benzalkonium Chloride 0.12%.

Inactive Ingredients: Flavor, Polyethylene Glycol 400, Propylene Glycol, Sodium Saccharin, Tannic Acid.

Indications: For temporary relief of pain from mouth sores, canker sores, fever blisters and gum irritations.

Warnings: If the condition for which this preparation is used persists or if a rash or irritation develops, discontinue use and consult a physician. Use as indicated but not for more than 5 consecutive days. Not for prolonged use. Avoid getting into eyes. Do not use if you have a history of allergy to local anesthetics such as procaine, butacaine, benzocaine, or other "caine" anesthetics. KEEP OUT OF THE REACH OF CHILDREN. In case of accidental ingestion, seek professional assistance or contact a Poison Control Center immediately. Do not use if imprinted bottle cap safety seal is broken or missing prior to opening.

Dosage and Administration: Apply with cotton or cotton swab to affected area not more than 3 to 4 times daily.

How Supplied: Available in 0.45 fl. oz. (13 ml) glass bottle.
Shown in Product Identification Guide, page 408

EDUCATIONAL MATERIAL

Teething Booklet From Baby Orajel®
Facts parents should know about tooth development and the teething process.
Free to physicians, pharmacists and patients
Fallacy and Fact Booklet From Pronto®
Answers questions about head lice control.
Free to physicians, pharmacists and patients.

Rx DRUG INFORMATION AT THE TOUCH OF A BUTTON
Join the thousands of doctors using the handheld, electronic *Pocket PDR.*
Use order form in front of book.

Effcon Laboratories, Inc.
P.O. BOX 7509
MARIETTA, GA 30065-1509

PIN-X®
Pinworm Treatment

Description: Each 1 mL of liquid for oral administration contains:
Pyrantel base .... 50 mg
(as Pyrantel Pamoate)

Indication: For the treatment of pinworms.

Warnings: Keep this and all drugs out of the reach of children. In case of accidental overdose, seek professional assistance or contact a poison control center immediately.
If you are pregnant or have liver disease, do not take this product unless directed by a doctor.

Directions for Use: Adults and children 2 years to under 12 years of age: oral dosage is a single dose of 5 milligrams of pyrantel base per pound, or 11 milligrams per kilogram, of body weight not to exceed 1 gram. Dosage information is summarized on the following dosing schedule:

Weight	Dosage
	(taken as a single dose)
25 to 37 lbs.	= ½ tsp.
38 to 62 lbs.	= 1 tsp.
63 to 87 lbs.	= 1½ tsp.
88 to 112 lbs.	= 2 tsp.
113 to 137 lbs.	= 2½ tsp.
138 to 162 lbs.	= 3 tsp. (1 tbsp.)
163 to 187 lbs.	= 3½ tsp.
188 lbs. & over	= 4 tsp.

SHAKE WELL BEFORE USING

How Supplied: Pin-X is supplied as a tan to yellowish, caramel-flavored suspension which contains 50 mg of pyrantel base (as pyrantel pamoate) per mL, in bottles of 30 mL (1 fl oz). NDC 55806-024-10
Store at controlled room temperature 15°–30°C (59°–86°F).
Manufactured for:
Effcon Laboratories Inc.
Marietta, GA 30065-1509
Manufactured by:
MIKART, INC.
Atlanta, GA 30318
Rev. 1/89
Code 587A00
Shown in Product Identification Guide, page 409

UNKNOWN DRUG?
Consult the
Product Identification Guide
(Gray Pages)
for full-color photos of
leading over-the-counter
medications

Fisons Corporation
P.O. BOX 1766
ROCHESTER, NY 14603

DELSYM® Cough Formula
[del 'sĭm]
(dextromethorphan polistirex)
Extended-Release Suspension
12-Hour Cough Relief

Active Ingredient: Each teaspoonful (5 mL) contains dextromethorphan polistirex equivalent to 30 mg dextromethorphan hydrobromide.

Inactive Ingredients: Citric acid, ethylcellulose, FD&C Yellow No. 6, flavor, high fructose corn syrup, methylparaben, polyethylene glycol 3350, polysorbate 80, propylene glycol, propylparaben, purified water, sucrose, tragacanth, vegetable oil, xanthan gum.

Indications: Temporarily relieves cough due to minor throat and bronchial irritation as may occur with the common cold or inhaled irritants.

Warnings: Do not take this product for persistent or chronic cough such as occurs with smoking, asthma, or emphysema, or if cough is accompanied by excessive phlegm (mucus) unless directed by a physician. A persistent cough may be a sign of a serious condition. If cough persists for more than 1 week, tends to recur, or is accompanied by fever, rash, or persistent headache, consult a physician. As with any drug, if you are pregnant or nursing a baby, seek the advice of a health professional before using this product. **Keep this and all drugs out of the reach of children.** In case of accidental overdose, seek professional assistance or contact a Poison Control Center immediately.

Drug Interaction Precaution: Do not use this product if you are now taking a prescription monoamine oxidase inhibitor (MAOI) (certain drugs for depression, psychiatric or emotional conditions, or Parkinson's disease), or for 2 weeks after stopping the MAOI drug. If you are uncertain whether your prescription drug contains an MAOI, consult a health professional before taking this product.

Directions: **Shake Bottle Well Before Using.** Dose as follows or as directed by a physician.
Adults and Children 12 years of age and over: 2 teaspoonfuls every 12 hours, not to exceed 4 teaspoonfuls in 24 hours.
Children 6 to under 12 years of age: 1 teaspoonful every 12 hours, not to exceed 2 teaspoonfuls in 24 hours.
Children 2 to under 6 years of age: ½ teaspoonful every 12 hours, not to exceed 1 teaspoonful in 24 hours.
Children under 2 years of age: Consult a physician.

How Supplied: 89 mL (3 fl oz) bottles NDC 0585-0842-61

FISONS **Pharmaceuticals**
Fisons Corporation
Rochester, NY 14623 U.S.A.
DELSYM is a registered trademark of Fisons Corporation.

Fleming & Company
1600 FENPARK DR.
FENTON, MO 63026

CHLOR-3
Medicinal Condiment

Active Ingredients: A troika of sodium chloride (50% 24.3 mEq/half tsp. iodized); potassium chloride (30% 11.5 mEq/half tsp.); magnesium chloride (20% 5.6 mEq/half tsp.).

Indications: The first medicinal condiment to restore needed K^+ & Mg^{++} lost during diuresis, at the expense of Na^+. To restore electrolytes lost by overcooking foods, or to add to diets that lack green vegetables, bananas, etc. And to replace conventional salting of foods in culinary and gourmet arts.

Symptoms and Treatment of Oral Overdosage: Hyperkalemia and hypermagnesemia are not end-stage results of usage.

How Supplied: In 8-oz plastic shaker, tamper-evident bottles.

IMPREGON Concentrate

Active Ingredient: Tetrachlorosalicylanilide 2%

Indications: Diaper Rash Relief, 'Staph' control, Mold inhibitor.

Actions: This is a bacteriostatic/fungistatic agent for home usage and hospital usage.

Warnings: Impregon should not be exposed to direct sunlight for long periods after applications.

Precaution: Addition of bleach prior to diaper treatment negates application effects.

Dosage and Administration: One capful (5ml) per gallon of water to impregnate diapers in the diaper pail. Dilutions for many home areas accompany the full package.

Note: For disposable-type diapers, add one teaspoonful to 8 oz of water to a 'Windex-type' sprayer. Spray middle half area of diapers until damp, and allow to dry before using, to prevent rashes.

How Supplied: Four ounce amber plastic bottles.

MAGONATE TABLETS
MAGONATE LIQUID
Magnesium Gluconate (Dihydrate)

Active Ingredients: Each tablet contains magnesium gluconate (dihydrate) 500mg (27mg of Mg^{++}). Each 5cc of Magonate Liquid contains magnesium gluconate (dihydrate) 1000mg (54mg of Mg^{++}).

Indications: For all patients in negative magnesium balance.

Precaution: Excessive dosage may cause loose stools.

Dosage and Administration: Magonate is recommended during and for three weeks after a course in chemotherapy, then monitored regularly.
Adults and children over 12 yrs.—one or two tablets or ½ to 1 teaspoon of liquid t.i.d. Under 12 yrs.—one tablet or ½ teaspoon of liquid t.i.d. Dosage may be increased in severe cases.

How Supplied: Magonate Tablets are supplied in bottles of 100 and 1000 tablets. Magonate Liquid is supplied in pints and gallons.

MARBLEN Suspension and Tablet

Composition: A modified 'Sippy Powder' antacid containing magnesium and calcium carbonates.

Action and Uses: The peach/apricot (pink) antacid suspension is sugar-free and neutralizes 18 mEq acid per teaspoonful with a low sodium content of 18mg per fl. oz. Each pink tablet consumes 18.0 mEq acid.

Administration and Dosage: One teaspoonful rather than a tablespoonful or one tablet to reduce patient cost by ⅔.

How Supplied: Plastic pints and bottles of 100 and 1000.

NEPHROX SUSPENSION
(aluminum hydroxide)
Antacid Suspension

Composition: A watermelon flavored aluminum hydroxide (320mg as gel)/mineral oil (10% by volume) antacid per teaspoonful.

Action and Uses: A sugar-free/saccharin-free pink suspension containing no magnesium and low sodium (19mg/oz). Extremely palatable and especially indicated in renal patients. Each teaspoon consumes 9 mEq acid.

Administration and Dosage: Two teaspoonfuls or as directed by a physician.

Caution: To be taken only at bedtime. Do not use at any other time or administer to infants, expectant women, and nursing mothers except upon the advice of a physician as this product contains mineral oil.

How Supplied: Plastic pints and gallons.

NICOTINEX Elixir
nicotinic acid

Composition: Contains niacin 50 mg./tsp. in a sherry wine base (amber color).

Action and Uses: Produces flushing when tablets fail. To increase micro-circulation of inner-ear in Meniere's, tinnitus and labyrinthine syndromes. For 'cold hands & feet', and as a vehicle for additives.

Administration and Dosage: One or two teaspoonsful on fasting stomach.

Side Effects: Patients should be warned of dermal flush. Ulcer and gout patients may be affected by 14% alcoholic content.

Contraindications: Severe hypotension and hemorrhage.

How Supplied: Plastic pints and gallons.

OCEAN MIST
(buffered saline)

Composition: A 0.65% special saline made isotonic by a dual preservative system and buffering excipients prevent nasal irritation.

Action and Uses: Rhinitis medicamentosa, rhinitis sicca and atrophic rhinitis. For patients 'hooked on nose drops' and glaucoma patients on diuretics having dry nasal capillaries. OCEAN may also be used as a mist or drop.

Administration and Dosage: One or two squeezes in each nostril P.R.N.

Supplied: Plastic 45cc spray bottles and pints.

PURGE
(flavored castor oil)

Composition: Contains 95% castor oil (USP) in a sweetened lemon flavored base that completely masks the odor and taste of the oil.

Indications: Preparation of the bowel for x-ray, surgery and proctological procedures, IVPs, and constipation.

Dosage: Infants—1–2 teaspoonfuls. Children—adjust between infant and adult dose. Adult—2–4 tablespoonfuls.

Precaution: Not indicated when nausea, vomiting, abdominal pain or symptoms of appendicitis occur. Pregnancy, use only on advice of physician.

Supplied: Plastic 1 oz. & 2 oz. bottles.

UNKNOWN DRUG?
Consult the
Product Identification Guide
(Gray Pages)
for full-color photos of
leading over-the-counter
medications

Gebauer Company
**9410 ST. CATHERINE AVENUE
CLEVELAND, OH 44104**

SALIVART®
[sal 'ĭ-vart]
Saliva Substitute

Description: Prompt, lasting relief of dryness of the mouth or throat (hyposalivation, xerostomia).

Contains:

	%W/W
Sodium carboxymethyl-cellulose	1.000
Sorbitol	3.000
Sodium chloride	0.084
Potassium chloride	0.120
Calcium chloride, dihydrate	0.015
Magnesium chloride, hexahydrate	0.005
Potassium phosphate, dibasic	0.034
Preservative Free	
Propellant: Nitrogen	

Indications: For reduced salivary flow, caused by medications, radiation therapy near the mouth or throat, salivary gland infection, mouth or throat inflammation, dental or oral surgery, fever, emotional factors. Also for relieving nasal crusting and bad taste.

Actions: Moistens and lubricates the oral cavity like natural saliva to allow normal eating, swallowing, and talking. Improves adherence of dentures.

Warnings: Avoid spraying in eyes. Keep out of reach of children. Contents under pressure. Do not puncture or incinerate. Protect from direct sunlight and from heat above 50°C (120°F).

Dosage and Administration: Spray Salivart directly into the mouth or throat, for 1 or 2 seconds, using it as often as needed to maintain moistness, or as instructed by physician. Nasal crusting can be relieved by applying Salivart with a cotton swab.

How Supplied:
75 mL   NDC 0386-0009-75
25 mL   NDC 0386-0009-25
*Shown in Product Identification
Guide, page 409*

**IF YOU SUSPECT
AN INTERACTION...**
The 1,400-page
PDR Guide to Drug Interactions •
Side Effects • *Indications*
can help.
Use the order form
in the front of this book.

Herald Pharmacal, Inc.
**6503 WARWICK ROAD
RICHMOND, VA 23225
1-800-253-9499**

AQUA GLYCOLIC® Face Cream

Description: A luxurious formulation for the face, Aqua Glycolic® Face Cream is a moisturizer, protectant and gentle exfoliant. The restorative qualities of this scientifically advanced cream will help diminish the appearance of fine lines, balance uneven skin tones and maintain the skin's proper moisture level.

Ingredients: Purified Water, Cetyl Ricinoleate, C12-15 Alkyl Benzoate, Ammonium Glycolate (and) Glycolic Acid, Ceresin, Glyceryl Stearate (and) PEG-100 Stearate, Sorbitan Stearate, Sorbitol, Propylene Glycol, Magnesium Aluminum Silicate, Dimethicone, Hyaluronic Acid, Diazolidinyl Urea, Xanthan Gum, Methylparaben, Trisodium EDTA and Propylparaben.

How Supplied: 2 oz. jars
*Shown in Product Identification
Guide, page 409*

AQUA GLYCOLIC® Hand & Body Lotion

Description: Uniquely formulated to gently remove dead skin cells from the outer layer of skin. The product will help relieve hyperkeratotic skin conditions; soften dry, cracked or sun-damaged skin; balance uneven skin tones; and maintain the proper moisture level in healthy skin.

Ingredients: Purified Water, Glycolic Acid (and) Ammonium Glycolate, Cetyl Alcohol, Glyceryl Stearate & PEG-100 Stearate, C12-15 Alkyl Benzoate, Mineral Oil, Stearyl Alcohol, Magnesium Aluminum Silicate, Xanthan Gum, Methylparaben and Propylparaben.

How Supplied: 8 oz. bottles
4 oz. bottles
*Shown in Product Identification
Guide, page 409*

AQUA GLYCOLIC® Shampoo & Body Cleanser

Description: Developed especially to alleviate itching, scaling scalp conditions, Aqua Glycolic® Shampoo & Body Cleanser leaves the hair soft and manageable. This non-irritating formula effectively removes residue left from conditioners and styling aids. Recommended as a facial cleanser for oily skin and as an overall body cleanser in the bath or shower.

Ingredients: Purified Water, Ammonium Lauryl Sulfate, Glycolic Acid (and) Ammonium Glycolate, Glycerin, Co-

Continued on next page

Herald—Cont.

coamphocarboxyglycinate, Fragrance, Propylene Glycol (and) Diazolidinyl Urea (and) Methylparaben (and) Propylparaben.

How Supplied: 8 oz. bottles

Shown in Product Identification Guide, page 409

AQUA GLYDE® Astringent & Cleanser

Description: Designed to thoroughly cleanse oily skin where soap and water cannot reach, Aqua Glyde® Astringent & Cleanser leaves the skin free of excess oil, dirt and makeup. As a home care product, Aqua Glyde® Astringent and Cleanser is extremely effective for clearing clogged pores generally associated with oily or problem-prone skin. It also serves as an excellent topical vehicle for compounding and routing medications to specific areas.

Ingredients: Purified Water, SD Alcohol 40, Glycolic Acid (and) Ammonium Glycolate, Eucalyptus Oil and FD&C Green #3.

How Supplied: 8 oz. bottles

Shown in Product Identification Guide, page 409

AQUA GLYDE® Shave & Aftershave

Description: Pioneered by a leading dermatologist, this state-of-the-art skin care product is expressly formulated to soften hair and improve shaving comfort. Helps eliminate minor razor irritation, bumps and imperfections associated with shaving.

Ingredients: Purified Water, Glycolic Acid (and) Ammonium Glycolate, Cetyl Alcohol, Stearyl Alcohol, Sorbitol, Ammonium Lauryl Sulfate, Methylparaben and Propylparaben.

How Supplied: 4 oz. bottles

Shown in Product Identification Guide, page 409

AQUA LACTEN® LOTION

Description: Aqua Lacten Lotion is specially formulated with urea and a combination of two Alpha Hydroxy Acids to moisturize and soften dry, rough, chapped skin.

Ingredients: Purified Water, Urea, Mineral Oil, Petrolatum, Propylene Glycol Stearate, Sorbitan Stearate, Cetyl Alcohol, Glycolic Acid, Magnesium Aluminum Silicate, Sodium Lauryl Sulfate, Lactic Acid, Methylparaben and Propylparaben.

How Supplied: 8 oz. bottles
16 oz. bottles

AQUAMED® LOTION

Description: Aquamed Lotion provides moisture for the hands, face and body to relieve dryness and itching. Softens and soothes detergent hands, mechanics' hands, chapped or chafed skin, sunburn, winter-itch and aging, dry skin.

Ingredients: Purified Water, Mineral Oil, Petrolatum, Propylene Glycol Stearate, Sorbitan Stearate, Cetyl Alcohol, Sodium Lauryl Sulfate, Methylparaben and Propylparaben.

How Supplied: 8 oz. bottles
16 oz. bottles

AQUARAY® SUNSCREEN

Description: Aquaray Sunscreen is an SPF 20 sunscreen that provides broad spectrum UVA/UVB protection. This moisturizing formula is non-greasy, non-sensitizing, water-resistant and recommended for individuals with sensitive skin. Aquaray Sunscreen contains no PABA, Padimate O, Fragrance, Lanolin, Alcohol or Parabens.

Active Ingredients: Octyl Methoxycinnamate 7.5%, Oxybenzone 5%, Octyl Salicylate 5.0%.

How Supplied: 4 oz. bottles

CAM® LOTION

Description: CAM Lotion is a lipid-free cleanser, specially formulated to cleanse without the irritation commonly associated with harsh soaps and hot water. Ideal for patients with atopic dermatitis, diaper dermatitis and other forms of eczema. In addition, CAM Lotion is a superb shaving lotion for individuals with sensitive skin.

Ingredients: Purified Water, Cetyl Alcohol, Stearyl Alcohol, Sorbitol, Sodium Lauryl Sulfate, Methylparaben and Propylparaben.

How Supplied: 8 oz. bottles
16 oz. bottles

HERALD® TAR SHAMPOO

Description: Herald Tar Shampoo offers therapeutic relief from symptoms commonly associated with seborrhea and psoriasis, and leaves the hair soft and manageable.

Active Ingredient: Coal Tar 0.5%

Other Ingredients: Purified Water, Laureth 4, DEA Lauryl Sulfate (and) DEA Lauraminopropionate, Laureth 23, PEG 6 Lauramide and Tetrasoduim EDTA.

How Supplied: 8 oz. bottles
16 oz. bottles

MAPO® BATH OIL

Description: Mapo Bath Oil is a lanolinated-mineral oil preparation designed to relieve dry, flaky, itchy skin. Mapo Bath Oil is useful in cleansing and softening soap-intolerant skin.

Ingredients: Mineral Oil, PEG 4 Dilaurate, Lanolin Oil, Rose Oil and BHT.

How Supplied: 8 oz. bottles
16 oz. bottles

EDUCATIONAL MATERIAL

Samples-available to physician
Brochures-available to physician, pharmacist, consumer

Inter-Cal Corporation
533 MADISON AVENUE
PRESCOTT, AZ 86301

ESTER–C®
(Calcium Ascorbate)

Description: Each Ester-C tablet & caplet contains 500 mg Vitamin C in the form of Calcium Ascorbate 550 mg, vegetable-derived cellulose, stearic acid, and magnesium stearate. Ester-C contains no preservatives, sugars, artificial colorings, or flavorings.

As the calcium salt of L-ascorbic acid, Ester-C has an empirical formula of $CaC_{12}H_{14}O_{12}$ and a formula weight of 390.3.

Actions: Vitamin C has been found to be essential for the prevention of scurvy. In humans, an exogenous source of the vitamin is required for collagen formation and tissue repair. Ascorbate ion is reversibly oxidized to dehydroascorbate ion in the body. Both of these are active forms of the vitamin and are considered to play important roles in biochemical oxidation-reduction reactions. The vitamin is involved in tyrosine metabolism, carbohydrate metabolism, iron metabolism, folic acid-folinic acid conversion, synthesis of lipids and proteins, resistance to infections, and cellular respiration.

Indications and Usage: Vitamin C and its salts, such as Calcium Ascorbate, are recommended as nutritional supplements in the prevention of scurvy. In scurvy, collagenous structures are primarily affected, and lesions develop in blood vessels and bones. Symptoms of mild deficiency may include faulty development of teeth and bones, bleeding gums, gingivitis, and loose teeth. An increased need for the vitamin exists in febrile states, chronic illness and infection, e.g., rheumatic fever, pneumonia, tuberculosis, whooping cough, diphtheria, sinusitis, etc. Additional increases in the daily intake of ascorbate are indicated in burns, delayed healing of bone fractures and wounds, and hemovascular disorders. Immature and premature infants require relatively larger amounts of Vitamin C.

Contraindications: Because of its calcium content, Ester-C is contraindicated in hypercalcemic states, e.g., from dosing with parathyroid hormone or overdosage of Vitamin D.

Adverse Reactions: There are no known adverse reactions following ingestion of Ester-C tablets, caplets & powder. The gastric disturbances characteristic of large doses of ascorbic acid are absent or greatly diminished when the pH-neutral form of calcium ascorbate present in Ester-C tablets, caplets & powder are utilized as the source of Vitamin C supplementation.

Dosage and Administration: The minimum U.S. Recommended Daily Allowance for Vitamin C for the prevention of diseases such as scurvy is 60 mg per day. Optimum daily allowances, e.g., for the maintenance of increased plasma and cellular reserves, are significantly greater. For adults, the recommended average preventative dose of the vitamin is 70 to 150 mg daily. The recommended average optimum dose of Ester-C is 550 to 1650 mg (1 to 3 tablets or caplets) daily.

For frank scurvy, doses of 300 mg to one gram of Vitamin C daily have been recommended. Normal adults, however, have received as much as six grams of the vitamin without evidence of toxicity.

For enhancement of wound healing, doses of the vitamin approximating two Ester-C tablets, caplets and powder daily for a week or ten days both preoperatively and postoperatively are generally considered adequate, although considerably larger amounts may be recommended. In the treatment of burns, the daily number of Ester-C tablets, caplets and powder recommended is governed by the extent of tissue injury. For severe burns, daily doses of 2 to 4 tablets or caplets (approximately one to two grams of Vitamin C) are recommended.

In other conditions in which the need for increased Vitamin C is recognized, three to five times the optimum allowance appears to be adequate.

How Supplied: 550 mg tablets and caplets of Ester-C in plastic bottles of 100, 250, 90, and 225's. 4 oz. and 8 oz. powders, 275 mg tablet also available.
Store at room temperature.
U.S. Patent granted April 18, 1989; No. 4,822,816.
Literature revised: December, 1989.
Mfd. by Inter-Cal Corp.
Prescott, AZ 86301

**Rx DRUG INFORMATION
AT THE TOUCH OF A BUTTON**
Join the thousands of doctors using the handheld, electronic *Pocket PDR.*
Use order form in front of book.

Johnson & Johnson Consumer Products, Inc.
GRANDVIEW RD
SKILLMAN, NJ 08558

K-Y® BRAND JELLY PERSONAL LUBRICANT

Description: K-Y® Brand Jelly Personal Lubricant is a greaseless, water-soluble jelly which is clear, spreads easily, is non-irritating, and is safe to use with latex products.

Indications: K-Y® Jelly provides vaginal moisture, lubricates condoms and helps ease insertion of tampons, rectal thermometers, enemas, douches and other devices inserted into body cavities. K-Y® Jelly will not harm rubber, plastic, diaphragms or glass surfaces.

Actions: Helps lubricate body cavities for easier insertion. When used as a sexual lubricant, K-Y® Jelly helps overcome vaginal dryness from sexual intercourse, menopause, childbirth, lactation or stressful periods.

Directions: Squeeze tube to obtain desired amount of lubricant (a 1–2 inch strip should be sufficient). Reapply as needed.

Ingredients: Chlorhexidine Gluconate, Glucono Delta Lactone, Glycerin, Hydroxyethyl Cellulose, Methylparaben, Purified Water, Sodium Hydroxide

THIS PRODUCT IS NOT A CONTRACEPTIVE AND DOES NOT CONTAIN A SPERMICIDE. Store at room temperature.

How Supplied: K-Y® Jelly is available in 2 and 4 oz. tubes and a convenient 3-pack (containing 0.4 oz. tubes).
*Shown in Product Identification
Guide, page 409*

Johnson & Johnson • MERCK
Consumer Pharmaceuticals Co.
CAMP HILL ROAD
FORT WASHINGTON, PA 19034

ALternaGEL™   OTC
[*al-tern 'a-jel*]
Liquid
High-Potency Aluminum Hydroxide Antacid

Description: ALternaGEL is available as a white, pleasant-tasting, high-potency aluminum hydroxide liquid antacid.

Ingredients: Each 5 mL teaspoonful contains: Active: 600 mg aluminum hydroxide (equivalent to dried gel, USP) providing 16 milliequivalents (mEq) of acid-neutralizing capacity (ANC), and less than 2.5 mg (0.109 mEq) of sodium and no sugar. Inactive: butylparaben, flavors, propylparaben, purified water, simethicone, and other ingredients.

Indications: ALternaGEL is indicated for the symptomatic relief of hyperacidity associated with peptic ulcer, gastritis, peptic esophagitis, gastric hyperacidity, hiatal hernia, and heartburn.
ALternaGEL will be of special value to those patients for whom magnesium-containing antacids are undesirable, such as patients with renal insufficiency, patients requiring control of attendant GI complications resulting from steroid or other drug therapy, and patients experiencing the laxation which may result from magnesium or combination antacid regimens.

Directions: One to two teaspoonfuls, as needed, between meals and at bedtime, or as directed by a physician: May be followed by a sip of water if desired. Concentrated product. Shake well before using. Keep tightly closed.

Warnings: Keep this and all drugs out of the reach of children. ALternaGEL may cause constipation.
Except under the advice and supervision of a physician: do not take more than 18 teaspoonfuls in a 24-hour period, or use the maximum dose of ALternaGEL for more than two weeks. ALternaGEL may cause constipation.
Prolonged use of aluminum-containing antacids in patients with renal failure may result in or worsen dialysis osteomalacia. Elevated tissue aluminum levels contribute to the development of the dialysis encephalopathy and osteomalacia syndromes. Small amounts of aluminum are absorbed from the gastrointestinal tract and renal excretion of aluminum is impaired in renal failure. Aluminum is not well removed by dialysis because it is bound to albumin and transferrin, which do not cross dialysis membranes. As a result, aluminum is deposited in bone, and dialysis osteomalacia may develop when large amounts of aluminum are ingested orally by patients with imparied renal function.
Aluminum forms insoluble complexes with phosphate in the gastrointestinal tract, thus decreasing phosphate absorption. Prolonged use of aluminum-containing antacids by normophosphatemic patients may result in hypophosphatemia if phosphate intake is not adequate. In its more severe forms, hypophosphatemia can lead to anorexia, malaise, muscle weakness, and osteomalacia.

Drug Interaction Precaution: Antacids may interact with certain prescription drugs. If you are presently taking a prescription drug, do not take this product without checking with your physician or other health professional.

How Supplied: ALternaGEL is available in bottles of 12 fluid ounces and 5 fluid ounces, and 1 fluid ounce hospital unit doses. NDC 16837-860.
*Shown in Product Identification
Guide, page 409*

Continued on next page

J&J • Merck—Cont.

DIALOSE® Tablets
[di 'a-lose]
Stool Softener Laxative

Description: DIALOSE is a very low sodium, nonhabit forming, stool softener containing 100 mg docusate sodium per tablet.

The docusate in DIALOSE is a highly efficient surfactant which facilitates absorption of water by the stool to form a soft, easily evacuated mass. Unlike stimulant laxatives, DIALOSE does not interfere with normal peristalsis, neither does it cause griping nor sensations of urgency.

Ingredients: Active: Docusate Sodium, 100 mg per tablet.
Inactive: Colloidal Silicone Dioxide, Dextrates, Flavors, Hydroxypropyl Methylcellulose, Magnesium Stearate, Microcrystalline Cellulose, Polyethylene Glycol, Polysorbate 80, Pregelatinized Starch, Propylene Glycol, Sodium Starch Glycolate, Titanium Dioxide, D&C Red No. 28, D&C Red No. 27 Aluminum Lake, FD&C Blue No. 1, FD&C Blue No. 1 Aluminum Lake, FD&C Red No. 40.

Indications: DIALOSE is indicated for the relief of occasional constipation (irregularity).
DIALOSE is an effective aid to soften or prevent formation of hard stools in a wide range of conditions that may lead to constipation. DIALOSE helps to eliminate straining associated with obstetric, geriatric, cardiac, surgical, anorectal, or proctologic conditions. In cases of mild constipation, the fecal softening action of DIALOSE can prevent constipation from progressing and relieve painful defecation.

Directions: *Adults:* One tablet, one to three times daily; adjust dosage as needed.
Children 6 to under 12 years: One tablet daily as needed.
Children under 6 years: As directed by physician.
It is helpful to increase the daily intake of fluids by taking a glass of water with each dose.

Warnings: Unless directed by a physician: Do not use when abdominal pain, nausea, or vomiting are present. Do not use for a period longer than one week. Do not take this product if you are presently taking a prescription drug or mineral oil. As with any drug, if you are pregnant or nursing a baby, seek the advice of a health professional before using this product. Keep out of the reach of children.

How Supplied: Bottles of 36 and 100 pink tablets. Also available in 100 tablet unit dose boxes (10 strips of 10 tablets each). NDC-16837-870.
Shown in Product Identification Guide, page 409

DIALOSE® PLUS Tablets
[di 'a-lose Plus]
Stool Softener/Stimulant Laxative

Description: DIALOSE PLUS provides a very low sodium tablet formulation of 100 mg docusate sodium and 65 mg yellow phenolphthalein.

Ingredients: Each tablet contains: Actives: Docusate Sodium, 100 mg., yellow phenolphthalein, 65 mg.
Inactive: Dextrates, Dibasic Calcium Phosphate Dihydrate, Flavors, Hydroxypropyl Methylcellulose, Magnesium Stearate, Microcrystalline Cellulose, Polydextrose, Polythylene Glycol, Polysorbate 80, Propylene Glycol, Sodium Starch Glycolate, Titanium Dioxide, Triacetin, D&C Yellow NO. 10 Aluminum Lake, D&C Red NO. 28, FD&C Blue NO. 1, FD&C Red NO. 40, FD&C Red NO. 40 Aluminum Lake.

Indications: DIALOSE PLUS is indicated for the treatment of constipation characterized by lack of moisture in the intestinal contents, resulting in hardness of stool and decreased intestinal motility. DIALOSE PLUS combines the advantages of the stool softener, docusate sodium, with the peristaltic activating effect of yellow phenolphthalein.

Directions: *Adults:* One or two tablets daily as needed, at bedtime or on arising
Children 6 to under 12 years: One tablet daily as needed
Children under 6 years: As directed by physician.
It is helpful to increase the daily intake of fluids by taking a glass of water with each dose.

Warnings: Unless directed by a physician: Do not use when abdominal pain, nausea, or vomiting are present. Do not use for a period longer than one week. If skin rash appears do not use this product or any other preparation containing phenolphthalein. Frequent or prolonged use may result in dependence on laxatives. Do not take this product if you are presently taking a prescription drug or mineral oil.
As with any drug, if you are pregnant or nursing a baby, seek the advice of a health professional before using this Keep out of the reach of children.

How Supplied: Bottles of 36 and 100 yellow tablets. Also available in 100 capsule unit dose boxes (10 strips of 10 capsules each). NDC 16837-871.
Shown in Product Identification Guide, page 409

FERANCEE®
[fer 'an-see]
Chewable Hematinic

Ingredients:
[See table top of next column]
Active: ferrous fumarate, sodium ascorbate, ascorbic acid.
Inactive: confectioner's sugar, flavors, magnesium stearate, mannitol, povi-

TWO TABLETS DAILY PROVIDE: US RDA*

Iron	744%	104 mg
Vitamin C	500%	300 mg

*Percentage of US Recommended Daily Allowances for adults and children 4 or more years of age.

done, saccharin calcium, starch, Yellow 5 (tartrazine), Yellow 6.

Indications: A pleasant-tasting hematinic for iron deficiency anemias, well-tolerated FERANCEE is particularly useful when chronic blood loss, onset of menses, or pregnancy create additional demands for iron supplementation. Available information indicates a low incidence of staining of the teeth by ferrous fumarate, alone or in combination with ascorbic acid. The peach-cherry flavored chewable tablets dissolve quickly in the mouth and may be either chewed or swallowed.

Directions: *Adults:* Two tablets daily, or as directed by physician.
Children over 6 years of age: One tablet daily, or as directed by physician.
Children under 6 years of age: As directed by physician.
IMPORTANT: KEEP IN DRY PLACE. REPLACE CAP TIGHTLY.

Warnings: As with any drug, if you are pregnant or nursing a baby, seek the advice of a health professional before using this product. Keep out of the reach of children. In case of accidental overdose, seek professional assistance or contact a Poison Control Center immediately.

How Supplied: FERANCEE is supplied in bottles of 100 brown and yellow, two-layer tablets. A child-resistant cap is standard on each bottle as a safeguard against accidental ingestion by children. Keep in a dry place. Replace cap tightly. NDC 16837-650.
Shown in Product Identification Guide, page 409

FERANCEE®-HP Tablets
[fer 'an-see-hp]
High Potency Hematinic

Ingredients:
ONE TABLET DAILY PROVIDES: US RDA*

Iron	611%	110 mg
Vitamin C	1000%	600 mg

*Percentage of US Recommended Daily Allowances for adults and children 4 or more years of age.
Active: ascorbic acid, ferrous fumarate, sodium ascorbate. Inactive: flavor, hydrogenated vegetable oil, microcrystalline cellulose, povidone, Red 40, and other ingredients.

Indications: FERANCEE-HP is a high potency formulation of iron and vitamin C and is intended for use as either:
(1) a maintenance hematinic for those patients needing a daily iron supplement to maintain normal hemoglobin levels, or

(2) intensive therapy for the acute and/or severe iron deficiency anemia where a high intake of elemental iron is required.

The use of well-tolerated ferrous fumarate provides high levels of elemental iron with a low incidence of gastric distress. The inclusion of 600 mg of vitamin C per tablet serves to maintain more of the iron in the absorbable ferrous state.

Precautions: Because FERANCEE-HP contains 110 mg of elemental iron per tablet, it is recommended that its use be limited to adults i.e., not less than 12 years of age.

Directions: One tablet per day taken after a meal or as directed by a physician, should be sufficient to maintain normal hemoglobin levels in most patients with a history of recurring iron deficiency anemia. Not recommended for children under 12 years of age.

For acute and/or severe iron deficiency anemia, two or three tablets per day taken one tablet per dose after meals. (Each tablet provides 110 mg elemental iron).

Warnings: As with all medications, keep out of the reach of children. In case of accidental overdose, seek professional assistance or contact a Poison Control Center immediately.

How Supplied: FERANCEE-HP is supplied in bottles of 60 red, film-coated, oval-shaped tablets.
NDC 16837-863.
Note: A child-resistant safety cap is standard on each bottle of 60 tablets as a safeguard against accidental ingestion by children.
Shown in Product Identification Guide, page 409

INFANTS' MYLICON® Drops
[*my'li-con*]
Antiflatulent

Ingredients: Each 0.6 mL of drops contains: Active: simethicone, 40 mg. Inactive: carbomer 934P, citric acid, flavors, hydroxypropyl methylcellulose, purified water, Red 3, saccharin calcium, sodium benzoate, sodium citrate.

Indications: For relief of the painful symptoms of excess gas in the digestive tract. Such gas is frequently caused by excessive swallowing of air or by eating foods that disagree. The defoaming action of INFANTS' MYLICON® Drops relieves flatulence by dispersing and preventing the formation of mucus-surrounded gas pockets in the gastrointestinal tract. INFANTS' MYLICON® Drops act in the stomach and intestines to change the surface tension of gas bubbles enabling them to coalesce, thereby freeing and eliminating the gas more easily by belching or passing flatus.

Directions: Infants (under 2 years): 0.3 ml four times daily after meals and at bedtime, or as directed by a physician. The dosage can also be mixed with 1 oz of

cool water, infant formula or other suitable liquids to ease administration. Adults and children: 0.6 ml four times daily, after meals and at bedtime, or as directed by a physician.

Warnings: Do not exceed 12 doses per day except under the advice and supervision of a physician. Keep this and all drugs out of the reach of chldren.

How Supplied: INFANTS' MYLICON® Drops are available in bottles of 15 ml (0.5 fl oz) and 30 ml (1.0 fl oz) pink, pleasant tasting liquid. NDC 16837-630.
Shown in Product Identification Guide, page 409

MYLANTA® AND MYLANTA® DOUBLE STRENGTH
[*my-lan'ta*]
Aluminum, Magnesium and Simethicone
Liquid and Tablets
Antacid/Anti-Gas

Description: MYLANTA® and MYLANTA® Double Strength are well-balanced, pleasant-tasting, antacid/anti-gas medications that provide consistent, effective relief of symptoms associated with gastric hyperacidity and excess gas. Non-constipating and considered dietetically low sodium or sodium free, MYLANTA® and MYLANTA® Double Strength contain two proven antacids, aluminum hydroxide and magnesium hydroxide, plus simethicone for gas relief.

Active Ingredients: Each 5 mL tea-, spoon or one chewable tablet contains:

	MYLANTA®	MYLANTA® Double Strength
Aluminum Hydroxide	200 mg	400 mg
Magnesium Hydroxide	200 mg	400 mg
Simethicone	20 mg	40 mg

Inactive Ingredients:
TABLETS:
Colloidal silicon dioxide, dextrates, flavors, magnesium stearate, mannitol, saccharin sodium, sorbitol, FD & C Blue 1 or FD & C Yellow 10.
LIQUIDS:
Butylparaben, carboxymethylcellulose sodium, flavors, hydroxypropyl methylcellulose, microcrystalline cellulose, propylparaben, purified water, saccharin sodium, and sorbitol.

Sodium Content: Each 5 mL teaspoon or one chewable tablet contains the following amount of sodium:

	MYLANTA®	MYLANTA® Double Strength
Tablets	0.77 mg (0.33 mEq)*	1.3 mg (0.06 mEq)†
Liquid	0.68 mg (0.03 mEq)*	1.14 mg (0.05 mEq)*

* considered dietetically sodium free
† considered dietetically low sodium

Acid Neutralizing Capacity: Two teaspoonfuls or two chewable tablets have the following acid neutralizing capacity:

	MYLANTA®	MYLANTA® Double Strength
Tablets	23.0 mEq	46.0 mEq
Liquid	25.4 mEq	50.8 mEq

Indications: MYLANTA® and MYLANTA® Double Strength are indicated for the relief of acid indigestion, heartburn, sour stomach, and symptoms of gas and upset stomach associated with those conditions. MYLANTA® and MYLANTA® Double Strength are also indicated as antacids for the symptomatic relief of hyperacidity associated with the diagnosis of peptic ulcer, gastritis, peptic esophagitis, heartburn and hiatal hernia and as antiflatulents to alleviate the symptoms of mucus-entrapped gas, including postoperative gas pain.

Advantages: MYLANTA® and MYLANTA® Double Strength are homogenized for a smooth, creamy taste. The choice of three pleasant-tasting liquid flavors and the non-constipating formula encourage patient acceptance, thereby minimizing the skipping of prescribed doses. MYLANTA® and MYLANTA® Double Strength are also available in tablets, and both the liquid and tablet forms are considered dietetically low sodium or sodium free. MYLANTA® and MYLANTA® Double Strength provide consistent relief in patients suffering from distress associated with hyperacidity, mucus-entrapped gas, or swallowed air.

Directions:
Liquid:
Shake well. 2-4 teaspoonfuls between meals and at bedtime, or as directed by a physician.
Tablets:
2-4 tablets, well chewed, between meals and at bedtime, or as directed by physician.

Warnings: Keep this and all drugs out of the reach of children. Do not take more than 24 tsps/tablets of MYLANTA® or 12 tsps/tablets of MYLANTA® Double Strength in a 24-hour period or use the maximum dose of this product for more than two weeks, except under the advice and supervison of a physician. Do not use this product if you have kidney disease. Prolonged use of aluminum-containing antacids in patients with renal failure may result in or worsen dialysis osteomalacia. Elevated tissue aluminum levels contribute to the development of the dialysis encephalopathy and osteomalacia syndromes. Small amounts of aluminum are absorbed from the gastrointestinal tract and renal excretion of aluminum is impaired in renal failure. Aluminum is not well removed by dialysis because it is

Continued on next page

J&J • Merck—Cont.

bound to albumin and transferrin, which do not cross dialysis membranes. As a result, aluminum is deposited in bone, and dialysis osteomalacia may develop when large amounts of aluminum are ingested orally by patients with impaired renal function.

Aluminum forms insoluble complexes with phosphate in the gastrointestinal tract, thus decreasing phosphate absorption. Prolonged use of aluminum-containing antacids by normophosphatemic patients may result in hypophosphatemia if phosphate intake is not adequate. In its more severe forms, hypophosphatemia can lead to anorexia, malaise, muscle weakness, and osteomalacia.

Drug Interaction Precaution: Antacids may interact with certain prescription drugs. If you are presently taking a prescription drug, do not take this product without checking with your physician or other health professional.

How Supplied: MYLANTA® and MYLANTA® Double Strength are available as white liquid suspensions in pleasant-tasting flavors, Original, Cherry Creme and Cool Mint Creme, and as two-layer green and white Cool Mint Creme and two-layer pink and white Cherry Creme chewable tablets. Tablets are identified as either MYLANTA® or MYLANTA® DS. Liquids are supplied in bottles of 5 oz, 12 oz, and 24 oz. MYLANTA® tablets are supplied in bottles of 48 and 100 count sizes and in 12 tablet roll packs. MYLANTA® Double Strength tablets are supplied in bottles of 30 and 60 count sizes and in 8 tablet roll packs. Also available for hospital use in liquid unit dose bottles of 1 oz and bottles of 5 oz.

MYLANTA®
NDC 16837-610 ORIGINAL LIQUID
NDC 16837-629 COOL MINT CREME LIQUID
NDC 16837-621 CHERRY CREME LIQUID
NDC 16837-628 CHERRY CREME
NDC 16837-620 COOL MINT CREME TABLETS

MYLANTA® Double Strength
NDC 16837-652 ORIGINAL LIQUID
NDC 16837-624 COOL MINT CREME LIQUID
NDC 16837-622 CHERRY CREME LIQUID
NDC 16837-627 CHERRY CREME TABLETS
NDC 16837-651 COOL MINT CREME TABLETS

Professional Labeling

Indications: Stress-induced upper gastrointestinal hemorrhage: MYLANTA DOUBLE STRENGTH is indicated for the prevention of stress-induced upper gastrointestinal hemorrhage. Hypercidic conditions: As an antacid, for the symptomatic relief of hyperacidity associated with the diagnosis of peptic ulcer and other gastrointestinal conditions

where a high degree of acid neutralization is desired.

Directions: Prevention of stress-induced upper gastrointestinal hemorrhage: 1) Aspirate stomach via nasogastric tube* and record pH. 2) Instill 10 mL of MYLANTA DOUBLE STRENGTH followed by 30 mL of water via nasogastric tube. Clamp tube. 3) Wait one hour. Aspirate stomach and record pH. 4a) If pH equals or exceeds 4.0, apply drainage or intermittent suction for one hour, then repeat the cycle. 4b) If pH is less than 4.0, instill double (20 mL) MYLANTA DOUBLE STRENGTH followed by 30 mL of water. Clamp tube. 5) Wait one hour. If pH equals or exceeds 4.0, see number 7, if pH is still less than 4.0, instill double (40 mL) MYLANTA DOUBLE STRENGTH followed by 30 mL of water. Clamp tube. 6) Wait one hour. If pH equals or exceeds 4.0, see number 7. If pH is still less than 4.0, instill double (80 mL)† MYLANTA DOUBLE STRENGTH followed by 30 mL of water. 7) Drain for one hour and repeat cycle with the effective dosage of MYLANTA DOUBLE STRENGTH.

In hyperacid states for symptomatic relief: One or two teaspoonfuls as needed between meals and at bedtime or as directed by a physician. Higher dosage regimens may be employed under the direct supervision of a physician in the treatment of active peptic ulcer disease.

Precaution: Aluminum-magnesium hydroxide containing antacids should be used with caution in patients with renal impairment.

Adverse Effects: Occasional regurgitation and mild diarrhea have been reported with the dosage recommended for the prevention of stress-induced upper gastrointestinal hemorrhage.

References: 1. Zinner MJ, Zuidema GD, Smigh PL, Mignosa M: The prevention of upper gastrointestinal tract bleeding in patients in an intensive care unit. *Surg Gynecol Obster* 153:214–220, 1981. 2. Lucas CE, Sugawa C, Riddle J, et al.: Natural history and surgical dilemma of "stress" gastric bleeding. *Arch Surg* 102:266–273, 1971. 3. Hastings PR, Skillman JJ, Bushnell LS, Silen W: Antacid titration in the prevention of acute gastrointestinal bleeding: a controlled, randomized trial in 100 critically ill patients. *N Engl J Med* 298:1042–1045, 1978. 4. Day SB, MacMillan BG, Altemeier WA: *Curling's Ulcer, An Experience of Nature.* Springfield, IL, Charles C Thomas Co., 1972, p. 205. 5. Skillman JJ, Bushnell LS, Goldman H, Silen W: Respiratory failure, hypotension, sepsis, and

*If nasogastric tube is not in place, administer 20 mL of MYLANTA DOUBLE STRENGTH orally q2h.
†In a recent clinical study[1] 20 mL of MYLANTA DOUBLE STRENGTH, q2h, was sufficient in more than 85 percent of the patients. No patient studied required more than 80 mL of MYLANTA DOUBLE STRENGTH q2h.

jaundice. A clinical syndrome associated with lethal hemorrhage from acute stress ulceration of the stomach. *Am J Surg* 117:523–530, 1969. 6. Priebe HJ, Skillman J, Bushnell LS, et al. Antacid versus cimetidine in preventing acute gastrointestinal bleeding. *N Engl J Med* 302:426–430, 1980. 7. Silen W: The prevention and management of stress ulcers. *Hosp Pract* 15:93–97, 1980. 8. Herrmann V, Kaminski DL: Evaluation of intragastric pH in acutely ill patients. *Arch Surg* 114:511–514, 1979. 9. Martin LF, Staloch DK, Simonowitz DA, et al.: Failure of cimetidine prophylaxis in the critically ill. *Arch Surg* 114:492–496, 1979. 10. Zinner MJ, Turtinen L, Gurll NJ, Reynolds DG: The effect of metiamide on gastric mucosal injury in rat restraint. *Clin Res* 23:484A, 1975. 11. Zinner M, Turtinen BA, Gurll NJ: The role of acid and ischemia in production of stress ulcers during canine hemorrhagic shock. *Surgery* 77:807–816, 1975. 12. Winans CS: Prevention and treatment of stress ulcer bleeding: Antacids or cimetidine? *Drug Ther Bull* (hospital) 12:37–45, 1981.

Shown in Product Identification Guide, page 409

MYLANTA® GAS-40mg Tablets
MYLANTA® GAS Tablets
Maximum Strength MYLANTA® GAS Tablets
[*My-lan'-ta*]
Antiflatulent

Active Ingredients:
Each chewable tablet contains:

	Simethicone
MYLANTA® GAS-40mg	40 mg
MYLANTA® GAS	80 mg
Maximum Strength MYLANTA® GAS	125 mg

Inactive Ingredients: Dextrates, flavor, sorbitol, stearic acid, tricalcium phosphate. Cherry: Red 7.

Indications: For relief of the painful symptoms of excess gas in the digestive tract. Such gas is frequently caused by excessive swallowing of air or by eating foods that disagree. MYLANTA® GAS-40mg, MYLANTA® GAS, and Maximum Strength MYLANTA® GAS Tablets are high capacity antiflatulents for adjunctive treatment of many conditions in which the retention of gas may be a problem, such as the following: air swallowing, postoperative gaseous distention, peptic ulcer, spastic or irritable colon, diverticulosis. If condition persists, consult your physician.

MYLANTA® GAS-40mg, MYLANTA® GAS, and Maximum Strength MYLANTA®GAS Tablets have a defoaming action that relieves flatulence by dispersing and preventing the formation of mucus-surrounded gas pockets in the gastrointestinal tract. MYLANTA® GAS-40mg, MYLANTA® GAS, and Maximum Strength MYLANTA® GAS Tablets act in the stomach and intestines to change the surface tension of gas bubbles enabling them to coalesce, thereby freeing and eliminating the gas more easily by belching or passing flatus.

Directions:
MYLANTA® GAS-40 mg Tablets
One or two tablets four times daily after meals and at bedtime. May also be taken as needed up to twelve tablets daily or as directed by a physician.
MYLANTA® GAS Tablets
One tablet four times daily after meals and at bedtime. May also be taken as needed up to six tablets daily or as directed by a physician.
Maximum Strength MYLANTA® GAS Tablets
One tablet four times daily after meals and at bedtime or as directed by a physician.
TABLETS SHOULD BE CHEWED THOROUGHLY

Warnings: Keep this and all drugs out of the reach of children.

How Supplied: MYLANTA® GAS-40 mg Tablets are available in bottles of 100 white, scored, chewable tablets, identified "MYL GAS 40." Also available in 100 tablet unit dose boxes (10 strips of 10 tablets each). NDC 16837-450.
MYLANTA® GAS Tablets are available as white (mint) or pink (cherry) scored, chewable tablets identified "MYL GAS 80." Mint flavor is available in bottles of 60 and 100 tablets and individually wrapped 12 and 30 tablet packages. Cherry flavor is available in bottles of 60 tablets and packages of 12 individually wrapped tablets. Mint NDC 16837-858. Cherry NDC 16837-859.
Maximum Strength MYLANTA® GAS Tablets are available as white, scored, chewable tablets identified "MYL GAS 125" in individually wrapped 12 and 24 tablet packages and economical 48 tablet bottles. NDC 16837-455.

Shown in Product Identification Guide, page 409

MYLANTA® GELCAPS
[*my-lan 'ta*]
Antacid

Description: MYLANTA® GELCAPS are an easy-to-swallow, non-chalky alternative to liquid and tablet antacids. The gelcaps contain two antacid ingredients, calcium carbonate, and magnesium carbonate, have no chalky taste, are low in sodium and provide fast, effective acid pain relief.

Ingredients: Each gelcap contains: **Active:** Calcium Carbonate 311 mg and Magnesium Carbonate 232 mg. **Inactive:** Benzyl Alcohol, Butylparaben, Castor Oil, D&C Yellow 10, Disodium Calcium Edetate, FD&C Blue 1, Gelatin, Hydroxypropyl Cellulose, Magnesium Stearate, Methylparaben, Microcrystalline Cellulose, Propylparaben, Sodium Croscarmellose, Sodium Lauryl Sulfate, Sodium Propionate, Titanium Dioxide.

Sodium Content: MYLANTA® GELCAPS contain a very low amount of sodium per daily dose. Typical value is 2.5 mg (.1087 mEq) sodium per gelcap.
Acid Neutralizing Capacity: Two MYLANTA® GELCAPS have an acid neutralizing capacity of 23.0 mEq.

Indications: For the relief of acid indigestion, heartburn, sour stomach and upset stomach associated with these symptoms.

Advantages: MYLANTA® GELCAPS are easy to swallow, provide fast, effective relief, eliminate antacid taste and are low in sodium. Convenience of dosage in the unique gelcap form can promote patient compliance.

Directions: 2–4 gelcaps as needed or as directed by a physician.

Warnings: Keep this and all other drugs out of the reach of children. Do not take more than 24 gelcaps in a 24-hour period or use the maximum dosage for more than two weeks or use if you have kidney disease, except under the advice and supervision of a physician.

Drug Interaction Precaution: Antacids may interact with certain prescription drugs. If you are presently taking a prescription drug, do not take this product without checking with your physician or other health professional.

How Supplied: MYLANTA® GELCAPS are available as a blue and white gelcap in convenient blister packs in boxes of 24 solid gelcaps or in bottles of 50 and 100 solid gelcaps.
NDC 16837-850   1/93
Shown in Product Identification Guide, page 409

MYLANTA NATURAL FIBER SUPPLEMENT
[*my-lan 'ta*]
Natural Fiber Bulking Agent

Description: MYLANTA NATURAL FIBER SUPPLEMENT is an ultra smooth bulk laxative powder. Each rounded tablespoon (sugar) or teaspoon (sugar free) contains approximately 3.4 grams of psyllium hydrophilic mucilloid fiber. MYLANTA NATURAL FIBER SUPPLEMENT contains no chemical stimulants and is nonaddictive.

Ingredients: Active: Each dose contains approximately 3.4 grams of psyllium hydrocolloid mucilloid fiber per dose.
Inactives:
Sugar: ascorbic acid, citric acid, gum arabic (acacia gum), natural orange flavor, silicone dioxide, sucrose, D&C yellow no. 10, FD&C yellow no.6.
Sugar-free: ascorbic acid, aspartame, citric acid, gum arabic (acacia gum), maltodextrin, natural orange flavor, silicone dioxide, D&C yellow no. 10, FD&C yellow no.6.

Indications: MYLANTA NATURAL FIBER SUPPLEMENT is indicated to restore normal bowel habits in chronic constipation, to promote normal elimination in irritable bowel syndrome, and to ease the passage of stools in presence of anorectal disorders. MYLANTA NATURAL FIBER SUPPLEMENT produces a soft, lubricating bulk which promotes natural elimination. MYLANTA NATURAL FIBER SUPPLEMENT is not a one-dose, fast-acting bowel regulator. Administration for several days may be needed to establish regularity.

Directions: *Adults:* One rounded tablespoon of the sugar-containing product or one rounded teaspoon of the sugar-free product, in a glass of water one to three times a day, or as directed by a physician. *Children:* Consult your doctor.
MIX THIS PRODUCT (CHILD OR ADULT DOSE) WITH AT LEAST 8 OUNCES (A FULL GLASS) OF WATER OR OTHER FLUID. TAKING THIS PRODUCT WITHOUT ENOUGH LIQUID MAY CAUSE CHOKING. SEE WARNINGS.

Instructions: Pour MYLANTA NATURAL FIBER SUPPLEMENT into a *dry* glass, add approximately 8 oz. of water and stir briskly. Replace cap tightly. Keep in a dry place.

Warning: TAKING THIS PRODUCT WITHOUT ADEQUATE FLUID MAY CAUSE IT TO SWELL AND BLOCK YOUR THROAT OR ESOPHAGUS AND MAY CAUSE CHOKING. DO NOT TAKE THIS PRODUCT IF YOU HAVE DIFFICULTY IN SWALLOWING. IF YOU EXPERIENCE CHEST PAIN, VOMITING, OR DIFFICULTY IN SWALLOWING OR BREATHING AFTER TAKING THIS PRODUCT, SEEK IMMEDIATE MEDICAL ATTENTION. Avoid inhalation. May cause a potentially severe reaction when inhaled by persons sensitive to psyllium powder or suffering from respiratory disorders. As with all medications, keep out of the reach of children.

How Supplied: Bottles of 13 oz (sugar) and 10 oz (sugar-free) tan, granular instant mix powder.
NDC 16837-881 (sugar-free)
NDC 16837-880 (sugar)
Shown in Product Identification Guide, page 410

MYLANTA® SOOTHING LOZENGES
[*mi-lan 'ta*]
ANTACID

Description: MYLANTA® SOOTHING LOZENGES are a dietically sodium free calcium rich antacid which dissolve in your mouth to quickly soothe your heartburn pain or acid indigestion.

Ingredients: Each MYLANTA® SOOTHING LOZENGE contains:

Continued on next page

J&J • Merck—Cont.

Active: Calcium Carbonate, 600 mg

Inactive: Citric Acid, Corn Syrup, FD&C Red 40, Flavor, Propylene Glycol, Soybean Oil, Sucrose, Titanium Dioxide

Indications: For the relief of heartburn, acid indigestion, sour stomach and upset stomach associated with these symptoms.

Acid Neutralizing Capacity: Each MYLANTA® SOOTHING LOZENGE has an acid neutralizing capacity of 11.4 mEq.

Directions: Allow 1 lozenge to dissolve in your mouth and if necessary, follow with a second. Repeat as needed or as directed by a physician.

Warnings: Keep this and all other drugs out of the reach of children. Do not take more than 12 lozenges in a 24-hour period or use the maximum dosage for more than two weeks, except under the advice and supervision of a physician.

Drug Interaction Precaution: Antacids may interact with certain prescription drugs. If you are presently taking a prescription drug, do not take this product without checking with your physician or other health professional.

How Supplied: MYLANTA® SOOTHING LOZENGES are available as green Cool Mint Creme flavored lozenges, and as pink Cherry Creme flavored lozenges identified as "M". Lozenges supplied in 18 count boxes and 50 count bottles. NDC 16837-876 (Cherry Creme) NDC 16837-875 (Cool Mint Creme)
Shown in Product Identification Guide, page 410

THE STUART FORMULA®
Tablets
Multivitamin/Multimineral
Supplement

ONE TABLET DAILY PROVIDES:

VITAMINS:	US RDA*	
A	100%	5,000 IU
D	100%	400 IU
E	33%	10 IU
C	83%	50 mg
Folic Acid	25%	100 mcg
B$_1$ (thiamin)	100%	1.5 mg
B$_2$ (riboflavin)	100%	1.7 mg
Niacin	100%	20 mg
B$_6$	50%	1.0 mg
(pyridoxine hydrochloride)		
B$_{12}$	50%	3 mcg
(cyanocobalamin)		

MINERALS:	US RDA	
Calcium	12.5%	125 mg
Copper	50%	1 mg
Iodine	100%	150 mcg
Iron	27.8%	5 mg

*Percentage of US Recommended Daily Allowances for adults and children 4 or more years of age.

Ingredients: Dibasic Calcium Phosphate, Microcrystalline Cellulose, Ascorbic Acid, Ferrous Fumarate, Niacinamide, dl-alpha Tocopheryl Acetate, Sodium Starch Glycolate, Magnesium Stearate, Vitamin A Acetate, Hydroxypropyl Methylcellulose, Colloidal Silicon Dioxide, Vitamin D3, Copper Sulfate, Thiamine Mononitrate, Riboflavin, Pyridoxine Hydrochloride, Cyanocobalamin, Iodine, Folic Acid, Carnauba Wax, Flavors, FD&C Red #40.

May Also Contain: Propylene Glycol, Polysorbate 80

Indications: The STUART FORMULA tablet provides a well-balanced multivitamin/multimineral formula intended for use as a daily dietary supplement for adults and children over age four.

Directions: One tablet daily or as directed by physician.

Warnings: Keep this and all drugs out of the reach of children. In case of accidental overdose, seek professional assistance or contact a Poison Control Center immediately.

How Supplied: Bottles of 100 and 250 white, round tablets. Child-resistant safety caps are standard on both bottles as a safeguard against accidental ingestion by children.
NDC 16837-866.
Shown in Product Identification Guide, page 410

STUARTINIC® Tablets
[stu "are-tin 'ic]
Hematinic

**ONE TABLET DAILY PROVIDES:
US RDA***

Iron	556%	100 mg
VITAMINS:		
C	833%	500 mg
Thiamin	327%	4.9 mg
Riboflavin	353%	6 mg
Niacin	100%	20 mg
B$_6$	40%	0.8 mg
B$_{12}$	417%	25 mcg
PantothenicAcid	92%	9.2 mg

*Percentage of US Recommended Daily Allowances for adults and children 4 or more years of age.

Ingredients: Active: ferrous fumarate, ascorbic acid, sodium ascorbate, niacinamide, calcium pantothenate, thiamin mononitrate, riboflavin, pyridoxine hydrochloride, cyanocobalamin.
Inactive: flavor, hydrogenated vegetable oil, microcrystalline cellulose, povidone, Yellow 6, Yellow 10, and other ingredients.

Indications: STUARTINIC is a complete hematinic for patients with history of iron deficiency anemia who also lack proper amounts of vitamin C and B-complex vitamins due to inadequate diet. The use of well-tolerated ferrous fumarate in STUARTINIC provides a high level of elemental iron with a low incidence of gastric distress. The inclusion of 500 mg of vitamin C per tablet serves to maintain more of the iron in the absorbable ferrous state. The B-complex vitamins improve nutrition where B-complex deficient diets contribute to the anemia.

Warnings: As with any drug, if you are pregnant or nursing a baby, seek the advice of a health professional before using this product. Keep out of the reach of children. In case of accidental overdose, seek professional assistance or contact a Poison Control Center immediately.

Dosage: One tablet daily taken after a meal or as directed by physician. Because of the high amount of iron per tablet, STUARTINIC is not recommended for children under 12 years of age.

How Supplied: STUARTINIC is supplied in bottles of 60 yellow, film-coated, oval-shaped tablets. NDC 16837-862.
Note: A child-resistant safety cap is standard on each 60 tablet bottle as a safeguard against accidental ingestion by children.
Shown in Product Identification Guide, page 410

Konsyl Pharmaceuticals, Inc.
**4200 S. HULEN
FORT WORTH, TX 76109**

KONSYL® POWDER
**(psyllium hydrophilic mucilloid)
Sugar Free, Sugar Substitute Free.
6.0 grams of psyllium per
TEASPOON**

Description: Konsyl is a bulk-forming natural therapeutic fiber for restoring and maintaining regularity. Konsyl contains 100% hydrophilic mucilloid, a highly efficient dietary fiber derived from the husk of the psyllium seed. Konsyl contains no chemical stimulants and is non-addictive. Each dose contains 6.0 grams of psyllium compared to 3.4 grams of psyllium in most other products.

Inactive Ingredients: None. Each 6 gram dose provides 3 calories. Konsyl is sodium free. Since Konsyl is sugar free, it is excellent for diabetics who require a bowel normalizer.

Actions: Konsyl provides bulk that promotes normal elimination. The product is uniform, instantly miscible, palatable, and non-irritative in the gastrointestinal tract.

Indications: Konsyl is indicated in the management of chronic constipation, irritable bowel syndrome, as adjunctive therapy in the constipation of diverticular disease, bowel management of patients with hemorrhoids, and for constipation during pregnancy, convalescence, and senility. Konsyl is also indicated for other indications as prescribed by physician.

Contraindications: Intestinal obstruction, fecal impaction.

Warnings: Keep this and all drugs out of the reach of children. Taking this product without adequate fluid may cause it to swell and block your throat or esophagus and may cause choking. Do not take this product if you have difficulty in swallowing. If you experience chest pain, vomiting or difficulty in swallowing or breathing after taking this product, seek immediate medical attention.

Precautions: May cause allergic reaction in people sensitive to inhaled or ingested psyllium powder.

Dosage and Administration:
Mix this product (child or adult dose) with at least 8 ounces of water or other fluid. Taking this product without enough liquid may cause choking. See Warnings.
ADULTS: Place one rounded teaspoon (6.0 grams) into a dry shaker cup or container that can be closed. Add 8 oz. of juice, cold water or your favorite beverage. Shake, don't stir, for 3–5 seconds. Drink promptly. If mixture thickens, add more liquid and shake. Follow with an 8 oz. glass of juice or water to aid product action. Konsyl can be taken one to three times daily, depending on need and response. Konsyl generally produces results within 12–72 hours. Take Konsyl at any convenient time, morning or evening; before or after meals. When taking Konsyl, one should drink several 8 oz. glasses of water a day to aid product action.
CHILDREN: (6–12 years old) Use ½ adult dose in 8 oz. of liquid, 1–3 times daily.

New Users: Easy Does It. Medical research shows that higher fiber intake is important for good digestive health. To help the body adjust and avoid minor gas and bloating sometimes associated with high fiber intake, it may be necessary to take one half dose over several days and then slowly increase the dosage over several days. Always follow with 8 oz. of liquid.
How Supplied: Powder, containers of 10.6 oz. (300 g), 15.9 oz. (450 g) and 30 single dose (6.0 g) packets.

Is this product OTC? Yes.

KONSYL-D® POWDER
(Psyllium hydrophilic mucilloid)
3.4 grams of psyllium per
TEASPOON with dextrose added

Description: Konsyl-D is a bulk-forming natural therapeutic fiber for restoring and maintaining regularity. Konsyl-D contains 3.4 grams of psyllium hydrophilic mucilloid, a highly efficient dietary fiber derived from the husk of the psyllium seed. Konsyl-D contains no chemical stimulants and is non-addictive. Each teaspoon dose contains 3.4 grams of psyllium which is unflavored and can be mixed with a variety of juices.

Inactive Ingredients: Dextrose. Each 6.5 gram dose provides 14 calories. Konsyl-D is sodium free.

Actions: See Konsyl description of Actions.

Indications: See Konsyl description of Indications.

Contraindications: Intestinal obstruction, fecal impaction.

Warnings: See Konsyl description of Warnings.

Precaution: May cause allergic reaction in people sensitive to inhaled or ingested psyllium powder.

Dosage and Administration:
Mix this product (child or adult dose) with at least 8 ounces (a full glass) of water or other fluid. Taking this product without enough liquid may cause choking. See Warnings.
ADULTS: Place one rounded teaspoon (6.5 grams) into a dry glass. Add 8 oz. of juice or other beverage. Stir for 3–5 seconds. Drink promptly. Follow with an 8 oz. glass of juice or water to aid product action. Konsyl-D can be taken one to three times daily, depending on need and response. Konsyl-D generally produces results within 12–72 hours. Take Konsyl-D at any convenient time, morning or evening; before or after meals. When taking Konsyl-D, one should drink several 8 oz. glasses of water a day to aid product action.
CHILDREN: (6–12 years old) ½ adult dose in 8 oz. of liquid, 1–3 times daily.

New Users: See Konsyl instructions for New Users.

How Supplied: Powder, containers of 11.5 oz (325 g), 17.6 oz (500 g) and 30 single dose (6.5 g) packets.

Is the Product OTC? Yes.

KONSYL®-ORANGE POWDER
(psyllium hydrophilic mucilloid)
Ultra Fine Texture ... Easy to Mix
Formula
3.4 grams of psyllium per
TABLESPOON

Description: Konsyl-Orange is a bulk-forming natural therapeutic fiber for restoring and maintaining regularity. Konsyl-Orange contains 3.4 grams of psyllium hydrophilic mucilloid, a highly efficient dietary fiber derived from the husk of the psyllium seed. Konsyl-Orange contains no chemical stimulants and is non-addictive. Each TABLESPOON dose contains 3.4 grams of psyllium which is ultrafine texture for easy mixing.

Inactive Ingredients: Sucrose, citric acid, FD&C Yellow #6 and D&C Yellow #10 and flavoring. Each 12 gram dose provides 35 calories. Konsyl-Orange is sodium free.

Actions: See Konsyl description of Actions.

Indications: See Konsyl description of Indication.

Contraindications: Intestinal obstruction, fecal impaction.

Precaution: May cause allergic reaction in people sensitive to inhaled or ingested psyllium powder.

Warnings: See Konsyl description of Warnings.

Dosage and Administration:
Mix this product (child or adult dose) with at least 8 ounces (a full glass) of water or other fluid. Taking this product without enough liquid may cause choking. See Warnings.
ADULTS: Place one rounded tablespoon (12.0 grams) into a dry glass. Add 8 oz. of water or other beverage. Stir 3–5 seconds. Drink promptly. Follow with an 8 oz. glass of water to aid product action. Konsyl-Orange can be taken one to three times daily, depending on need and response. Konsyl Orange generally produces results within 12–72 hours. Take Konsyl Orange at any convenient time, morning or evening; before or after meals. When taking Konsyl-Orange, one should drink several 8 oz. glasses of water daily to aid product action.
CHILDREN: (6–12 years old) ½ adult dose in 8 oz. of liquid, 1–3 times daily.

New Users: See Konsyl instructions for New Users.

How Supplied: Ultra fine powder container of 19 oz (538 g) and 30 single dose (12.0 g) packets.

Is the product OTC? Yes.

Lactaid, Inc.
PLEASANTVILLE, NJ 08232

LACTAID® Caplets
(lactase enzyme)

PRODUCT OVERVIEW

Key Facts: Lactaid® lactase enzyme hydrolyzes lactose into two digestible simple sugars: glucose and galactose. Lactaid Caplets are taken orally for *in vivo* hydrolysis of lactose.

Major Uses: Lactase insufficiency, suspected from gastrointestinal discomfort (ie, gas, bloating, flatulence, cramps, and diarrhea) after the ingestion of milk or lactose-containing products.

PRESCRIBING INFORMATION

Description: Each Lactaid Caplet contains 3000 FCC (Food Chemical Codex) units of lactase enzyme (derived from *Aspergillus oryzae*).

Action: Lactase enzyme hydrolyzes the lactose sugar (a double sugar) into its simple sugar components, glucose and galactose.

Indications:
Lactase insufficiency, suspected from gastrointestinal discomfort (ie, gas, bloating, flatulence, cramps, and diar-

Continued on next page

Lactaid—Cont.

rhea) after the ingestion of milk or lactose-containing products.

Usual Dosage: These convenient, portable caplets are easy to swallow or chew and can be used with milk or any dairy food. We recommend swallowing or chewing 3 caplets with the first bite of dairy food. Take no more than 6 caplets at a time. Don't be discouraged if at first Lactaid does not work to your satisfaction. Because the degree of enzyme deficiency naturally varies from person to person and from food to food, you may have to adjust the number of caplets up or down to find your own level of comfort. Lactaid Caplets are nonhabit-forming, and because they work only on the food as you eat it, use them every time you enjoy dairy foods.

Warning: If you experience any discomfort which is unusual or seems unrelated to the condition for which you took this product, consult a doctor before taking any more of it. Do not use if you've had an allergic reaction to Lactaid products. If abdominal discomfort from dairy foods persists after using Lactaid, consult your physician. Do not use if carton is opened or if printed plastic neckwrap is broken.

Inactive Ingredients: Dextrates, Dibasic Calcium Phosphate, Microcrystalline Cellulose, Croscarmellose Sodium, Hydrogenated Vegetable Oil and Cornstarch.

Nutritional Information: Serving size: 3 Caplets: Calories: 4. Protein: Less than 1 g. Fat: Less than 1 g. Sodium: 5 mg. Percentage U.S. Recommended Daily Allowances (U.S.RDA): Contains less than 2% of the U.S. RDA of Protein, Vitamin A, Vitamin C and Thiamine.

How Supplied: Lactaid Caplets are available in bottles of 12, 50, and 100 counts. Store at or below room temperature (below 77°F) but do not refrigerate. Keep away from heat.

Shown in Product Identification Guide, page 411

LACTAID® Drops   OTC
(lactase enzyme)

PRODUCT OVERVIEW

Key Facts: Lactaid® lactase enzyme hydrolyzes lactose into two digestible simple sugars: glucose and galactose. Lactaid Drops are added to milk for *in vitro* hydrolysis of lactose.

Major Uses: Lactase insufficiency, suspected from gastrointestinal discomfort (ie, gas, bloating, flatulence, cramps, and diarrhea) after the ingestion of milk.

PRESCRIBING INFORMATION

Description: Each 5 drop dosage contains sufficient lactase enzyme (derived from *Kluyveromyces lactis*) to hydrolyze 70% of lactose from a quart of milk.

Action: The lactase enzyme hydrolyzes the lactose sugar (a double sugar) into its simple sugar components, glucose and galactose.

Indications: Lactase insufficiency, suspected from gastrointestinal discomfort (ie, gas, bloating, flatulence, cramps, and diarrhea) after the ingestion of milk.

Usual Dosage: Lactaid drops are a liquid form of the natural lactase enzyme that makes milk more digestible. To use, add Lactaid drops to a quart of milk, shake gently and refrigerate for 24 hours. We recommend starting with 5–7 drops per quart of milk but because sensitivity to lactose can vary you may have to adjust the number of drops you use. If you are still experiencing discomfort after consuming milk with 5–7 Lactaid drops per quart, you may want to add 10 drops per quart or even 15 drops per quart. 15 drops per quart should remove nearly all of the lactose in the milk. Lactaid can be used with any kind of milk: whole, 1%, 2%, non-fat, skim, powdered and chocolate milk.

Warning: If you experience any discomfort which is unusual or seems unrelated to the condition for which you took this product, consult a doctor before taking any more of it. Do not use if you've had an allergic reaction to Lactaid products. If abdominal discomfort from dairy foods persists after using Lactaid, consult your physician. Do not use if carton is opened or if printed plastic neckwrap is broken.

Inactive Ingredients: Glycerin, Water

Nutrutional Information: Serving size: 5 drops; Servings per container: 75. Calories: 0; Protein: 0g; Carbohydrate: 0g; Fat: 0g; Sodium: 0 mg. Percentage of U.S. Recommended Daily Allowances (U.S. RDA): Contains less than 2% of the U.S. RDA of Protein, Vitamin A, Vitamin C and Thiamine.

How Supplied: Lactaid Drops are available in .09 fl. oz. (12 quart supply), .22 fl. oz. (30 quart supply), and .53 fl. oz. (75 quart supply). Store at or below room temperature (below 77°F). Refrigerate after opening.

Shown in Product Identification Guide, page 411

**IF YOU SUSPECT
AN INTERACTION...**
The 1,400-page
*PDR Guide to Drug Interactions ●
Side Effects ● Indications*
can help.
Use the order form
in the front of this book.

Lavoptik Company, Inc.
**661 WESTERN AVENUE N.
ST. PAUL, MN 55103**

LAVOPTIK® Eye Wash

Description: Isotonic LAVOPTIK Eye Wash is a buffered solution designed to help physically remove contaminants from the surface of the eye and lids. Formulated to buffer contaminants toward the safe range and help restore normal salts and water ratios in the tears.

Contents: Each 100 ml

Sodium Chloride	0.49	gram
Sodium Biphosphate	0.40	gram
Sodium Phosphate	0.45	gram
Preservative Agent		
Benzalkonium Chloride	0.005	gram

Precautions: If you experience severe eye pain, headache, rapid change in vision (side or straight ahead); sudden appearance of floating objects, acute redness of the eyes, pain on exposure to light or double vision consult a physician at once. If symptoms persist or worsen after use of this product, consult a physician. If solution changes color or becomes cloudy do not use. Keep this and all medicines out of reach of children. Keep container tightly closed. Do not use if safety seal is broken at time of purchase.

Administration: 6 ounce size with Eye Cup.
Rinse cup with clean water immediately before and after each use, avoid contamination of rim and inside surfaces of cup. Apply cup, half-filled with LAVOPTIK Eye Wash tightly to the eye. Tilt head backward. Open eyelids wide, rotate eyeball and blink several times to insure thorough washing. Discard washings. Repeat other eye. Tightly cap bottle.
32 ounce size.
Break seal as you remove cap and pour directly on contaminated area.

How Supplied: 6 ounce bottle with eyecup, NDC 10651-01040.
32 ounce bottle, NDC 10651-01019.

Lederle Laboratories
**A Division of American
Cyanamid Co.
ONE CYANAMID PLAZA
WAYNE, NJ 07470**

LEDERMARK®
Product Identification Code

Many Lederle tablets and capsules bear an identification code. A current listing appears in the Product Information Section of the 1994 PDR for prescription drugs.

CALTRATE® 600
[căl-trāte]
**High Potency Calcium Supplement
Nature's Most Concentrated Form
of Calcium™
No Sugar, No Salt, No Lactose,
No Cholesterol, No Preservatives,
Film-Coated for Easy Swallowing**

Inactive Ingredients: Croscarmellose
Sodium, Hydroxypropyl Methylcellu-
lose, Magnesium Stearate, Microcrystal-
line Cellulose, PVPP, Sodium Lauryl
Sulfate, and Titanium Dioxide.
TWO TABLETS DAILY PROVIDE:

**For Adults—
Percentage of US
Recommended Daily
Allowance (US RDA)**

3000 mg Calcium
Carbonate which
provides 1200 mg
elemental calcium   120%

Recommended Intake: One or two
tablets daily or as directed by the
physician.
Warning: Keep out of the reach of
children.
How Supplied: Bottle of 60—
NDC 0005-5510-19
Store at Room Temperature.
© 1990   11643-91
                                          D15

*Shown in Product Identification
Guide, page 410*

CALTRATE® 600+Iron & Vitamin D
[căl-trāte]
**High Potency Calcium Supplement
Nature's Most Concentrated Form
of Calcium™
No Sugar, No Salt, No Lactose, No
Cholesterol, Film-Coated for Easy
Swallowing**

Inactive Ingredients: Blue 2, Croscarmellose Sodium, Hydroxypropyl Cellulose, Magnesium Stearate, Microcrystalline Cellulose, Polysorbate 80, Povidone,
PVPP, Red 40, Sodium Lauryl Sulfate,
Titanium Dioxide, and Triethyl Citrate.
• CALTRATE + Iron contains pure
calcium and time-release iron for
diets deficient in both minerals.
• Plus Vitamin D to help absorb
calcium.
ONE TABLET DAILY CONTAINS:

**For Adults—
Percentage of US
Recommended Daily
Allowance (US RDA)**

1500 mg Calcium Carbonate
which provides 600 mg
elemental calcium   60%
18 mg elemental Iron in
the Optisorb® Time-
Release System
(as ferrous fumarate)   100%
125 IU Vitamin D   31%

Recommended Intake: One or two
tablets daily or as directed by the
physician.
Warning: Keep out of the reach of
children.
How Supplied: Bottle of 60—
NDC 0005-5523-19
Store at Room Temperature.
© 1991   11602-91
                                          D9

*Shown in Product Identification
Guide, page 410*

CALTRATE® 600 + Vitamin D
[căl-trāte]
**High Potency Calcium Supplement
Nature's Most Concentrated Form
of Calcium™
No Sugar, No Salt, No Lactose, No
Cholesterol, Film-Coated for Easy
Swallowing**

Inactive Ingredients: Blue 2, Croscarmellose Sodium, FD&C Yellow No. 6, Hydroxypropyl Methylcellulose, Magnesium Stearate, Microcrystalline Cellulose, Povidone, PVPP, Red 40, Sodium
Lauryl Sulfate, and Titanium Dioxide.
TWO TABLETS DAILY PROVIDE:

**For Adults—
Percentage of US
Recommended Daily
Allowance (US RDA)**

3000 mg Calcium Carbonate
which provides 1200 mg
elemental calcium   120%
250 IU Vitamin D   62%

Recommended Intake: One or two
tablets daily or as directed by the physician.
Warning: Keep out of the reach of
children.
How Supplied: Bottle of 60—
NDC-0005-5509-19
Store at Room Temperature.
© 1990   11642-91
                                          D12

*Shown in Product Identification
Guide, page 410*

CENTRUM®
[sĕn-trŭm]
**High Potency
Multivitamin-Multimineral Formula,
Advanced Formula
From A to Zinc®
Including the Complete Antioxidant
Group**

Each tablet contains:
[See table top of next column]

Inactive Ingredients: FD&C Yellow
No. 6, Hydroxypropyl Methylcellulose,
Lactose, Magnesium Stearate, Micro-
crystalline Cellulose, Polysorbate 80,
Polyvinylpyrrolidone, Stearic Acid, Tita-
nium Dioxide, and Triethyl Citrate.

Recommended Intake: Adults, 1 tablet daily.

**For Adults—
Percentage of US
Recommended Daily
Allowance (US RDA)**

VITAMINS		
Vitamin A	5000 IU	(100%)
(as Acetate and Beta Carotene)		
Vitamin D	400 IU	(100%)
Vitamin E	30 IU	(100%)
Vitamin K_1	25 mcg*	
Vitamin C	60 mg	(100%)
Folic Acid	400 mcg	(100%)
Vitamin B_1	1.5 mg	(100%)
Vitamin B_2	1.7 mg	(100%)
Niacinamide	20 mg	(100%)
Vitamin B_6	2 mg	(100%)
Vitamin B_{12}	6 mcg	(100%)
Pantothenic Acid	10 mg	(100%)
Biotin	30 mcg	(10%)
MINERALS		
Calcium	162 mg	(16%)
Phosphorus	109 mg	(11%)
Iodine	150 mcg	(100%)
Iron	18 mg	(100%)
Magnesium	100 mg	(25%)
Copper	2 mg	(100%)
Zinc	15 mg	(100%)
Manganese	2.5 mg*	
Potassium	40 mg*	
Chloride	36.3 mg*	
Chromium	25 mcg*	
Molybdenum	25 mcg*	
Selenium	20 mcg*	
Nickel	5 mcg*	
Tin	10 mcg*	
Silicon	2 mg*	
Vanadium	10 mcg*	
Boron	150 mcg*	

*No US RDA established.

How Supplied:
Light peach, engraved CENTRUM C1.
Bottle of 60—NDC 0005-4239-19
Combopack†—NDC 0005-4239-30
†Bottles of 100 plus 30
Store at Room Temperature.
                                      22513-92
                                          D38

*Shown in Product Identification
Guide, page 410*

CENTRUM® Liquid
**High Potency
Multivitamin-Multimineral Formula
Advanced Formula**

Each 15 mL (1 tablespoon) contains:
[See table top of next column]

Inactive Ingredients: Alcohol 6.6%,
Artificial and Natural Flavors, Citric
Acid, Glycerin, Polysorbate 80, Sodium
Benzoate, and Sucrose.

Recommended Intake: Adults, 1 tablespoonful (15 mL) daily.

Warning: Keep this and all medication
out of the reach of children.

How Supplied: 8 oz Bottle—
NDC 0005-4343-61
Store at Controlled Room Temperature
15°–30°C (59°–86°F).

Continued on next page

Lederle—Cont.

**For Adults—
Percentage of US
Recommended
Daily
Allowance
(US RDA)**

Vitamin A (as Palmitate)	2500 IU	(50%)
Vitamin E (as dl-Alpha Tocopheryl Acetate)	30 IU	(100%)
Vitamin C (as Ascorbic Acid)	60 mg	(100%)
Vitamin B$_1$ (as Thiamine Hydrochloride)	1.5 mg	(100%)
Vitamin B$_2$ (as Riboflavin)	1.7 mg	(100%)
Niacinamide	20 mg	(100%)
Vitamin B$_6$ (as Pyridoxine Hydrochloride)	2 mg	(100%)
Vitamin B$_{12}$ (as Cyanocobalamin)	6 mcg	(100%)
Vitamin D$_2$	400 IU	(100%)
Biotin	300 mcg	(100%)
Pantothenic Acid (as Panthenol)	10 mg	(100%)
Iodine (as Potassium Iodide)	150 mcg	(100%)
Iron (as Ferrous Gluconate)	9 mg	(50%)
Zinc (as Zinc Gluconate)	3 mg	(20%)
Manganese (as Manganese Chloride)	2.5 mg	*
Chromium (as Chromium Chloride)	25 mcg	*
Molybdenum (as Sodium Molybdate)	25 mcg	*

*No US RDA established.

PROTECT FROM FREEZING.

23317
D3

*Shown in Product Identification
Guide, page 410*

CENTRUM, JR.®

[sĕn-trŭm]
**Shamu and his Crew™
+ EXTRA C
Children's Chewable
Vitamin/Mineral Formula
Nutritional Support From Head to
Toe®**

[See table at right]

Inactive Ingredients: Artificial Flavorings, Aspartame,† Blue 2, Citric Acid, FD&C Yellow No. 6, Lactose, Magnesium Stearate, Microcrystalline Cellulose, Pregelatinized Starch, Red 40, Silica Gel, Sorbitol, Stearic Acid, and Sucrose.
† **Phenylketonurics: Contains Phenylalanine.**

Warnings: CONTAINS IRON, WHICH CAN BE HARMFUL IN LARGE DOSES. CLOSE TIGHTLY AND KEEP OUT OF THE REACH OF CHILDREN. IN CASE OF ACCIDENTAL OVERDOSE, CONTACT A PHY-

SICIAN OR POISON CONTROL CENTER IMMEDIATELY.

Recommended Intake: Children 2 to 4 years of age: Chew approximately one-half tablet daily. Children over 4 years of age: Chew one tablet daily.

How Supplied: Bottle of 60—NDC 0005-4249-19

Tamper Resistant Feature: Bottle sealed with clear band printed LEDERSEAL®. Do not accept if band is not below the label panel or if it is missing or broken.
Store at Room Temperature.
© 1993   32302-93
                          D11
Sea World Characters ©1993 Sea World, Inc. All Rights Reserved.
Shamu and his Crew™ are trademarks and copyrights of Sea World, Inc. CENTRUM, JR.®, The Spectrum Design and all other marks and indicia are trademarks and copyrights of Lederle.

*Shown in Product Identification
Guide, page 410*

CENTRUM, JR.®

[sĕn-trŭm]
**Shamu and his Crew™
+EXTRA CALCIUM
Children's Chewable
Vitamin/Mineral Formula
Nutritional Support From Head to
Toe®**

[See table on next page.]

Inactive Ingredients: Artificial Flavorings, Aspartame,† Blue 2, Citric Acid, FD&C Yellow No. 6, Lactose, Magnesium Stearate, Microcrystalline Cellulose, Pregelatinized Starch, Red 40, Silica Gel, Sorbitol, Stearic Acid, and Sucrose.

† **Phenylketonurics: Contains Phenylalanine.**

Warnings: CONTAINS IRON, WHICH CAN BE HARMFUL IN LARGE DOSES. CLOSE TIGHTLY AND KEEP OUT OF THE REACH OF CHILDREN. IN CASE OF ACCIDENTAL OVERDOSE, CONTACT A PHYSICIAN OR POISON CONTROL CENTER IMMEDIATELY.

Recommended Intake: Children 2 to 4 years of age: chew approximately one-half tablet daily. Children over 4 years of age: chew one tablet daily.

How Supplied: Bottle of 60—NDC 0005-4222-19

Tamper Resistant Feature: Bottle sealed with clear band printed LEDERSEAL®. Do not accept if band is not below the label panel or if it is missing or broken.
Store at Room Temperature.
© 1993   32303-93
                          D9
Sea World Characters ©1993 Sea World, Inc. All Rights Reserved.
Shamu and his Crew™ are trademarks and copyrights of Sea World, Inc. CENTRUM, JR.®, The Spectrum Design and all other marks and indicia are trademarks and copyrights of Lederle.

*Shown in Product Identification
Guide, page 410*

**CENTRUM, JR.® + EXTRA C
Children's Chewable
Vitamin/Mineral Formula**

EACH TABLET CONTAINS:	Quantity per tablet	Percentage of US Recommended Daily Allowance (US RDA)	
		For Children 2 to 4 (½ tablet)	For Children Over 4 (1 tablet)
VITAMINS			
Vitamin A (as Acetate and Beta Carotene)	5,000 IU	(100%)	(100%)
Vitamin D	400 IU	(50%)	(100%)
Vitamin E	30 IU	(150%)	(100%)
Vitamin C	300 mg	(375%)	(500%)
Folic Acid	400 mcg	(100%)	(100%)
Biotin	45 mcg	(15%)	(15%)
Thiamine	1.5 mg	(107%)	(100%)
Pantothenic Acid	10 mg	(100%)	(100%)
Riboflavin	1.7 mg	(107%)	(100%)
Niacinamide	20 mg	(111%)	(100%)
Vitamin B$_6$	2 mg	(143%)	(100%)
Vitamin B$_{12}$	6 mcg	(100%)	(100%)
Vitamin K$_1$	10 mcg*		
MINERALS			
Iron	18 mg	(90%)	(100%)
Magnesium	40 mg	(10%)	(10%)
Iodine	150 mcg	(107%)	(100%)
Copper	2 mg	(100%)	(100%)
Phosphorus	50 mg	(3.12%)	(5.0%)
Calcium	108 mg	(6.75%)	(10.8%)
Zinc	15 mg	(93%)	(100%)
Manganese	1 mg*		
Molybdenum	20 mcg*		
Chromium	20 mcg*		

*Recognized as essential in human nutrition but no US RDA established.

CENTRUM, JR.® + EXTRA CALCIUM
Children's Chewable
Vitamin/Mineral Formula

EACH TABLET CONTAINS:	Quantity per tablet		Percentage of US Recommended Daily Allowance (US RDA)	
			For Children 2 to 4 (½ tablet)	For Children Over 4 (1 tablet)
VITAMINS				
Vitamin A (as Acetate and Beta Carotene)	5,000	IU	(100%)	(100%)
Vitamin D	400	IU	(50%)	(100%)
Vitamin E	30	IU	(150%)	(100%)
Vitamin C	60	mg	(75%)	(100%)
Folic Acid	400	mcg	(100%)	(100%)
Biotin	45	mcg	(15%)	(15%)
Thiamine	1.5	mg	(107%)	(100%)
Pantothenic Acid	10	mg	(100%)	(100%)
Riboflavin	1.7	mg	(107%)	(100%)
Niacinamide	20	mg	(111%)	(100%)
Vitamin B_6	2	mg	(143%)	(100%)
Vitamin B_{12}	6	mcg	(100%)	(100%)
Vitamin K_1	10	mcg*		
MINERALS				
Iron	18	mg	(90%)	(100%)
Magnesium	40	mg	(10%)	(10%)
Iodine	150	mcg	(107%)	(100%)
Copper	2	mg	(100%)	(100%)
Phosphorus	50	mg	(3.12%)	(5.0%)
Calcium	160	mg	(10%)	(16%)
Zinc	15	mg	(93%)	(100%)
Manganese	1	mg*		
Molybdenum	20	mcg*		
Chromium	20	mcg*		

*Recognized as essential in human nutrition but no US RDA established.

CENTRUM, JR.® + IRON
Children's Chewable
Vitamin/Mineral Formula

EACH TABLET CONTAINS:	Quantity per tablet		Percentage of US Recommended Daily Allowance (US RDA)	
			For Children 2 to 4 (½ tablet)	For Children Over 4 (1 tablet)
VITAMINS				
Vitamin A (as Acetate and Beta Carotene)	5,000	IU	(100%)	(100%)
Vitamin D	400	IU	(50%)	(100%)
Vitamin E	30	IU	(150%)	(100%)
Vitamin C	60	mg	(75%)	(100%)
Folic Acid	400	mcg	(100%)	(100%)
Biotin	45	mcg	(15%)	(15%)
Thiamine	1.5	mg	(107%)	(100%)
Pantothenic Acid	10	mg	(100%)	(100%)
Riboflavin	1.7	mg	(107%)	(100%)
Niacinamide	20	mg	(111%)	(100%)
Vitamin B_6	2	mg	(143%)	(100%)
Vitamin B_{12}	6	mcg	(100%)	(100%)
Vitamin K_1	10	mcg*		
MINERALS				
Iron	18	mg	(90%)	(100%)
Magnesium	40	mg	(10%)	(10%)
Iodine	150	mcg	(107%)	(100%)
Copper	2	mg	(100%)	(100%)
Phosphorus	50	mg	(3.12%)	(5.0%)
Calcium	108	mg	(6.75%)	(10.8%)
Zinc	15	mg	(93%)	(100%)
Manganese	1	mg*		
Molybdenum	20	mcg*		
Chromium	20	mcg*		

*Recognized as essential in human nutrition but no US RDA established.

Continued on next page

Lederle—Cont.

CENTRUM, JR.®
[sĕn-trŭm]
Shamu and his Crew™
+ IRON
Children's Chewable
Vitamin/Mineral Formula
Nutritional Support From Head
to Toe®

[See table on preceding page]

Inactive Ingredients: Artificial Flavorings, Aspartame,† Blue 2, Citric Acid, FD&C Yellow No. 6, Lactose, Magnesium Stearate, Microcrystalline Cellulose, Pregelatinized Starch, Red 40, Silica Gel, Sorbitol, Stearic Acid, and Sucrose.

† **Phenylketonurics: Contains Phenylalanine.**

Warnings: CONTAINS IRON, WHICH CAN BE HARMFUL IN LARGE DOSES. CLOSE TIGHTLY AND KEEP OUT OF THE REACH OF CHILDREN. IN CASE OF ACCIDENTAL OVERDOSE, CONTACT A PHYSICIAN OR POISON CONTROL CENTER IMMEDIATELY.

Recommended Intake: Children 2 to 4 years of age: Chew approximately one-half tablet daily. Children over 4 years of age: Chew one tablet daily.

How Supplied: Assorted Flavors—Uncoated Tablet—Partially Scored—Engraved Lederle C2 and CENTRUM, JR. Bottle of 60—NDC 0005-4234-19

Tamper Resistant Feature: Bottle sealed with clear band printed LEDERSEAL®. Do not accept if band is not below the label panel or if it is missing or broken.

Store at Room Temperature.
© 1993   32304-93
                                            D12
Sea World Characters ©1993 Sea World, Inc. All Rights Reserved.
Shamu and his Crew™ are trademarks and copyrights of Sea World, Inc. CENTRUM, JR.®, The Spectrum Design and all other marks and indicia are trademarks and copyrights of Lederle.
Shown in Product Identification Guide, page 410

CENTRUM SILVER®
Specially Formulated
Multivitamin-Multimineral for Adults
50+
Complete
From A to Zinc®

Each tablet contains:
[See table top of next column]
Inactive Ingredients: Blue 2, Crospovidone, FD&C Yellow No. 6, Hydroxypropyl Methylcellulose, Lactose, Magnesium Stearate, Microcrystalline Cellulose, Polyethylene Glycol, Polysorbate 80, Red 40, Silica Gel, Stearic Acid, and Titanium Dioxide.

	For Adults—Percentage of US Recommended Daily Allowance (US RDA)	
Vitamin A	6000 IU	(120%)
(as Acetate and Beta Carotene)		
Vitamin B_1	1.5 mg	(100%)
Vitamin B_2	1.7 mg	(100%)
Vitamin B_6	3 mg	(150%)
Vitamin B_{12}	25 mcg	(416%)
Biotin	30 mcg	(10%)
Folic Acid	200 mcg	(50%)
Niacinamide	20 mg	(100%)
Pantothenic Acid	10 mg	(100%)
Vitamin C	60 mg	(100%)
Vitamin D	400 IU	(100%)
Vitamin E	45 IU	(150%)
Vitamin K_1	10 mcg*	
Calcium	200 mg	(20%)
Copper	2 mg	(100%)
Iodine	150 mcg	(100%)
Iron	9 mg	(50%)
Magnesium	100 mg	(25%)
Phosphorus	48 mg	(5%)
Zinc	15 mg	(100%)
Chloride	72 mg*	
Chromium	100 mcg*	
Manganese	2.5 mg*	
Molybdenum	25 mcg*	
Nickel	5 mcg*	
Potassium	80 mg*	
Selenium	20 mcg*	
Silicon	10 mcg*	
Vanadium	10 mcg*	
Boron	150 mcg*	

*No US RDA established.

Recommended Intake:
Adults, 1 tablet daily.

How Supplied: Bottle of 60—NDC 0005-4177-19
Bottle of 100—NDC 0005-4177-23
Store at Room Temperature.
© 1991   11630-91
                                            D3
Shown in Product Identification Guide, page 411

Dual Action
FERRO–SEQUELS®
[fĕrrō-sēquals]
High Potency Iron Supplement
Time-Release Iron Plus
Clinically Proven Anticonstipant
Easy-to-Swallow Tablets
Low Sodium, No Sugar

Active Ingredients: Each tablet contains 150 mg of ferrous fumarate equivalent to 50 mg of elemental iron and 100 mg of docusate sodium (DSS).

Inactive Ingredients: Blue 1, Corn Starch, Crospovidone, Hydroxypropyl Methylcellulose, Lactose, Magnesium Stearate, Microcrystalline Cellulose, Modified Food Starch, Povidone, Silica Gel, Sodium Lauryl Sulfate, Titanium Dioxide, and Yellow 10.

Warnings: As with any drug, if you are pregnant or nursing a baby, seek the advice of a health professional before using this product. Keep this and all medications out of the reach of children. In case of accidental overdose, seek professional assistance or contact a Poison Control Center immediately.

Recommended Intake: One tablet, once or twice daily or as prescribed by a physician.

How Supplied: Green, capsule-shaped, film-coated tablets engraved LL and F2. Boxes of 30—
NDC 0005-5267-68
Bottle of 30—NDC 0005-5267-13
Bottle of 100—NDC 0005-5267-23
Bottle of 1000—NDC 0005-5267-34
Unit Dose Pack 10×10—
NDC 0005-5267-60
Store at Room Temperature.
                                            27533
                                            D3
Shown in Product Identification Guide, page 411

FIBERCON®
[fī-bĕr-cŏn]
Calcium Polycarbophil
Bulk-Forming Fiber Laxative

Less than one calorie per caplet,
Sodium- and Preservative-free,
Film-coated for easy swallowing,
Calcium rich, No chemical
stimulants, Non-habit forming.

Active Ingredient: Each caplet contains 625 mg calcium polycarbophil equivalent to 500 mg polycarbophil.

Inactive Ingredients: Calcium Carbonate, Caramel, Crospovidone, Hydroxypropyl Methylcellulose, Magnesium Stearate, Microcrystalline Cellulose, Povidone, and Silica Gel.

Indications: Relief of constipation. FIBERCON restores and maintains regularity and promotes normal function of the bowel.

Actions: FIBERCON works naturally so continued use for 1 to 3 days is normally required to provide full benefit.

Warnings: Any sudden change in bowel habits may indicate a more serious condition than constipation. Consult your physician if symptoms such as nausea, vomiting, abdominal pain, or rectal bleeding occur or if this product has no effect within 1 week.
For chronic or continued constipation consult your physician.

Interaction Precaution: If you are taking any form of tetracycline antibiotic, FIBERCON should be taken at least 1 hour before or 2 hours after you have taken the antibiotic.

KEEP THIS AND ALL MEDICINES OUT OF THE REACH OF CHILDREN.

STORE AT CONTROLLED ROOM TEMPERATURE 15°–30°C (59°–86°F). PROTECT CONTENTS FROM MOISTURE.

Recommended Intake: FIBERCON dosage will vary according to diet, exercise, previous laxative use or severity of constipation. Recommended adult starting dose: 2 or 4 caplets daily. May be increased up to eight caplets daily. Children 6 to 12 years: swallow one caplet one to three times a day. Children under 6 years: consult a physician.
A FULL GLASS (8 fl oz) OF LIQUID SHOULD BE TAKEN WITH EACH DOSE. See package insert for additional information.

How Supplied:
Film-coated caplets, scored, engraved LL and F66.
Package of 36 caplets, NDC 0005-2500-02
Package of 60 caplets, NDC 0005-2500-86
Package of 90 caplets, NDC 0005-2500-33
Bottle of 150 caplets, NDC 0005-2500-58
Bottle of 500 caplets, NDC 0005-2500-31
Unit Dose Pkg, NDC 0005-2500-28
10995-91
D8

Shown in Product Identification Guide, page 411

GEVRABON®
[*jĕv-ra băn*]
Vitamin-Mineral Supplement

Composition: Each fluid ounce (30 mL) contains:

For Adults—Percentage of US Recommended Daily Allowance (US RDA)

Vitamin B_1 (as Thiamine Hydrochloride)..................5 mg (333%)
Vitamin B_2 (as Riboflavin-5-Phosphate Sodium)....2.5 mg (147%)
Niacinamide.........................50 mg (250%)
Vitamin B_6 (Pyridoxine Hydrochloride)..............1 mg (50%)
Vitamin B_{12} (as Cyanocobalamin)...............1 mcg (17%)
Pantothenic Acid (as D-Pantothenyl Alcohol).....10 mg (100%)
Iodine (as Potassium Iodide)..............................100 mcg (67%)
Iron (as Ferrous Gluconate) ....15 mg (83%)
Magnesium (as Magnesium Chloride)....................2 mg (0.5%)
Zinc (as Zinc Chloride)..........2 mg (13%)
Choline (as Tricholine Citrate)....................................100 mg*
Manganese (as Manganese Chloride)..............................2 mg*
*Recognized as essential in human nutrition but no U.S. RDA established.
Alcohol 18%

Inactive Ingredients: Alcohol, Citric Acid, Glycerin, Sherry Wine, Sucrose.

Indications: For use as a nutritional supplement. Shake well.

Warnings: As with any drug, if you are pregnant or nursing a baby, seek the advice of a health professional before using

INCREMIN®

		Percentage of US Recommended Daily Allowance (US RDA)	
		Children Under 4	Children Over 4 and Adults
Vitamin B_1 (as Thiamine Hydrochloride)	5 mg	714%	333%
Vitamin B_6	5 mg	714%	250%
Vitamin B_{12} (as Cyanocobalamin)	25 mcg	833%	417%
Iron (as Ferric Pyrophosphate)	30 mg	300%	167%
*L-Lysine Hydrochloride	300 mg		

*No US RDA established.

this product. Keep this preparation out of the reach of children.

Administration and Dosage: Adult: One ounce (30 mL) daily or as prescribed by the physician as a nutritional supplement.

Important Note: In time a slight natural deposit, characteristic of the sherry wine base, may occur. This does not indicate in any way a loss of quality.

How Supplied: Syrup (sherry flavor) decanters of 16 fl oz—NDC 0005-5250-35
Keep Out of Direct Sunlight.
Store at Room Temperature, 15°–30°C (59°–86°F).

DO NOT FREEZE.
16520
D4

GEVRAL® T
[*jĕv-ral t*]
High Potency Multivitamin and Multimineral Supplement Tablets

Each tablet contains:

For Adults—Percentage of US Recommended Daily Allowance (US RDA)

Vitamin A	5000 IU	(100%)
Vitamin E	45 IU	(150%)
Vitamin C	90 mg	(150%)
Folic Acid	0.4 mg	(100%)
Vitamin B_1	2.25 mg	(150%)
Vitamin B_2	2.6 mg	(153%)
Niacinamide	30 mg	(150%)
Vitamin B_6	3 mg	(150%)
Vitamin B_{12}	9 mcg	(150%)
Vitamin D_2	400 IU	(100%)
Calcium	162 mg	(16%)
Phosphorus	125 mg	(13%)
Iodine	225 mcg	(150%)
Iron	27 mg	(150%)
Magnesium	100 mg	(25%)
Copper	1.5 mg	(75%)
Zinc	22.5 mg	(150%)

Inactive Ingredients: Blue 2, Crospovidone, Hydroxypropyl Methylcellulose, Lactose, Magnesium Stearate, Microcrystalline Cellulose, Mineral Oil, Red 40, Silicon Dioxide, Sodium Lauryl Sulfate, Stearic Acid, and Titanium Dioxide.

Recommended Intake: 1 tablet daily or as prescribed by physician.

Warning: Keep this and all medications out of the reach of children.

How Supplied: Tablets (film-coated, maroon). Engraved LL and G2.
Bottle of 100—NDC 0005-4286-23
Store at Room Temperature.
A SPECTRUM® Product   21268-92
D8

INCREMIN®
[*ĭn-cre-mĭn*]
**WITH IRON SYRUP
Vitamins + Iron
DIETARY SUPPLEMENT
(Cherry Flavored)**

Composition: Each teaspoonful (5 mL) contains:
[See table above.]

Inactive Ingredients: Alcohol 0.75%, Cherry Flavor, Red 33, Sodium Benzoate, Sodium Hydroxide, Sorbic Acid, and Sorbitol.

Indications: For the prevention of iron deficiency anemia in children and adults.

Warnings: As with any drug, if you are pregnant or nursing a baby, seek the advice of a health professional before using this product.
Keep this and all medications out of the reach of children.

Recommended Dosages (or as prescribed by a physician):
Children: One teaspoonful (5 mL) daily for the prevention of iron deficiency anemia.
Adults: One teaspoonful (5 mL) daily for the prevention of iron deficiency anemia.

Notice: To protect from light always dispense in this container or in an amber bottle.
Store at Room Temperature.

How Supplied: Syrup (cherry flavor)—Bottles of 4 fl oz—NDC 0005-5604-58
20421-92
DS15

PROTEGRA™
[*prō-tĕg-ră*]
Antioxidant Vitamin & Mineral Supplement

Each softgel contains:
[See table top of next column]

Inactive Ingredients: Gelatin, cottonseed oil, glycerin, dibasic calcium

Continued on next page

Lederle—Cont.

For Adults– Percentage of US Recommended Daily Allowance (US RDA)		
Vitamin E	200 IU	667%
Vitamin C	250 mg	417%
Beta Carotene	3 mg	100%*
Zinc	7.5 mg	50%
Copper	1 mg	50%
Selenium	15 mcg	**
Manganese	1.5 mg	**

*US RDA for Vitamin A.
**No US RDA established.

phosphate, lecithin, partially hydrogenated cottonseed and soybean oils, beeswax, titanium dioxide, FD&C Yellow #6, and FD&C Red #40.

Recommended Intake: Adults: One softgel daily or as directed by a physician. PROTEGRA™ can be taken by itself or with a multiple vitamin.

How Supplied: Bottle of 50—NDC-0005-4377-18
Store at Controlled Room Temperature 15°–30°C (59°–86°F)
Warning: Keep out of the reach of children. 20156-92

Shown in Product Identification Guide, page 411

STRESSTABS® Advanced Formula
[strĕss-tăbs]
High Potency
Stress Formula Vitamins

Each tablet contains:

For Adults– Percentage of US Recommended Daily Allowance (US RDA)		
Vitamin E	30 IU	(100%)
Vitamin C	500 mg	(833%)
B VITAMINS		
Folic Acid	400 mcg	(100%)
Vitamin B₁	10 mg	(667%)
Vitamin B₂	10 mg	(588%)
Niacinamide	100 mg	(500%)
Vitamin B₆	5 mg	(250%)
Vitamin B₁₂	12 mcg	(200%)
Biotin	45 mcg	(15%)
Pantothenic Acid	20 mg	(200%)

Inactive Ingredients: Calcium Carbonate, FD&C Yellow No. 6, Magnesium Stearate, Microcrystalline Cellulose, Modified Food Starch, Silica Gel, and Stearic Acid.

Recommended Intake: Adults, 1 tablet daily or as directed by the physician.

How Supplied: Capsule-shaped tablet (film-coated, orange, scored). Engraved LL and S3.
Bottle of 30—NDC 0005-4124-13
Bottle of 60—NDC 0005-4124-19
Store at Room Temperature. 22505-92
D21
Shown in Product Identification Guide, page 411

STRESSTABS® + IRON
Advanced Formula
[strĕss-tăbs]
High Potency
Stress Formula Vitamins

Each tablet contains:

For Adults– Percentage of US Recommended Daily Allowance (US RDA)		
Vitamin E	30 IU	(100%)
Vitamin C	500 mg	(833%)
B VITAMINS		
Folic Acid	400 mcg	(100%)
Vitamin B₁	10 mg	(667%)
Vitamin B₂	10 mg	(588%)
Niacinamide	100 mg	(500%)
Vitamin B₆	5 mg	(250%)
Vitamin B₁₂	12 mcg	(200%)
Biotin	45 mcg	(15%)
Pantothenic Acid	20 mg	(200%)
Iron	18 mg	(100%)

Inactive Ingredients: Calcium Carbonate, FD&C Yellow No. 6, Magnesium Stearate, Microcrystalline Cellulose, Modified Food Starch, Red 40, Silica Gel, and Stearic Acid.

Recommended Intake: Adults, 1 tablet daily or as directed by the physician.

How Supplied: Capsule-shaped tablets (film-coated, orange-red, scored). Engraved LL and S2.
Bottle of 60—NDC 0005-4126-19
Store at Room Temperature. 22512-92
D19

Shown in Product Identification Guide, page 411

STRESSTABS® + ZINC
Advanced Formula
[strĕss-tăbs]
High Potency
Stress Formula Vitamins

Each tablet contains:

For Adults— Percentage of US Recommended Daily Allowance (US RDA)		
Vitamin E	30 IU	(100%)
Vitamin C	500 mg	(833%)
B VITAMINS		
Folic Acid	400 mcg	(100%)
Vitamin B₁	10 mg	(667%)
Vitamin B₂	10 mg	(588%)
Niacinamide	100 mg	(500%)
Vitamin B₆	5 mg	(250%)
Vitamin B₁₂	12 mcg	(200%)
Biotin	45 mcg	(15%)
Pantothenic Acid	20 mg	(200%)
Copper	3 mg	(150%)
Zinc	23.9 mg	(159%)

Inactive Ingredients: Calcium Carbonate, FD&C Yellow No. 6, Magnesium Stearate, Microcrystalline Cellulose, Modified Food Starch, Silica Gel, and Stearic Acid.

Recommended Intake: Adults, 1 tablet daily or as directed by the physician.

How Supplied: Capsule-shaped tablet (film-coated, peach color, scored). Engraved LL and S3.
Bottle of 60—NDC 0005-4125-19
Store at Room Temperature. 22509-92
D21
Shown in Product Identification Guide, page 411

ZINCON®
[zinc-ŏn]
Dandruff Shampoo

Contains: Pyrithione Zinc (1%), Water, Sodium Methyl Cocoyl Taurate, Cocamide MEA, Sodium Chloride, Magnesium Aluminum Silicate, Sodium Cocoyl Isethionate, Fragrance, Glutaraldehyde, D&C Green #5, Citric Acid or Sodium Hydroxide to adjust pH if necessary.

Indications: Relieves the itching and scalp flaking associated with dandruff. Relieves the itching, irritation, and skin flaking associated with seborrheic dermatitis of the scalp.

Directions: For best results use twice a week. Wet hair, apply to scalp and massage vigorously. Rinse and repeat.
SHAKE WELL BEFORE USING.

Warnings: Keep this and all drugs out of the reach of children. For external use only. Avoid contact with the eyes—if this happens, rinse thoroughly with water. If condition worsens or does not improve after regular use of this product as directed, consult a doctor. Do not use on children under 2 years of age except as directed by a doctor.

How Supplied:
4 oz Bottle—NDC 0005-5455-58
8 oz Bottle—NDC 0005-5455-61
13918
D4
Shown in Product Identification Guide, page 411

If desired, additional information on any Lederle product will be provided by contacting Lederle Professional Services Dept.

EDUCATIONAL MATERIAL

Calcium Supplements: The Differences Are Real
8-page pamphlet describing why today's women need to supplement their diet with calcium.
Important Vitamin News
6-page pamphlet explaining the importance of antioxidants in a healthy diet and good sources of antioxidants in food and vitamin supplements.
Write to: Lederle Promotional Center
2200 Bradley Hill Road
Blauvelt, NY 10913

Lever Brothers Company
390 PARK AVENUE
NEW YORK, NY 10022

DOVE® BAR AND LIQUID DOVE® BEAUTY WASH

Active Ingredients: Sodium Cocoyl Isethionate, Stearic Acid, Sodium Tallowate, Water, Sodium Isethionate, Coconut Acid, Sodium Stearate, Sodium Dodecylbenzenesulfonate, Sodium Cocoate, Fragrance, Sodium Chloride, Titanium Dioxide.

Actions and Uses: Dove is specially formulated to be predictably gentle to all kinds of skin—dry, oily, normal skin, as well as sensitive pediatric or senescent skin. The mildness of Dove is suitable for patients on drying topical acne medications and Dove is nonacnegenic and noncomedogenic.

Directions: Instruct patients to use Dove as they would any other cleanser.

How Supplied: Original Dove 3.5 oz. and 4.75 bars; Unscented Dove 4.75 oz.; 6 oz. pump dispenser—Liquid Dove beauty wash.
Shown in Product Identification Guide, page 411

LEVER 2000®

Active Ingredients: Triclosan, sodium tallowate, sodium cocoyl isethionate, water, sodium cocoate, stearic acid, sodium isethionate, coconut fatty acid, fragrance, titanium dioxide, sodium chloride, tetrasodium EDTA, disodium phosphate, trisodium etidronate, BHT.

Actions and Uses: Lever 2000® is the mildest antibacterial bar soap available. Lever 2000® offers broad spectrum antibacterial activity against both gram-negative and gram-positive pathogens. It is a useful adjunct to any therapeutic regimen that fights topical bacterial infection. It is also milder to the skin than any other antibacterial or deodorant bar soap. Lever 2000® has been proven mild enough for children's tender skin as young as 18 months and can also be used by adolescents and adults.

Directions: Instruct patients to use Lever 2000® as they would any other mild antibacterial or deodorant soap.

How Supplied: Original Lever 2000 3.5 oz, 5.0 oz bars; Liquid Lever 2000 7 oz pump, 14 oz and 64 oz refills; 28 oz Wall Dispenser; Unscented Lever 2000 5.0 oz bar.
Shown in Product Identification Guide, page 411

3M
BUILDING 270-3N-07
ST PAUL, MN 55144-1000

TITRALAC™ REGULAR AND EXTRA STRENGTH
[T ĭ' tră lăc]

Active Ingredients: Calcium Carbonate: *Regular:* 420mg./tablet (168 mg. elemental calcium). *Extra Strength:* 750mg/tablet (300 mg. elemental calcium).

Inactive Ingredients: Glycine, Magnesium Stearate, Saccharin, Spearmint Oil, Starch.

Indications: A spearmint flavored non-chalky antacid tablet which quickly relieves heartburn, sour stomach, acid indigestion and upset stomach associated with these symptoms.

Dosage and Administration: *Regular:* Two tablets every two or three hours as symptoms occur or as directed by a physician. Tablets can be chewed, swallowed or allowed to melt in the mouth. *Extra Strength:* One or two tablets every two or three hours as symptoms occur or as directed by a physician. Tablets can be chewed or allowed to melt in the mouth.

Warnings: *Regular:* Do not take more than 19 tablets in a 24-hour period or use maximum dosage for more than two weeks, except under the advise and supervision of a physician. *Extra Strength:* Do not take more than ten tablets in a 24-hour period or use maximum dosage for more than two weeks, except under the advice and supervision of a physician. **Keep this and all medication out of the reach of children**

Dietary Guidelines: Titralac™ Antacid is sodium free and sugar free. Also aluminum free.

How Supplied: *Regular:* Available in bottles of 40, 100, 1000 tablets. *Extra Strength:* Available in bottles of 100 tablets.
Shown in Product Identification Guide, page 411

TITRALAC PLUS ANTACID
[T ĭ 'tră lăc]
TITRALAC PLUS™ LIQUID AND TABLETS

Active Ingredients: *Tablets:* Calcium Carbonate: 420 mg/tablet (168 mg elemental calcium), Simethicone: 21 mg/tablet. *Liquid:* Calcium Carbonate: 1000 mg/2 teaspoons (10 ml.) (400 mg elemental calcium), Simethicone: 40 mg/2 teaspoons (10 ml.)

Inactive Ingredients: *Tablets:* Glycine, Magnesium Stearate, Saccharin, Spearmint Oil, Starch. May also contain Croscarmellose Sodium. *Liquid:* Benzyl Alcohol, Colloidal Silicon Dioxide, Glyceryl Laurate, Methylparaben, Potassium Benzoate, Propylparaben, Saccharin, Sorbitol, Spearmint Flavor, Water, Xanthan Gum.

Indications: A spearmint flavored non-chalky antacid which quickly relieves heartburn, sour stomach, acid indigestion, and accompanying gas often associated with these symptoms.

Dosage and Administration: *Tablets:* Two tablets every two or three hours as symptoms occur or as directed by a physician. Tablets can be chewed, swallowed or allowed to melt in the mouth. *Liquid:* Two teaspoons, between meals and at bedtime or as directed by a physician. Shake well before using.

Warnings: *Tablets:* Do not take more than 19 tablets in a 24-hour period or use maximum dosage for more than two weeks, except under the advice and supervision of a physician. *Liquid:* do not take more than 16 teaspoons in a 24-hour period, or use maximum dosage for more than two weeks, except under the advice and supervision of a physician. Keep this and all medication out of the reach of children.

Dietary Guidelines: Tablets and liquid are sodium free, sugar free, and aluminum free.

How Supplied: *Tablets:* Available in bottles of 100 tablets. *Liquid:* Available in 12 fl. oz. bottles.
Shown in Product Identification Guide, page 411

Marlyn Health Care
14851 N. SCOTTSDALE RD
SCOTTSDALE, AZ 85254

MARLYN FORMULA 50®

PRODUCT OVERVIEW

Key Facts: MARLYN FORMULA 50 is a combination of amino acids and B6 in a gelatin capsule which provides protein "building blocks" important to growth and development of all protein containing tissue including nails, hair and skin.

Major Uses: Dermatologists recommend Formula 50 not only for splitting, peeling nails but also prescribe it in conjunction with their favorite topical cream for control of nail fungus. OB-Gyn's recommend it for help in controlling excessive hair fall-out after child birth.
The recommended daily dose is six capsules daily.

Safety Information: There are no known contraindications or adverse reactions.

PRESCRIBING INFORMATION
MARLYN FORMULA 50®

Composition: Each capsule contains:
Amino Acids.................................0.3 Gm*
Vitamin B6 (pyridoxine HCl)......1.0 mg.
*Approximate analysis of the amino acids: indispensable amino acids (lysine, tryptophan, phenylalanine, methio-

Continued on next page

Marlyn—Cont.

nine, threonine, leucine, isoleucine, valine), 35.30%; semi-dispensable amino acids (arginine, histidine, tyrosine, cystine, glycine), 19.18%; dispensable amino acids (glutamic acid, alanine, aspartic acid, serine, proline), 45.56%.
Amino acids: Protein "building blocks" important to growth and development of all protein containing tissue including nails, hair, and skin.

Dosage and Administration: The recommended daily dose is 6 capsules daily.

Supply: Bottles of 100, 250 and 1000 capsules.

WOBENZYM N™

[wō-bĕn-zy-m]

Manufactured by Mucos Pharma GMbH in Germany. Exclusively distributed by Maryln Co., Scottsdale, AZ USA.

Description: Each enteric coated Wobenzym N tablet contains:
Pancreatin 8 NF .... 100 mg
Trypsin 720 FIP-U .... 24 mg
Chymotrypsin 300 FIP-U .... 1 mg
Bromelain 225 FIP-U .... 45 mg
Papain 164 FIP-U .... 60 mg
Rutosid 3 H_2O .... 50 mg

Dosage and Administration: Take 2 (two) tablets 3 (three) times daily after each meal.

How Supplied: Tamper-resistant blister packs of either 40 enteric coated tablets or 200 enteric coated tablets. Available without a prescription.

McNeil Consumer Products Company
Division of McNeil-PPC, Inc.
FORT WASHINGTON, PA 19034

IMODIUM® A–D
(loperamide hydrochloride)

Description: Each 5 ml (teaspoon) of Imodium A-D liquid contains loperamide hydrochloride 1 mg. Imodium A-D liquid is stable, cherry flavored, and clear in color.
Each caplet of Imodium AD contains 2 mg of loperamide and is scored and colored green.

Actions: Imodium A-D contains a clinically proven antidiarrheal medication. Loperamide HCl acts by slowing intestinal motility and by affecting water and electrolyte movement through the bowel.

Indication: Imodium A-D is indicated for the control and symptomatic relief of acute nonspecific diarrhea, including travelers' diarrhea.

Usual Dosage: Adults: Take four teaspoonfuls or two caplets after first loose bowel movement. If needed, take two teaspoonfuls or one caplet after each subse-

quent loose bowel movement. Do not exceed eight teaspoonfuls or four caplets in any 24 hour period, unless directed by a physician.
9–11 years old (60–95 lbs.): Two teaspoonfuls or one caplet after first loose bowel movement, followed by one teaspoonful or one-half caplet after each subsequent loose bowel movement. Do not exceed six teaspoonfuls or three caplets a day.
6–8 years old (48–59 lbs.): Two teaspoonfuls or one caplet after first loose bowel movement, followed by one teaspoonful or one-half caplet after each subsequent loose bowel movement. Do not exceed four teaspoonfuls or two caplets a day.
Professional Dosage Schedule for children two-five years old (24–47 lbs): one teaspoon after first loose bowel movement, followed by one after each subsequent loose bowel movement. Do not exceed three teaspoonfuls a day.

Warnings: DO NOT USE FOR MORE THAN TWO DAYS UNLESS DIRECTED BY A PHYSICIAN. Do not use if diarrhea is accompanied by high fever (greater than 101°F), or if blood or mucus is present in the stool, or if you have had a rash or other allergic reaction to loperamide HCl. If you are taking antibiotics or have a history of liver disease, consult a physician before using this product. As with any drug, if you are pregnant or nursing a baby, seek the advice of a physician before using this product. Keep this and all drugs out of the reach of children. In case of accidental overdose, seek professional assistance or contact a poison control center immediately. Store at room temperature.

Overdosage: Overdosage of loperamide HCl in man may result in constipation, CNS depression and nausea. A slurry of activated charcoal administered promptly after ingestion of loperamide hydrochloride can reduce the amount of drug which is absorbed. If vomiting occurs spontaneously upon ingestion, a slurry of 100 grams of activated charcoal should be administered orally as soon as fluids can be retained. If vomiting has not occurred, and CNS depression is evident, gastric lavage should be performed followed by administration of 100 gms of the activated charcoal slurry through the gastric tube. In the event of overdosage, patients should be monitored for signs of CNS depression for at least 24 hours. Children may be more sensitive to central nervous system effects than adults. If CNS depression is observed, naloxone may be administered. If responsive to naloxone, vital signs must be monitored carefully for recurrence of symptoms of drug overdose for at least 24 hours after the last dose of naloxone.

Inactive Ingredients: Liquid: Alcohol (5.25%), citric acid, flavors, glycerin, methylparaben, propylparaben and purified water.
Caplets: Corn starch, lactose, magnesium stearate, microcrystalline cellulose, FD&C Blue #1 and D&C yellow #10.

How Supplied: Cherry flavored liquid (clear) 2 fl. oz., 3 fl. oz., and 4 fl. oz. tamper resistant bottles with child resistant safety caps and special dosage cups. Green Scored caplets in 6's and 12's and 18's blister packaging which is tamper resistant and child resistant.
Shown in Product Identification Guide, page 411

PEDIACARE® Cold-Allergy Chewable Tablets
PEDIACARE® Cough-Cold Liquid and Chewable Tablets
PEDIACARE® NightRest Cough-Cold Liquid
PEDIACARE® Infants' Decongestant Drops

Description: Each PEDIACARE Cold-Allergy Chewable Tablet contains chlorpheniramine maleate 1 mg and pseudoephedrine hydrochloride 15 mg. Each 5 ml of PEDIACARE Cough-Cold Liquid contains pseudoephedrine hydrochloride 15 mg, chlorpheniramine maleate 1 mg and dextromethorphan hydrobromide 5 mg. Each Pediacare Cough-Cold Formula Chewable Tablet contains pseudoephedrine hydrochloride 15 mg, chlorpheniramine maleate 1 mg and dextromethorphan hydrobromide 5 mg. Each 0.8 ml oral dropper of PEDIACARE Infants' Oral Decongestant Drops contains pseudoephedrine hydrochloride 7.5 mg. PEDIACARE NightRest Cough-Cold liquid contains pseudoephedrine hydrochloride 15 mg, chlorpheniramine maleate 1 mg and dextromethorphan hydrobromide 7.5 mg per 5 ml. PEDIACARE Cough-Cold Liquid and Infants' Drops are stable, cherry flavored and red in color. PEDIACARE Cold-Allergy Chewable Tablets are fruit flavored and pink in color. PEDIACARE Cough-Allergy Chewable Tablets are fruit flavored and pink in color.

Actions: PEDIACARE Products are available in four different formulas, allowing you to select the ideal product to temporarily relieve the patient's symptoms. PEDIACARE Cold-Allergy Chewable Tablets contain an antihistamine and a nasal decongestant to relieve children's cold and allergy symptoms. PEDIACARE Cough-Cold liquid and 6–12 Chewable Tablets contain both of the above ingredients plus a cough suppressant, dextromethorphan hydrobromide, to provide temporary relief of nasal congestion, runny nose, sneezing and coughing due to the common cold, hay fever or other upper respiratory allergies. PEDIACARE NightRest Cough-Cold Liquid contains a decongestant, pseudoephedrine hydrochloride, an antihistamine, chlorpheniramine maleate, and a cough suppressant, dextromethorphan hydrobromide, to provide temporary relief of coughs, nasal congestion, runny nose and sneezing due to the common cold. PEDIACARE NightRest may be used day or night to relieve cough and cold symptoms. PEDIACARE Infants'

Age Group	0–3 mos	4–11 mos	12–23 mos	2–3 yrs	4–5 yrs	6–8 yrs	9–10 yrs	11 yrs	Dosage
Weight (lbs)	6–11 lb	12–17 lb	18–23 lb	24–35 lb	36–47 lb	48–59 lb	60–71 lb	72–95 lb	
PEDIACARE Infants' Drops*	½ dropper (0.4 ml)	1 dropper (0.8 ml)	1½ droppers (1.2 ml)	2 droppers (1.6 ml)					q4–6h
PEDIACARE Cold-Allergy Chewable Tablets**				1 tabs	1½ tabs	2 tabs	2½ tabs	3 tabs	q4–6h
PEDIACARE Cough-Cold Liquid**				1 tsp	1½ tsp	2 tsp	2½ tsp	3 tsp	q4–6h
and Chewable Tablets**				1 tabs	1½ tabs	2 tabs	2½ tabs	3 tabs	q4–6h
PEDIACARE NightRest Liquid**				1 tsp	1½ tsp	2 tsp	2½ tsp	3 tsp	q6–8h

*Administer to children under 2 years only on the advice of a physician.
**Administer to children under 6 years only on the advice of a physician.

Oral Decongestant Drops contain a decongestant, pseudoephedrine hydrochloride, to provide temporary relief of nasal congestion due to the common cold, hay fever or other upper respiratory allergies.

Professional Dosage: A calibrated dosage cup is provided for accurate dosing of the PEDIACARE Liquid formulas. A calibrated oral dropper is provided for accurate dosing of PEDIACARE Infants' Drops. All doses of PEDIACARE Cold-Allergy Chewable Tablets, PEDIACARE Cough-Cold Liquid and Chewable Tablets, as well as PEDIACARE Infants' Drops may be repeated every 4–6 hours, not to exceed 4 doses in 24 hours. PEDIACARE NightRest Liquid may be repeated every 6–8 hrs, not to exceed 4 doses in 24 hours.

[See table above.]

WARNINGS: Do not use if carton is opened, or if printed plastic bottle wrap or foil inner seal is broken. Keep this and all medication out of the reach of children. In case of accidental overdosage, contact a physician or poison control center immediately.

The following information appears on the appropriate package labels:

PEDIACARE Cold-Allergy Chewable Tablets: PHENYLKETONURICS: CONTAINS PHENYALANINE 8MG PER TABLET. Do not exceed recommended dosage because at higher doses nervousness, dizziness or sleeplessness may occur. Do not give this product to children for more than 7 days. If symptoms do not improve, or are accompanied by fever, consult a physician. May cause excitability, especially in children. May cause drowsiness. Sedatives and tranquilizers may increase the drowsiness effect. Do not give this product to children who are taking sedatives or tranquilizers, without first consulting the child's physician. Do not give this product to children who have a breathing problem such as chronic bronchitis, or who have glaucoma, heart disease, high blood pressure, thyroid disease, or diabetes, without first consulting the child's physician.

PEDIACARE Cough-Cold Liquid, NightRest Cough-Cold Liquid and Chewable Tablets: Do not exceed recommended dosage because at higher doses nervousness, dizziness or sleeplessness may occur. Do not give this product to children for more than 7 days. If symptoms do not improve, or are accompanied by fever, consult a physician. A persistent cough may be a sign of a serious condition. If cough persists for more than one week, tends to recur or is accompanied by fever, rash, or persistent headache, consult a physician. Do not give this product for persistent or chronic cough such as occurs with asthma or if cough is accompanied by excessive phlegm (mucus) unless directed by a physician. May cause excitability especially in children. [May cause drowsiness. Sedatives and tranquilizers may increase the drowsiness effect. Do not give this product to children who are taking sedatives or tranquilizers without first consulting the child's physician.] Do not give this product to children who have a breathing problem such as chronic bronchitis, or who have glaucoma, heart disease, high blood pressure, thyroid disease or diabetes, without first consulting the child's physician.

Drug Interaction Precaution: Do not give this product to a child who is taking a prescription drug for high blood pressure or to a child who is taking a prescription monoamine oxidase inhibitor (MAOI) (certain drugs for depression, psychiatric or emotional conditions) or for 2 weeks after stopping the MAOI drug. If you are uncertain whether your child's prescription drug contains an MAOI, consult a health professional before giving this product.

PEDIACARE Infants' Oral Decongestant Drops: Do not exceed the recommended dosage because at higher doses nervousness, dizziness or sleeplessness may occur. Do not give this product to children who have heart disease, high blood pressure, thyroid disease or diabetes unless directed by a physician. Do not give this product to children for more than seven days. If symptoms do not improve or are accompanied by fever, consult a physician. Do not give this product to children who are taking a prescription drug for high blood pressure or depression without first consulting a physician. Take by mouth only. Not for nasal use.

PEDIACARE Cold-Allergy Chewable Tablets also contain the warning, "Phenylketonurics: Contains phenylalanine 8 mg per tablet", and the inactive ingredient listing, "Inactive Ingredients: Aspartame, Cellulose, Citric Acid, Corn Starch, Flavors, Mannitol, Colloidal Silicon Dioxide, Stearic Acid, and Red #7."

PEDIACARE Cough-Cold Liquid: Inactive Ingredients: Benzoic acid, citric acid, flavors, glycerin, polyethylene glycol, propylene glycol, sodium benzoate, sorbitol, sucrose, purified water, Red #33, Blue #1 and Red #40.

PEDIACARE NightRest Cough-Cold Liquid: Inactive ingredients: Benzoic acid, citric acid, flavors, glycerin, polyethylene glycol. proplene glycol, sodium benzoate, sorbitol, sucrose, purified water. Red #33, blue #1 and Red #40.

PEDIACARE Cough-Cold Chewable Tablets also contain the warning, "Phenylketonurics: contains phenylalanine 6 mg per tablet", and the inactive ingredient listing, "Inactive Ingredients: Aspartame, cellulose, citric acid, flavors, magnesium stearate, magnesium trisilicate, mannitol, starch and Red #7."

PEDIACARE Infants' Oral Decongestant Drops: Inactive Ingredients: Benzoic acid, citric acid, flavors, glycerin, polyethylene glycol, propylene glycol, purified water, sodium benzoate, sorbitol, sucrose and Red #40.

Overdosage: Acute dextromethorphan overdose usually does not result in serious signs and symptoms unless massive amounts have been ingested. Signs and symptoms of a substantial overdose may include nausea and vomiting, visual disturbances, CNS disturbances, and urinary retention. Symptoms from pseudoephedrine overdose consist most often of mild anxiety, tachycardia and/or mild hypertension. Symptoms usually appear within 4 to 8 hours of ingestion and are transient, usually requiring no treatment. Chlorpheniramine toxicity should be treated as you would an antihistamine/anticholinergic overdose and is likely to be present within a few hours after acute ingestion.

Continued on next page

McNeil Consumer—Cont.

How Supplied: PEDIACARE Cough-Cold Liquid and NightRest Cough-Cold Liquid (colored red)—bottles of 4 fl. oz. with child-resistant safety cap and calibrated dosage cup. PEDIACARE Cold-Allergy Chewable Tablets (pink, scored)—blister packs of 16. PEDIACARE Cough-Cold Chewable Tablets (pink, scored)—blister packs of 16. PEDIACARE Infants' Drops (colored red)—bottles of ½ fl. oz with calibrated dropper.

Shown in Product Identification Guide, pages 411 and 412

MAXIMUM STRENGTH SINE-AID®
Sinus Headache Gelcaps, Caplets and Tablets

Description: Each MAXIMUM STRENGTH SINE-AID® Gelcap, Caplet or Tablet contains acetaminophen 500 mg and pseudoephedrine hydrochloride 30 mg.

Actions: MAXIMUM STRENGTH SINE-AID® Gelcaps, Caplets and Tablets contain a clinically proven analgesic-antipyretic and a decongestant. Maximum allowable non-prescription levels of acetaminophen and pseudoephedrine provide temporary relief of sinus congestion and pain. Acetaminophen is equal to aspirin in analgesic and antipyretic effectiveness and it is unlikely to produce many of the side effects associated with aspirin and aspirin-containing products. Acetaminophen produces analgesia by elevation of the pain threshold and antipyresis through action on the hypothalamic heat-regulating center. Pseudoephedrine hydrochloride is a sympathomimetic amine that promotes sinus cavity drainage by reducing nasopharyngeal mucosal congestion.

Indications: MAXIMUM STRENGTH SINE-AID® Gelcaps, Caplets and Tablets provide effective symptomatic relief from sinus headache pain and congestion. SINE-AID® is particularly well-suited in patients with aspirin allergy, hemostatic disturbances (including anticoagulant therapy), and bleeding diatheses (e.g. hemophilia) and upper gastrointestinal disease (e.g. ulcer, gastritis, hiatus hernia).

Precautions: If a rare sensitivity occurs, the drug should be discontinued. Although pseudoephedrine is virtually without pressor effect in normotensive patients, it should be used with caution in hypertensives.

Usual Dosage: Adult dosage: Two gelcaps, caplets or tablets every four to six hours. Do not exceed eight gelcaps, caplets or tablets in any 24 hour period.
Warning: Do not administer to children under 12 or exceed the recommended dosage because at higher doses nervousness, dizziness or sleeplessness may occur. Do not take this product for more than 7 days. If symptoms do not improve or are accompanied by a fever, consult a physician. Do not take this product if you have heart disease, high blood pressure, thyroid disease, diabetes or difficulty in urination due to enlargement of the prostate gland unless directed by a doctor. Do not use with other products containing acetaminophen.

Drug Interaction Precaution: Do not take this product if you are presently taking a prescription drug for high blood pressure or depression without first consulting your doctor.

Do not use if carton is open or if blister unit is broken, or if printed neck wrap or printed foil inner seal is broken. Keep this and all medication out of the reach of children. As with any drug, if you are pregnant or nursing a baby, seek the advice of a health professional before using this product. In case of accidental overdosage, contact a physician or poison control center immediately.

Overdosage: Acetaminophen in massive overdosage may cause hepatic toxicity in some patients. In adults and adolescents, hepatic toxicity has rarely been reported following ingestion of acute overdoses of less than 10 grams. Fatalities are infrequent (less than 3–4% of untreated cases) and have rarely been reported with overdoses of less than 15 grams. In children, an acute overdosage of less than 150 mg/kg has not been associated with hepatic toxicity.
Early symptoms following a potentially hepatotoxic overdose may include: nausea, vomiting, diaphoresis and general malaise. Clinical and laboratory evidence of hepatic toxicity may not be apparent until 48 to 72 hours postingestion. In adults and adolescents, regardless of the quantity of acetaminophen reported to have been ingested, administer MUCOMYST® acetylcysteine immediately if 24 hours or less have elapsed from the reported time of ingestion. For full prescribing information, refer to the MUCOMYST package insert. Do not await results of assays for acetaminophen level before initiating treatment with MUCOMYST acetylcysteine. The following additional procedures are recommended: The stomach should be emptied promptly by lavage or by induction of emesis with syrup of ipecac. A serum acetaminophen assay should be obtained as early as possible, but no sooner than four hours following ingestion. Liver function studies should be obtained initially and repeated at 24-hour intervals.
Serious toxicity or fatalities are extremely infrequent in children, possibly due to differences in the way they metabolize acetaminophen. In children, the maximum potential amount ingested can be more easily estimated. If more than 150 mg/kg or an unknown amount was ingested, obtain an acetaminophen plasma level. The acetaminophen plasma level should be obtained as soon as possible, but no sooner than 4 hours following the ingestion. Induce emesis using syrup of ipecac. If the plasma level is obtained and falls above the broken line on the acetaminophen overdose nomogram, the MUCOMYST acetylcysteine therapy should be initiated and continued for a full course of therapy. If acetaminophen plasma assay capability is not available, and the estimated acetaminophen ingestion exceeds 150 mg/kg, MUCOMYST acetylcysteine therapy should be initiated and continued for a full course of therapy.
For additional emergency information, call your regional poison center or call the Rocky Mountain Poison Center toll-free, (1-800-525-6115).
Symptoms from pseudoephedrine overdose consist most often of mild anxiety, tachycardia and/or mild hypertension. Symptoms usually appear within 4 to 8 hours of ingestion and are transient, usually requiring no treatment.

Inactive Ingredients: Gelcaps: Benzyl Alcohol, Butylparaben, Castor Oil, Cellulose, Corn Starch, Edetate Calcium Disodium, Gelatin, Hydroxypropyl Methylcellulose, Iron Oxide Black, Magnesium Stearate, Methylparaben, Propylparaben, Sodium Lauryl Sulfate, Sodium Propionate, Sodium Starch Glycolate, Titanium Dioxide, FD&C Red #40.
Caplets: Cellulose, Corn Starch, Hydroxypropyl Methylcellulose, Magnesium Stearate, Polyethylene Glycol, Sodium Starch Glycolate, Titanium Dioxide, Blue #1 and Red #40.
Tablets: Cellulose, Corn Starch, Magnesium Stearate and Sodium Starch Glycolate.

How Supplied: Gelcaps (colored red and white imprinted "SINE-AID")—blister package of 20 and tamper resistant bottle of 40.
Caplets (colored white imprinted "Maximum SINE-AID")—blister package of 24 and tamper resistant bottle of 50.
Tablets (colored white embossed "Sine-Aid")—blister package of 24 and tamper resistant bottle of 50.

Shown in Product Identification Guide, page 413

CHILDREN'S TYLENOL®
acetaminophen
Chewable Tablets, Elixir, Drops
Suspension Liquid, Drops

Description: Infants' TYLENOL acetaminophen Drops are stable, alcohol-free, fruit-flavored and orange in color. Infants' TYLENOL Suspension Drops are alcohol-free, grape-flavored and purple in color. Each 0.8 ml (one calibrated dropperful) contains 80 mg acetaminophen. Children's TYLENOL Elixir is stable and alcohol-free, cherry-flavored, and red in color or grape-flavored, and purple in color. Children's TYLENOL Suspension Liquid is alcohol-free, cherry-flavored and red in color. Each 5 ml contains 160 mg acetaminophen. Each Children's TYLENOL Chewable Tablet contains 80 mg acetaminophen in a grape- or fruit-flavored tablet.

Actions: Acetaminophen is a clinically proven analgesic/antipyretic. Acetaminophen produces analgesia by elevation of the pain threshold and antipyresis through action on the hypothalamic heat regulating center. Acetaminophen is equal to aspirin in analgesic and antipyretic effectiveness and it is unlikely to produce many of the side effects associated with aspirin and aspirin containing products.

Indications: Children's TYLENOL Chewable Tablets, Elixir, Drops, Suspension Liquid and Suspension Drops are designed for treatment of infants and children with conditions requiring temporary relief of fever and discomfort due to colds and "flu," and of simple pain and discomfort due to teething, immunizations and tonsillectomy.

Precautions: If a rare sensitivity reaction occurs, the drug should be stopped.

Usual Dosage: All dosages may be repeated every 4 hours, but not more than 5 times daily. Administer to children under 2 years only on the advice of a physician. Children's TYLENOL Chewable Tablets: 2–3 years: two tablets. 4–5 years: three tablets, 6–8 years: four tablets. 9–10 years: five tablets. 11–12 years: six tablets.
Children's TYLENOL Elixir and Suspension Liquid: (special cup for measuring dosage is provided) 4–11 months: one-half teaspoon. 12–23 months: three-quarters teaspoon, 2–3 years: one teaspoon. 4–5 years: one and one-half teaspoons. 6–8 years: 2 teaspoons. 9–10 years: two and one-half teaspoons. 11–12 years: three teaspoons.
Infants' TYLENOL Drops and Suspension Drops: 0–3 months: 0.4 ml. 4–11 months: 0.8 ml. 12–23 months: 1.2 ml. 2–3 years: 1.6 ml. 4–5 years: 2.4 ml.

Warning: Keep this and all medication out of reach of children. In case of accidental overdose, contact a physician or poison control center immediately. Consult your physician if fever persists for more than 3 days or if pain continues for more than 5 days. Store at room temperature.
NOTE: In addition to the above:
Children's TYLENOL® Drops and Suspension Drops—Do not use if printed carton overwrap or printed plastic bottle wrap is broken or missing or if carton is opened.
Children's TYLENOL Elixir and Suspension Liquid—Do not use if printed carton overwrap is broken or missing or if carton is opened. Do not use if printed plastic bottle wrap or printed foil inner seal is broken. Not a USP elixir.
Children's TYLENOL Chewables—Do not use if carton is opened or if printed plastic bottle wrap or printed foil inner seal is broken. Phenylketonurics: contains phenylalanine 3mg per tablet. Do not use with other products containing acetaminophen.

Overdosage: Acetaminophen in massive overdosage may cause hepatic toxicity in some patients. In adults and adolescents, hepatic toxicity has rarely been reported following ingestion of acute overdoses of less than 10 grams. Fatalities are infrequent (less than 3–4% of untreated cases) and have rarely been reported with overdoses of less than 15 grams. In children, an acute overdosage of less than 150 mg/kg has not been associated with hepatic toxicity.
Early symptoms following a potentially hepatotoxic overdose may include: nausea, vomiting, diaphoresis and general malaise. Clinical and laboratory evidence of hepatic toxicity may not be apparent until 48 to 72 hours postingestion. In adults and adolescents, regardless of the quantity of acetaminophen reported to have been ingested, administer MUCOMYST® acetylcysteine immediately if 24 hours or less have elapsed from the reported time of ingestion. For full prescribing information, refer to the MUCOMYST package insert. Do not await results of assays for acetaminophen level before initiating treatment with MUCOMYST acetylcysteine. The following additional procedures are recommended: The stomach should be emptied promptly by lavage or by induction of emesis with syrup of ipecac. A serum acetaminophen assay should be obtained as early as possible, but no sooner than four hours following ingestion. Liver function studies should be obtained initially and repeated at 24-hour intervals.
Serious toxicity or fatalities are extremely infrequent in children, possibly due to differences in the way they metabolize acetaminophen. In children, the maximum potential amount ingested can be more easily estimated. If more than 150 mg/kg or an unknown amount was ingested, obtain an acetaminophen plasma level. The acetaminophen plasma level should be obtained as soon as possible, but no sooner than 4 hours following the ingestion. Induce emesis using syrup of ipecac. If the plasma level is obtained and falls above the broken line on the acetaminophen overdose nomogram, the MUCOMYST acetylcysteine therapy should be initiated and continued for a full course of therapy. If acetaminophen plasma assay capability is not available, and the estimated acetaminophen ingestion exceeds 150 mg/kg, MUCOMYST acetylcysteine therapy should be initiated and continued for a full course of therapy.
For additional emergency information, call your regional poison center or call the Rocky Mountain Poison Center toll free, (1-800-525-6115).

Inactive Ingredients: Children's TYLENOL Chewable Tablets—Aspartame, Cellulose, Citric Acid, Ethylcellulose, Flavors, Hydroxypropyl Methylcellulose, Mannitol, Starch, Magnesium Stearate, Red #7 and Blue #1 (Grape only). Children's TYLENOL Elixir—Benzoic Acid, Citric Acid, Flavors, Glycerin, Polyethylene Glycol, Propylene Glycol, Sodium Benzoate, Sorbitol, Sucrose, Purified Water, Red #40. In addition to the above ingredients cherry flavored elixir contains Red #33 and grape flavored elixir contains malic acid and Blue #1. Children's TYLENOL Suspension Liquid—Butylparaben, Cellulose, Citric Acid, Corn Syrup, Flavors, Glycerin, Propylene Glycol, Purified Water, Sodium Benzoate, Sorbitol, Xanthan Gum, FD&C Red #40.
Infant's TYLENOL Drops—Butylparaben, Citric Acid, Flavors, Glycerin, Polyethylene Glycol, Propylene Glycol, Saccharin, Sodium Citrate, purified water and yellow #6.
Infant's TYLENOL Suspension Drops—Butylparaben, Cellulose, Citric Acid, Corn Syrup, Flavors, Glycerin, Propylene Glycol, Purified Water, Sodium Benzoate, Sorbitol, Xanthan Gum, FD&C Red #33 and FD&C Blue #1.

How Supplied: Chewable Tablets (pink colored fruit, purple colored grape, scored, imprinted "TYLENOL")—Bottles of 30 and child resistant blister packs of 48 (fruit only). Elixir (cherry colored red and grape colored purple) Suspension liquid (cherry flavored colored red)—bottles of 2 and 4 fl. oz. Drops (colored orange)—bottles of ½ oz. (15 ml.) and 1 oz. (30 ml.) with calibrated plastic dropper. Suspension drops (grape flavored colored purple)—bottles of ½ oz (15 ml) with calibrated plastic dropper.
All packages listed above have child-resistant safety caps.

Shown in Product Identification Guide, page 412

CHILDREN'S TYLENOL COLD®
Multi Symptom Chewable Tablets and Liquid

Description: Each Children's Tylenol Cold MULTI SYMPTOM Chewable Grape-Flavored Tablet contains acetaminophen 80 mg, chlorpheniramine maleate 0.5 mg and pseudoephedrine hydrochloride 7.5 mg. Children's Tylenol Cold MULTI SYMPTOM Liquid is grape flavored and contains no alcohol. Each teaspoon (5 ml) contains acetaminophen 160 mg, chlorpheniramine maleate 1 mg, and pseudoephedrine hydrochloride 15 mg.

Actions: Children's Tylenol Cold MULTI SYMPTOM Chewable Tablets and Liquid combine the analgesic-antipyretic acetaminophen with the decongestant pseudoephedrine hydrochloride and the antihistamine chlorpheniramine maleate to help relieve nasal congestion, dry runny noses and prevent sneezing as well as to relieve the fever, aches, pains and general discomfort associated with colds and upper respiratory infections. Acetaminophen is equal to aspirin in analgesic and antipyretic effectiveness and it is unlikely to produce the side effects often associated with aspirin or aspirin-containing products.

Continued on next page

McNeil Consumer—Cont.

Indications: Provides fast, effective temporary relief of nasal congestion, runny nose, sore throat, sneezing, minor aches and pains, headaches and fever due to the common cold, hay fever or other upper respiratory allergies.

Usual Dosage: Administer to children under 6 years only on the advice of a physician. Children's Tylenol Cold Chewable Tablets: 2–5 years—2 tablets, 6–11 years—4 tablets.

Children's Tylenol Cold Liquid Formula: 2–5 years—1 teaspoonful; 6–11 years—2 teaspoonful. Measuring cup is provided and marked for accurate dosing.

Doses may be repeated every 4-6 hours as needed, not to exceed 4 doses in 24 hours. The Warnings are identical for the two dosage forms except the Liquid Cold Formula does not contain the phenylketonurics statement since the product does not contain aspartame.

WARNING: DO NOT USE IF CARTON IS OPENED, OR IF PRINTED PLASTIC BOTTLE WRAP OR PRINTED FOIL INNER SEAL IS BROKEN. KEEP THIS AND ALL MEDICATION OUT OF THE REACH OF CHILDREN. IN CASE OF ACCIDENTAL OVERDOSAGE, CONTACT A PHYSICIAN OR POISON CONTROL CENTER IMMEDIATELY. Phenylketonurics: contains phenylalanine, 4 mg per tablet. Do not exceed recommended dosage because at higher doses nervousness, dizziness or sleeplessness may occur. Do not give this product to children for more than 7 days. If fever persists for more than 3 days, or if symptoms do not improve or new ones occur within 5 days or are accompanied by fever, consult a physician before continuing use. If sore throat is severe, persists for more than 2 days, is accompanied or followed by fever, headache, rash, nausea or vomiting, consult a physician promptly. May cause excitability especially in children. Do not give this product to children who have a breathing problem such as chronic bronchitis, or who have glaucoma, heart disease, high blood pressure, thyroid disease or diabetes without first consulting the child's physician. May cause drowsiness. Sedatives and tranquilizers may increase the drowsiness effect. Do not give this product to children who are taking sedatives or tranquilizers, without first consulting the child's physician. Do not use with other products containing acetaminophen.

Drug Interaction Precaution: Do not give this product to a child who is taking a prescription drug for high blood pressure or depression without first consulting the child's physician.

Overdosage: Acetaminophen in massive overdosage may cause hepatic toxicity in some patients. In adults and adolescents, hepatic toxicity has rarely been reported following ingestion of acute overdosage of less than 10 grams. Fatalities are infrequent (less than 3–4% of untreated cases) and have rarely been reported with overdoses of less than 15 grams. In children, an acute overdosage of less than 150 mg/kg has not been associated with hepatic toxicity.

Early symptoms following a potentially hepatotoxic overdose may include: nausea, vomiting, diaphoresis and general malaise. Clinical and laboratory evidence of hepatic toxicity may not be apparent until 48 to 72 hours postingestion. In adults and adolescents, regardless of the quantity of acetaminophen reported to have been ingested, administer MUCOMYST® acetylcysteine immediately if 24 hours or less have elapsed from the reported time of ingestion. For full prescribing information, refer to the MUCOMYST package insert. Do not await the results of assays for acetaminophen level before initiating treatment with MUCOMYST acetylcysteine. The following additional procedures are recommended: The stomach should be emptied promptly by lavage or by induction of emesis with syrup of ipecac. A serum acetaminophen assay should be obtained as early as possible, but no sooner than four hours following ingestion. Liver function studies should be obtained initially and repeated at 24-hour intervals.

Serious toxicity or fatalities are extremely infrequent in children, possibly due to differences in the way they metabolize acetaminophen. In children, the maximum potential amount ingested can be more easily estimated. If more than 150 mg/kg or an unknown amount was ingested, obtain an acetaminophen plasma level. The acetaminophen plasma level should be obtained as soon as possible, but no sooner than 4 hours following the ingestion. Induce emesis using syrup of ipecac. If the plasma level is obtained and falls above the broken line on the acetaminophen overdose nomogram, the MUCOMYST acetylcysteine therapy should be initiated and continued for a full course of therapy. If acetaminophen plasma assay capability is not available, and the estimated acetaminophen ingestion exceeds 150 mg/kg, MUCOMYST acetylcysteine therapy should be initiated and continued for a full course of therapy.

For additional emergency information, call your regional poison center or call the Rocky Mountain Poison Center toll-free, (1-800-525-6115).

Chlorpheniramine toxicity should be treated as you would an antihistamine/anticholinergic overdose and is likely to be present within a few hours after acute ingestion.

Symptoms from pseudoephedrine overdose consist most often of mild anxiety, tachycardia and/or mild hypertension. Symptoms usually appear within 4 to 8 hours of ingestion and are transient, usually requiring no treatment.

Inactive Ingredients: Chewable Tablets—Aspartame, citric acid, corn starch, ethylcellulose, flavors, magnesium stearate, mannitol, microcrystalline cellulose, sucrose, Blue #1 and Red #7.

Liquid—Benzoic acid, citric acid, flavors, glycerin, malic acid, polyethylene glycol, propylene glycol, sodium benzoate, sorbitol, sucrose, purified water, Blue #1 and Red #40.

How Supplied: Chewable Tablets (colored purple, scored, imprinted "Tylenol Cold") on one side and "TC" on opposite side—bottles of 24. Cold Formula—bottles (colored purple) of 4 fl. oz.

Shown in Product Identification Guide, page 412

CHILDREN'S TYLENOL® COLD PLUS COUGH
Multi Symptom Liquid

Description: Children's Tylenol Cold MULTI SYMPTOM Plus Cough Liquid is cherry flavored and contains no alcohol. Each teaspoon (5 ml) contains acetaminophen 160 mg, chlorpheniramine maleate 1 mg, dextromethorphan hydrobromide 5 mg and pseudoephedrine hydrochloride 15 mg.

Actions: Children's Tylenol Cold MULTI SYMPTOM Plus Cough Liquid combines the analgesic-antipyretic acetaminophen with the decongestant pseudoephedrine hydrochloride, the cough suppressant dextromethorphan hydrobromide, and the antihistamine chlorpheniramine maleate to help relieve coughs, nasal congestion, and sore throat, dry runny noses, and prevent sneezing as well as to relieve the fever, aches, pains and general discomfort associated with colds and upper respiratory infections.

Acetaminophen is equal to aspirin in analgesic and antipyretic effectiveness and it is unlikely to produce the side effects often associated with aspirin or aspirin-containing products.

Indications: Provides fast, effective temporary relief of coughs, nasal congestion, runny nose, sore throat, sneezing, minor aches and pains, headaches and fever due to the common cold, hay fever or other upper respiratory allergies.

Usual Dosage: Administer to children under 6 years only on the advice of a physician.

Children's Tylenol Cold Plus Cough Liquid Formula: 2–5 years—1 teaspoonful; 6–11 years—2 teaspoonsful. Measuring cup is provided and marked for accurate dosing.

Doses may be repeated every 4-6 hours as needed, not to exceed 4 doses in 24 hours.

WARNING: DO NOT USE IF CARTON IS OPENED, OR IF PRINTED PLASTIC BOTTLE WRAP OR PRINTED FOIL INNER SEAL IS BROKEN. KEEP THIS AND ALL MEDICATION OUT OF THE REACH OF CHILDREN. IN CASE OF ACCIDENTAL OVERDOSAGE, CONTACT A PHYSICIAN OR POISON CONTROL CENTER IMMEDIATELY. Do not exceed

recommended dosage because at higher doses nervousness, dizziness or sleeplessness may occur. Do not give this product to children for more than 7 days. If fever persists for more than 3 days, or if symptoms do not improve or new ones occur within 5 days or are accompanied by fever, consult a physician before continuing use. If sore throat is severe, persists for more than 2 days, is accompanied or followed by fever, headache, rash, nausea or vomiting, consult physician promptly. May cause excitability especially in children. Do not give this product to children who have a breathing problem such as chronic bronchitis, or who have glaucoma, heart disease, high blood pressure, thyroid disease or diabetes without first consulting the child's physician. May cause drowsiness. Sedatives and tranquilizers may increase the drowsiness effect. Do not give this product to children who are taking sedatives or tranquilizers, without first consulting the child's physician. A persistent cough may be a sign of a serious condition. If cough persists for more than 1 week, tends to recur, or is accompanied by fever, rash or persistent headache, consult a physician. Do not give this product for persistent or chronic cough such as occurs with asthma or if cough is accompanied by excessive phlegm (mucus) unless directed by a physician. Do not use with other products containing acetaminophen.

Drug Interaction Precaution: Do not give this product to a child who is taking a prescription drug for high blood pressure or to a child who is taking a prescription monoamine oxidase inhibitor (MAOI) (certain drugs for depression, psychiatric or emotional conditions), or for 2 weeks after stopping the MAOI drug. If you are uncertain whether your child's prescription drug contains an MAOI, consult a health professional before giving this product.

Overdosage: Acetaminophen in massive overdose may cause hepatic toxicity in some patients. In adults and adolescents, hepatic toxicity has rarely been reported following ingestion of acute overdosage of less than 10 grams. Fatalities are infrequent (less than 3-4% of untreated cases) and have rarely been reported with overdoses of less than 15 grams. In children, an acute overdosage of less than 150 mg/kg has not been associated with hepatic toxicity. Early symptoms following a potentially hepatotoxic overdose may include: nausea, vomiting, diaphoresis and general malaise. Clinical and laboratory evidence of hepatic toxicity may not be apparent until 48 to 72 hours postingestion. In adults and adolescents, regardless of the quantity of acetaminophen reported to have been ingested, administer MUCOMYST® acetylcysteine immediately if 24 hours or less have elapsed from the reported time of ingestion. For

full prescribing information, refer to the MUCOMYST package insert. Do not await the results of assays for acetaminophen level before initiating treatment with MUCOMYST acetylcysteine. The following additional procedures are recommended: The stomach should be emptied promptly by lavage or by induction of emesis with syrup of ipecac. A serum acetaminophen assay should be obtained as early as possible, but no sooner than four hours following ingestion. Liver function studies should be obtained initially and repeated at 24-hour intervals.

Serious toxicity or fatalities are extremely infrequent in children, possibly due to differences in the way they metabolize acetaminophen. In children, the maximum potential amount ingested can be more easily estimated. If more than 150 mg/kg or an unknown amount was ingested, obtain an acetaminophen plasma level. The acetaminophen plasma level should be obtained as soon as possible, but no sooner than 4 hours following the ingestion. Induce emesis using syrup of ipecac. If the plasma level is obtained and falls above the broken line on the acetaminophen overdose nomogram, the MUCOMYST acetylcysteine therapy should be initiated and continued for a full course of therapy. If acetaminophen plasma assay capability is not available, and the estimated acetaminophen ingestion exceeds 150 mg/kg, MUCOMYST acetylcysteine therapy should be initiated and continued for a full course of therapy.

For additional emergency information, call your regional poison center or call the Rocky Mountain Poison Center toll-free, (1-800-525-6115).

Chlorpheniramine toxicity should be treated as you would an antihistamine/anticholinergic overdose and is likely to be present within a few hours after acute ingestion.

Symptoms from pseudoephedrine overdose consist most often of mild anxiety, tachycardia and/or mild hypertension. Symptoms usually appear within 4 to 8 hours of ingestion and are transient, usually requiring no treatment.

Inactive Ingredients: Citric Acid, Corn Syrup, Flavors, Polyethylene Glycol, Propylene Glycol, Sodium Benzoate, Sodium Carboxymethylcellulose, Sorbitol, Purified Water, Red #33 and Red #40.

How Supplied: Cold Plus Cough Formula—bottles (red colored) of 4 fl. oz.
Shown in Product Identification Guide, page 412

**Effervescent Formula
TYLENOL® Cold Medication
Tablets**

Description: Each Effervescent Formula TYLENOL Cold Medication Tablet contains acetaminophen 325 mg., chlorpheniramine maleate 2 mg., and phenylpropanolamine hydrochloride 12.5 mg.

Actions: Effervescent Formula TYLENOL Cold Medication Tablets contain a clinically proven analgesic-antipyretic, decongestant and antihistamine. Acetaminophen produces analgesia by elevation of the pain threshold and antipyresis through action on the hypothalamic heat-regulating center. Acetaminophen is equal to aspirin in analgesic and antipyretic effectiveness and it is unlikely to produce many of the side effects associated with aspirin and aspirin-containing products. Phenylpropanolamine is a sympathomimetic amine which provides temporary relief of nasal congestion. Chlorpheniramine is an antihistamine which helps provide temporary relief of runny nose, sneezing and watery and itchy eyes.

Indications: Effervescent Formula TYLENOL Cold Medication provides effective temporary relief of runny nose, sneezing, watery and itchy eyes, nasal congestion, sore throat and aches, pains, and fever due to a cold or "flu."

Precautions: If a rare sensitivity reaction occurs, the drug should be stopped. Although phenylpropanolamine is virtually without pressor effect in normotensive patients, it should be used with caution in hypertensives.

Usual Dosage: Effervescent Formula TYLENOL® Cold must be dissolved in water before taking.
ADULTS (12 years and over): 2 tablets every 4 hours, not to exceed 12 tablets in 24 hours.
CHILDREN (6–11): 1 tablet every 4 hours, not to exceed 6 tablets in 24 hours.
WARNINGS: Do not administer to children under 6. Do not take this product for more than 7 days (Adults) or 5 days (children) or for fever for more than 3 days unless directed by a doctor. If symptoms do not improve or are accompanied by fever, consult a doctor. If sore throat is severe, persists for more than 2 days, is accompanied or followed by fever, headache, rash, nausea or vomiting, consult a doctor promptly. Do not exceed recommended dosage because at higher doses, nervousness, dizziness or sleeplessness may occur. May cause excitability especially in children. Do not take this product, unless directed by a doctor, if you have a breathing problem such as emphysema or chronic bronchitis, or if you have glaucoma or difficulty in urination due to enlargement of the prostate gland. Do not take this product if you have heart disease, high blood pressure, thyroid disease or diabetes unless directed by a doctor. May cause drowsiness; alcohol, sedatives and tranquilizers may increase the drowsiness effect. Avoid alcoholic beverages while taking this product. Do not take this product if you are taking sedatives or tranquilizers without first consulting your doctor. Use caution when driving a motor vehicle or operating machinery. Do not use with other products containing acetamino-

Continued on next page

McNeil Consumer—Cont.

phen. DO NOT USE IF GLUED CARTON FLAP IS OPENED OR IF FOIL PACK IS TORN OR BROKEN. **KEEP THIS AND ALL MEDICATION OUT OF THE REACH OF CHILDREN. AS WITH ANY DRUG, IF YOU ARE PREGNANT OR NURSING A BABY, SEEK THE ADVICE OF A HEALTH PROFESSIONAL BEFORE USING THIS PRODUCT. IN CASE OF ACCIDENTAL OVERDOSAGE, CONTACT A DOCTOR OR POISON CONTROL CENTER IMMEDIATELY. DO NOT TAKE THIS PRODUCT IF YOU ARE ON A SODIUM RESTRICTED DIET, EXCEPT UNDER THE ADVICE AND SUPERVISION OF A DOCTOR. EACH TABLET CONTAINS 525 MG. OF SODIUM.**

Drug Interaction Precaution: Do not take this product if you are presently taking a prescription drug for high blood pressure or depression without first consulting your doctor.

Overdosage: Acetaminophen in massive overdosage may cause hepatic toxicity in some patients. In adults and adolescents, hepatic toxicity has rarely been reported following ingestion of acute overdosage of less than 10 grams. Fatalities are infrequent (less than 3–4% of untreated cases) and have rarely been reported with overdoses of less than 15 grams. In children, an acute overdosage of less than 150 mg/kg has not been associated with hepatic toxicity. Early symptoms following a potentially hepatotoxic overdose may include: nausea, vomiting, diaphoresis and general malaise. Clinical and laboratory evidence of hepatic toxicity may not be apparent until 48 to 72 hours postingestion. In adults and adolescents, regardless of the quantity of acetaminophen reported to have been ingested, administer MUCOMYST® acetylcysteine immediately if 24 hours or less have elapsed from the reported time of ingestion. For full prescribing information, refer to the MUCOMYST package insert. Do not await results of assays for acetaminophen level before initiating treatment with MUCOMYST acetylcysteine. The following additional procedures are recommended: The stomach should be emptied promptly by lavage or by induction of emesis with syrup of ipecac. A serum acetaminophen assay should be obtained as early as possible, but no sooner than four hours following ingestion. Liver function studies should be obtained initially and repeated at 24-hour intervals.

Serious toxicity or fatalities are extremely infrequent in children, possibly due to differences in the way they metabolize acetaminophen. In children, the maximum potential amount ingested can be more easily estimated. If more than 150 mg/kg or an unknown amount was ingested, obtain an acetaminophen plasma level. The acetaminophen plasma level should be obtained as soon as possible, but no sooner than 4 hours following the ingestion. Induce emesis using syrup of ipecac. If the plasma level is obtained and falls above the broken line on the acetaminophen overdose nomogram, the MUCOMYST acetylcysteine therapy should be initiated and continued for a full course of therapy. If acetaminophen plasma assay capability is not available, and the estimated acetaminophen ingestion exceeds 150 mg/kg, MUCOMYST acetylcysteine therapy should be initiated and continued for a full course of therapy.

For additional emergency information, call your regional poison center or call the Rocky Mountain Poison Center toll-free, (1-800-525-6115).

Symptoms from phenylpropanolamine overdose consist most often of mild anxiety, tachycardia and/or mild hypertension. Symptoms usually appear within 4 to 8 hours of ingestion and are transient, usually requiring no treatment.

Inactive Ingredients: Citric Acid, Flavor, Potassium Benzoate, Povidone, Saccharin, Sodium Bicarbonate, Sodium Carbonate, Sodium Docusate, Sorbitol.

How Supplied: Tablets: carton of 20 tablets in 10 foil twin packs.

Shown in Product Identification Guide, page 413

TYLENOL® Cold
Night Time Medication
Liquid

Description: Each 30 ml (1 fl. oz.) of TYLENOL Cold Night Time Medication Liquid contains acetaminophen 650 mg., diphenhydramine hydrochloride 50 mg., pseudoephedrine hydrochloride 60 mg., (alcohol 10%).

Actions: TYLENOL Cold Night Time Medication Liquid contains a clinically proven analgesic-antipyretic, decongestant, cough suppressant and antihistamine. Acetaminophen produces analgesia by elevation of the pain threshold and antipyresis through action on the hypothalamic heat-regulating center. Acetaminophen is equal to aspirin in analgesic and antipyretic effectiveness and it is unlikely to produce many of the side effects associated with aspirin and aspirin-containing products. Pseudoephedrine hydrochloride is a sympathomimetic amine which provides temporary relief of nasal congestion. Diphenhydramine is an antihistamine which helps provide temporary relief of runny nose, sneezing and watery and itchy eyes.

Indications: TYLENOL Cold Night Time Medication Liquid provides effective temporary relief of runny nose, sneezing, watery and itchy eyes, nasal congestion, and aches, pains, sore throat and fevers due to a cold or "flu."

Precautions: If a rare sensitivity reaction occurs, the drug should be stopped. Although pseudoephedrine is virtually without pressor effect in normotensive patients, it should be used with caution in hypertensives.

Usual Dosage: Measuring cup is provided and marked for accurate dosing. Adults (12 years and over): 1 fluid ounce (2 tbsp.) in measuring cup provided every 6 hours, not to exceed 4 doses in 24 hours. Not recommended for children.

WARNINGS: Do not administer to children under 12. Do not take this product for more than 7 days or for fever for more than 3 days unless directed by a doctor. If symptoms do not improve or are accompanied by fever, consult a doctor. If sore throat is severe, persists for more than 2 days, is accompanied or followed by fever, headache, rash, nausea or vomiting, consult a doctor promptly. Do not exceed recommended dosage because at higher doses nervousness, dizziness or sleeplessness may occur. May cause excitability, especially in children. Do not take this product unless directed by a doctor, if you have a breathing problem, such as emphysema or chronic bronchitis, or if you have glaucoma or difficulty in urination due to enlargement of the prostate gland. Do not take this product if you have heart disease, high blood pressure, thyroid disease or diabetes unless directed by a doctor. May cause marked drowsiness; alcohol, sedatives and tranquilizers may increase the drowsiness effect. Avoid alcoholic beverages while taking this product. Do not take this product if you are taking sedatives or tranquilizers without first consulting your doctor. Use caution when driving a motor vehicle or operating machinery. Do not use with other products containing acetaminophen.

DO NOT USE IF CARTON IS OPENED OR IF PRINTED PLASTIC WRAP OR PRINTED FOIL INNER SEAL IS BROKEN. KEEP THIS AND ALL MEDICATION OUT OF THE REACH OF CHILDREN. AS WITH ANY DRUG, IF YOU ARE PREGNANT OR NURSING A BABY, SEEK THE ADVICE OF A HEALTH PROFESSIONAL BEFORE USING THIS PRODUCT. IN CASE OF ACCIDENTAL OVERDOSAGE, CONTACT A DOCTOR OR POISON CONTROL CENTER IMMEDIATELY.

Drug Interaction Precaution: Do not take this product if you are presently taking a prescription drug for high blood pressure or depression without first consulting your doctor.

Overdosage: Acetaminophen in massive overdosage may cause hepatic toxicity in some patients. In adults and adolescents, hepatic toxicity has rarely been reported following ingestion of acute overdosage of less than 10 grams. Fatalities are infrequent (less than 3–4% of untreated cases) and have rarely been reported with overdoses of less than 15 grams. In children, an acute overdosage of less than 150 mg/kg has not been associated with hepatic toxicity. Early symptoms following a potentially hepatotoxic overdose may include: nausea, vomiting, diaphoresis and general malaise. Clinical and laboratory evidence of hepatic toxicity may not be apparent until 48 to 72 hours postingestion. In adults and adolescents, regardless of the quantity of acetaminophen reported to have been ingested, administer MUCOMYST® acetylcysteine immediately if 24 hours or less have elapsed from the reported time of ingestion. For full prescribing information, refer to the MUCOMYST package insert. Do not await results of assays for acetaminophen level before initiating treatment with MUCOMYST acetylcysteine. The following additional procedures are recommended: The stomach should be emptied promptly by lavage or by induction of emesis with syrup of ipecac. A serum acetaminophen assay should be obtained as early as possible, but no sooner than four hours following ingestion. Liver function studies should be obtained initially and repeated at 24-hour intervals.

Serious toxicity or fatalities are extremely infrequent in children, possibly due to differences in the way they metabolize acetaminophen. In children, the maximum potential amount ingested can be more easily estimated. If more than 150 mg/kg or an unknown amount was ingested, obtain an acetaminophen plasma level. The acetaminophen plasma level should be obtained as soon as possible, but no sooner than 4 hours following the ingestion. Induce emesis using syrup of ipecac. If the plasma level is obtained and falls above the broken line on the acetaminophen overdose nomogram, the MUCOMYST acetylcysteine therapy should be initiated and continued for a full course of therapy. If acetaminophen plasma assay capability is not available, and the estimated acetaminophen ingestion exceeds 150 mg/kg, MUCOMYST acetylcysteine therapy should be initiated and continued for a full course of therapy.

For additional emergency information, call your regional poison center or call the Rocky Mountain Poison Center toll-free, (1-800-525-6115).

Diphenhydramine toxicity should be treated as you would an antihistamine/anticholinergic overdose and is likely to be present within a few hours after acute ingestion.

Symptoms from pseudoephedrine overdose consist most often of mild anxiety, tachycardia and/or mild hypertension. Symptoms usually appear within 4 to 8 hours of ingestion and are transient, usually requiring no treatment.

Inactive Ingredients: Alcohol (10%), Citric Acid, Flavors, Glycerin, Polyethylene Glycol, Purified Water, Sodium Benzoate, Sucrose, Red #40, Red #33 and Blue #1.

How Supplied: Cherry flavored (colored red) in 5 oz. bottles with child-resistant safety cap, special dosage cup graded in ounces and tablespoons, and tamper-resistant packaging.

Shown in Product Identification Guide, page 413

Extra-Strength TYLENOL® acetaminophen Adult Liquid Pain Reliever

Description: Each 15 ml. (½ fl. oz. or one tablespoonful) of Extra-Strength TYLENOL® acetaminophen adult Liquid Pain Reliever contains 500 mg. acetaminophen (alcohol 7%).

Actions: TYLENOL acetaminophen is a clinically proven analgesic and antipyretic. Acetaminophen produces analgesia by elevation of the pain threshold and antipyresis through action on the hypothalamic heat-regulating center. Acetaminophen is equal to aspirin in analgesic and antipyretic effectiveness and it is unlikely to produce many of the side effects associated with aspirin and aspirin-containing products.

Indications: Acetaminophen provides temporary relief of minor aches, pains, headaches and fevers.

Precautions: If a rare sensitivity reaction occurs, the drug should be discontinued.

Usual Dosage: Extra-Strength TYLENOL Adult Liquid Pain Reliever is an adult preparation for those adults who prefer liquids or can't swallow solid medication. Not for use in children under 12. Measuring cup is marked for accurate dosage. Extra-Strength Dose—1 fl. oz. (30 ml or 2 tablespoonsful, 1000 mg), which is equivalent to two 500 mg Extra-Strength TYLENOL Tablets, Caplets, Gelcaps or Geltabs. Take every 4–6 hours, no more than 4 doses in any 24-hour period.

Warning: Do not take for pain for more than 10 days or for fever for more than 3 days unless directed by a doctor. Severe or recurrent pain or high or continued fever may be indicative of serious illness. Under these conditions, consult a physician. **Do not use if printed plastic overwrap or printed foil inner seal is broken. Keep this and all medication out of the reach of children. As with any drug, if you are pregnant or nursing a baby, seek the advice of a health professional before using this product. In case of accidental overdosage, contact a doctor or poison control center immediately. Do not use with other products containing acetaminophen.**

Overdosage: Acetaminophen in massive overdosage may cause hepatic toxicity in some patients. In adults and adolescents, hepatic toxicity has rarely been reported following ingestion of acute overdosage of less than 10 grams. Fatalities are infrequent (less than 3–4% of untreated cases) and have rarely been reported with overdoses of less than 15 grams. In children, an acute overdosage of less than 150 mg/kg has not been associated with hepatic toxicity. Early symptoms following a potentially hepatotoxic overdose may include: nausea, vomiting, diaphoresis and general malaise. Clinical and laboratory evidence of hepatic toxicity may not be ap-

parent until 48 to 72 hours postingestion. In adults and adolescents, regardless of the quantity of acetaminophen reported to have been ingested, administer MUCOMYST® acetylcysteine immediately if 24 hours or less have elapsed from the reported time of ingestion. For full prescribing information, refer to the MUCOMYST package insert. Do not await the results of assays for acetaminophen level before initiating treatment with MUCOMYST acetylcysteine. The following additional procedures are recommended: The stomach should be emptied promptly by lavage or by induction of emesis with syrup of ipecac. A serum acetaminophen assay should be obtained as early as possible, but no sooner than four hours following ingestion. Liver function studies should be obtained initially and repeated at 24-hour intervals.

Serious toxicity or fatalities are extremely infrequent in children, possibly due to differences in the way they metabolize acetaminophen. In children, the maximum potential amount ingested can be more easily estimated. If more than 150 mg/kg or an unknown amount was ingested, obtain an acetaminophen plasma level. The acetaminophen plasma level should be obtained as soon as possible, but no sooner than 4 hours following the ingestion. Induce emesis using syrup of ipecac. If the plasma level is obtained and falls above the broken line on the acetaminophen overdose nomogram, the MUCOMYST acetylcysteine therapy should be initiated and continued for a full course of therapy. If acetaminophen plasma assay capability is not available, and the estimated acetaminophen ingestion exceeds 150 mg/kg, MUCOMYST acetylcysteine therapy should be initiated and continued for a full course of therapy.

For additional emergency information, call your regional poison center or call the Rocky Mountain Poison Center toll-free, (1-800-525-6115).

Inactive Ingredients: Alcohol (7%), Citric Acid, Flavors, Glycerin, Polyethylene Glycol, Purified Water, Sodium Benzoate, Sorbitol, Sucrose, Yellow #6 (Sunset Yellow), Yellow #10 and Blue #1.

How Supplied: Mint-flavored liquid (colored green), 8 fl. oz. tamper-resistant bottle with child resistant safety cap and special dosage cup.

EXTRA STRENGTH TYLENOL® Headache Plus Pain Reliever with Antacid Caplets

Description: Each Extra Strength TYLENOL® Headache Plus Pain Reliever with Antacid caplet contains acetaminophen 500 mg. and calcium carbonate 250 mg.

Indications: TYLENOL® Headache Plus provides temporary relief of minor

Continued on next page

McNeil Consumer—Cont.

aches and pains with heartburn or acid indigestion and upset stomach associated with these symptoms.

Actions: TYLENOL® Headache Plus contains a clinically proven analgesic and antacid. Acetaminophen produces analgesia by elevation of the pain threshold. Acetaminophen is equal to aspirin in analgesic effectiveness, and it is unlikely to produce many of the side effects associated with aspirin and aspirin-containing products. The antacid, calcium carbonate, provides fast relief of heartburn or acid indigestion and upset stomach associated with these symptoms.

Usual Dosage: Adults and children 12 years of age and older: Two caplets every 6 hours. No more than a total of 8 caplets in any 24 hour period or as directed by a physician.

Precautions: If a rare sensitivity reaction occurs, the drug should be stopped.

Warning: Do not give this product to children under 12 years of age. Do not use the maximum dosage of this product for more than 10 days except under the advice and supervision of a physician. Do not take the product for pain for more than 10 days, or for fever for more than 3 days unless directed by a physician. If pain or fever persists or gets worse, if new symptoms occur, or if redness or swelling is present, consult a physician because these could be signs of a serious condition. Do not use with other products containing acetaminophen. **Do not use if carton is opened, or if printed neck wrap or printed foil seal is broken. Keep this and all medication out of the reach of children. As with any drug, if you are pregnant or nursing a baby, seek the advice of a health professional before using this product. In the case of accidental overdose, seek professional assistance or contact a poison control center immediately. Prompt medical attention is critical for adults as well as for children even if you do not notice any signs or symptoms.**

Drug Interaction Precaution: Antacids may interact with certain prescription drugs. If you are presently taking a prescription drug, do not take this product without checking with your physician or other health professional.

Overdosage: Acetaminophen in massive overdosage may cause hepatic toxicity in some patients. In adults and adolescents, hepatic toxicity has rarely been reported following ingestion of acute overdosage of less than 10 grams. Fatalities are infrequent (less than 3–4% of untreated cases) and have rarely been reported with overdoses of less than 15 grams. In children, an acute overdosage of less than 150 mg/kg has not been associated with hepatic toxicity. Early symptoms following a potentially hepatotoxic overdose may include: nau-

sea, vomiting, diaphoresis and general malaise. Clinical and laboratory evidence of hepatic toxicity may not be apparent until 48 to 72 hours postingestion. In adults and adolescents, regardless of the quantity of acetaminophen reported to have been ingested, administer MUCOMYST® acetylcysteine immediately if 24 hours or less have elapsed from the reported time of ingestion. For full prescribing information, refer to the MUCOMYST package insert. Do not await results of assays for acetaminophen level before initiating treatment with MUCOMYST acetylcysteine. The following additional procedures are recommended: The stomach should be emptied promptly by lavage or by induction of emesis with syrup of ipecac. A serum acetaminophen assay should be obtained as early as possible, but no sooner than four hours following ingestion. Liver function studies should be obtained initially and repeated at 24-hour intervals.

Serious toxicity or fatalities are extremely infrequent in children, possibly due to differences in the way they metabolize acetaminophen. In children, the maximum potential amount ingested can be more easily estimated. If more than 150 mg/kg or an unknown amount was ingested, obtain an acetaminophen plasma level. The acetaminophen plasma level should be obtained as soon as possible, but no sooner than 4 hours following the ingestion. Induce emesis using syrup of ipecac. If the plasma level is obtained and falls above the broken line on the acetaminophen overdose nomogram, the MUCOMYST acetylcysteine therapy should be initiated and continued for a full course of therapy. If acetaminophen, plasma assay capability is not available, and the estimated acetaminophen ingestion exceeds 150 mg/kg, MUCOMYST acetylcysteine therapy should be initiated and continued for a full course of therapy.

For additional emergency information, call your regional poison center or call the Rocky Mountain Poison Center toll-free (1-800-525-6115).

Inactive Ingredients: Acacia, Cellulose, Corn Starch, Croscarmellose Sodium, Hydroxypropyl Methylcellulose, Magnesium Stearate, Maltodextrin, Propylene Glycol, Sodium Starch Glycolate, Titanium Dioxide, Triacetin, Blue #1 and Blue #2.

How Supplied: Caplets (white with royal blue imprinted "TYLENOL Headache Plus"). Tamper resistant bottles of 24, 50 and 100.

Shown in Product Identification Guide, page 413

EXTRA STRENGTH TYLENOL® PM
Pain Reliever/Sleep Aid
(Gelcaps, Caplets and Tablets)

Description: Each EXTRA STRENGTH TYLENOL® PM Gelcap, Caplet or Tab-

let contains acetaminophen 500 mg and diphenhydramine HCl 25 mg.

Actions: EXTRA STRENGTH TYLENOL® PM gelcaps, caplets and tablets contain a clinically proven analgesic-antipyretic and an antihistamine. Maximum allowable non-prescription levels of acetaminophen and diphenhydramine provide temporary relief of occasional headaches and minor aches and pains accompanying sleeplessness. Acetaminophen is equal to aspirin in analgesic and antipyretic effectiveness and it is unlikely to produce many of the side effects associated with aspirin containing products. Acetaminophen produces analgesia by elevation of the pain threshold. Diphenhydramine HCl is an antihistamine with sedative properties.

Indications: EXTRA STRENGTH TYLENOL® PM gelcaps, caplets and tablets provide effective symptomatic relief from occasional headaches and minor aches and pains with accompanying sleeplessness.

Precautions: If a rare sensitivity occurs, the drug should be discontinued.

Usual Dosage: Adults and Children 12 years of Age and Older: Two gelcaps, caplets or tablets at bedtime or as directed by physician. Do not exceed recommended dosage.

Warnings: Do not give to children under 12 years of age or use for more than 10 days unless directed by a physician. Consult your physician if symptoms persist or new ones occur, or if fever persists for more than 3 days, or if sleeplessness persists continuously for more than 2 weeks. Insomnia may be a symptom of serious underlying medical illness. Do not take this product if you have asthma, glaucoma, emphysema, chronic pulmonary disease, shortness of breath, difficulty in breathing or difficulty in urination due to enlargement of the prostate gland unless directed by a physician. Avoid alcoholic beverages while taking this product. Do not take if you are taking sedatives or tranquilizers without first consulting your physician. **Do not use if carton is open or if printed neck wrap or printed foil inner seal is broken. Keep this and all medications out of the reach of children. In case of accidental overdose, contact a physician or poison control center immediately. As with any drug, if you are pregnant or nursing a baby, seek the advice of a health professional before using this product. Do not use with other products containing acetaminophen.**

Caution: This product will cause drowsiness. Do not drive a motor vehicle or operate machinery after use.

Overdosage: Acetaminophen in massive overdosage may cause hepatic toxicity in some patients. In adults and adolescents, hepatic toxicity has rarely been reported following ingestion of acute overdosage of less than 10 grams. Fatalities are infrequent (less than 3–4% of un-

malaise. Clinical and laboratory evidence of hepatic toxicity may not be apparent until 48 to 72 hours postingestion. In adults and adolescents, regardless of the quantity of acetaminophen reported to have been ingested, administer MUCOMYST® acetylcysteine immediately if 24 hours or less have elapsed from the reported time of ingestion. For full prescribing information, refer to the MUCOMYST package insert. Do not await results of assays for acetaminophen level before initiating treatment with MUCOMYST acetylcysteine. The following additional procedures are recommended: The stomach should be emptied promptly by lavage or by induction of emesis with syrup of ipecac. A serum acetaminophen assay should be obtained as early as possible, but no sooner than four hours following ingestion. Liver function studies should be obtained initially and repeated at 24-hour intervals.

Serious toxicity or fatalities are extremely infrequent in children, possibly due to differences in the way they metabolize acetaminophen. In children, the maximum potential amount ingested can be more easily estimated. If more than 150 mg/kg or an unknown amount was ingested, obtain an acetaminophen plasma level. The acetaminophen plasma level should be obtained as soon as possible, but no sooner than 4 hours following the ingestion. Induce emesis using syrup of ipecac. If the plasma level is obtained and falls above the broken line on the acetaminophen overdose nomogram, the MUCOMYST acetylcysteine therapy should be initiated and continued for a full course of therapy. If acetaminophen plasma assay capability is not available, and the estimated acetaminophen ingestion exceeds 150 mg/kg, MUCOMYST acetylcysteine therapy should be initiated and continued for a full course of therapy.

For additional emergency information, call your regional poison center or call the Rocky Mountain Poison Center toll-free, (1-800-525-6115).

Diphenhydramine toxicity should be treated as you would an antihistamine/anticholinergic overdose and is likely to be present within a few hours after acute ingestion.

Symptoms from pseudoephedrine overdose consist most often of mild anxiety, tachycardia and/or mild hypertension. Symptoms usually appear within 4 to 8 hours of ingestion and are transient, usually requiring no treatment.

Inactive Ingredients: Alcohol (10%), Citric Acid, Flavors, Glycerin, Polyethylene Glycol, Purified Water, Sodium Benzoate, Sucrose, Red #40, Red #33 and Blue #1.

How Supplied: Cherry flavored (colored red) in 5 oz. bottles with child-resistant safety cap, special dosage cup graded in ounces and tablespoons, and tamper-resistant packaging.

Shown in Product Identification Guide, page 413

Extra-Strength
TYLENOL® acetaminophen
Adult Liquid Pain Reliever

Description: Each 15 ml. (½ fl. oz. or one tablespoonful) of Extra-Strength TYLENOL® acetaminophen adult Liquid Pain Reliever contains 500 mg. acetaminophen (alcohol 7%).

Actions: TYLENOL acetaminophen is a clinically proven analgesic and antipyretic. Acetaminophen produces analgesia by elevation of the pain threshold and antipyresis through action on the hypothalamic heat-regulating center. Acetaminophen is equal to aspirin in analgesic and antipyretic effectiveness and it is unlikely to produce many of the side effects associated with aspirin and aspirin-containing products.

Indications: Acetaminophen provides temporary relief of minor aches, pains, headaches and fevers.

Precautions: If a rare sensitivity reaction occurs, the drug should be discontinued.

Usual Dosage: Extra-Strength TYLENOL Adult Liquid Pain Reliever is an adult preparation for those adults who prefer liquids or can't swallow solid medication. Not for use in children under 12. Measuring cup is marked for accurate dosage. Extra-Strength Dose—1 fl. oz. (30 ml or 2 tablespoonsful, 1000 mg), which is equivalent to two 500 mg Extra-Strength TYLENOL Tablets, Caplets, Gelcaps or Geltabs. Take every 4–6 hours, no more than 4 doses in any 24-hour period.

Warning: Do not take for pain for more than 10 days or for fever for more than 3 days unless directed by a doctor. Severe or recurrent pain or high or continued fever may be indicative of serious illness. Under these conditions, consult a physician. **Do not use if printed plastic overwrap or printed foil inner seal is broken. Keep this and all medication out of the reach of children. As with any drug, if you are pregnant or nursing a baby, seek the advice of a health professional before using this product. In case of accidental overdosage, contact a doctor or poison control center immediately. Do not use with other products containing acetaminophen.**

Overdosage: Acetaminophen in massive overdosage may cause hepatic toxicity in some patients. In adults and adolescents, hepatic toxicity has rarely been reported following ingestion of acute overdosage of less than 10 grams. Fatalities are infrequent (less than 3–4% of untreated cases) and have rarely been reported with overdoses of less than 15 grams. In children, an acute overdosage of less than 150 mg/kg has not been associated with hepatic toxicity. Early symptoms following a potentially hepatotoxic overdose may include: nausea, vomiting, diaphoresis and general malaise. Clinical and laboratory evidence of hepatic toxicity may not be ap-

parent until 48 to 72 hours postingestion. In adults and adolescents, regardless of the quantity of acetaminophen reported to have been ingested, administer MUCOMYST® acetylcysteine immediately if 24 hours or less have elapsed from the reported time of ingestion. For full prescribing information, refer to the MUCOMYST package insert. Do not await the results of assays for acetaminophen level before initiating treatment with MUCOMYST acetylcysteine. The following additional procedures are recommended: The stomach should be emptied promptly by lavage or by induction of emesis with syrup of ipecac. A serum acetaminophen assay should be obtained as early as possible, but no sooner than four hours following ingestion. Liver function studies should be obtained initially and repeated at 24-hour intervals.

Serious toxicity or fatalities are extremely infrequent in children, possibly due to differences in the way they metabolize acetaminophen. In children, the maximum potential amount ingested can be more easily estimated. If more than 150 mg/kg or an unknown amount was ingested, obtain an acetaminophen plasma level. The acetaminophen plasma level should be obtained as soon as possible, but no sooner than 4 hours following the ingestion. Induce emesis using syrup of ipecac. If the plasma level is obtained and falls above the broken line on the acetaminophen overdose nomogram, the MUCOMYST acetylcysteine therapy should be initiated and continued for a full course of therapy. If acetaminophen plasma assay capability is not available, and the estimated acetaminophen ingestion exceeds 150 mg/kg, MUCOMYST acetylcysteine therapy should be initiated and continued for a full course of therapy.

For additional emergency information, call your regional poison center or call the Rocky Mountain Poison Center toll-free, (1-800-525-6115).

Inactive Ingredients: Alcohol (7%), Citric Acid, Flavors, Glycerin, Polyethylene Glycol, Purified Water, Sodium Benzoate, Sorbitol, Sucrose, Yellow #6 (Sunset Yellow), Yellow #10 and Blue #1.

How Supplied: Mint-flavored liquid (colored green), 8 fl. oz. tamper-resistant bottle with child resistant safety cap and special dosage cup.

EXTRA STRENGTH
TYLENOL® Headache Plus
Pain Reliever with Antacid
Caplets

Description: Each Extra Strength TYLENOL® Headache Plus Pain Reliever with Antacid caplet contains acetaminophen 500 mg. and calcium carbonate 250 mg.

Indications: TYLENOL® Headache Plus provides temporary relief of minor

Continued on next page

McNeil Consumer—Cont.

aches and pains with heartburn or acid indigestion and upset stomach associated with these symptoms.

Actions: TYLENOL® Headache Plus contains a clinically proven analgesic and antacid. Acetaminophen produces analgesia by elevation of the pain threshold. Acetaminophen is equal to aspirin in analgesic effectiveness, and it is unlikely to produce many of the side effects associated with aspirin and aspirin-containing products. The antacid, calcium carbonate, provides fast relief of heartburn or acid indigestion and upset stomach associated with these symptoms.

Usual Dosage: Adults and children 12 years of age and older: Two caplets every 6 hours. No more than a total of 8 caplets in any 24 hour period or as directed by a physician.

Precautions: If a rare sensitivity reaction occurs, the drug should be stopped.

Warning: Do not give this product to children under 12 years of age. Do not use the maximum dosage of this product for more than 10 days except under the advice and supervision of a physician. Do not take the product for pain for more than 10 days, or for fever for more than 3 days unless directed by a physician. If pain or fever persists or gets worse, if new symptoms occur, or if redness or swelling is present, consult a physician because these could be signs of a serious condition. Do not use with other products containing acetaminophen. **Do not use if carton is opened, or if printed neck wrap or printed foil seal is broken. Keep this and all medication out of the reach of children. As with any drug, if you are pregnant or nursing a baby, seek the advice of a health professional before using this product. In the case of accidental overdose, seek professional assistance or contact a poison control center immediately. Prompt medical attention is critical for adults as well as for children even if you do not notice any signs or symptoms.**

Drug Interaction Precaution: Antacids may interact with certain prescription drugs. If you are presently taking a prescription drug, do not take this product without checking with your physician or other health professional.

Overdosage: Acetaminophen in massive overdosage may cause hepatic toxicity in some patients. In adults and adolescents, hepatic toxicity has rarely been reported following ingestion of acute overdosage of less than 10 grams. Fatalities are infrequent (less than 3–4% of untreated cases) and have rarely been reported with overdoses of less than 15 grams. In children, an acute overdosage of less than 150 mg/kg has not been associated with hepatic toxicity. Early symptoms following a potentially hepatotoxic overdose may include: nau-

sea, vomiting, diaphoresis and general malaise. Clinical and laboratory evidence of hepatic toxicity may not be apparent until 48 to 72 hours postingestion. In adults and adolescents, regardless of the quantity of acetaminophen reported to have been ingested, administer MUCOMYST® acetylcysteine immediately if 24 hours or less have elapsed from the reported time of ingestion. For full prescribing information, refer to the MUCOMYST package insert. Do not await results of assays for acetaminophen level before initiating treatment with MUCOMYST acetylcysteine. The following additional procedures are recommended: The stomach should be emptied promptly by lavage or by induction of emesis with syrup of ipecac. A serum acetaminophen assay should be obtained as early as possible, but no sooner than four hours following ingestion. Liver function studies should be obtained initially and repeated at 24-hour intervals.

Serious toxicity or fatalities are extremely infrequent in children, possibly due to differences in the way they metabolize acetaminophen. In children, the maximum potential amount ingested can be more easily estimated. If more than 150 mg/kg or an unknown amount was ingested, obtain an acetaminophen plasma level. The acetaminophen plasma level should be obtained as soon as possible, but no sooner than 4 hours following the ingestion. Induce emesis using syrup of ipecac. If the plasma level is obtained and falls above the broken line on the acetaminophen overdose nomogram, the MUCOMYST acetylcysteine therapy should be initiated and continued for a full course of therapy. If acetaminophen, plasma assay capability is not available, and the estimated acetaminophen ingestion exceeds 150 mg/kg, MUCOMYST acetylcysteine therapy should be initiated and continued for a full course of therapy.

For additional emergency information, call your regional poison center or call the Rocky Mountain Poison Center toll-free (1-800-525-6115).

Inactive Ingredients: Acacia, Cellulose, Corn Starch, Croscarmellose Sodium, Hydroxypropyl Methylcellulose, Magnesium Stearate, Maltodextrin, Propylene Glycol, Sodium Starch Glycolate, Titanium Dioxide, Triacetin, Blue #1 and Blue #2.

How Supplied: Caplets (white with royal blue imprinted "TYLENOL Headache Plus"). Tamper resistant bottles of 24, 50 and 100.

Shown in Product Identification Guide, page 413

EXTRA STRENGTH TYLENOL® PM
Pain Reliever/Sleep Aid
(Gelcaps, Caplets and Tablets)

Description: Each EXTRA STRENGTH TYLENOL® PM Gelcap, Caplet or Tab-

let contains acetaminophen 500 mg and diphenhydramine HCl 25 mg.

Actions: EXTRA STRENGTH TYLENOL® PM gelcaps, caplets and tablets contain a clinically proven analgesic-antipyretic and an antihistamine. Maximum allowable non-prescription levels of acetaminophen and diphenhydramine provide temporary relief of occasional headaches and minor aches and pains accompanying sleeplessness. Acetaminophen is equal to aspirin in analgesic and antipyretic effectiveness and it is unlikely to produce many of the side effects associated with aspirin containing products. Acetaminophen produces analgesia by elevation of the pain threshold. Diphenhydramine HCl is an antihistamine with sedative properties.

Indications: EXTRA STRENGTH TYLENOL® PM gelcaps, caplets and tablets provide effective symptomatic relief from occasional headaches and minor aches and pains with accompanying sleeplessness.

Precautions: If a rare sensitivity occurs, the drug should be discontinued.

Usual Dosage: Adults and Children 12 years of Age and Older: Two gelcaps, caplets or tablets at bedtime or as directed by physician. Do not exceed recommended dosage.

Warnings: Do not give to children under 12 years of age or use for more than 10 days unless directed by a physician. Consult your physician if symptoms persist or new ones occur, or if fever persists for more than 3 days, or if sleeplessness persists continuously for more than 2 weeks. Insomnia may be a symptom of serious underlying medical illness. Do not take this product if you have asthma, glaucoma, emphysema, chronic pulmonary disease, shortness of breath, difficulty in breathing or difficulty in urination due to enlargement of the prostate gland unless directed by a physician. Avoid alcoholic beverages while taking this product. Do not take if you are taking sedatives or tranquilizers without first consulting your physician. **Do not use if carton is open or if printed neck wrap or printed foil inner seal is broken. Keep this and all medications out of the reach of children. In case of accidental overdose, contact a physician or poison control center immediately. As with any drug, if you are pregnant or nursing a baby, seek the advice of a health professional before using this product. Do not use with other products containing acetaminophen.**

Caution: This product will cause drowsiness. Do not drive a motor vehicle or operate machinery after use.

Overdosage: Acetaminophen in massive overdosage may cause hepatic toxicity in some patients. In adults and adolescents, hepatic toxicity has rarely been reported following ingestion of acute overdosage of less than 10 grams. Fatalities are infrequent (less than 3–4% of untreated cases) and have rarely been reported with overdoses of less than 15 grams. In children, an acute overdosage of less than 150 mg/kg has not been associated with hepatic toxicity.

Early symptoms following a potentially hepatotoxic overdose may include: nausea, vomiting, diaphoresis and general malaise. Clinical and laboratory evidence of hepatic toxicity may not be apparent until 48 to 72 hours postingestion. In adults and adolescents, regardless of the quantity of acetaminophen reported to have been ingested, administer MUCOMYST® acetylcysteine immediately if 24 hours or less have elapsed from the reported time of ingestion. For full prescribing information, refer to the MUCOMYST package insert. Do not await results of assays for acetaminophen level before initiating treatment with MUCOMYST acetylcysteine. The following additional procedures are recommended: The stomach should be emptied promptly by lavage or by induction of emesis with syrup of ipecac. A serum acetaminophen assay should be obtained as early as possible, but no sooner than four hours following ingestion. Liver function studies should be obtained initially and repeated at 24-hour intervals. Serious toxicity or fatalities are extremely infrequent in children, possibly due to differences in the way they metabolize acetaminophen. In children, the maximum potential amount ingested can be more easily estimated. If more than 150 mg/kg or an unknown amount was ingested, obtain an acetaminophen plasma level. The acetaminophen plasma level should be obtained as soon as possible, but no sooner than 4 hours following the ingestion. Induce emesis using syrup of ipecac. If the plasma level is obtained and falls above the broken line on the acetaminophen overdose nomogram, the MUCOMYST acetylcysteine therapy should be initiated and continued for a full course of therapy. If acetaminophen plasma assay capability is not available, and the estimated acetaminophen ingestion exceeds 150 mg/kg, MUCOMYST acetylcysteine therapy should be initiated and continued for a full course of therapy.

For additional emergency information, call your regional poison center or call the Rocky Mountain Poison Center toll-free, (1-800-525-6115).

Diphenhydramine toxicity should be treated as you would an antihistamine/anticholinergic overdose and is likely to be present within a few hours after acute ingestion.

Inactive Ingredients: Gelcaps: Benzyl Alcohol, Butylparaben, Castor Oil, Cellulose, Cornstarch, Edetate Calcium Disodium, Gelatin, Hydroxypropyl Methylcellulose, Magnesium Stearate, Propylparaben, Sodium Lauryl Sulfate, Sodium Citrate, Sodium Propionate, Sodium Starch Glycolate, Titanium Dioxide, Blue #1 and Red #28.

Tablets:

Inactive Ingredients: Cellulose, Cornstarch, Magnesium Stearate or Stearic Acid and Colloidal Silicon Dioxide, Polysorbate 80, Sodium Citrate, Sodium Starch Glycolate, Titanium Dioxide and Blue #1. May contain Hydroxypropyl Methylcellulose.

Caplets:

Inactive Ingredients: Cellulose, Cornstarch, Hydroxypropyl Methylcellulose, Magnesium Stearate or Stearic Acid and Colloidal Silicon Dioxide, Polyethylene Glycol, Polysorbate 80, Sodium Citrate, Sodium Starch Glycolate, Titanium Dioxide, Blue #1 and Blue #2.

How Supplied: Gelcaps (colored blue and white imprinted "TYLENOL PM") tamper-resistant bottles of 20 and 40. Caplets (colored light blue imprinted "Tylenol PM") tamper-resistant bottles of 24 and 50. Tablets (colored light blue embossed with "Tylenol" on one side and "PM" on the other) tamper-resistant bottles of 24 and 50.

Shown in Product Identification Guide, page 413

Extra Strength TYLENOL® acetaminophen Gelcaps, Geltabs; Caplets, Tablets

Description: Each Extra Strength TYLENOL Gelcap, Geltabs, Caplet or Tablet contains acetaminophen 500 mg.

Actions: Acetaminophen is a clinically proven analgesic and antipyretic. Acetaminophen produces analgesia by elevation of the pain threshold and antipyresis through action on the hypothalamic heat-regulating center. Acetaminophen is equal to aspirin in analgesic and antipyretic effectiveness and it is unlikely to produce many of the side effects associated with aspirin and aspirin-containing products.

Indications: For the temporary relief of minor aches, pains, headaches and fever.

Precautions: If a rare sensitivity reaction occurs, the drug should be discontinued.

Usual Dosage: Adults and children 12 years of Age and Older: Two Gelcaps, Geltabs, Caplets or Tablets 3 or 4 times daily. No more than a total of 8 Gelcaps, Geltabs, Caplets or Tablets in any 24-hour period.

Warning: Do not take for pain for more than 10 days or for fever for more than 3 days unless directed by a doctor. Severe or recurrent pain or high or continued fever may be indicative of serious illness. Under these conditions, consult a doctor. **Do not use if printed red neck wrap or printed foil inner seal is broken. Keep this and all medication out of the reach of children. As with any drug, if you are pregnant or nursing a baby, seek the advice of a health professional before using this product. In case of accidental overdosage, contact a doctor or poison control center immediately. Do not use with other products containing acetaminophen.**

Overdosage: Acetaminophen in massive overdosage may cause hepatic toxicity in some patients. In adults and adolescents, hepatic toxicity has rarely been reported following ingestion of acute overdosage of less than 10 grams. Fatalities are infrequent (less than 3–4% of untreated cases) and have rarely been reported with overdoses of less than 15 grams. In children, an acute overdosage of less than 150 mg/kg has not been associated with hepatic toxicity.

Early symptoms following a potentially hepatotoxic overdose may include: nausea, vomiting, diaphoresis and general malaise. Clinical and laboratory evidence of hepatic toxicity may not be apparent until 48 to 72 hours postingestion. In adults and adolescents, regardless of the quantity of acetaminophen reported to have been ingested, administer MUCOMYST® acetylcysteine immediately if 24 hours or less have elapsed from the reported time of ingestion. For full prescribing information, refer to the MUCOMYST package insert. Do not await the results of assays for acetaminophen level before initiating treatment with MUCOMYST acetylcysteine. The following additional procedures are recommended: The stomach should be emptied promptly by lavage or by induction of emesis with syrup of ipecac. A serum acetaminophen assay should be obtained as early as possible, but no sooner than four hours following ingestion. Liver function studies should be obtained initially and repeated at 24-hour intervals.

Serious toxicity or fatalities are extremely infrequent in children, possibly due to differences in the way they metabolize acetaminophen. In children, the maximum potential amount ingested can be more easily estimated. If more than 150 mg/kg or an unknown amount was ingested, obtain an acetaminophen plasma level. The acetaminophen plasma level should be obtained as soon as possible, but no sooner than 4 hours following the ingestion. Induce emesis using syrup of ipecac. If the plasma level is obtained and falls above the broken line on the acetaminophen overdose nomogram, the MUCOMYST acetylcysteine therapy should be initiated and continued for a full course of therapy. If acetaminophen plasma assay capability is not available, and the estimated acetaminophen ingestion exceeds 150 mg/kg, MUCOMYST acetylcysteine therapy should be initiated and continued for a full course of therapy.

For additional emergency information, call your regional poison center or call the Rocky Mountain Poison Center toll-free, (1-800-525-6115).

Inactive Ingredients: Tablets—Magnesium Stearate, Cellulose, Sodium

Continued on next page

McNeil Consumer—Cont.

Starch Glycolate and Starch. Caplets—Cellulose, Hydroxypropyl Methylcellulose, Magnesium Stearate, Polyethylene Glycol, Sodium Starch Glycolate, Starch and Red #40.

Gelcaps—Benzyl Alcohol, Butylparaben, Castor Oil, Cellulose, Edetate Calcium Disodium, Gelatin, Hydroxypropyl Methylcellulose, Magnesium Stearate, Methylparaben, Propylparaben, Sodium Lauryl Sulfate, Sodium Propionate, Sodium Starch Glycolate, Starch, Titanium Dioxide, Blue #1 and #2, Red #40 and Yellow #10. Geltabs—Benzyl Alcohol, Butylparaben, Castor Oil, Cellulose, Corn Starch, Edetate Calcium Disodium, Gelatin, Hydroxypropyl Methylcellulose, Magnesium Stearate, Methylparaben, Propylparaben, Sodium Lauryl Sulfate, Sodium Propionate, Sodium Starch Glycolate, Titanium Dioxide, Blue #1 and #2, Red #40, and Yellow #10.

How Supplied: Tablets (colored white, imprinted "TYLENOL" and "500")—vials of 10 and tamper-resistant bottles of 30, 60, 100, and 200. Caplets (colored white, imprinted "TYLENOL 500 mg")—vials of 10 and tamper-resistant bottles of 24, 50, 100, 175, and 250's. Gelcaps (colored yellow and red, imprinted "Tylenol 500") tamper-resistant bottles of 24, 50, 100, and 150 and Fast Cap Package of 72. Geltabs (colored yellow and red, imprinted "Tylenol 500") tamper-resistant bottles of 24, 50, and 100. For adults who prefer liquids or can't swallow solid medication, Extra-Strength TYLENOL® Adult Liquid Pain Reliever, mint flavored, is also available (colored green; 1 fl. oz. = 1000 mg.).

Shown in Product Identification Guide, page 412

Hot Medication TYLENOL® Cold & Flu Medication Packets

Description: Each packet of Hot Medication TYLENOL Cold & Flu Medication contains acetaminophen 650 mg., chlorpheniramine maleate 4 mg., pseudoephedrine hydrochloride 60 mg. and dextromethorphan hydrobromide 30 mg.

Actions: Hot Medication TYLENOL Cold and Flu Medication contains a clinically proven analgesic-antipyretic, decongestant, cough suppressant and antihistamine. Acetaminophen produces analgesia by elevation of the pain threshold and antipyresis through action on the hypothalamic heat-regulating center. Acetaminophen is equal to aspirin in analgesic and antipyretic effectiveness and it is unlikely to produce many of the side effects associated with aspirin and aspirin-containing products. Pseudoephedrine hydrochloride is a sympathomimetic amine which provides temporary relief of nasal congestion. Dextromethorphan is a cough suppressant which provides temporary relief of coughs due to

minor throat irritations that may occur with the common cold. Chlorpheniramine is an antihistamine which helps provide temporary relief of runny nose, sneezing and watery and itchy eyes.

Indications: Hot Medication TYLENOL Cold and Flu Medication provides effective temporary relief of runny nose, sneezing, watery and itchy eyes, nasal congestion, sore throat, coughing, and aches, pains, and fever due to a cold or "flu."

Precautions: If a rare sensitivity reaction occurs, the drug should be stopped. Although pseudoephedrine is virtually without pressor effect in normotensive patients, it should be used with caution in hypertensives.

Usual Dosage: Adults (12 years and over): Dissolve one packet in 6 oz. cup of hot water. Sip while hot. Sweeten to taste, if desired. May repeat every 6 hours, not to exceed 4 doses in 24 hours.

Warnings: Do not administer to children under 12. Do not take this product for more than 7 days or for fever for more than 3 days unless directed by a doctor. If symptoms do not improve or are accompanied by fever, consult a doctor. If sore throat is severe, persists for more than 2 days, is accompanied or followed by fever, headache, rash, nausea or vomiting, consult a doctor promptly. A persistent cough may be a sign of a serious condition. If cough persists for more than 1 week, tends to recur or is accompanied by fever, rash or persistent headache, consult a doctor. Do not take this product for persistent or chronic cough such as occurs with smoking, asthma, emphysema or if cough is accompanied by excessive phlegm (mucus) unless directed by a doctor. Do not exceed recommended dosage because at higher doses, nervousness, dizziness or sleeplessness my occur. May cause excitability especially in children. Do not take this product, unless directed by a doctor, if you have a breathing problem such as emphysema or chronic bronchitis, or if you have glaucoma or difficulty in urination due to enlargement of the prostate gland. Do not take this product if you have heart disease, high blood pressure, thyroid disease or diabetes unless directed by a doctor. May cause drowsiness; alcohol, sedatives and tranquilizers may increase the drowsiness effect. Avoid alcoholic beverages while taking this product. Do not take this product if you are taking sedatives or tranquilizers without first consulting your doctor. Use caution when driving a motor vehicle or operating machinery. Do not use with other products containing acetaminophen. **DO NOT USE IF GLUED CARTON FLAP IS OPENED OR IF FOIL PACKET IS TORN OR BROKEN. KEEP THIS AND ALL MEDICATION OUT OF THE REACH OF CHILDREN. AS WITH ANY DRUG, IF YOU ARE PREGNANT OR NURSING A BABY, SEEK THE ADVICE OF A HEALTH PROFESSIONAL BEFORE USING**

THIS PRODUCT. IN CASE OF ACCIDENTAL OVERDOSAGE, CONTACT A DOCTOR OR POISON CONTROL CENTER IMMEDIATELY. PHENYLKETONURICS: CONTAINS PHENYLALANINE 11 MG PER PACKET.

Drug Interaction Precaution: Do not take this product if you are presently taking a prescription drug for high blood pressure or you are now taking a prescription monoamine oxidase inhibitor (MAOI) (certain drugs for depression, psychiatric or emotional conditions, or Parkinson's disease), or for 2 weeks after stopping the MAOI drug. If you are uncertain whether your prescription drug contains an MAOI, consult a health professional before taking this product.

Overdosage: Acetaminophen in massive overdosage may cause hepatic toxicity in some patients. In adults and adolescents, hepatic toxicity has rarely been reported following ingestion of acute overdosage of less than 10 grams. Fatalities are infrequent (less than 3–4% of untreated cases) and have rarely been reported with overdoses of less than 15 grams. In children, an acute overdosage of less than 150 mg/kg has not been associated with hepatic toxicity.

Early symptoms following a potentially hepatotoxic overdose may include: nausea, vomiting, diaphoresis and general malaise. Clinical and laboratory evidence of hepatic toxicity may not be apparent until 48 to 72 hours postingestion. In adults and adolescents, regardless of the quantity of acetaminophen reported to have been ingested, administer MUCOMYST® acetylcysteine immediately if 24 hours or less have elapsed from the reported time of ingestion. For full prescribing information, refer to the MUCOMYST package insert. Do not await results of assays for acetaminophen level before initiating treatment with MUCOMYST acetylcysteine. The following additional procedures are recommended: The stomach should be emptied promptly by lavage or by induction of emesis with syrup of ipecac. A serum acetaminophen assay should be obtained as early as possible, but no sooner than four hours following ingestion. Liver function studies should be obtained initially and repeated at 24-hour intervals.

Serious toxicity or fatalities are extremely infrequent in children, possibly due to differences in the way they metabolize acetaminophen. In children, the maximum potential amount ingested can be more easily estimated. If more than 150 mg/kg or an unknown amount was ingested, obtain an acetaminophen plasma level. The acetaminophen plasma level should be obtained as soon as possible, but no sooner than 4 hours following the ingestion. Induce emesis using syrup of ipecac. If the plasma level is obtained and falls above the broken line on the acetaminophen overdose nomogram, the MUCOMYST acetylcysteine therapy should be initiated and continued for a full course of therapy. If acetaminophen plasma assay capability is not available, and the estimated acetaminophen ingestion exceeds 150 mg/kg, MUCOMYST acetylcysteine therapy should be initiated and continued for a full course of therapy.

For additional emergency information, call your regional poison center or call the Rocky Mountain Poison Center toll-free, (1-800-525-6115).

Symptoms from pseudoephedrine overdose consist most often of mild anxiety, tachycardia and/or mild hypertension. Symptoms usually appear within 4 to 8 hours of ingestion and are transient, usually requiring no treatment.

Acute dextromethorphan overdose usually does not result in serious signs and symptoms unless massive amounts have been ingested. Signs and symptoms of a substantial overdose may include nausea and vomiting, visual disturbances, CNS disturbances, and urinary retention.

Chlorpheniramine toxicity should be treated as you would an antihistamine/anticholinergic overdose and is likely to be present within a few hours after acute ingestion.

Inactive Ingredients: Aspartame, Citric Acid, Flavors, Sodium Citrate, Starch, Sucrose, Red #40 and Yellow #10.

How Supplied: Packets of powder (yellow colored) in cartons of 6 tamper-resistant foil packets.

Shown in Product Identification Guide, page 413

**Junior Strength TYLENOL®
acetaminophen
Coated Caplets and
Chewable Tablets**

Description: Each Junior Strength Tylenol Coated Caplet or Chewable tablet contains 160 mg acetaminophen in a small, coated, capsule shaped tablet or grape or fruit chewable tablet.

Actions: Acetaminophen is a clinically proven analgesic/antipyretic. Acetaminophen produces analgesia by elevation of the pain threshold and antipyresis through action on the hypothalamic heat-regulating center. Acetaminophen is equal to aspirin in analgesic and antipyretic effectiveness and it is unlikely to produce many of the side effects associated with aspirin and aspirin-containing products.

Indications: Junior Strength TYLENOL Caplets are designed for easy swallowability in older children and young adults. Both Junior Strength TYLENOL Caplets and Junior Strength Chewable Tablets provide fast, effective temporary relief of fever and discomfort due to colds and "flu," and pain and discomfort due to simple headaches, minor muscle aches, sprains and overexertion.

Precautions: If a rare sensitivity reaction occurs, the drug should be stopped.

Usual Dosage: Caplets should be taken with liquid. Chewable tablets should be well chewed. All dosages may be repeated every 4 hours, but not more than 5 times daily. For ages: 6–8 years: two Caplets or tablets, 9–10 years: two and one-half Caplets or tablets, 11 years: three Caplets or tablets, 12 years: four Caplets or tablets.

Warning: Do not use if carton is opened or if a blister unit is broken. Keep this and all medications out of the reach of children. In case of accidental overdosage, contact a physician or poison control center immediately. Consult your physician if fever persists for more than three days or if pain continues for more than five days. As with any drug, if you are pregnant or nursing a baby, seek the advice of a health professional before using this product. In addition the caplet package states: Not for children who have difficulty swallowing tablets. In addition the chewable tablet package states: Phenylketonurics: contains phenylalanine 5 mg per tablet. Do not use with other products containing acetaminophen.

Overdosage: Acetaminophen in massive overdosage may cause hepatic toxicity in some patients. In adults and adolescents, hepatic toxicity has rarely been reported following ingestion of acute overdosage of less than 10 grams. Fatalities are infrequent (less than 3–4% of untreated cases) and have rarely been reported with overdoses of less than 15 grams. In children, an acute overdose of less than 150 mg/kg has not been associated with hepatic toxicity.

Early symptoms following a potentially hepatotoxic overdose may include: nausea, vomiting, diaphoresis and general malaise. Clinical and laboratory evidence of hepatic toxicity may not be apparent until 48 to 72 hours postingestion. In adults and adolescents, regardless of the quantity of acetaminophen reported to have been ingested, administer MUCOMYST® acetylcysteine immediately if 24 hours or less have elapsed from the reported time of ingestion. For full prescribing information, refer to the MUCOMYST package insert. Do not await the results of assays for acetaminophen level before initiating treatment with MUCOMYST acetylcysteine. The following additional procedures are recommended: The stomach should be emptied promptly by lavage or by induction of emesis with syrup of ipecac. A serum acetaminophen assay should be obtained as early as possible, but no sooner than four hours following ingestion. Liver function studies should be obtained initially and repeated at 24-hour intervals.

Serious toxicity or fatalities are extremely infrequent in children, possibly due to differences in the way they metabolize acetaminophen. In children, the maximum potential amount ingested can be more easily estimated. If more than 150 mg/kg or an unknown amount was ingested, obtain an acetaminophen

plasma level. The acetaminophen plasma level should be obtained as soon as possible, but no sooner than 4 hours following the ingestion. Induce emesis using syrup of ipecac. If the plasma level is obtained and falls above the broken line on the acetaminophen overdose nomogram, the MUCOMYST acetylcysteine therapy should be initiated and continued for a full course of therapy. If acetaminophen plasma assay capability is not available, and the estimated acetaminophen ingestion exceeds 150 mg/kg, MUCOMYST acetylcysteine therapy should be initiated and continued for a full course of therapy.

For additional emergency information, call your regional poison center or call the Rocky Mountain Poison Center toll-free (1-800-525-6115).

Inactive Ingredients: Caplets: Cellulose, Ethylcellulose, Magnesium Stearate, Sodium Lauryl Sulfate, Sodium Starch Glycolate, Starch.

Tablets: Aspartame, Cellulose, Citric Acid, Ethylcellulose, Flavors, Magnesium Stearate, Mannitol, Starch, Blue #1 and Red #7.

How Supplied: Coated Caplets, (colored white, coated, scored, imprinted "TYLENOL 160") Package of 30. Chewable tablets (colored purple or pink, imprinted "TYLENOL 160") Package of 24. All packages are safety sealed and use child resistant blister packaging.

Shown in Product Identification Guide, pages 412 and 413

**Maximum-Strength
TYLENOL® Allergy Sinus
Medication Caplets, Gelcaps**

Description: Each Maximum Strength TYLENOL® Allergy Sinus Caplet or Gelcap contains acetaminophen 500 mg, chlorpheniramine maleate 2 mg, and pseudoephedrine hydrochloride 30 mg.

Actions: Maximum Strength TYLENOL® Allergy Sinus Caplets or Gelcaps contain a clinically proven analgesic-antipyretic, decongestant, and antihistamine. Acetaminophen produces analgesia by elevation of the pain threshold and antipyresis through action on the hypothalamic heat-regulating center. Acetaminophen is equal to aspirin in analgesic and antipyretic effectiveness, and it is unlikely to produce many of the side effects associated with aspirin and aspirin-containing products. Pseudoephedrine hydrochloride is a sympathomimetic amine which provides temporary relief of nasal congestion. Chlorpheniramine is an antihistamine which helps provide temporary relief of runny nose, sneezing and watery and itchy eyes.

Indications: TYLENOL® Allergy Sinus provides effective temporary relief of these upper respiratory allergy, hay fever and sinusitis symptoms: sneezing,

Continued on next page

McNeil Consumer—Cont.

itchy, watery eyes, runny nose, itching of the nose or throat, nasal and sinus congestion and sinus pain and headaches.

Precautions: If a rare sensitivity reaction occurs, the drug should be stopped. Although pseudoephedrine is virtually without pressor effect in normotensive patients, it should be used with caution in hypertensives.

Usual Dosage: Adults: Two caplets or gelcaps every 6 hours, not to exceed 8 caplets or gelcaps in 24 hours.
WARNING: Do not administer to children under 12 or exceed the recommended dosage because nervousness, dizziness, or sleeplessness may occur. May cause excitability, especially in children. This preparation may cause drowsiness; alcohol may increase the drowsiness effect. Avoid alcoholic beverages when taking this product. Use caution when driving a motor vehicle or operating machinery. Do not take this product if you have heart disease, high blood pressure, thyroid disease, diabetes, asthma, glaucoma, emphysema, chronic pulmonary disease, shortness of breath, difficulty in breathing or difficulty in urination due to enlargement of prostate gland unless directed by a doctor. Do not take this product for more than 7 days. If symptoms do not improve or are accompanied by a high fever, consult a physician." **DO NOT USE IF CARTON IS OPEN OR IF A BLISTER UNIT IS BROKEN. KEEP THIS AND ALL MEDICATION OUT OF THE REACH OF CHILDREN. AS WITH ANY DRUG, IF YOU ARE PREGNANT OR NURSING A BABY, SEEK THE ADVICE OF A HEALTH PROFESSIONAL BEFORE USING THIS PRODUCT. IN THE CASE OF ACCIDENTAL OVERDOSE, CONTACT A PHYSICIAN OR POISON CONTROL CENTER IMMEDIATELY. Do not use with other products containing acetaminophen.**

Drug Interaction Precaution: Do not take this product if you are presently taking a prescription drug for high blood pressure or depression without first consulting your doctor.

Overdosage: Acetaminophen in massive overdosage may cause hepatic toxicity in some patients. In adults and adolescents, hepatic toxicity has rarely been reported following ingestion of acute overdose of less than 10 grams. Fatalities are infrequent (less than 3–4% of untreated cases) and have rarely been reported with overdoses of less than 15 grams. In children, an acute overdosage of less than 150 mg/kg has not been associated with hepatic toxicity.
Early symptoms following a potentially hepatotoxic overdose may include: nausea, vomiting, diaphoresis and general malaise. Clinical and laboratory evidence of hepatic toxicity may not be apparent until 48 to 72 hours postingestion.

In adults and adolescents, regardless of the quantity of acetaminophen reported to have been ingested, administer MUCOMYST® acetylcysteine immediately if 24 hours or less have elapsed from the reported time of ingestion. For full prescribing information, refer to the MUCOMYST package insert. Do not await results of assays for acetaminophen level before initiating treatment with MUCOMYST acetylcysteine. The following additional procedures are recommended: The stomach should be emptied promptly by lavage or by induction of emesis with syrup of ipecac. A serum acetaminophen assay should be obtained as early as possible, but no sooner than four hours following ingestion. Liver function studies should be obtained initially and repeated at 24-hour intervals.
Several toxicity or fatalities are extremely infrequent in children, possibly due to differences in the way they metabolize acetaminophen. In children, the maximum potential amount ingested can be easily estimated. If more than 150 mg/kg or an unknown amount was ingested, obtain an acetaminophen plasma level. The acetaminophen plasma level should be obtained as soon as possible, but no sooner than 4 hours following ingestion. Induce emesis using syrup of ipecac. If the plasma level is obtained and falls above the broken line on the acetaminophen overdose nomogram, the MUCOMYST acetylcysteine therapy should be initiated and continued for a full course of therapy. If acetaminophen plasma assay capability is not available, and the estimated acetaminophen ingestion exceeds 150 mg/kg, MUCOMYST acetylcysteine therapy should be initiated and continued for a full course of therapy.
For additional emergency information, call your regional poison center or call the Rocky Mountain Poison Control Center toll-free, (1-800-525-6115).
Chlorpheniramine toxicity should be treated as you would an antihistamine/anticholinergic overdose and is likely to be present within a few hours after acute ingestion.
Symptoms from pseudophedrine overdose consist most often of mild anxiety, tachycardia and/or hypertension. Symptoms usually appear within 4 to 8 hours of ingestion and are transient, usually requiring no treatment.

Inactive Ingredients: CAPLET: Cellulose, hydroxypropyl cellulose, hydroxypropyl methylcellulose, magnesium stearate, polyethylene glycol, sodium starch glycolate, corn starch, titanium dioxide, blue #1, yellow #6, yellow #10.
GELCAP: Benzyl Alcohol, Butylparaben, Castor oil, Cellulose, Edetate Calcium Disodium, Gelatin, Hydroxypropyl Methylcellulose, Magnesium Stearate, Methylparaben, Propylparaben, Sodium Lauryl Sulfate, Sodium Propionate, Sodium Starch Glycolate, Starch, Titanium Dioxide Blue #1 and #2 and Yellow #10.

How Supplied: Caplets: (dark yellow, imprinted "TYLENOL Allergy Sinus")—Blister packs of 24 and tamper-resistant bottles of 50.
Gelcaps: (dark green and dark yellow, imprinted "TYLENOL A/S")—Blister packs of 20 and tamper-resistant bottles of 40.
Shown in Product Identification Guide, page 413

MAXIMUM STRENGTH TYLENOL® COUGH MEDICATION

Description: Each 20 ml (4 tsp.) adult dose contains dextromethorphan HBr 30 mg., and acetaminophen 1,000mg.

Actions: MAXIMUM STRENGTH TYLENOL® COUGH Medication Liquid contains a clinically proven cough suppressant and analgesic-antipyretic. Acetaminophen produces analgesia by elevation of the pain threshold and antipyresis through action on the hypothalamic heat-regulating center. Dextromethorphan is a cough suppressant which provides temporary relief of coughs due to minor throat irritations that may occur with the common cold.

Indications: MAXIMUM STRENGTH TYLENOL® COUGH Medication provides effective, temporary relief of coughing, and the aches, pains and sore throat that may accompany a cough due to a cold.

Usual Dosage: A specially marked dosage cup is provided for accurate dosing. Adults: (12 years and older) 4 teaspoons or 20ml as marked on dosage cup every 6–8 hours, not to exceed 4 doses in 24 hours. Children: (ages 6–11) 1 1/4 teaspoons or 6.25ml as marked on dosage cup every 4 hours, not to exceed 5 doses in 24 hours. Not recommended for children under 6 years.
WARNING: Do not take this product for more than 10 days or for fever for more than 3 days unless directed by a physician. Severe or recurrent pain or high or continued fever may be indicative of serious illness. Under these conditions, consult a physician. A persistent cough may be a sign of a serious condition. If cough persists for more than 1 week, tends to recur or is accompanied by fever, rash or persistent headache, consult a doctor. Do not take this product for persistent or chronic cough such as occurs with smoking, asthma, emphysema, or if cough is accompanied by excessive phlegm (mucus) unless directed by a doctor. If sore throat is severe, persists for more than 2 days, is accompanied or followed by fever, headache, rash, nausea or vomiting, consult a doctor promptly. Do not use with other products containing acetaminophen.
Do not use if carton is opened or if printed neck wrap (under dosage cup) or printed foil inner seal is broken. Keep this and all medication out of the reach of children. As with any drug, if you are

pregnant or nursing a baby, seek the advice of a health professional before using this product. In case of accidental overdosage, contact a doctor or poison control center immediately.

Drug Interaction Precaution: Do not take this product if you are presently taking a prescription drug for high blood pressure or depression without first consulting your doctor.

Do not use this product if you are now taking a prescription monoamine oxidase inhibitor (MAOI) (certain drugs for depression, psychiatric or emotional conditions, or Parkinson's disease), or for 2 weeks after stopping the MAOI drug. If you are uncertain whether your prescription drug contains an MAOI, consult a health professional before taking this product.

Overdosage: Acetaminophen in massive dosage may cause hepatic toxicity in some patients. In adults and adolescents, hepatic toxicity has rarely been reported following ingestion of acute overdosage of less than 10 grams. Fatalities are infrequent (less than 3–4% of untreated cases) and have rarely been reported with overdoses of less than 15 grams. In children, an acute overdosage of less than 150mg/kg has not been associated with hepatic toxicity.

Early symptoms following a potentially hepatotoxic overdose may include: nausea, vomiting, diaphoresis and general malaise. Clinical and laboratory evidence of hepatic toxicity may not be apparent until 48 to 72 hours postingestion. In adults and adolescents, regardless of the quantity of acetaminophen reported to have been ingested, administer MUCOMYST® acetylcysteine immediately if 24 hours or less have elapsed from the reported time of ingestion. For full prescribing information, refer to the MUCOMYST package insert. Do not await results of assays for acetaminophen level before initiating treatment with MUCOMYST acetylcysteine. The following additional procedures are recommended: The stomach should be emptied by lavage or by induction of emesis with syrup of ipecac. A serum acetaminophen assay should be obtained as early as possible, but no sooner than four hours following ingestion. Liver function studies should be obtained initially and repeated at 24-hour intervals.

Serious toxicity or fatalities are extremely infrequent in children, possibly due to differences in the way they metabolize acetaminophen. In children, the maximum potential amount ingested can be more easily estimated. If more than 150mg/kg or an unknown amount was ingested, obtain an acetaminophen plasma level. The acetaminophen plasma level should be obtained as soon as possible, but no sooner than 4 hours following the ingestion. Induce emesis using syrup of ipecac. If the plasma level is obtained and falls above the broken line on the acetaminophen overdose nomogram, the MUCOMYST acetylcysteine therapy should be initiated and con-

tinued for a full course of therapy. If acetaminophen plasma assay capability is not available, and the estimated acetaminophen ingestion exceeds 150mg/kg, MUCOMYST acetycysteine therapy should be initiated and continued for a full course of therapy.

For additional emergency information, call your regional poison center or call the Rocky Mountain Poison Center toll free (1-800-525-6115).

Acute dextromethorphan overdose usually does not result in serious signs and symptoms unless massive amounts have been ingested. Signs and symptoms of a substantial overdose may include nausea and vomiting, visual disturbances, CNS disturbances, and urinary retention.

Inactive Ingredients: Alcohol (10%), Citric Acid, Flavors, Glycerin, Polyethylene Glycol, Purified Water, Sodium Benzoate, Sodium Carboxymethylcellulose, Sodium Saccharin, Sorbitol, Sucrose, Red #33, and Red #40.

How Supplied: MAXIMUM STRENGTH TYLENOL® COUGH is available in a 4 oz. bottle with child-resistant safety cap, special dosing cup marked in ml, and tamper resistant packaging.

Shown in Product Identification Guide, page 413

MAXIMUM STRENGTH TYLENOL® COUGH MEDICATION WITH DECONGESTANT

Description: Each 20 ml (4 tsp.) adult dose contains dextromethorphan HBr 30 mg., and acetaminophen 1,000mg, and pseudoephedrine HCl 60mg.

Actions: MAXIMUM STRENGTH TYLENOL® COUGH Medication with Decongestant Liquid contains a clinically proven cough suppressant, an analgesic-antipyretic, and decongestant. Acetaminophen produces analgesia by elevation of the pain threshold and antipyresis through action on the hypothalamic heat-regulating center. Dextromethorphan is a cough suppressant which provides temporary relief of coughs due to minor throat irritations that may occur with the common cold. Pseudoephedrine hydrochloride is a sympathomimetic amine which provides temporary relief of nasal congestion.

Indications: MAXIMUM STRENGTH TYLENOL® COUGH Medication with Decongestant provides effective, temporary relief of coughing, nasal congestion and the aches, pains and sore throat that may accompany a cough due to a cold.

Usual Dosage: A specially marked dosage cup is provided for accurate dosing. Adults: (12 years and older) 4 teaspoons or 20ml as marked on dosage cup every 6–8 hours, not to exceed 4 doses in 24 hours. Children: (ages 6–11) 1 1/4 teaspoons or 6.25ml as marked on dosage cup every 4 hours, not to exceed 5 doses

in 24 hours. Not recommended for children under 6 years.

WARNING: Do not take this product for more than 7 days or for fever for more than 3 days unless directed by a doctor. If symptoms do not improve or are accompanied by fever, consult a physician. A persistent cough may be a sign of a serious condition. If cough persists for more than 1 week, tends to recur or is accompanied by fever, rash or persistent headache, consult a doctor. Do not take this product for persistent or chronic cough such as occurs with smoking, asthma, emphysema, or if cough is accompanied by excessive phlegm (mucus) unless directed by a doctor. Do not exceed the recommended dosage because at higher doses nervousness, dizziness or sleeplessness may occur. Do not take this product if you have heart disease, high blood pressure, thyroid disease, diabetes or difficulty in urination due to enlargement of the prostate gland unless directed by a doctor. If sore throat is severe, persists for more than 2 days, is accompanied or followed by fever, headache, rash, nausea or vomiting, consult a doctor promptly. Do not use with other products containing acetaminophen.

Do not use if carton is opened or if printed neck wrap (under dosage cup) or printed foil inner seal is broken. Keep this and all medication out of the reach of children. As with any drug, if you are pregnant or nursing a baby, seek the advice of a health professional before using this product. In case of accidental overdosage, contact a doctor or poison control center immediately.

Drug Interaction Precaution: Do not take this product if you are presently taking a prescription drug for high blood pressure or you are now taking a prescription monoamine oxidase inhibitor (MAOI) (certain drugs for depression, psychiatric or emotional conditions, or Parkinson's disease), or for 2 weeks after stopping the MAOI drug. If you are uncertain whether your prescription drug contains an MAOI, consult a health professional before taking this product.

Overdosage: Acetaminophen in massive dosage may cause hepatic toxicity in some patients. In adults and adolescents, hepatic toxicity has rarely been reported following ingestion of acute overdosage of less than 10 grams. Fatalities are infrequent (less than 3–4% of untreated cases) and have rarely been reported with overdoses of less than 15 grams. In children, an acute overdosage of less than 150mg/kg has not been associated with hepatic toxicity.

Early symptoms following a potentially hepatotoxic overdose may include: nausea, vomiting, diaphoresis and general malaise. Clinical and laboratory evidence of hepatic toxicity may not be apparent until 48 to 72 hours postingestion. In adults and adolescents, regardless of the quantity of acetaminophen reported to have been ingested, administer

Continued on next page

McNeil Consumer—Cont.

MUCOMYST® acetylcysteine immediately if 24 hours or less have elapsed from the reported time of ingestion. For full prescribing information, refer to the MUCOMYST package insert. Do not await results of assays for acetaminophen level before initiating treatment with MUCOMYST acetylcysteine. The following additional procedures are recommended: The stomach should be emptied by lavage or by induction of emesis with syrup of ipecac. A serum acetaminophen assay should be obtained as early as possible, but no sooner than four hours following ingestion. Liver function studies should be obtained initially and repeated at 24-hour intervals.

Serious toxicity or fatalities are extremely infrequent in children, possibly due to differences in the way they metabolize acetaminophen. In children, the maximum potential amount ingested can be more easily estimated. If more than 150mg/kg or an unknown amount was ingested, obtain an acetaminophen plasma level. The acetaminophen plasma level should be obtained as soon as possible, but no sooner than 4 hours following the ingestion. Induce emesis using syrup of ipecac. If the plasma level is obtained and falls above the broken line on the acetaminophen overdose nomogram, the MUCOMYST acetylcysteine therapy should be initiated and continued for a full course of therapy. If acetaminophen plasma assay capability is not available, and the estimated acetaminophen ingestion exceeds 150mg/kg, MUCOMYST acetycysteine therapy should be initiated and continued for a full course of therapy. For additional emergency information, call your regional poison center or call the Rocky Mountain Poison Center toll free (1-800-525-6115).

Acute dextromethorphan overdose usually does not result in serious signs and symptoms unless massive amounts have been ingested. Signs and symptoms of a substantial overdose may include nausea and vomiting, visual disturbances, CNS disturbances, and urinary retention.

Symptoms from pseudoephedrine overdose consist most often of mild anxiety, tachycardia and/or mild hypertension. Symptoms usually appear within 4 to 8 hours of ingestion and are transient, usually requiring no treatment.

Inactive Ingredients: Alcohol (10%), Citric Acid, Flavors, Glycerin, Polyethylene Glycol, Purified Water, Sodium Benzoate, Sodium Carboxymethylcellulose, Sodium Saccharin, Sorbitol, Sucrose, Red #33, Red #40 and Blue #1.

How Supplied: MAXIMUM STRENGTH TYLENOL COUGH with Decongestant is available in a 4 oz. bottle with child-resistant safety cap, special dosing cup marked in ml, and tamper resistant packaging.

Shown in Product Identification Guide, page 413

Maximum Strength TYLENOL Flu Medication
No Drowsiness Formula
Gelcaps

Description: Each Maximum Strength TYLENOL Flu Medication No Drowsiness Formula Gelcap contains acetaminophen 500 mg., pseudoephedrine hydrochloride 30 mg., and dextromethorphan hydrobromide 15 mg.

Actions: Maximum Strength TYLENOL Flu Medication No Drowsiness Formula Gelcaps contain a clinically proven analgesic-antipyretic, decongestant and cough suppressant. Acetaminophen produces analgesia by elevation of the pain threshold and antipyresis through action on the hypothalamic heat-regulating center. Acetaminophen is equal to aspirin in analgesic and antipyretic effectiveness and it is unlikely to produce many of the side effects associated with aspirin and aspirin-containing products. Pseudoephedrine hydrochloride is a sympathomimetic amine which provides temporary relief of nasal congestion. Dextromethorphan is a cough suppressant which provides temporary relief of coughs due to minor throat irritations that may occur with the common cold.

Indications: Maximum Strength TYLENOL Flu Medication No Drowsiness Formula provides effective temporary relief of body aches, headaches, fever, sore throat, coughing and nasal congestion due to a cold or "flu."

Precautions: If a rare sensitivity reaction occurs, the drug should be stopped. Although pseudoephedrine is virtually without pressor effect in normotensive patients, it should be used with caution in hypertensives.

Usual Dosage: Adults (12 Years and older): Two gelcaps every 6 hours, not to exceed 8 gelcaps in 24 hours.

Warning: Do not administer to children under 12. Do not take this product for more than 7 days or for fever for more than 3 days unless directed by a doctor. If symptoms do not improve or are accompanied by fever, consult a doctor. A persistant cough may be a sign of a serious condition. If cough persists for more than 1 week, tends to recur or is accompanied by fever, rash or persistent headache, consult a doctor. Do not take this product for persistent or chronic cough such as occurs with smoking, asthma, emphysema or if cough is accompanied by excessive phlegm (mucus) unless directed by a doctor. If sore throat is severe, persists for more than 2 days, is accompanied or followed by fever, headache, rash, nausea or vomiting, consult a doctor promptly. Do not exceed recommended dosage because at higher doses, nervousness, dizziness or sleeplessness may occur. Do not take this product if you have heart disease, high blood pressure, thyroid disease, diabetes, or difficulty in urination due to enlargement of the prostate gland unless directed by a doctor. Do not use with other products containing acetaminophen.

DO NOT USE IF CARTON IS OPENED OR IF A BLISTER UNIT IS BROKEN. KEEP THIS AND ALL MEDICATION OUT OF THE REACH OF CHILDREN. AS WITH ANY DRUG, IF YOU ARE PREGNANT OR NURSING A BABY, SEEK THE ADVICE OF A HEALTH PROFESSIONAL BEFORE USING THIS PRODUCT. IN CASE OF ACCIDENTAL OVERDOSE, CONTACT A DOCTOR OR POISON CONTROL CENTER IMMEDIATELY.

Drug Interaction Precaution: Do not take this product if you are presently taking a prescription drug for high blood pressure or you are now taking a prescription monoamine oxidase inhibitor (MAOI) (certain drugs for depression, psychiatric or emotional conditions, or Parkinson's disease), or for 2 weeks after stopping the MAOI drug. If you are uncertain whether your prescription drug contains an MAOI, consult a health professional before taking this product.

Overdosage: Acetaminophen in massive overdosage may cause hepatic toxicity in some patients. In adults and adolescents, hepatic toxicity has rarely been reported following ingestion of acute overdosage of less than 10 grams. Fatalities are infrequent (less than 3–4% of untreated cases) and have rarely been reported with overdosage of less than 15 grams. In children, an acute overdosage of less than 150 mg/kg has not been associated with hepatic toxicity.

Early symptoms following a potentially hepatotoxic overdose may include: nausea, vomiting, diaphoresis and general malaise. Clinical and laboratory evidence of hepatic toxicity may not be apparent until 48 to 72 hours postingestion. In adults and adolescents, regardless of the quantity of acetaminophen reported to have been ingested, administer MUCOMYST® acetylcysteine immediately if 24 hours or less have elapsed from the reported time of ingestion. For full prescribing information, refer to the MUCOMYST package insert. Do not await results of assays for acetaminophen level before initiating treatment with MUCOMYST acetyleysteine. The following additional procedures are recommended: The stomach should be emptied promptly by lavage or by induction of emesis with syrup of ipecac. A serum acetaminophen assay should be obtained as early as possible, but not sooner than four hours following ingestion. Liver function studies should be obtained initially and repeated at 24-hour intervals.

Serious toxicity or fatalities are extremely infrequent in children, possibly due to differences in the way they metabolize acetaminophen. In children, the maximum potential amount ingested can be more easily estimated. If more than 150 mg/kg or an unknown amount was ingested, obtain an acetaminophen plasma level. The acetaminophen plasma level should be obtained as soon as possible, but no sooner than 4 hours following the ingestion. Induce emesis using syrup of ipecac. If the plasma level is obtained and falls above the broken line on the acetaminophen overdose nomogram, the MUCOMYST acetyleysteine therapy should be initiated and continued for a full course of therapy. If acetaminophen plasma assay capability is not available, and the estimated acetaminophen ingestion exceeds 150 mg/kg, MUCOMYST acetyleysteine therapy should be initiated and continued for a full course of therapy.

For additional emergency information, call your regional poison center or call the Rocky Mountain Poison Center tollfree, (1-800-525-6115).

Symptoms from pseudoephedrine overdose consist most often of mild anxiety, tachycardia and/or mild hypertension. Symptoms usually appear within 4 to 8 hours of ingestion and are transient, usually requiring no treatment.

Acute dextromethorphan overdose usually does not result in serious signs and symptoms unless massive amounts have been ingested. Signs and symptoms of a substantial overdose may include nausea and vomiting, visual disturbances, CNS disturbances, and urinary retention.

Inactive Ingredients: Benzyl Alcohol, Butylparaben, Castor Oil, Cellulose, Corn Starch, Edetate Calcium Disodium, Gelatin, Hydroxypropyl Methylcellulose, Iron Oxide Black, Magnesium Stearate, Methylparaben, Propylparaben, Sodium Lauryl Sulfate, Sodium Propionate, Sodium Starch Glycolate, Titanium Dioxide, Red #40 and Blue #1.

How Supplied: Gelcaps (colored burgundy and white, imprinted "TYLENOL FLU") in blister packs of 10 and 20.

Shown in Product Identification Guide, page 413

**Maximum-Strength
TYLENOL® Sinus Medication
Gelcaps, Caplets and Tablets**

Description: Each Maximum-Strength TYLENOL® Sinus Medication Gelcap, Caplet or Tablet contains acetaminophen 500 mg and pseudoephedrine hydrochloride 30 mg.

Actions: Maximum-Strength TYLENOL Sinus Medication contains a clinically proven analgesic-antipyretic and a decongestant. Maximum allowable nonprescription levels of acetaminophen and pseudoephedrine provide temporary relief of sinus headache and congestion. Acetaminophen is equal to aspirin in analgesic and antipyretic effectiveness and it is unlikely to produce many of the side effects associated with aspirin and aspirin-containing products.

Acetaminophen produces analgesia by elevation of the pain threshold and antipyresis through action on the hypothalamic heat-regulating center. Pseudoephedrine hydrochloride is a sympathomimetic amine which promotes sinus cavity

drainage by reducing nasopharyngeal mucosal congestion.

Indications: Maximum-Strength TYLENOL Sinus Medication provides effective symptomatic relief from sinus headache pain and congestion. Maximum-Strength TYLENOL Sinus Medication is particularly well-suited in patients with aspirin allergy, hemostatic disturbances (including anticoagulant therapy), and bleeding diatheses (e.g., hemophilia) and upper gastrointestinal disease (e.g., ulcer, gastritis, hiatus hernia).

Precautions: If a rare sensitivity occurs, the drug should be discontinued. Although pseudoephedrine is virtually without pressor effect in normotensive patients, it should be used with caution in hypertensives.

Usual Dosage: Adults and Children 12 years of Age and Older: Two Tablets, Caplets or Gelcaps every 4–6 hours. Do not exceed eight Tablets, Caplets or Gelcaps in any 24-hour period. WARNING: Do not administer to children under 12 or exceed the recommended dosage because at higher doses nervousness, dizziness, or sleeplessness may occur. Do not take this product for more than 7 days. If symptoms do not improve or are accompanied by fever, consult a physician. Do not take this product if you have heart disease, high blood pressure, thyroid disease, diabetes, or difficulty in urination due to enlargement of the prostate gland unless directed by a doctor. Do not use with other products containing acetaminophen.

Drug Interaction Precaution: Do not take this product if you are presently taking a prescription drug for high blood pressure or depression without first consulting your doctor. **Do not use if carton is opened or if blister unit is broken or if printed green neck wrap or printed foil inner seal is broken. Keep this and all medication out of the reach of children. As with any drug, if you are pregnant or nursing a baby, seek the advice of a health professional before using this product. In case of accidental overdosage, contact a physician or poison control center immediately.**

Overdosage: Acetaminophen in massive overdosage may cause hepatic toxicity in some patients. In adults and adolescents, hepatic toxicity has rarely been reported following ingestion of acute overdosage of less than 10 grams. Fatalities are infrequent (less than 3–4% of untreated cases) and have rarely been reported with overdoses of less than 15 grams. In children, an acute overdosage of less than 150 mg/kg has not been associated with hepatic toxicity. Early symptoms following a potentially hepatotoxic overdose may include: nausea, vomiting, diaphoresis and general malaise. Clinical and laboratory evidence of hepatic toxicity may not be apparent until 48 to 72 hours postingestion. In adults and adolescents, regardless of

the quantity of acetaminophen reported to have been ingested, administer MUCOMYST® acetylcysteine immediately if 24 hours or less have elapsed from the reported time of ingestion. For full prescribing information, refer to the MUCOMYST package insert. Do not await the results of assays for acetaminophen level before initiating treatment with MUCOMYST acetylcysteine. The following additional procedures are recommended: The stomach should be emptied promptly by lavage or by induction of emesis with syrup of ipecac. A serum acetaminophen assay should be obtained as early as possible, but no sooner than four hours following ingestion. Liver function studies should be obtained initially and repeated at 24-hour intervals.

Serious toxicity or fatalities are extremely infrequent in children, possibly due to differences in the way they metabolize acetaminophen. In children, the maximum potential amount ingested can be more easily estimated. If more than 150 mg/kg or an unknown amount was ingested, obtain an acetaminophen plasma level. The acetaminophen plasma level should be obtained as soon as possible, but no sooner than 4 hours following the ingestion. Induce emesis using syrup of ipecac. If the plasma level is obtained and falls above the broken line on the acetaminophen overdose nomogram, the MUCOMYST acetylcysteine therapy should be initiated and continued for a full course of therapy. If acetaminophen plasma assay capability is not available, and the estimated acetaminophen ingestion exceeds 150 mg/kg, MUCOMYST acetylcysteine therapy should be initiated and continued for a full course of therapy.

For additional emergency information, call your regional poison center or call the Rocky Mountain Poison Center tollfree, (1-800-525-6115).

Symptoms from pseudoephedrine overdose consist most often of mild anxiety, tachycardia and/or mild hypertension. Symptoms usually appear within 4 to 8 hours of ingestion and are transient, usually requiring no treatment.

Inactive Ingredients: Caplets—Cellulose, Hydroxypropyl Methylcellulose, Magnesium Stearate, Polyethylene Glycol, Polysorbate 80, Sodium Starch Glycolate, Starch, Titanium Dioxide, Blue #1, Red #40 and Yellow #10. Tablets—Cellulose, Magnesium Stearate, Sodium Starch Glycolate Starch, Yellow #6, Yellow #10, and Blue #1. Gelcaps—Benzyl alcohol, butylparaben, castor oil, cellulose, edetate calcium disodium, gelatin, hydroxypropyl methylcellulose, iron oxide black, magnesium stearate, methylparaben, propylparaben, sodium lauryl sulfate, sodium propionate, sodium starch glycolate, starch, titanium dioxide, Blue #1 and Yellow #10.

Continued on next page

McNeil Consumer—Cont.

How Supplied: Tablets (colored light green, imprinted "Maximum-Strength TYLENOL Sinus")—in blister packs of 24 and tamper-resistant bottles of 50. Caplets (light green coating, printed "TYLENOL Sinus" in dark green) in blister packs of 24 and tamper-resistant bottles of 50.

Gelcaps (colored green and white), printed "TYLENOL Sinus" in blister packs of 24 and tamper-resistant bottles of 50.

Shown in Product Identification Guide, page 414

Multisymptom Formula TYLENOL® Cold Medication Tablets and Caplets

Description: Each Multi-Symptom Formula TYLENOL Cold Tablet or Caplet contains acetaminophen 325 mg., chlorpheniramine maleate 2 mg., pseudoephedrine hydrochloride 30 mg. and dextromethorphan hydrobromide 15 mg.

Actions: Multi-Symptom Formula TYLENOL Cold Medication Tablets and Caplets contain a clinically proven analgesic-antipyretic, decongestant, cough suppressant and antihistamine. Acetaminophen produces analgesia by elevation of the pain threshold and antipyresis through action on the hypothalamic heat-regulating center. Acetaminophen is equal to aspirin in analgesic and antipyretic effectiveness and it is unlikely to produce many of the side effects associated with aspirin and aspirin-containing products. Pseudoephedrine hydrochloride is a sympathomimetic amine which provides temporary relief of nasal congestion. Dextromethorphan is a cough suppressant which provides temporary relief of coughs due to minor throat irritations that may occur with the common cold. Chlorpheniramine is an antihistamine which helps provide temporary relief of runny nose, sneezing and watery and itchy eyes.

Indications: Multi-Symptom Formula TYLENOL Cold Medication provides effective temporary relief of runny nose, sneezing, watery and itchy eyes, nasal congestion, sore throat, coughing, and aches, pains and fever due to a cold or "flu."

Precautions: If a rare sensitivity reaction occurs, the drug should be stopped. Although pseudoephedrine is virtually without pressor effect in normotensive patients, it should be used with caution in hypertensives.

Usual Dosage: Adults: Two tablets or caplets every 6 hours, not to exceed 8 tablets or caplets in 24 hours. Children (6–12 years): One caplet or tablet every 6 hours, not to exceed 4 tablets or caplets in 24 hours for 5 days.

WARNING: Do not administer to children under 6. Do not take this product for more than 7 days or for fever for more than 3 days unless directed by a doctor. If symptoms do not improve or are accompanied by fever, consult a doctor. If sore throat is severe, persists for more than 2 days, is accompanied or followed by fever, headache, rash, nausea or vomiting, consult a doctor promptly. A persistent cough may be a sign of a serious condition. If cough persists for more than 1 week, tends to recur or is accompanied by fever, rash or persistent headache, consult a doctor. Do not take this product for persistent or chronic cough such as occurs with smoking, asthma, emphysema or if cough if accompanied by excessive phlegm (mucus) unless directed by a doctor. Do not exceed recommended dosage because at higher doses, nervousness, dizziness or sleeplessness may occur. May cause excitability especially in children. Do not take this product, unless directed by a doctor, if you have a breathing problem such as emphysema or chronic bronchitis, or if you have glaucoma or difficulty in urination due to enlargement of the prostate gland. Do not take this product if you have heart disease, high blood pressure, thyroid disease or diabetes unless directed by a doctor. May cause drowsiness; alcohol, sedatives and tranquilizers may increase the drowsiness effect. Avoid alcoholic beverages while taking this product. Do not take this product if you are taking sedatives or tranquilizers without first consulting your doctor. Use caution when driving a motor vehicle or operating machinery. Do not use with other products containing acetaminophen.

DO NOT USE IF CARTON IS OPENED OR IF A BLISTER UNIT IS BROKEN. KEEP THIS AND ALL MEDICATION OUT OF THE REACH OF CHILDREN. AS WITH ANY DRUG, IF YOU ARE PREGNANT OR NURSING A BABY, SEEK THE ADVICE OF A HEALTH PROFESSIONAL BEFORE USING THIS PRODUCT. IN THE CASE OF ACCIDENTAL OVER-DOSAGE CONTACT A DOCTOR OR POISON CONTROL CENTER IMMEDIATELY.

Drug Interaction Precaution: Do not take this product if you are presently taking a prescription drug for high blood pressure or you are now taking a prescription monoamine oxidase inhibitor (MAOI) (certain drugs for depression, psychiatric or emotional conditions, or Parkinson's disease), or for 2 weeks after stopping the MAOI drug. If you are uncertain whether your prescription drug contains an MAOI, consult a health professional before taking this product.

Overdosage: Acetaminophen in massive overdosage may cause hepatic toxicity in some patients. In adults and adolescents, hepatic toxicity has rarely been reported following ingestion of acute overdosage of less than 10 grams. Fatalities are infrequent (less than 3–4% of untreated cases) and have rarely been reported with overdoses of less than 15 grams. In children, an acute overdosage of less than 150 mg/kg has not been associated with hepatic toxicity.

Early symptoms following a potentially hepatotoxic overdose may include: nausea, vomiting, diaphoresis and general malaise. Clinical and laboratory evidence of hepatic toxicity may not be apparent until 48 to 72 hours postingestion. In adults and adolescents, regardless of the quantity of acetaminophen reported to have been ingested, administer MUCOMYST® acetylcysteine immediately if 24 hours or less have elapsed from the reported time of ingestion. For full prescribing information, refer to the MUCOMYST package insert. Do not await results of assays for acetaminophen level before initiating treatment with MUCOMYST acetylcysteine. The following additional procedures are recommended: The stomach should be emptied promptly by lavage or by induction of emesis with syrup of ipecac. A serum acetaminophen assay should be obtained as early as possible, but no sooner than four hours following ingestion. Liver function studies should be obtained initially and repeated at 24-hour intervals.

Serious toxicity or fatalities are extremely infrequent in children, possibly due to differences in the way they metabolize acetaminophen. In children, the maximum potential amount ingested can be more easily estimated. If more than 150 mg/kg or an unknown amount was ingested, obtain an acetaminophen plasma level. The acetaminophen plasma level should be obtained as soon as possible, but no sooner than 4 hours following the ingestion. Induce emesis using syrup of ipecac. If the plasma level is obtained and falls above the broken line on the acetaminophen overdose nomogram, the MUCOMYST acetylcysteine therapy should be initiated and continued for a full course of therapy. If acetaminophen plasma assay capability is not available, and the estimated acetaminophen ingestion exceeds 150 mg/kg, MUCOMYST acetylcysteine therapy should be initiated and continued for a full course of therapy.

For additional emergency information, call your regional poison center or call the Rocky Mountain Poison Center toll-free, (1-800-525-6115).

Chlorpheniramine toxicity should be treated as you would an antihistamine/anticholinergic overdose and is likely to be present within a few hours after acute ingestion.

Symptoms from pseudoephedrine overdose consist most often of mild anxiety, tachycardia and/or mild hypertension. Symptoms usually appear within 4 to 8 hours of ingestion and are transient, usually requiring no treatment.

Acute dextromethorphan overdose usually does not result in serious signs and symptoms unless massive amounts have been ingested. Signs and symptoms of a substantial overdose may include nausea and vomiting, visual disturbances, CNS disturbances, and urinary retention.

Inactive Ingredients: Tablets: Cellulose, Starch, Magnesium Stearate, Yellow #6 and Yellow #10. Caplets: Cellulose, Glyceryl Triacetate, Hydroxypropyl Methylcellulose, Magnesium Stearate, Sodium Starch Glycolate, Corn Starch, Titanium Dioxide, Blue #1 and Yellow #6 & #10.

How Supplied: Tablets (colored yellow, imprinted "TYLENOL Cold")—blister packs of 24 and tamper-resistant bottles of 50. Caplets (light yellow, imprinted "TYLENOL Cold")—blister packs of 24 and tamper-resistant bottles of 50.

Shown in Product Identification Guide, page 413

**TYLENOL® Cold Medication
No Drowsiness Formula
Caplets and Gelcaps**

Description: Each TYLENOL Cold Medication No Drowsiness Formula Caplet and Gelcap contains acetaminophen 325 mg., pseudoephedrine hydrochloride 30 mg. and dextromethorphan hydrobromide 15 mg.

Actions: TYLENOL Cold Medication No Drowsiness Formula Caplets and Gelcaps contain a clinically proven analgesic-antipyretic, decongestant and cough suppressant. Acetaminophen produces analgesia by elevation of the pain threshold and antipyresis through action on the hypothalamic heat-regulating center. Acetaminophen is equal to aspirin in analgesic and antipyretic effectiveness and it is unlikely to produce many of the side effects associated with aspirin and aspirin-containing products. Pseudoephedrine hydrochloride is a sympathomimetic amine which provides temporary relief of nasal congestion. Dextromethorphan is a cough suppressant which provides temporary relief of coughs due to minor throat irritations that may occur with the common cold.

Indications: TYLENOL Cold Medication No Drowsiness Formula provides effective temporary relief of the nasal congestion, sore throat, coughing, and aches, pains and fever due to a cold or "flu."

Precautions: If a rare sensitivity reaction occurs, the drug should be stopped. Although pseudoephedrine is virtually without pressor effect in normotensive patients, it should be used with caution in hypertensives.

Usual Dosage: Adults (12 years and older): Two caplets or gelcaps every 6 hours, not to exceed 8 caplets or gelcaps in 24 hours. Children (6–12 years): One caplet or gelcap every 6 hours, not to exceed 4 caplets or gelcaps in 24 hours for 5 days.
WARNING: Do not administer to children under 6. Do not take this product for more than 7 days or for fever for more than 3 days unless directed by a doctor. If symptoms do not improve or are accompanied by fever, consult a doctor. If sore throat is severe, persists for more than 2 days, is accompanied or followed by fever, headache, rash, nausea or vomiting, consult a doctor promptly. A persistent cough may be a sign of a serious condition. If cough persists for more than 1 week, tends to recur or is accompanied by fever, rash or persistent headache, consult a doctor. Do not take this product for persistent or chronic cough such as occurs with smoking, asthma, emphysema or if cough is accompanied by excessive phlegm (mucus) unless directed by a doctor. Do not exceed recommended dosage because at higher doses, nervousness, dizziness or sleeplessness may occur. Do not take this product if you have heart disease, high blood pressure, thyroid disease, diabetes or difficulty in urination due to enlargement of the prostate gland unless directed by a doctor. Do not use with other products containing acetaminophen.
DO NOT USE IF CARTON IS OPENED OR IF A BLISTER UNIT IS BROKEN. KEEP THIS AND ALL MEDICATION OUT OF THE REACH OF CHILDREN. AS WITH ANY DRUG, IF YOU ARE PREGNANT OR NURSING A BABY, SEEK THE ADVICE OF A HEALTH PROFESSIONAL BEFORE USING THIS PRODUCT. IN THE CASE OF ACCIDENTAL OVERDOSAGE CONTACT A DOCTOR OR POISON CONTROL CENTER IMMEDIATELY.
Drug Interaction Precaution: Do not take this product if you are presently taking a prescription drug for high blood pressure or you are now taking a prescription monoamine oxidase inhibitor (MAOI) (certain drugs for depression, psychiatric or emotional conditions, or Parkinson's disease), or for 2 weeks after stopping the MAOI drug. If you are uncertain whether your prescription drug contains an MAOI, consult a health professional before taking this product.

Overdosage: Acetaminophen in massive overdosage may cause hepatic toxicity in some patients. In adults and adolescents, hepatic toxicity has rarely been reported following ingestion of acute overdosage of less than 10 grams. Fatalities are infrequent (less than 3–4% of untreated cases) and have rarely been reported with overdosage of less than 15 grams. In children, an acute overdosage of less than 150 mg/kg has not been associated with hepatic toxicity.
Early symptoms following a potentially hepatotoxic overdose may include: nausea, vomiting, diaphoresis and general malaise. Clinical and laboratory evidence of hepatic toxicity may not be apparent until 48 to 72 hours postingestion. In adults and adolescents, regardless of the quantity of acetaminophen reported to have been ingested, administer MUCOMYST® acetylcysteine immediately if 24 hours or less have elapsed from the reported time of ingestion. For full prescribing information, refer to the MUCOMYST package insert. Do not await results of assays for acetaminophen level before initiating treatment with MUCOMYST acetylcysteine. The following additional procedures are recommended: The stomach should be emptied promptly by lavage or by induction of emesis with syrup of ipecac. A serum acetaminophen assay should be obtained as early as possible, but no sooner than four hours following ingestion. Liver function studies should be obtained initially and repeated at 24–hour intervals.
Serious toxicity or fatalities are extremely infrequent in children, possibly due to differences in the way they metabolize acetaminophen. In children, the maximum potential amount ingested can be more easily estimated. If more than 150 mg/kg or an unknown amount was ingested, obtain an acetaminophen plasma level. The acetaminophen plasma level should be obtained as soon as possible, but no sooner than 4 hours following the ingestion. Induce emesis using syrup of ipecac. If the plasma level is obtained and falls above the broken line on the acetaminophen overdose nomogram, the MUCOMYST acetylcysteine therapy should be initiated and continued for a full course of therapy. If acetaminophen plasma assay capability is not available, and the estimated acetaminophen ingestion exceeds 150 mg/kg. MUCOMYST acetylcysteine therapy should be initiated and continued for a full course of therapy.
For additional emergency information, call your regional poison center or call the Rocky Mountain Poison Center toll-free, (1-800-525-6115).
Symptoms from pseudoephedrine overdose consist most often of mild anxiety, tachycardia and/or mild hypertension. Symptoms usually appear within 4 to 8 hours of ingestion and are transient, usually requiring no treatment.
Acute dextromethorphan overdose usually does not result in serious signs and symptoms unless massive amounts have been ingested. Signs and symptoms of a substantial overdose may include nausea and vomiting, visual disturbances, CNS disturbances, and urinary retention.

Inactive Ingredients: Caplet: Cellulose, Glyceryl Triacetate, Hydroxypropyl Methylcellulose, Magnesium Stearate, Sodium Starch Glycolate, Starch, Titanium Dioxide, Blue #1 and Yellow #10. Gelcap: Benzyl Alcohol, Butylparaben, Castor Oil, Cellulose, Corn Starch, Edetate Calcium Disodium, Gelatin, Hydroxypropyl Methylcellulose, Magnesium Stearate, Methylparaben, Propylparaben, Sodium Propionate, Sodium Lauryl Sulfate, Sodium Starch Glycolate, Titanium Dioxide, Red #40 and Yellow #10.

How Supplied: Caplets (colored white, imprinted "TYLENOL COLD")—blister packs of 24 and tamper-resistant bottles of 50.

Continued on next page

McNeil Consumer—Cont.

Gelcaps (colored red and tan, imprinted "TYLENOL COLD")—blister packs of 20 and tamper-resistant bottles of 40.

Shown in Product Identification Guide, page 413

No Drowsiness Formula TYLENOL® Cold & Flu Hot Medication Packets

Description: Each packet of No Drowsiness TYLENOL Cold & Flu contains acetaminophen 650 mg., pseudoephedrine hydrochloride 60 mg and dextromethorphan hydrobromide 30 mg.

Actions: No Drowsiness TYLENOL Cold and Flu Hot Medication contains a clinically proven analgesic-antipyretic, decongestant, and cough suppressant. Acetaminophen produces analgesia by elevation of the pain threshold and antipyresis through action on the hypothalamic heat-regulating center. Acetaminophen is equal to aspirin in analgesic and antipyretic effectiveness and it is unlikely to produce many of the side effects associated with aspirin and aspirin-containing products. Pseudoephedrine hydrochloride is a sympathomimetic amine which provides temporary relief of nasal congestion. Dextromethorphan is a cough suppressant which provides temporary relief of coughs due to minor throat irritations that may occur with the common cold.

Indications: No Drowsiness TYLENOL Cold and Flu Hot Medication provides effective temporary relief of nasal congestion, sore throat, coughing, and aches, pains, and fever due to a cold or "flu."

Precautions: If a rare sensitivity reaction occurs, the drug should be stopped. Although pseudoephedrine is virtually without pressor effect in normotensive patients, it should be used with caution in hypertensives.

Usual Dosage: Adults (12 years and over): Dissolve one packet in 6 oz. cup of hot water. Sip while hot. Sweeten to taste, if desired. May repeat every 6 hours, not to exceed 4 doses in 24 hours.

WARNINGS: Do not administer to children under 12. Do not take this product for more than 7 days or for fever for more than 3 days unless directed by a doctor. If symptoms do not improve or are accompanied by fever, consult a doctor. If sore throat is severe, persists for more than 2 days, is accompanied or followed by fever, headache, rash, nausea or vomiting, consult a doctor promptly. A persistent cough may be a sign of a serious condition. If cough persists for more than 1 week, tends to recur or is accompanied by fever, rash or persistent headache, consult a doctor. Do not take this product for persistent or chronic cough such as occurs with smoking, asthma, emphysema, or if cough is accompanied by excessive phlegm (mucus) unless directed by a doctor. Do not exceed recommended dosage because at higher doses nervousness, dizziness, or sleeplessness may occur. Do not take this product if you have heart disease, high blood pressure, thyroid disease, diabetes or difficulty in urinination due to enlargement of the prostate gland unless directed by a doctor. Do not use with other products containing acetaminophen. **DO NOT USE IF GLUED CARTON FLAP IS OPENED OR IF FOIL PACKET IS TORN OR BROKEN. KEEP THIS AND ALL MEDICATION OUT OF THE REACH OF CHILDREN. AS WITH ANY DRUG, IF YOU ARE PREGNANT OR NURSING A BABY, SEEK THE ADVICE OF A HEALTH PROFESSIONAL BEFORE USING THIS PRODUCT. IN CASE OF ACCIDENTAL OVERDOSAGE, CONTACT A DOCTOR OR POISON CONTROL CENTER IMMEDIATELY. PHENYLKETONURICS: CONTAINS PHENYLALANINE 11 MG PER PACKET.**

Drug Interaction Precaution: Do not take this product if you are presently taking a prescription drug for high blood pressure or you are now taking a prescription monoamine oxidase inhibitor (MAOI) (certain drugs for depression, psychiatric or emotional conditions, or Parkinson's disease), or for 2 weeks after stopping the MAOI drug. If you are uncertain whether your prescription drug contains an MAOI, consult a health professional before taking this product.

Overdosage: Acetaminophen in massive overdosage may cause hepatic toxicity in some patients. In adults and adolescents, hepatic toxicity has rarely been reported following ingestion of acute overdosage of less than 10 grams. Fatalities are infrequent (less than 3–4% of untreated cases) and have rarely been reported with overdoses of less than 15 grams. In children, an acute overdosage of less than 150 mg/kg has not been associated with hepatic toxicity.
Early symptoms following a potentially hepatotoxic overdose may include: nausea, vomiting, diaphoresis and general malaise. Clinical and laboratory evidence of hepatic toxicity may not be apparent until 48 to 72 hours postingestion. In adults and adolescents, regardless of the quantity of acetaminophen reported to have been ingested, administer MUCOMYST® acetylcysteine immediately if 24 hours or less have elapsed from the reported time of ingestion. For full prescribing information, refer to the MUCOMYST package insert. Do not await results of assays for acetaminophen level before initiating treatment with MUCOMYST acetylcysteine. The following additional procedures are recommended. The stomach should be emptied promptly by lavage or by induction of emesis with syrup of ipecac. A serum acetaminophen assay should be obtained as early as possible, but no sooner than four hours following ingestion. Liver function studies should be obtained initially and repeated at 24-hour intervals.
Serious toxicity or fatalities are extremely infrequent in children, possibly due to differences in the way they metabolize acetaminophen. In children, the maximum potential amount ingested can be more easily estimated. If more than 150 mg/kg or an unknown amount was ingested, obtain an acetaminophen plasma level. The acetaminophen plasma level should be obtained as soon as possible, but not sooner than 4 hours following the ingestion. Induce emesis using syrup of ipecac. If the plasma level is obtained and falls above the broken line on the acetaminophen overdose nomogram, the MUCOMYST acetylcysteine therapy should be initiated and continued for a full course of therapy. If acetaminophen plasma assay capability is not available, and the estimated acetaminophen ingestion exceeds 150 mg/kg, MUCOMYST acetylcysteine therapy should be initiated and continued for a full course of therapy.
For additional emergency information, call your regional poison center or call the Rocky Mountain Poison Control toll-free, (1-800-525-6115).
Symptoms from pseudoephedrine overdose consist most often of mild anxiety, tachycardia and/or mild hypertension. Symptoms usually appear within 4 to 8 hours of ingestion and are transient, usually requiring no treatment.
Acute dextromethorphan overdose usually does not result in serious signs and symptoms unless massive amounts have been ingested. Signs and symptoms of a substantial overdose may include nausea and vomiting, visual disturbances. CNS disturbances and urinary retention.

Inactive Ingredients: Aspartame, Citric Acid, Flavors, Sodium Citrate, Starch, Sucrose, Red #40 and Yellow #10.

How Supplied: Packets of powder (yellow colored) in cartons of 6 tamper-resistant foil packets.

Shown in Product Identification Guide, page 413

Regular Strength TYLENOL® acetaminophen Caplets and Tablets   OTC

Description: Each Regular Strength TYLENOL Tablet or Caplet contains acetaminophen 325 mg.

Actions: Acetaminophen is a clinically proven analgesic and antipyretic. Acetaminophen produces analgesia by elevation of the pain threshold and antipyresis through action on the hypothalamic heat-regulating center. Acetaminophen is equal to aspirin in analgesic and antipyretic effectiveness and it is unlikely to produce many of the side effects associated with aspirin and aspirin-containing products.

Indications: Acetaminophen acts safely and quickly to provide temporary relief from: simple headache; minor muscular aches; the minor aches and pains associated with bursitis, neuralgia, sprains, overexertion, menstrual cramps; and from the discomfort of fever due to colds and "flu". Also for temporary relief of minor aches and pains of arthritis and rheumatism.

Precautions: If a rare sensitivity reaction occurs, the drug should be discontinued.

Usual Dosage: Adults and Children 12 years of Age and Older: 1 to 2 tablets or caplets 3 or 4 times daily. Children (6-12): $\frac{1}{2}$ to 1 tablet or caplet 3 or 4 times daily. Consult a physician for use by children under 6.
WARNING: DO NOT USE IF PRINTED RED NECK WRAP IS BROKEN OR MISSING. DO NOT TAKE FOR PAIN FOR MORE THAN 10 DAYS OR FOR FEVER FOR MORE THAN 3 DAYS UNLESS DIRECTED BY A PHYSICIAN. SEVERE OR RECURRENT PAIN OR HIGH OR CONTINUED FEVER MAY BE INDICATIVE OF SERIOUS ILLNESS. UNDER THESE CONDITIONS, CONSULT A PHYSICIAN. KEEP THIS AND ALL MEDICATION OUT OF THE REACH OF CHILDREN. AS WITH ANY DRUG, IF YOU ARE PREGNANT OR NURSING A BABY, SEEK THE ADVICE OF A HEALTH PROFESSIONAL BEFORE USING THIS PRODUCT. IN THE CASE OF ACCIDENTAL OVERDOSAGE, CONTACT A PHYSICIAN OR POISON CONTROL CENTER IMMEDIATELY. Do not use with other products containing acetaminophen.

Overdosage: Acetaminophen in massive overdosage may cause hepatic toxicity in some patients. In adults and adolescents, hepatic toxicity has rarely been reported following ingestion of acute overdoses of less than 10 grams. Fatalities are infrequent (less than 3–4% of untreated cases) and have rarely been reported with overdoses of less than 15 grams. In children, an acute overdosage of less than 150 mg/kg has not been associated with hepatic toxicity.
Early symptoms following a potentially hepatotoxic overdose may include: nausea, vomiting, diaphoresis and general malaise. Clinical and laboratory evidence of hepatic toxicity may not be apparent until 48 to 72 hours postingestion. In adults and adolescents, regardless of the quantity of acetaminophen reported to have been ingested, administer MUCOMYST® acetylcysteine immediately if 24 hours or less have elapsed from the reported time of ingestion. For full prescribing information, refer to the MUCOMYST package insert. Do not await results of assays for acetaminophen level before initiating treatment with MUCOMYST acetylcysteine. The following additional procedures are recommended: The stomach should be emptied promptly by lavage or by induction of emesis with syrup of ipecac. A serum acetaminophen assay should be obtained as early as possible, but no sooner than four hours following ingestion. Liver function studies should be obtained initially and repeated at 24-hour intervals.

Serious toxicity or fatalities are extremely infrequent in children, possibly due to differences in the way they metabolize acetaminophen. In children, the maximum potential amount ingested can be more easily estimated. If more than 150 mg/kg or an unknown amount was ingested, obtain an acetaminophen plasma level. The acetaminophen plasma level should be obtained as soon as possible, but no sooner than 4 hours following the ingestion. Induce emesis using syrup of ipecac. If the plasma level is obtained and falls above the broken line on the acetaminophen overdose nomogram, the MUCOMYST acetylcysteine therapy should be initiated and continued for a full course of therapy. If acetaminophen plasma assay capability is not available, and the estimated acetaminophen ingestion exceeds 150 mg/kg, MUCOMYST acetylcysteine therapy should be initiated and continued for a full course of therapy.
For additional emergency information, call your regional poison center or call the Rocky Mountain Poison Center toll-free (1-800-525-6115).

Inactive Ingredients: Tablets—Magnesium Stearate, Cellulose, Docusate Sodium, Sodium Benzoate or Sodium Lauryl Sulfate, and Starch. Caplets—Cellulose, Hydroxypropyl Methylcellulose, Magnesium Stearate, Polyethylene Glycol, Sodium Starch Glycolate, Starch and Red #40 .

How Supplied: Tablets (colored white, scored, imprinted "TYLENOL")—tins of 12, and tamper-resistant bottles of 24, 50, 100 and 200. Caplets (colored white, "TYLENOL")—tamper-resistant bottles of 24, 50, 100. For additional pain relief, Extra-Strength TYLENOL® Gelcaps, Geltabs, Caplets and Tablets, 500 mg, and Extra-Strength TYLENOL® Adult Liquid Pain Reliever are available (colored green; 1 fl. oz. = 1000 mg.)
Shown in Product Identification Guide, page 412

Mead Johnson Pediatrics
Mead Johnson & Company
A Bristol-Myers Squibb Company
2400 W. LLOYD EXPRESSWAY
EVANSVILLE, IN 47721

Enfamil® Infant Formula[1]
Enfamil® With Iron Infant Formula[1]
Enfamil® Infant Formula Nursette®
Enfamil® Premature Formula
Enfamil® Premature Formula With Iron
Enfamil® Human Milk Fortifier
Fer-In-Sol® Iron Supplement Drops, Syrup, Capsules

Nutramigen® Hypoallergenic Protein Hydrolysate Formula[1]
Poly-Vi-Sol® Vitamins, Chewable Tablets and Drops (without Iron)
Poly-Vi-Sol® Vitamins, Peter Rabbit[2] Shaped Chewable Tablets (without Iron)
Poly-Vi-Sol® Vitamins with Iron, Peter Rabbit[2] Shaped Chewable Tablets
Poly-Vi-Sol® Vitamins with Iron, Drops
ProSobee® Soy Formula[1]
ProSobee® Soy Formula Nursette®[1]

[1]Concentrated liquid, powder, and ready to use

[2]Registered trademark of F. Warne & Co., Inc.

Special Metabolic Diets:
Lofenalac® Iron Fortified Low Phenylalanine Diet Powder
Low Methionine Diet Powder (Product 3200K)
Low PHE/TYR Diet Powder (Product 3200AB)
Mono- and Disaccharide-Free Diet Powder (Product 3232A)
MSUD Diet Powder
Phenyl-Free® Phenylalanine-Free Diet Powder
Pregestimil® Iron Fortified Protein Hydrolysate Formula with Medium Chain Triglycerides
Ricelyte® Oral Electrolyte Maintenance Solution Made With Rice Syrup Solids
Special Metabolic Modules:
HIST 1
HIST 2
HOM 1
HOM 2
LYS 1
LYS 2
MSUD 1
MSUD 2
OS 1
OS 2
PKU 1
PKU 2
PKU 3
Protein-Free Diet Powder (Product 80056)
TYR 1
TYR 2
UCD 1
UCD 2
Tempra® 1 Acetaminophen Infant Drops
Tempra® 2 Acetaminophen Toddlers Syrup
Tempra® 3 Chewable Tablets, Regular or Double-Strength
Trind® Liquid, Antihistamine, Nasal Decongestant, Sugar-Free
Trind-DM® Liquid, Cough Suppressant, Antihistamine, Nasal Decongestant, Sugar-Free
Tri-Vi-Sol® Vitamin Drops
Tri-Vi-Sol® Vitamin Drops with Iron
Detailed information may be obtained by contacting Mead Johnson Pediatrics Medical Affairs Department at (812) 429-7900.

Miles Inc.
P. O. BOX 340
ELKHART, IN 46515

ALKA–MINTS® Chewable Antacid Rich in Calcium

Active Ingredient: Each ALKA-MINTS Chewable Antacid tablet contains calcium carbonate 850 mg. (340 mg of elemental calcium). Each tablet contains less than .5 mg sodium per tablet, and is dietarily sodium free.

Inactive Ingredients: Dioctyl sodium sulfosuccinate, flavor, hydrolyzed cereal solids, magnesium stearate, polyethylene glycol, sorbitol, sugar (compressible).

Indications: ALKA-MINTS is an antacid for occasional use for relief of acid indigestion, heartburn and sour stomach.

Actions: ALKA-MINTS has a natural, clean, spearmint taste that leaves the mouth feeling refreshed. Measured by the in-vitro standard established by the Food and Drug Administration, one ALKA-MINTS tablet neutralizes 15.9 mEq of acid.

Warnings: Do not take more than 9 tablets in a 24 hour period, or use the maximum dosage of this product for more than 2 weeks, except under the advice and supervision of a physician. May cause constipation. As with any drug, if you are pregnant or nursing a baby, seek the advice of a health professional before using this product. Keep this and all drugs out of the reach of children.

Dosage and Administration: Chew 1 or 2 tablets every 2 hours or as directed by a physician.

How Supplied: Cartons of 30's. Each carton contains convenient pocket-sized packs with individually sealed tablets so ALKA-MINTS stay fresh wherever you go.

Product Identification Mark:
ALKA-MINTS embossed on each tablet.
Shown in Product Identification Guide, page 414

ALKA–SELTZER® Effervescent Antacid & Pain Reliever With Specially Buffered Aspirin

Active Ingredients: Each tablet contains: aspirin 325 mg., heat treated sodium bicarbonate 1916 mg., citric acid 1000 mg. ALKA-SELTZER® in water contains principally the antacid sodium citrate and the analgesic sodium acetylsalicylate. Buffered pH is between 6 and 7.

Inactive Ingredients: None.

Indications: ALKA-SELTZER® Effervescent Antacid & Pain Reliever is an analgesic and an antacid and is indicated for relief of sour stomach, acid indigestion or heartburn with headache or body aches and pains. Also for fast relief of upset stomach with headache from overindulgence in food and drink—especially recommended for taking before bed and again on arising. Effective for pain relief alone: headache or body and muscular aches and pains.

Actions: When the ALKA-SELTZER® Effervescent Antacid & Pain Reliever tablet is dissolved in water, the acetylsalicylate ion differs from acetylsalicylic acid chemically, physically and pharmacologically. Being fat insoluble, it is not absorbed by the gastric mucosal cells. Studies and observations in animals and man including radiochrome determinations of fecal blood loss, measurement of ion fluxes and direct visualization with gastrocamera, have shown that, as contrasted with acetylsalicylic acid, the acetylsalicylate ion delivered in the solution does not alter gastric mucosal permeability to permit back-diffusion of hydrogen ion, and gastric damage and acute gastric mucosal lesions are therefore not seen after administration of the product. ALKA-SELTZER® Effervescent Antacid & Pain Reliever has the capacity to neutralize gastric hydrochloric acid quickly and effectively. In-vitro, 154 ml. of 0.1 N hydrochloric acid are required to decrease the pH of one tablet of ALKA-SELTZER® Effervescent Antacid & Pain Reliever in solution to 4.0. Measured against the in vitro standard established by the Food and Drug Administration one tablet neutralizes 17.2 mEq of acid. In vivo, the antacid activity of two ALKA-SELTZER® Antacid & Pain Reliever tablets is comparable to that of 10 ml. of milk of magnesia. ALKA-SELTZER® Effervescent Antacid & Pain Reliever is able to resist pH changes caused by the continuing secretion of acid in the normal individual and to maintain an elevated pH until emptying occurs.
ALKA-SELTZER® Effervescent Antacid & Pain Reliever provides highly water soluble acetylsalicylate ions which are fat insoluble. Acetylsalicylate ions are not absorbed from the stomach. They empty from the stomach and thereby become available for absorption from the duodenum. Thus, fast drug absorption and high plasma acetylsalicylate levels are achieved. Plasma levels of salicylate following the administration of ALKA-SELTZER® Effervescent Antacid & Pain Reliever solution (acetylsalicylate ion equivalent to 648 mg. acetylsalicylic acid) can reach 29 mg./liter in 10 minutes and rise to peak levels as high as 55 mg./liter within 30 minutes.

Warnings: Children and teenagers should not use this medicine for chicken pox or flu symptoms before a doctor is consulted about Reye syndrome, a rare but serious illness reported to be associated with aspirin. As with any drug, if you are pregnant or nursing a baby, seek the advice of a health professional before using this product. IT IS ESPECIALLY IMPORTANT NOT TO USE ASPIRIN DURING THE LAST 3 MONTHS OF PREGNANCY UNLESS SPECIFI-CALLY DIRECTED TO DO SO BY A DOCTOR BECAUSE IT MAY CAUSE PROBLEMS IN THE UNBORN CHILD OR COMPLICATIONS DURING DELIVERY. Except under the advice and supervision of a physician, do not take more than, Adults: 8 tablets in a 24 hour period. (60 years of age or older: 4 tablets in a 24 hour period), or use the maximum dosage for more than 10 days. Do not use if you are allergic to aspirin or have asthma, if you have bleeding problems, or if you are on a sodium restricted diet. Each tablet contains 567 mg. of sodium. If ringing in the ears or a loss of hearing occurs, consult a doctor before taking any more of this product.
Do not take this product for pain for more than 10 days unless directed by a doctor. If pain persists or gets worse, if new symptoms occur, or if redness or swelling is present, consult a doctor because these could be signs of a serious condition.
Keep this and all drugs out of the reach of children.

Drug Interaction Precaution: Do not take this product if you are taking a prescription drug for anticoagulation (thinning the blood), diabetes, gout or arthritis unless directed by a doctor.

Dosage and Administration:
ALKA-SELTZER® must be dissolved in water before taking.
Adults: 2 tablets every 4 hours.
CAUTION: If symptoms persist or recur frequently, or if you are under treatment for ulcer, consult your physician.

Professional Labeling:

ASPIRIN FOR MYOCARDIAL INFARCTION

Indication: The Aspirin contained in ALKA-SELTZER® is indicated to reduce the risk of death and/or non-fatal myocardial infarction in patients with a previous infarction or unstable angina pectoris.

Clinical Trials: The indication is supported by the results of six, large, randomized multicenter, placebo-controlled studies[1–7] involving 10,816, predominantly male, post-myocardial infarction (MI) patients and one randomized placebo-controlled study of 1,266 men with unstable angina. Therapy with aspirin was begun at intervals after the onset of acute MI varying from less than 3 days to more than 5 years and continued for periods of from less than one year to four years. In the unstable angina study, treatment was started within 1 month after the onset of unstable angina and continued for 12 weeks and complicating conditions such as congestive heart failure were not included in the study.
Aspirin therapy in MI patients was associated with about a 20 percent reduction in the risk of subsequent death and/or non-fatal reinfarction, a median absolute decrease of 3 percent from the 12 to 22 percent event rates in the placebo groups. In aspirin-treated unstable angina patients the reduction in risk was

about 50 percent, a reduction in event rate of 5 percent from the 10 percent rate in the placebo group over the 12 weeks of the study.

Daily dosage of aspirin in the post-myocardial infarction studies was 300 mg in one study and 900 to 1500 mg in five studies. A dose of 325 mg was used in the study of unstable angina.

Adverse Reactions: Gastrointestinal Reactions: Symptoms and signs of gastrointestinal irritation were not significantly increased in subjects treated for unstable angina with buffered aspirin in solution (ALKA-SELZER®). Doses of 1000 mg per day of aspirin tablets caused gastrointestinal symptoms and bleeding that in some cases were clinically significant. In the largest post-infarction study (the Aspirin Myocardial Infarction Study (AMIS) with 4,500 people), the percentage incidences of gastrointestinal symptoms for the aspirin (1000 mg of a standard, solid-tablet formulation) and placebo-treated subjects, respectively, were: stomach pain (14.5%; 4.4%); heartburn (11.9%; 4.8%); nausea and/or vomiting (7.6%; 2.1%); hospitalization for gastrointestinal disorder (4.9%; 3.5%). In the AMIS and other trials, aspirin treated patients had increased rates of gross gastrointestinal bleeding. As with all aspirin products ALKA-SELTZER is contraindicated in patients with aspirin sensitivity, with asthma, or with coagulation disease.

Cardiovascular and Biochemical: In the AMIS trial, the dosage of 1000 mg per day of aspirin was associated with small increases in systolic blood pressure (BP) (average 1.5 to 2.1 mm) and diastolic BP (0.5 to 0.6 mm), depending upon whether maximal or last available readings were used. Blood urea nitrogen and uric acid levels were also increased, but by less than 1.0 mg%. Subjects with marked hypertension or renal insufficiency had been excluded from the trial so that the clinical importance of these observations for such subjects or for any subjects treated over more prolonged periods is not known. It is recommended that patients placed on long-term aspirin treatment, even at doses of 300 mg per day, be seen at regular intervals to assess changes in these measurements.

Sodium in Buffered Aspirin for Solution Formulations: One tablet daily of buffered aspirin in solution adds 567 mg of sodium to that in the diet and may not be tolerated by patients with active sodium-retaining states such as congestive heart or renal failure. This amount of sodium adds about 30 percent to the 70 to 90 meq intake suggested as appropriate for dietary treatment of essential hypertension in the 1984 Report of the Joint National Committee on Detection, Evaluation, and Treatment of High Blood Pressure.[8]

Dosage and Administration: Although most of the studies used dosages exceeding 300 mg, daily, two trials used only 300 mg and pharmacologic data indicate that this dose inhibits platelet function fully. Therefore, 300 mg or a conventional 325 mg aspirin dose daily is a reasonable, routine dose that would minimize gastrointestinal adverse reactions. This use of aspirin applies to both solid, oral dosage forms (buffered and plain aspirin) and buffered aspirin in solution.

References:
(1) Elwood, P. C., et al., A Randomized Controlled Trial of Acetysalicylic Acid in the Secondary Prevention of Mortality from Myocardial Infarction," *British Medical Journal* 1:436–440, 1974.
(2) The Coronary Drug Project Research Group, "Aspirin in Coronary Heart Disease," *Journal of Chronic Diseases*, 29:625–642, 1976.
(3) Breddin K., et al., "Secondary Prevention of Myocardial Infarction: A Comparison of Acetylsalicylic Acid, Phenprocoumon or Placebo," *International Congress Series* 470:263–268, 1979.
(4) Aspirin Myocardial Infarction Study Research Group, "A Randomized, Controlled Trial of Aspirin in Persons Recovered from Myocardial Infarction," *Journal American Medical Association* 245:661–669, 1980.
(5) Elwood, P. C., and P. M. Sweetnam, "Aspirin and Secondary Mortality after Myocardial Infarction," *Lancet* pp. 1313–1315, December 22–29, 1979.
(6) The Persantine-Aspirin Reinfarction Study Research Group, "Persantine and Aspirin in Coronary Heart Disease," *Circulation*, 62: 449–460, 1980.
(7) Lewis, H. D., et al., "Protective Effects of Aspirin Against Acute Myocardial Infarction and Death in Men with Unstable Angina, Results of a Veterans Administration Cooperative Study," *New England Journal of Medicine* 309:396–403, 1983.
(8) "1984 Report of the Joint National Committee on Detection, Evaluation, Treatment of High Blood Pressure," U.S. Department of Health and Human Services and United States Public Health Service, National Institutes of Health.

How Supplied: Tablets: foil sealed; box of 12 in 6 foil twin packs; box of 24 in 12 foil twin packs; box of 36 tablets in 18 foil twin packs; 100 tablets in 50 foil twin packs; carton of 72 tablets in 36 foil twin packs. Product Identification Mark: "ALKA-SELTZER" embossed on each tablet.

Shown in Product Identification Guide, page 414

ALKA–SELTZER® Extra Strength Antacid & Pain Reliever

Active Ingredients: Each tablet contains: Aspirin 500mg, heat treated sodium bicarbonate 1985mg, citric acid 1000mg. Alka-Seltzer in water contains principally the antacid sodium citrate and the analgesic sodium acetylsalicylate.

Inactive Ingredient: Flavors

Indications: For fast relief of acid indigestion, sour stomach or heartburn with headache or body aches and pains. Also, for fast relief of upset stomach with headache from overindulgence in food and drink—especially recommended for taking before bed and again on arising. Effective for pain relief alone: headache or body and muscular aches and pains.

Warnings: Children and teenagers should not use this medicine for chicken pox or flu symptoms before a doctor is consulted about Reye syndrome, a rare but serious illness reported to be associated with aspirin. As with any drug, if you are pregnant or nursing a baby, seek the advice of a health professional before using this product. IT IS ESPECIALLY IMPORTANT NOT TO USE ASPIRIN DURING THE LAST 3 MONTHS OF PREGNANCY UNLESS SPECIFICALLY DIRECTED TO DO SO BY A DOCTOR BECAUSE IT MAY CAUSE PROBLEMS IN THE UNBORN CHILD OR COMPLICATIONS DURING DELIVERY. Except under the advice and supervision of a physician, do not take more than, Adults: 7 tablets in a 24-hour period (60 years of age or older, 4 tablets in a 24-hour period), or use the daily maximum dosage for more than 10 days. Do not use if you are allergic to aspirin or have asthma, if you have bleeding problems, or if you are on a sodium restricted diet. Each tablet contains 588mg of sodium. If ringing in the ears or a loss of hearing occurs, consult a doctor before taking any more of this product.
Do not take this product for pain for more than 10 days unless directed by a doctor. If pain persists or gets worse, if new symptoms occur, or if redness or swelling is present, consult a doctor because these could be signs of a serious condition. Keep this and all drugs out of the reach of children.

Drug Interaction Precaution: Do not take this product if you are taking a prescription drug for anticoagulation (thinning the blood), diabetes, gout, or arthritis unless directed by a doctor.

Dosage and Administration: Extra Strength Alka-Seltzer must be dissolved in water before taking. Adults: 2 tablets every 4 hours. Caution: If symptoms persist, or recur frequently, or if you are under treatment for ulcer, consult your physician.

How Supplied: Foil sealed effervescent tablets in cartons of 12's in 6 foil twin packs; 24's in 12 foil twin packs.
Shown in Product Identification Guide, page 414

Continued on next page

Miles—Cont.

ALKA–SELTZER® GOLD
Effervescent Antacid

Active Ingredients: Each tablet contains heat treated sodium bicarbonate 958 mg., citric acid 832 mg., potassium bicarbonate 312 mg. ALKA-SELTZER® Effervescent Antacid in water contains principally the antacids sodium citrate and potassium citrate.

Inactive Ingredient: A tableting aid. Does not contain aspirin.

Indications: ALKA-SELTZER® Effervescent Antacid is indicated for relief of acid indigestion, sour stomach or heartburn.

Actions: The ALKA-SELTZER® Effervescent Antacid solution provides quick and effective neutralization of gastric acid. Measured by the in vitro standard established by the Food and Drug Administration one tablet will neutralize 10.6 mEq of acid.

Warnings: Except under the advice and supervision of a physician, do not take more than: Adults: 8 tablets in a 24 hour period (60 years of age or older: 7 tablets in a 24 hour period), Children: 4 tablets in a 24 hour period; or use the maximum dosage of this product for more than 2 weeks.
Do not use this product if you are on a sodium restricted diet. Each tablet contains 311 mg. of sodium.
Keep this and all drugs out of the reach of children. As with any drug, if you are pregnant or nursing a baby, seek the advice of a health professional before using this product.

Dosage and Administration: Adults: Take 2 tablets fully dissolved in water every 4 hours. Children: ½ the adult dosage.

How Supplied: Boxes of 20 tablets in 10 foil twin packs; 36 tablets in 18 foil twin packs.
Shown in Product Identification Guide, page 414

Lemon Lime ALKA-SELTZER®
Effervescent Antacid & Pain Reliever

Active Ingredients: Each tablet contains: Aspirin 325 mg, heat treated sodium bicarbonate 1710 mg, citric acid 1220 mg. Alka-Seltzer in water contains principally the antacid sodium citrate and the analgesic sodium acetylsalicylate.

Inactive Ingredients: Flavors, Saccharin Sodium.

Indications: For fast relief of ACID INDIGESTION, SOUR STOMACH or HEARTBURN with HEADACHE, or BODY ACHES AND PAINS. Also for fast relief of UPSET STOMACH with HEADACHE from overindulgence in food and drink—especially recommended for taking before bed and again on arising. EFFECTIVE FOR PAIN RELIEF ALONE: HEADACHE or BODY and MUSCULAR ACHES and PAINS.

Warnings: Children and teenagers should not use this medicine for chicken pox or flu symptoms before a doctor is consulted about Reye syndrome, a rare but serious illness reported to be associated with aspirin.
As with any drug, if you are pregnant or nursing a baby, seek the advice of a health professional before using this product. IT IS ESPECIALLY IMPORTANT NOT TO USE ASPIRIN DURING THE LAST 3 MONTHS OF PREGNANCY UNLESS SPECIFICALLY DIRECTED TO DO SO BY A DOCTOR BECAUSE IT MAY CAUSE PROBLEMS IN THE UNBORN CHILD OR COMPLICATIONS DURING DELIVERY.
Except under the advice and supervision of a physician: Do not take more than, ADULTS: 6 tablets in a 24-hour period, (60 years of age or older: 4 tablets in a 24-hour period), or use the daily maximum dosage for more than 10 days. Do not use if you are allergic to aspirin or have asthma, if you have bleeding problems, or if you are on a sodium restricted diet. Each tablet contains 506 mg of sodium. If ringing in the ears or a loss of hearing occurs, consult a doctor before taking any more of this product.
Do not take this product for pain for more than 10 days unless directed by a doctor. If pain persists or gets worse, if new symptoms occur, or if redness or swelling is present, consult a doctor because these could be signs of a serious condition.
Keep this and all drugs out of the reach of children.

Drug Interaction Precaution: Do not take this product if you are taking a prescription drug for anticoagulation (thinning the blood), diabetes, gout, or arthritis unless directed by a doctor.

Directions: Alka-Seltzer must be dissolved in water before taking. ADULTS: 2 tablets every 4 hours. CAUTION: If symptoms persist or recur frequently or if you are under treatment for ulcer, consult your physician.

Professional Labeling:

ASPIRIN FOR MYOCARDIAL INFARCTION

Indication: The Aspirin contained in Alka-Seltzer is indicated to reduce the risk of death and/or non-fatal myocardial infarction in patients with a previous infarction or unstable angina pectoris.

Clinical Trials: The indication is supported by the results of six, large, randomized multicenter, placebo-controlled studies[1-7] involving 10,816, predominantly male, post-myocardial infarction (MI) patients and one randomized placebo-controlled study of 1,266 men with unstable angina. Therapy with aspirin was begun at intervals after the onset of acute MI varying from less than 3 days to more than 5 years and continued for periods of from less than one year to four years. In the unstable angina study, treatment was started within 1 month after the onset of unstable angina and continued for 12 weeks and complicating conditions such as congestive heart failure were not included in the study.
Aspirin therapy in MI patients was associated with about a 20 percent reduction in the risk of subsequent death and/or non-fatal reinfarction, a median absolute decrease of 3 percent from the 12 to 22 percent event rates in the placebo groups. In aspirin-treated unstable angina patients the reduction in risk was about 50 percent, a reduction in event rate of 5 percent from the 10 percent rate in the placebo group over the 12 weeks of the study.
Daily dosage of aspirin in the post-myocardial infarction studies was 300 mg in one study and 900 to 1500 mg in five studies. A dose of 325 mg was used in the study of unstable angina.

Adverse Reactions: Gastrointestinal Reactions: Symptoms and signs of gastrointestinal irritation were not significantly increased in subjects treated for unstable angina with buffered aspirin in solution (ALKA-SELTZER®). Doses of 1000 mg per day of aspirin tablets caused gastrointestinal symptoms and bleeding that in some cases were clinically significant. In the largest post-infarction study (the Aspirin Myocardial Infarction Study (AMIS) with 4,500 people), the percentage incidences of gastrointestinal symptoms for the aspirin (1000 mg of a standard, solid-tablet formulation) and placebo-treated subjects, respectively, were: stomach pain (14.5%; 4.4%); heartburn (11.9%; 4.8%); nausea and/or vomiting (7.6%; 2.1%); hospitalization for gastrointestinal disorder (4.9%; 3.5%). In the AMIS and other trials, aspirin treated patients had increased rates of gross gastrointestinal bleeding. As with all aspirin products Alka-Seltzer is contraindicated in patients with aspirin sensitivity, with asthma, or with coagulation disease.

Cardiovascular and Biochemical: In the AMIS trial, the dosage of 1000 mg per day of aspirin was associated with small increases in systolic blood pressure (BP) (average 1.5 to 2.1 mm) and diastolic BP (0.5 to 0.6 mm), depending upon whether maximal or last available readings were used. Blood urea nitrogen and uric acid levels were also increased, but by less than 1.0 mg%. Subjects with marked hypertension or renal insufficiency had been excluded from the trial so that the clinical importance of these observations for such subjects or for any subjects treated over more prolonged periods is not known. It is recommended that patients placed on long-term aspirin treatment, even at doses of 300 mg per day, be seen at regular intervals to assess changes in these measurements.

Sodium in Buffered Aspirin for Solution Formulations: One tablet daily of flavored buffered aspirin in solution adds

506 mg of sodium to that in the diet and may not be tolerated by patients with active sodium-retaining states such as congestive heart or renal failure. This amount of sodium adds about 30 percent to the 70 to 90 meq intake suggested as appropriate for dietary treatment of essential hypertension in the 1984 Report of the Joint National Committee on Detection, Evaluation, and Treatment of High Blood Pressure.[8]

Dosage and Administration: Although most of the studies used dosages exceeding 300 mg, daily, two trials used only 300 mg and pharmacologic data indicate that this dose inhibits platelet function fully. Therefore, 300 mg or a conventional 325 mg aspirin dose daily is a reasonable, routine dose that would minimize gastrointestinal adverse reactions. This use of aspirin applies to both solid, oral dosage forms (buffered and plain aspirin) and buffered aspirin in solution.

References:
(1) Elwood, P. C., et al., A Randomized Controlled Trial of Acetysalicylic Acid in the Secondary Prevention of Mortality from Myocardial Infarction," *British Medical Journal* 1:436–440, 1974.
(2) The Coronary Drug Project Research Group, "Aspirin in Coronary Heart Disease," *Journal of Chronic Diseases,* 29:625–642, 1976.
(3) Breddin K., et al., "Secondary Prevention of Myocardial Infarction: A Comparison of Acetylsalicylic Acid, Phenprocoumon or Placebo," *International Congress Series* 470:263–268, 1979.
(4) Aspirin Myocardial Infarction Study Research Group, "A Randomized, Controlled Trial of Aspirin in Persons Recovered from Myocardial Infarction," *Journal American Medical Association* 245:661–669, 1980.
(5) Elwood, P. C., and P. M. Sweetnam, "Aspirin and Secondary Mortality after Myocardial Infarction," *Lancet* pp. 1313–1315, December 22–29, 1979.
(6) The Persantine-Aspirin Reinfarction Study Research Group, "Persantine and Aspirin in Coronary Heart Disease," *Circulation,* 62: 449–460, 1980.
(7) Lewis, H. D., et al., "Protective Effects of Aspirin Against Acute Myocardial Infarction and Death in Men with Unstable Angina, Results of a Veterans Administration Cooperative Study," *New England Journal of Medicine* 309:396–403, 1983.
(8) "1984 Report of the Joint National Committee on Detection, Evaluation, Treatment of High Blood Pressure," U.S. Department of Health and Human Services and United States Public Health Service, National Institutes of Health.

How Supplied: Foil sealed effervescent tablets in cartons of 12's in 6 foil twin packs; 24's in 12 foil twin packs; 36's in 18 foil twin packs.

Shown in Product Identification Guide, page 414

ALKA-SELTZER PLUS®
Cold Medicine

Active Ingredients:
Each dry ALKA-SELTZER PLUS® Cold Tablet contains the following active ingredients: Phenylpropanolamine bitartrate 24.08 mg., chlorpheniramine maleate 2 mg., aspirin 325 mg. The product is dissolved in water prior to ingestion and the aspirin is converted into its soluble ionic form, sodium acetylsalicylate.

Inactive Ingredients: Citric acid, flavors, sodium bicarbonate.

Indications: Provides temporary relief of these major cold and flu symptoms: nasal and sinus congestion, runny nose, sneezing, headache, scratchy sore throat, fever, body aches and pains.

Warnings: Children and teenagers should not use this medicine for chicken pox or flu symptoms before a doctor is consulted about Reye syndrome, a rare but serious illness reported to be associated with aspirin. If sore throat is severe, persists for more than 2 days, is accompanied by high fever, headache, nausea or vomiting, consult a physician promptly. As with any drug, if you are pregnant or nursing a baby, seek the advice of a health professional before using this product. **IT IS ESPECIALLY IMPORTANT NOT TO USE ASPIRIN DURING THE LAST 3 MONTHS OF PREGNANCY UNLESS SPECIFICALLY DIRECTED TO DO SO BY A DOCTOR BECAUSE IT MAY CAUSE PROBLEMS IN THE UNBORN CHILD OR COMPLICATIONS DURING DELIVERY.**
Do not exceed recommended dosage because at higher doses nervousness, dizziness or sleeplessness may occur. May cause excitability, especially in children. Do not take this product unless directed by a doctor if you are allergic to aspirin, have a breathing problem such as emphysema or chronic bronchitis, asthma, glaucoma, difficulty in urination due to enlargement of the prostate gland, heart disease, high blood pressure, diabetes, thyroid disease, bleeding problems or on a sodium restricted diet. Each tablet contains 506 mg of sodium.
May cause drowsiness; alcohol, sedatives and tranquilizers may increase drowsiness effect. Avoid alcoholic beverages while taking this product. Do not take this product if you are taking sedatives or tranquilizers without first consulting your doctor. Use caution when driving a motor vehicle or operating machinery. Do not take this product for more than 7 days. If symptoms do not improve or are accompanied by fever or if fever persists for more than 3 days, consult a doctor. Keep this and all drugs out of the reach of children.

Drug Interaction Precaution: Do not take this product if you are presently taking a prescription drug for anticoagulation (thinning the blood), diabetes, gout, arthritis, high blood pressure or are presently taking monoamine oxidase inhibitor (MAOI) for depression or for 2 weeks after stopping use of a MAOI without first consulting your doctor.

Dosage and Administration:
ALKA-SELTZER PLUS® is taken in solution; 2 tablets dissolved in approximately 4 ounces of water. Adults: two tablets every 4 hours up to 8 tablets in 24 hours.

How Supplied: Tablets: carton of 12 tablets in 6 foil twin packs; 20 tablets in 10 foil twin packs; carton of 36 tablets in 18 foil twin packs; carton of 48 tablets in 24 foil twin packs.

Product Identification Mark:
"Alka-Seltzer Plus" embossed on each tablet.

Shown in Product Identification Guide, page 414

ALKA–SELTZER PLUS®
Night-Time Cold Medicine

Active Ingredients: Each tablet contains aspirin 500 mg, brompheniramine maleate 2 mg, phenylpropanolamine bitartrate 20 mg, dextromethorphan hydrobromide 10 mg. In water the aspirin is converted into its soluble ionic form, sodium acetylsalicylate.

Inactive Ingredients: Aspartame, citric acid, flavor, sodium bicarbonate, tableting aids.

Indications: For temporary relief of these major cold and flu symptoms: coughing, nasal and sinus congestion, body aches and pains, runny nose, headache, sneezing, fever, scratchy sore throat so you can get the rest you need.

Warning: Children and teenagers should not use this medicine for chicken pox or flu symptoms before a doctor is consulted about Reye syndrome, a rare but serious illness reported to be associated with aspirin. If sore throat is severe, persists for more than 2 days, is accompanied by high fever, headache, nausea or vomiting, consult a physician promptly. As with any drug, if you are pregnant or nursing a baby, seek the advice of a health professional before using this product. **IT IS ESPECIALLY IMPORTANT NOT TO USE ASPIRIN DURING THE LAST 3 MONTHS OF PREGNANCY UNLESS SPECIFICALLY DIRECTED TO DO SO BY A DOCTOR BECAUSE IT MAY CAUSE PROBLEMS IN THE UNBORN CHILD OR COMPLICATIONS DURING DELIVERY.**
Do not exceed recommended dosage because at higher doses nervousness, dizziness or sleeplessness may occur. May cause excitability, especially in children. Do not take this product unless directed by a doctor if you are allergic to aspirin, have a breathing problem such as em-

Continued on next page

Miles—Cont.

physema or chronic bronchitis, asthma, glaucoma, difficulty in urination due to enlargement of the prostate gland, heart disease, high blood pressure, diabetes, thyroid disease, bleeding problems or on a sodium restricted diet. Each tablet contains 506 mg of sodium.

May cause marked drowsiness; alcohol, sedatives and tranquilizers may increase drowsiness effect. Avoid alcoholic beverages while taking this product. Do not take this product if you are taking sedatives or tranquilizers without first consulting your doctor. Use caution when driving a motor vehicle or operating machinery. Do not take this product for persistent or chronic cough such as occurs with smoking, asthma, emphysema, or if cough is accompanied by excessive phlegm (mucus), unless directed by a doctor. A persistent cough may be a sign of a serious condition. If cough persists for more than 1 week, tends to recur or is accompanied by fever, rash, or persistent headache, consult a doctor. Do not take this product for more than 7 days. If symptoms do not improve or are accompanied by fever or if fever persists for more than 3 days, consult a doctor. Keep this and all drugs out of the reach of children.

Phenylketonurics: Contains Phenylalanine 9 mg per tablet.

Drug Interaction Precaution: Do not take this product if you are presently taking a prescription drug for anticoagulation (thinning the blood), diabetes, gout, arthritis, high blood pressure or are presently taking a monoamine oxidase inhibitor (MAOI) for depression or for 2 weeks after stopping use of a MAOI without first consulting your doctor.

Dosage and Administration: Adults: Take 2 tablets fully dissolved in 4 ounces of water (use more or less water to taste). Additional fluid intake is encouraged for cold sufferers. Repeat every 4 hours, not to exceed 8 tablets in any 24-hour period.

How Supplied: Tablets: carton of 12 tablets in 6 foil twin packs; carton of 20 tablets in 10 foil twin packs; carton of 36 tablets in 18 foil twin packs.

Product Identification Mark: "A/S PLUS NIGHT-TIME" etched on each tablet

Shown in Product Identification Guide, page 414

ALKA–SELTZER PLUS®
Sinus Allergy Medicine

Active Ingredients: Phenylpropanolamine bitartrate 24.08 mg, brompheniramine maleate 2 mg, aspirin 500 mg. In water the aspirin is converted into its soluble ionic form, sodium acetylsalicylate.

Inactive Ingredients: Aspartame, citric acid, flavors, heat-treated sodium bicarbonate, tableting aids

Indications: For the temporary relief of these major sinusitis, allergic rhinitis or hay fever symptoms: nasal congestion sinus pain and pressure, runny nose, headache, itchy, watery eyes and sneezing.

Warnings: Children and teenagers should not use this medicine for chicken pox or flu symptoms before a doctor is consulted about Reye syndrome, a rare but serious illness reported to be associated with aspirin. As with any drug, if you are pregnant or nursing a baby, seek the advice of a health professional before using this product. **IT IS ESPECIALLY IMPORTANT NOT TO USE ASPIRIN DURING THE LAST 3 MONTHS OF PREGNANCY UNLESS SPECIFICALLY DIRECTED TO DO SO BY A DOCTOR BECAUSE IT MAY CAUSE PROBLEMS IN THE UNBORN CHILD OR COMPLICATIONS DURING DELIVERY.**

Do not exceed recommended dosage because at higher doses nervousness, dizziness or sleeplessness may occur. May cause excitability, especially in children. Do not take this product unless directed by a doctor if you are allergic to aspirin, have a breathing problem such as emphysema or chronic bronchitis, asthma, glaucoma, difficulty in urination due to enlargement of the prostate gland, heart disease, high blood pressure, diabetes, thyroid disease, bleeding problems or on a sodium restricted diet. Each tablet contains 506 mg of sodium.

May cause drowsiness; alcohol, sedatives and tranquilizers may increase the drowsiness effect. Avoid alcoholic beverages while taking this product. Do not take this product if you are taking sedatives or tranquilizers without first consulting your doctor. Use caution when driving a motor vehicle or operating machinery. Do not take this product for more than 7 days. If symptoms do not improve or are accompanied by fever or if fever persists for more than 3 days, consult a doctor. Keep this and all drugs out of the reach of children.

Phenylketonurics: Contains Phenylalanine 8.98 mg per tablet.

Drug Interaction Precaution: Do not take this product if you are presently taking a prescription drug for anticoagulation (thinning of the blood), diabetes, gout, arthritis, high blood pressure or are presently taking a monamine oxidase inhibitor (MAOI) for depression or for 2 weeks after stopping use of a MAOI without first consulting your doctor.

Directions: Adults: Take 2 tablets dissolved in approximately 4 ounces (½ glass) of water every 4 hours. Do not exceed 8 tablets in any 24-hour period.

How Supplied: Boxes of 32 tablets in 16 foil twin packs; 16 tablets in 8 foil twin packs

Product Identification Mark: "AS + Sinus Allergy" embossed on each tablet.

Shown in Product Identification Guide, page 414

ALKA-SELTZER PLUS® COLD & COUGH MEDICINE

Active Ingredients: Each ALKA-SELTZER PLUS® COLD AND COUGH tablet contains the following active ingredients: Aspirin 500 mg, Chlorpheniramine Maleate 2 mg, Phenylpropanolamine Bitartrate 24.08 mg, Dextromethorphan Hydrobromide 10 mg. In water the aspirin is converted into its soluble ionic form, sodium acetylsalicylate.

Inactive Ingredients: Aspartame, Citric Acid, Flavor, Sodium Bicarbonate, Tableting Aids.

Indications: Provides temporary relief of these major symptoms of colds and flu with cough: nasal and sinus congestion, body aches and pains, runny nose, coughing, headache, scratchy sore throat, sneezing, fever.

Warning: Children and teenagers should not use this medicine for chicken pox or flu symptoms before a doctor is consulted about Reye syndrome, a rare but serious illness reported to be associated with aspirin. If sore throat is severe, persists for more than 2 days, is accompanied by high fever, headache, nausea or vomiting, consult a physician promptly. As with any drug, if you are pregnant or nursing a baby, seek the advice of a health professional before using this product. **IT IS ESPECIALLY IMPORTANT NOT TO USE ASPIRIN DURING THE LAST 3 MONTHS OF PREGNANCY UNLESS SPECIFICALLY DIRECTED TO DO SO BY A DOCTOR BECAUSE IT MAY CAUSE PROBLEMS IN THE UNBORN CHILD OR COMPLICATIONS DURING DELIVERY.**

Do not exceed recommended dosage because at higher doses nervousness, dizziness or sleeplessness may occur. May cause excitability, especially in children. Do not take this product unless directed by a doctor if you are allergic to aspirin, have a breathing problem such as emphysema or chronic bronchitis, asthma, glaucoma, difficulty in urination due to enlargement of the prostate gland, heart disease, high blood pressure, diabetes, thyroid disease, bleeding problems or on a sodium restricted diet. Each tablet contains 506 mg of sodium.

May cause marked drowsiness; alcohol, sedatives and tranquilizers may increase drowsiness effect. Avoid alcoholic beverages while taking this product. Do not take this product if you are taking sedatives or tranquilizers without first consulting your doctor. Use caution when driving a motor vehicle or operating machinery. Do not take this product for persistent or chronic cough such as occurs with smoking, asthma, emphysema, or if cough is accompanied by excessive phlegm (mucus) unless directed by a doctor. A persistent cough may be a sign of a serious condition. If cough persists for more than 1 week, tends to recur or is accompanied by fever, rash, or persistent headache, consult a doctor. Do not take this product for more than 7 days. If symptoms do not improve or are accompanied by fever or if fever persists for more than 3 days, consult a doctor. Keep this and all drugs out of the reach of children.

Phenylketonurics: Contains Phenylalanine 7 mg per tablet.

Drug Interaction Precaution: Do not take this product if you are presently taking a prescription drug for anticoagulation (thinning the blood), diabetes, gout, arthritis, high blood pressure or are presently taking a monoamine oxidase inhibitor (MAOI) for depression or for 2 weeks aftr stopping use of a MAOI without first consulting your doctor.

Dosage and Administration: ALKA-SELTZER PLUS® COLD & COUGH MEDICINE is taken in solution; approximately 4 ounces of water. Additional fluid intake is encouraged for cold sufferers. Adults: 2 tablets every 4 hours up to 8 tablets in 24 hours.

How Supplied: Tablets: carton of 36 tablets in 18 foil twin packs: carton of 20 tablets in 10 foil twin packs: carton of 48 tablets in 24 foil packs, carton of 12 tablets in 6 foil packs.

Product Identification Mark: "AS + Cold Cough" embossed on each tablet.
Shown in Product Identification Guide, page 414

BACTINE® Antiseptic·Anesthetic First Aid Liquid

Active Ingredients: Benzalkonium Chloride 0.13% w/w, Lidocaine HCl 2.5% w/w.

Inactive Ingredients: Edetate Disodium, Fragrances, Octoxynol 9, Propylene Glycol, Purified Water.

Indications: First aid to help prevent bacterial contamination or skin infection and for the temporary relief of pain and itching in minor cuts, scrapes and burns.

Warnings: FOR EXTERNAL USE ONLY. Do not use in the eyes or apply over large areas of the body. In case of deep or puncture wounds, animal bites, or serious burns, consult a doctor. Stop use and consult a doctor if the condition persists or gets worse. Do not use longer than 1 week unless directed by a doctor. Do not use in large quantities, particularly over raw surfaces or blistered areas. Keep this and all drugs out of the reach of children. In case of accidental ingesion, seek professional assistance or contact a Poison Control Center immediately.

Directions: For adults and children 2 years of age and older. Clean the affected area. Apply a small amount of this product on the area 1 to 3 times daily. May be covered with a sterile bandage. If bandaged, let dry first.

How Supplied: 2 oz., 4 oz. and 16 oz. liquid, and 3.5 oz. pump spray.
Shown in Product Identification Guide, page 414

BUGS BUNNY™ Children's Chewable Vitamins Plus Iron (Sugar Free)
FLINTSTONES® Children's Chewable Vitamins Plus Iron
One Tablet Provides

Vitamins	Quantity	% of U.S. RDA For Children 2 to 4 Years of Age	For Adults and Children over 4 Years of Age
Vitamin A (as Acetate and Beta Carotene)	2500 I.U.	100	50
Vitamin D	400 I.U.	100	100
Vitamin E	15 I.U.	150	50
Vitamin C	60 mg.	150	100
Folic Acid	0.3 mg.	150	75
Thiamine	1.05 mg.	150	70
Riboflavin	1.20 mg.	150	70
Niacin	13.50 mg.	150	67
Vitamin B$_6$	1.05 mg.	150	52
Vitamin B$_{12}$	4.5 mcg.	150	75
Mineral:			
Iron (Elemental)	15 mg.	150	83

BACTINE® First Aid Antibiotic Plus Anesthetic Ointment

Active Ingredients: Each gram contains Polymyxin B Sulfate 5000 units; Bacitracin 400 units; Neomycin Sulfate 5 mg (equivalent to 3.5 mg Neomycin base); Diperodon HCl 10 mg (pain reliever).

Inactive Ingredients: Mineral Oil, White Petrolatum.

Indications: First aid to help prevent infection, guard against bacterial contamination, relieve pain and itching in minor cuts, scrapes and burns.

Warning: For external use only. Do not use in the eyes or apply over large areas of the body. In case of deep or puncture wounds, animal bites or serious burns, consult a physician. Stop use and consult a physician if the condition persists or gets worse. Do not use longer than one (1) week unless directed by a physician. Keep this and all medicines out of children's reach. In case of accidental ingestion, seek professional assistance or contact a Poison Control Center immediately.

Directions: Clean the affected area. Apply a small amount of this product (an amount equal to the surface area of the tip of a finger) one to three times daily. May be covered with a sterile bandage.

How Supplied: ½ oz. tube.
Shown in Product Identification Guide, page 414

BACTINE® 1.0% Hydrocortisone Anti-Itch Cream

Active Ingredient: Hydrocortisone 1.0%.

Inactive Ingredients: Aluminum Sulfate, Beeswax, Calcium Acetate, Cetearyl Alcohol, Dextrin, Glycerin, Hydrocortisone Alcohol, Light Mineral Oil, Methylparaben, Purified Water, Sodium Lauryl Sulfate, White Petrolatum.

Indications: For the temporary relief of itching associated with minor skin irritations, inflammation and rashes.

Warnings: For external use only. Avoid contact with the eyes. If condition worsens or if symptoms persist for more than seven days or clear up and occur again within a few days, stop use of this product and do not begin use of any other hydrocortisone product unless you have consulted a physician. Do not use for the treatment of diaper rash. Consult a physician.
Keep this and all drugs out of the reach of children. In case of accidental ingestion, seek professional assistance or contact a Poison Control Center immediately.

Directions: For Adults and Children 2 years of age and older. Apply to affected area not more than 3 or 4 times daily. Children under 2 years of age: Do not use, consult a physician.
Shown in Product Identification Guide, page 414

BUGS BUNNY™ Children's Chewable Vitamins Plus Iron (Sugar Free)
FLINTSTONES® Children's Chewable Vitamins
FLINTSTONES® Children's Chewable Vitamins Plus Iron

Vitamin Ingredients: Each multivitamin supplement with iron contains the ingredients listed in the chart below: [See table above.]
FLINTSTONES® Children's Chewable Vitamins provide the same quantities of vitamins, but do not provide iron.

Indication: Dietary supplementation.

Dosage and Administration: One chewable tablet daily. For adults and children two years and older; tablet must be chewed.

Warning For Bugs Bunny Only: Phenylketonurics: Contains Phenylalanine.

Precaution:
IRON SUPPLEMENTS ONLY.
Contains iron, which can be harmful in large doses. Close tightly and keep out

Continued on next page

Miles—Cont.

of reach of children. In case of overdose contact a Poison Control Center immediately.

How Supplied: Flintstones are supplied in bottles of 60 and 100, Bugs Bunny in bottles of 60 with child-resistant caps.

Shown in Product Identification Guide, pages 414 and 415

FLINTSTONES® Plus Extra C
Children's Chewable Vitamins
BUGS BUNNY™ With Extra C
Children's Chewable Vitamins
(Sugar Free)

Vitamin Ingredients: Each multivitamin supplement contains the ingredients listed in the chart below:

Indication: Dietary supplementation.

Dosage and Administration: One tablet daily for adults and children two years and older; tablet must be chewed.

Warning For Bugs Bunny Only: Phenylketonurics: Contains Phenylalanine.

How Supplied: Flintstones in bottles of 60's & 100's, Bugs Bunny in bottles of 60 with child-resistant caps.

Shown in Product Identification Guide, pages 414 and 415

FLINTSTONES® COMPLETE
With Iron, Calcium & Minerals
Children's Chewable Vitamins

BUGS BUNNY™ COMPLETE
Children's Chewable
Vitamins + Minerals
With Iron and Calcium
(Sugar Free)

Ingredients: Each supplement provides the ingredients listed in the chart above.

FLINTSTONES® COMPLETE
Children's Chewable Vitamins
BUGS BUNNY™ COMPLETE
Children's Chewable
Vitamins + Minerals
(Sugar Free)

Vitamins	Quantity Per Tablet	Percentage of U.S. Recommended Daily Allowance (U.S. RDA) For Children 2 to 4 Years of Age (½ tablet)	For Adults & Children Over 4 Years of Age (1 tablet)
Vitamin A (as Acetate and Beta Carotene)	5000 I.U.	100	100
Vitamin D	400 I.U.	50	100
Vitamin E	30 I.U.	150	100
Vitamin C	60 mg.	75	100
Folic Acid	0.4 mg.	100	100
Vitamin B-1 (Thiamine)	1.5 mg.	107	100
Vitamin B-2 (Riboflavin)	1.7 mg.	106	100
Niacin	20 mg.	111	100
Vitamin B-6 (Pyridoxine)	2 mg.	143	100
Vitamin B-12 (Cyanocobalamin)	6 mcg.	100	100
Biotin	40 mcg.	13	13
Pantothenic Acid	10 mg.	100	100

Minerals	Quantity	Percent U.S. RDA	
Iron (elemental)	18 mg.	90	100
Calcium	100 mg.	6	10
Copper	2 mg.	100	100
Phosphorus	100 mg.	6	10
Iodine	150 mcg.	107	100
Magnesium	20 mg.	5	5
Zinc	15 mg.	94	100

Indication: Dietary Supplementation.

Dosage and Administration: 2–4 years of age: Chew one-half tablet daily. Over 4 years of age: Chew one tablet daily.

Warning: Phenylketonurics: Contains Phenylalanine.

Precaution: Contains iron, which can be harmful in large doses. Close tightly and keep out of reach of children. In case of overdose, contact a physician or Poison Control Center immediately.

How Supplied: Bottles of 60's with child-resistant caps.

Shown in Product Identification Guide, pages 414 and 415

FLINTSTONES® PLUS CALCIUM
with Beta Carotene
Children's Chewable Vitamins

Ingredients: Calcium Carbonate, Sorbitol, Starch, Sodium Ascorbate, Gelatin, Stearic Acid, Magnesium Stearate, Natural and Artificial Flavors. Vitamin E Acetate, Artificial Colors (including Yellow 6), Silica, Glycerides of Stearic and Palmitic Acids, Malic Acid, Aspartame* (a sweetener), Pyridoxine Hydrochloride, Riboflavin, Thiamine Mononitrate, Vitamin A Acetate, Beta Carotene, Monoammonium Glycyrrhizinate, Folic Acid, Vitamin D, Vitamin B12.
*Phenylketonurics: Contains Phenylalanine

CHEW ONE TABLET DAILY

One Tablet Daily Provides: Vitamins	Quantity Per Tablet	Percent U.S. RDA For Children 2 to 4 Years of Age	For Adults and Children Over 4 Years of Age
Vitamin A (as Acetate and Beta Carotene)	2500 I.U.	100	50
Vitamin D	400 I.U.	100	100
Vitamin E	15 I.U.	150	50
Vitamin C	60 mg	150	100
Folic Acid	0.3 mg	150	75
Thiamine	1.05 mg	150	70
Riboflavin	1.20 mg	150	70
Niacin	13.50 mg	150	67
Vitamin B-6	1.05 mg	150	52
Vitamin B-12	4.5 mcg	150	75

BUGS BUNNY™ With Extra C
Children's Chewable Vitamins
(Sugar Free)
FLINTSTONES® Plus Extra C
Children's Chewable Vitamins

Vitamins One Tablet Provides	Quantity	% of U.S. RDA For Children 2 To 4 Years of Age	For Adults and Children Over 4 Years of Age
Vitamin A (as Acetate and Beta Carotene)	2500 I.U.	100	50
Vitamin D	400 I.U.	100	100
Vitamin E	15 I.U.	150	50
Vitamin C	250 mg.	625	417
Folic Acid	0.3 mg.	150	75
Thiamine	1.05 mg.	150	70
Riboflavin	1.20 mg.	150	70
Niacin	13.50 mg.	150	67
Vitamin B_6	1.05 mg.	150	52
Vitamin B_{12}	4.5 mcg.	150	75

Minerals	Quantity	Percent	U.S. RDA
Calcium	200 mg	25	20

FOR ADULTS AND CHILDREN 2 YEARS AND OLDER; TABLET MUST BE CHEWED

KEEP OUT OF REACH OF CHILDREN.

Do not use this product if safety seal bearing Miles logo under cap is torn or missing.
Child Resistant Cap

How Supplied: Bottle of 60 Tablets

Shown in Product Identification Guide, page 415

DOMEBORO® Astringent Solution Powder Packets

Active Ingredients: Each powder packet, when dissolved in water and ready to use, provides the active ingredient aluminum acetate resulting from the reaction of calcium acetate 938 mg, and aluminum sulfate 1191 mg. The resulting astringent solution is buffered to an acid pH.

Inactive Ingredient: Dextrin

Indications: For temporary relief of minor skin irritations due to poison ivy, poison oak, poison sumac, insect bites, athlete's foot or rashes caused by soaps, detergents, cosmetics or jewelry.

Actions: DOMEBORO provides soothing, effective relief of minor skin irritations. For over 50 years, doctors have been recommending DOMEBORO ASTRINGENT SOLUTION to help relieve minor skin irritations.

Warnings: If condition worsens or symptoms persist for more than 7 days, discontinue use of the product and consult a doctor. For external use only. Avoid contact with the eyes. Do not cover compress or wet dressing with plastic to prevent evaporation. Keep this and all drugs out of the reach of children. In case of accidental ingestion, seek professional assistance or contact a Poison Control Center immediately.

Directions: One packet dissolved in 16 ounces of water makes a modified Burow's Solution approximately equivalent to a 1:40 dilution; two packets, a 1:20 dilution; and four packets, a 1:10 dilution. Dissolve one or two packets in water and stir the solution until fully dissolved. Do not strain or filter the solution. Can be used as a compress, wet dressing or as a soak. AS A COMPRESS OR WET DRESSING: Saturate a clean, soft, white cloth or gauze in the solution; gently squeeze and apply loosely to the affected area. Saturate the cloth in the solution every 15 to 30 minutes and apply to the affected area. Repeat as often as necessary. Discard remaining solution after use. AS A SOAK: Soak affected area in the solution for 15 to 30 minutes. Repeat 3 times a day. Discard remaining solution after use.

How Supplied: Boxes of 12 or 100 powder packets.
Shown in Product Identification Guide, page 414

DOMEBORO® Astringent Solution Effervescent Tablets

Active Ingredients: Each effervescent tablet, when dissolved in water and ready to use, provides the active ingredient aluminum acetate resulting from the reaction of calcium acetate 604 mg, and aluminum sulfate 878 mg. The resulting astringent solution is buffered to an acid pH.

Inactive Ingredients: Dextrin, polyethylene glycol, sodium bicarbonate

Indications: For temporary relief of minor skin irritations due to poison ivy, poison oak, poison sumac, insect bites, athlete's foot or rashes caused by soaps, detergents, cosmetics or jewelry.

Actions: DOMEBORO provides soothing, effective relief of minor skin irritations. For over 50 years doctors have been recommending DOMEBORO ASTRINGENT SOLUTION to help relieve minor skin irritations.

Warnings: If conditions worsens or symptoms persist for more than 7 days, discontinue use of the product and consult a doctor. For external use only. Avoid contact with the eyes. Do not cover compress or wet dressing with plastic to prevent evaporation. Keep this and all drugs out of the reach of children. In case of accidental ingestion, seek professional assistance or contact a Poison Control Center immediately.

Directions: One tablet dissolved in 12 ounces of water makes a modified Burow's Solution approximately equivalent to a 1:40 dilution; two tablets, a 1:20 dilution; and four tablets, a 1:10 dilution. Dissolve one or two tablets in water and stir the solution until fully dissolved. Do not strain or filter the solution. Can be used as a compress, wet dressing or as a soak. AS A COMPRESS OR WET DRESSING: Saturate a clean, soft, white cloth or gauze in the solution; gently squeeze and apply loosely to the affected area. Repeat as often as necessary. Discard remaining solution after use. AS A SOAK: Soak affected area in the solution for 15 to 30 minutes. Repeat 3 times a day. Discard remaining solution after use.

How Supplied: Boxes of 12 or 100 effervescent tablets

MILES® Nervine Nighttime Sleep–Aid

Active Ingredient: Each capsule-shaped tablet contains diphenhydramine HCl 25 mg.

Inactive Ingredients: Calcium Phosphate Dibasic, Calcium Sulfate, Carboxymethylcellulose Sodium, Corn Starch, Magnesium Stearate, Microcrystalline Cellulose.

Indications: Miles® Nervine helps you fall asleep and relieves occasional sleeplessness.

Actions: Antihistamines act on the central nervous system and produce drowsiness.

Warnings: Do not give to children under 12 years of age. Avoid alcoholic beverages while taking this product. Do not take this product if you are taking sedatives or tranquilizers without first consulting your doctor. If sleeplessness persists continuously for more than 2 weeks, consult your doctor. Insomnia may be a symptom of serious underlying medical illness. Do not take this product if you have asthma, glaucoma, emphysema, chronic pulmonary disease, shortness of breath, difficulty in breathing or difficulty in urination due to enlargement of the prostate gland unless directed by a doctor. As with any drug, if you are pregnant or nursing a baby, seek the advice of a health professional before using this product. Keep this and all drugs out of the reach of children. In case of accidental overdose, seek professional assistance or contact a poison control center immediately.

Dosage and Administration: Two caplets once daily at bedtime or as directed by a physician.

How Supplied: Blister pack 12's, bottle of 30's with a child-resistant cap.
Shown in Product Identification Guide, page 415

MYCELEX® OTC CREAM ANTIFUNGAL

Active Ingredient: Clotrimazole 1%

Inactive Ingredients: Benzyl alcohol (1%) as a preservative, cetostearyl alcohol, cetyl esters wax, octyldodecanol, polysorbate 60, purified water, sorbitan monostearate.

Store between 2°–30°C (36°–86°F).

Continued on next page

Miles—Cont.

Indications: Cures athlete's foot (tinea pedis), jock itch (tinea cruris), and ringworm (tinea corporis). For effective relief of the itching, cracking, burning and discomfort which can accompany these conditions.

Warnings: For external use only. Do not use on children under 2 years of age except under the advice and supervision of a doctor. If irritation occurs or if there is no improvement within 4 weeks (for athlete's foot or ringworm) or within 2 weeks (for jock itch) discontinue use and consult a doctor or pharmacist. Keep this and all drugs out of the reach of children. In case of accidental ingestion seek professional assistance or contact a Poison Control Center immediately. Use only as directed.

Directions: Cleanse skin with soap and water and dry thoroughly. Apply a thin layer and gently massage over affected area morning and evening or as directed by a doctor. For athlete's foot, pay special attention to the spaces between the toes. It is also helpful to wear well-fitting, ventilated shoes and to change shoes and socks at least once daily. Best results in athlete's foot and ringworm are usually obtained with 4 weeks' use of this product and in jock itch with 2 weeks' use. If satisfactory results have not occurred within these times, consult a doctor or pharmacist. Children under 12 years of age should be supervised in the use of this product. This product is not effective on the scalp or nails.
FOR BEST RESULTS, FOLLOW DIRECTIONS AND CONTINUE TREATMENT FOR LENGTH OF TIME INDICATED.

How Supplied: Cream Tube 15 g (½ oz.)

MYCELEX® OTC SOLUTION ANTIFUNGAL

Active Ingredient: Clotrimazole 1%

Inactive Ingredient: Polyethylene glycol 400
Store between 2°–30°C (36°–86°F).

Indications: Cures athlete's foot (tinea pedis), jock itch (tinea cruris), and ringworm (tinea corporis). For effective relief of the itching, cracking, burning and discomfort which can accompany these conditions.

Warnings: For external use only. Do not use on children under 2 years of age except under the advice and supervision of a doctor. If irritation occurs or if there is no improvement within 4 weeks (for athlete's foot or ringworm) or within 2 weeks (for jock itch) discontinue use and consult a doctor or pharmacist. Keep this and all drugs out of the reach of children. In case of accidental ingestion seek pro-fessional assistance or contact a Poison Control Center immediately. Use only as directed.

Directions: Cleanse skin with soap and water and dry thoroughly. Apply a thin layer and gently massage over affected area morning and evening or as directed by a doctor. For athlete's foot, pay special attention to the spaces between the toes. It is also helpful to wear well-fitting, ventilated shoes and to change shoes and socks at least once daily. Best results in athlete's foot and ringworm are usually obtained with 4 weeks' use of this product and in jock itch with 2 weeks' use. If satisfactory results have not occurred within these times, consult a doctor or pharmacist. Children under 12 years of age should be supervised in the use of this product. This product is not effective on the scalp or nails.
FOR BEST RESULTS, FOLLOW DIRECTIONS AND CONTINUE TREATMENT FOR LENGTH OF TIME INDICATED.

How Supplied: Solution Bottle 10 mL (⅓ fluid ounce)

MYCELEX-7® VAGINAL CREAM ANTIFUNGAL

Active Ingredient: Clotrimazole 1%

Inactive Ingredients: Benzyl alcohol, cetostearyl alcohol, cetyl esters wax, octyldodecanol, polysorbate 60, purified water, sorbitan monostearate

Indications: For treatment of vaginal yeast (Candida) infection.

Actions: Cures most vaginal yeast infections. MYCELEX®-7 Antifungal Vaginal Cream can kill the yeast that may cause vaginal infection. It is greaseless and does not stain clothes.

Precautions: IF THIS IS THE **FIRST** TIME YOU HAVE HAD VAGINAL ITCH AND DISCOMFORT, CONSULT YOUR DOCTOR. IF YOU HAVE HAD A DOCTOR DIAGNOSE A VAGINAL YEAST INFECTION BEFORE AND HAVE THE SAME SYMPTOMS NOW, USE THIS CREAM AS DIRECTED FOR 7 CONSECUTIVE DAYS.

**WARNING: DO NOT USE IF YOU HAVE ABDOMINAL PAIN, FEVER, OR FOUL-SMELLING DISCHARGE. CONTACT YOUR DOCTOR IMMEDIATELY.
IF YOU DO NOT IMPROVE IN 3 DAYS OR IF YOU DO NOT GET WELL IN 7 DAYS, YOU MAY HAVE A CONDITION OTHER THAN A YEAST INFECTION. CONSULT YOUR DOCTOR.** If your symptoms return within two months or if you have infections that do not clear up easily with proper treatment, consult your doctor. You could be pregnant or there could be a serious underlying medical cause for your infections, including diabetes or a damaged immune system (including damage from infection with HIV-the virus that causes AIDS). (PLEASE READ PATIENT PACKAGE PAMPHLET). Do not use during pregnancy except under the advice and supervision of a doctor. Do not use tampons while using this medication. Keep this and all drugs out of the reach of children. In case of accidental ingestion, seek professional assistance or contact a Poison Control Center immediately. **NOT FOR USE IN CHILDREN LESS THAN 12 YEARS OF AGE.**

Dosage and Administration: Before using, read the enclosed pamphlet. **Directions:** Fill the applicator and insert one applicatorful of cream into the vagina, preferably at bedtime. Repeat this procedure daily for 7 consecutive days.

How Supplied: 1.5 oz. (45 g) tube and applicator. (7-Day Therapy)

Shown in Product Identification Guide, page 415

MYCELEX-7® VAGINAL INSERTS ANTIFUNGAL

Active Ingredient: Each insert contains 100 mg clotrimazole.

Inactive Ingredients: Corn starch, lactose, magnesium stearate, povidone.

Indications: For treatment of vaginal yeast (Candida) infection.

Actions: Cures most vaginal yeast infections. MYCELEX-7 Antifungal Vaginal Inserts can kill the yeast that may cause vaginal infection. They do not stain clothes.

Precautions: IF THIS IS THE **FIRST** TIME YOU HAVE HAD VAGINAL ITCH AND DISCOMFORT, CONSULT YOUR DOCTOR. IF YOU HAVE HAD A DOCTOR DIAGNOSE A VAGINAL YEAST INFECTION BEFORE AND HAVE THE SAME SYMPTOMS NOW, USE THESE INSERTS AS DIRECTED FOR 7 CONSECUTIVE DAYS.

**WARNING: DO NOT USE IF YOU HAVE ABDOMINAL PAIN, FEVER, OR FOUL-SMELLING DISCHARGE. CONTACT YOUR DOCTOR IMMEDIATELY.
IF YOU DO NOT IMPROVE IN 3 DAYS OR IF YOU DO NOT GET WELL IN 7 DAYS, YOU MAY HAVE A CONDITION OTHER THAN A YEAST INFECTION. CONSULT YOUR DOCTOR.** If your symptoms return within two months or if you have infections that do not clear up easily with proper treatment, consult your doctor. You could be pregnant or there could be a serious underlying medical cause for your infections, including diabetes or a damaged immune system (including damage from infection with HIV-the virus that causes AIDS). (PLEASE READ PATIENT PACKAGE PAMPHLET) Do not use during pregnancy except under the advice and supervi-

sion of a doctor. Do not use tampons while using this medication. Keep this and all drugs out of the reach of children. In case of accidental ingestion, seek professional assistance or contact a Poison Control Center immediately. **NOT FOR USE IN CHILDREN LESS THAN 12 YEARS OF AGE.**

Dosage and Administration: Before using, read the enclosed pamphlet. **Directions:** Unwrap one insert, place it in the applicator, and use the applicator to place the insert into the vagina, preferably at bedtime. Repeat this procedure daily for 7 consecutive days.

How Supplied: 7 vaginal inserts and applicator. (7-Day Therapy)

ONE–A–DAY® Essential Vitamins
11 Essential Vitamins

Ingredients: One tablet daily of ONE-A-DAY® Essential provides:

Vitamins	Quantity	U.S. RDA
Vitamin A (as Acetate and Beta Carotene)	5000 I.U.	100
Vitamin C	60 mg.	100
Thiamine (B$_1$)	1.5 mg.	100
Riboflavin (B$_2$)	1.7 mg.	100
Niacin	20 mg.	100
Vitamin D	400 I.U.	100
Vitamin E	30 I.U.	100
Vitamin B$_6$	2 mg.	100
Folic Acid	0.4 mg.	100
Vitamin B$_{12}$	6 mcg.	100
Pantothenic Acid	10 mg.	100

Indication: Dietary supplementation.

Dosage and Administration: One tablet daily for adults.

How Supplied: ONE-A-DAY® Essential, bottles of 75's and 130's.
Shown in Product Identification Guide, page 415

ONE-A-DAY® EXTRAS ANTIOXIDANT

Ingredients: Ascorbic Acid, Vitamin E Acetate, Gelatin, Glycerin, Soybean Oil, Selenium Yeast, Lecithin, Zinc Oxide, Vegetable Oil (Partially Hydrogenated Cottonseed and Soybean Oils), Yellow Wax (Beeswax, Yellow) Manganese Sulfate, Beta Carotene, Cupric Oxide, Titanium Dioxide, Artificial Colors including FD&C Yellow #5 (Tartrazine). **EXTRAS** individual supplements can be taken alone or with your everyday multivitamin.

Directions for Use: Adults take one softgel capsule daily. To preserve quality and freshness, keep bottle tightly closed.

VITAMINS	QUANTITY	% US RDA
Vitamin E	200 I.U.	667
Vitamin C	250 mg	417
Vitamin A (as Beta Carotene)	5000 I.U.	100

MINERALS	QUANTITY	% US RDA
Zinc	7.5 mg	50
Copper	1.0 mg	50
Selenium	15.0 mcg	*
Manganese	1.5 mg	*

*No. U.S. RDA established

Indications: ONE-A-DAY EXTRAS ANTIOXIDANT is specially formulated to create a *high potency* **antioxidant supplement that meets a wide range of dietary needs. Antioxidants** may neutralize the effects of free radicals (oxidants) which many scientists believe can be a cause of cell damage. ONE-A-DAY EXTRAS ANTIOXIDANT formula combines the antioxidant nutrients with the essential trace minerals necessary for antioxidant enzyme activity. Easy to swallow softgel capsule.

CHILD RESISTANT CAP
Do not use this product if safety seal bearing Miles logo under cap is torn or missing.

How Supplied: Bottle of 50 softgels.
Shown in Product Identification Guide, page 415

ONE-A-DAY® EXTRAS GARLIC

Ingredients: Garlic Oil Macerate, Gelatin, Glycerin, Sorbitol, Xylose. **EXTRAS** individual supplements can be taken alone or with your everyday multivitamin.

Directions For Use: Adults take one softgel capsule daily. Do not chew. Swallow whole to ensure maximum strength and breath freshness. To preserve quality and freshness, keep bottle tightly closed.

KEEP OUT OF REACH OF CHILDREN

Indications: ONE-A-DAY EXTRAS GARLIC contains 600 mg of concentrated garlic which is equivalent to one garlic clove. Provides the benefits of fresh garlic in one softgel capsule. Easy to swallow high potency softgel capsule.

CHILD RESISTANT CAP
Do not use this product if safety seal bearing Miles logo under cap is torn or missing.

How Supplied: Bottles of 45 softgels
Shown in Product Identification Guide, page 415

ONE-A-DAY® EXTRAS VITAMIN C

Ingredients: Ascorbic Acid, Starch, Cellulose, Stearic Acid, Crospovidone, Lactose, Magnesium Stearate. **EXTRAS** individual supplements can be taken alone or with your everyday multivitamin.

Directions for Use:
Adults take one tablet daily.

VITAMINS	QUANTITY	% U.S. RDA
Vitamin C	500 mg	833

KEEP OUT OF REACH OF CHILDREN

Indications: ONE-A-DAY® EXTRAS VITAMIN C is formulated to give you 500 mg of Vitamin C. Contains high potency level of Vitamin C in one tablet. Vitamin C is an antioxidant nutrient which may neutralize the effects of free radicals (oxidants) which many scientists believe can be a cause of cell damage.

CHILD RESISTANT CAP
Do not use this product if safety seal bearing Miles logo under cap is torn or missing.

How Supplied: Bottle of 100 Tablets
Shown in Product Identification Guide, page 415

ONE-A-DAY® EXTRAS VITAMIN E

Ingredients: Vitamin E Acetate, Gelatin, Glycerin.
EXTRAS individual supplements can be taken alone or with your everyday multivitamin.

Directions for Use:
Adults take one softgel capsule daily. To preserve quality and freshness, keep bottle tightly closed.

VITAMIN	QUANTITY	% U.S. RDA
Vitamin E	400 I.U.	1,333

KEEP OUT OF REACH OF CHILDREN

Indications: ONE-A-DAY EXTRAS VITAMIN E is formulated to give you 400 I.U. of Vitamin E. High potency level of Vitamin E in one easy to swallow softgel capsule. Vitamin E is an antioxidant nutrient which may neutralize the effects of free radicals (oxidants) which many scientists believe can be a cause of cell damage.

CHILD RESISTANT CAP
Do not use this product if safety seal bearing Miles logo under cap is torn or missing.

How Supplied: Bottle of 60 Softgels.
Shown in Product Identification Guide, page 415

ONE-A-DAY® Maximum Multivitamin/Multimineral Supplement for Adults

Ingredients: Dicalcium Phosphate, Magnesium Hydroxide, Cellulose, Potassium Chloride, Ascorbic Acid, Gelatin, Ferrous Fumarate, Zinc Sulfate, Modified Cellulose Gum, Vitamin E Acetate, Citric Acid, Niacinamide, Hydroxypropyl Methylcellulose, Magnesium Stea-

Continued on next page

Miles—Cont.

rate, Calcium Pantothenate, Selenium Yeast, Artificial Color, Polyvinylpyrrolidone, Hydroxypropylcellulose, Manganese Sulfate, Silica, Copper Sulfate, Chromium Yeast, Molybdenum Yeast, Pyridoxine Hydrochloride, Riboflavin, Thiamine Mononitrate, Beta Carotene, Vitamin A Acetate, Folic Acid, Potassium Iodide, Sodium Hexametaphosphate, Biotin, Vitamin D, Vitamin B-12, Lecithin.

One tablet daily of ONE-A-DAY® Maximum provides:

Vitamins	Quantity	% of U.S. RDA
Vitamin A (as Acetate and Beta Carotene)	5000 I.U.	100
Vitamin C	60 mg.	100
Thiamine (B₁)	1.5 mg.	100
Riboflavin (B₂)	1.7 mg.	100
Niacin	20 mg.	100
Vitamin D	400 I.U.	100
Vitamin E	30 I.U.	100
Vitamin B₆	2 mg.	100
Folic Acid	0.4 mg.	100
Vitamin B₁₂	6 mcg.	100
Biotin	30 mcg.	10
Pantothenic Acid	10 mg.	100

Minerals	Quantity	% of U.S. RDA
Iron (Elemental)	18 mg.	100
Calcium (Elemental)	130 mg.	13
Phosphorus	100 mg.	10
Iodine	150 mcg.	100
Magnesium	100 mg.	25
Copper	2 mg.	100
Zinc	15 mg.	100
Chromium	10 mcg.	*
Selenium	10 mcg.	*
Molybdenum	10 mcg.	*
Manganese	2.5 mg.	*
Potassium	37.5 mg.	*
Chloride	34 mg.	*

*No U.S. RDA established

Indication: Dietary supplementation.

Dosage and Administration: One tablet daily for adults.

Precaution: Contains iron, which can be harmful in large doses. Close tightly and keep out of reach of children. In case of overdose, contact a physician or Poison Control Center immediately.

How Supplied: Bottles of 60, and 100 with child-resistant caps.
Shown in Product Identification Guide, page 415

ONE-A-DAY® MEN'S
MULTIVITAMIN SUPPLEMENT

Ingredients: Ascorbic Acid, Calcium Carbonate, Gelatin, Vitamin E Acetate, Starch, Niacinamide, Cellulose, Calcium Silicate, Calcium Pantothenate, Hydroxypropyl Methylcellulose, Artificial Color (FD&C Yellow #6), Hydroxypropylcellulose, Magnesium Stearate, Pyridoxine Hydrochloride, Riboflavin, Thiamine Mononitrate, Vitamin A Acetate, Beta Carotene, Folic Acid, Sodium Hexametaphosphate, Vitamin D, Vitamin B-12, Lecithin.

Directions for Use: Adults take one tablet daily.

Vitamins	Quantity	% U.S. RDA
Vitamin A (as Acetate and Beta Carotene)	5000 I.U.	100
Vitamin C	200 mg	333
Thiamine (B-1)	2.25 mg	150
Riboflavin (B-2)	2.55 mg	150
Niacin	20 mg	100
Vitamin D	400 I.U.	100
Vitamin E	45 I.U.	150
Vitamin B-6	3 mg	150
Folic Acid	0.4 mg	100
Vitamin B-12	9 mcg	150
Pantothenic Acid	10 mg	100

KEEP OUT OF REACH OF CHILDREN

Indications: ONE-A-DAY MEN'S is formulated with 11 essential vitamins plus Extra C, E and B-Vitamins, and contains no iron.
CHILD RESISTANT CAP
Do not use this product if safety seal bearing Miles logo under cap is torn or missing.

How Supplied: Bottles of 60's & 100's
Shown in Product Identification Guide, page 415

ONE-A-DAY® WOMEN'S
Multivitamin/Mineral Supplement
A formula which gives
you 11 essential vitamins plus
extra iron, and calcium & zinc.

Ingredients: One tablet daily of ONE-A-DAY® WOMEN'S FORMULA provides:

Vitamins	Quantity	% of U.S. RDA
Vitamin A (as Acetate and Beta Carotene)	5000 I.U.	100
Vitamin C	60 mg.	100
Thiamine (B₁)	1.5 mg.	100
Riboflavin (B₂)	1.7 mg.	100
Niacin	20 mg.	100
Vitamin D	400 I.U.	100
Vitamin E	30 I.U.	100
Vitamin B₆	2 mg.	100
Folic Acid	0.4 mg.	100
Vitamin B₁₂	6 mcg.	100
Pantothenic Acid	10 mg.	100

Minerals	Quantity	% of U.S. RDA
Iron (Elemental)	27 mg.	150
Calcium (Elemental)	450 mg.	45
Zinc	15 mg.	100

Indication: Dietary supplementation.

Dosage and Administration: One tablet daily.

Precaution: Contains iron, which can be harmful in large doses. Close tightly and keep out of reach of children. In case of overdose, contact a physician or Poison Control Center immediately.

How Supplied: Bottles of 60 and 100 with child-resistant caps.
Shown in Product Identification Guide, page 415

Muro Pharmaceutical, Inc.
890 EAST STREET
TEWKSBURY, MA 01876-1496

BROMFED® SYRUP
Antihistamine-Nasal Decongestant
(alcohol free)
ORANGE-LEMON FLAVOR

Each 5 mL (1 teaspoonful) contains: 2 mg brompheniramine maleate and 30 mg pseudoephedrine hydrochloride; also contains citric acid, FD & C Yellow #6, flavor, glycerin, methyl paraben, sodium benzoate, sodium citrate, sodium saccharin, sorbitol, sucrose, purified water.

Indications: For temporary relief of nasal congestion, sneezing, itchy and watery eyes and running nose due to common cold, hay fever or other upper respiratory allergies.

Directions: Adults and children 12 years of age and over: 2 teaspoonfuls every 4–6 hours. Children 6 to 12 years of age: 1 teaspoonful every 4–6 hours. Do not exceed 4 doses in 24 hours. Children under 6 years of age, consult a physician.

Warnings: If symptoms do not improve within 7 days or are accompanied by high fever, consult a physician before continuing use. May cause drowsiness. May cause excitability especially in children. DO NOT exceed recommended daily dosage because at higher doses nervousness, dizziness, or sleeplessness may occur. **Except under the advice and supervision of a physician:** DO NOT give this product to children under 6 years. DO NOT take this product if you have asthma, glaucoma, difficulty in urination due to enlargement of the prostate gland, high blood pressure, heart disease, diabetes, or thyroid disease. As with any drug, if you are pregnant or nursing a baby, seek the advice of a health professional before using this product.

Caution: Avoid operating a motor vehicle or heavy machinery and alcoholic beverages while taking this product. Keep this and all drugs out of the reach of children.

Drug Interaction Precaution: Do not take this product if you are presently taking a prescription antihypertensive or antidepressant drug containing a monoamine oxidase inhibitor except under the advice and supervision of a physician.

Overdosage: In case of accidental overdose, seek professional assistance or contact a Poison Control Center immediately.

Store between 15° and 30°C (59° and 86°F). Dispense in tight, light resistant, child resistant containers as defined in USP.

How Supplied: NDC 0451-4201-16 For 16 fl. oz. (480 mL), NDC 0451-4201-04 For 4 fl. oz. (120 mL).

GUAIFED® SYRUP
Expectorant/Nasal Decongestant

A red colored, berry citrus flavored syrup.
Each 5mL (teaspoonful) contains:
Pseudoephedrine HCl, USP   30mg
Guaifenesin, USP   200mg
CONTAINS NO ANTIHISTAMINE which may cause drowsiness or excessive drying.

Guaifed® Syrup also contains inactive ingredients:
Benzoic Acid, Berry Citrus Flavor, Citric Acid, FD&C Red #40, Glycerin, Menthol, Polyethylene Glycol, Povidone, Purified Water, Saccharin Sodium, Sodium Citrate, Sorbitol, Vanillin.

Directions: Guaifed® Syrup—Adults and Children 12 years of age and over: Two teaspoonfuls every 4–6 hours, not to exceed eight teaspoonfuls in 24 hours. Children 6 to under 12 years of age: One teaspoonful every 4–6 hours, not to exceed four teaspoonfuls in 24 hours. Children 2 to under 6 years of age: ½ teaspoonful every 4–6 hours, not to exceed two teaspoonfuls in 24 hours. Children under 2 years of age: consult a physician.

How Supplied: Guaifed® Syrup is a red colored, berry citrus flavored syrup supplied in 473 mL bottles (NDC #0451-2601-16) and 118 mL bottles (NDC #0451-2601-04).
Store at controlled room temperature between 15°C and 30°C (59°F and 86°F). Dispense in Child Resistant, tight and light resistant containers.

GUAITAB® TABLETS
Expectorant/Nasal Decongestant

A purple layered tablet
Each tablet contains:
Pseudoephedrine HCl   60mg
Guaifenesin   400mg

GUAITAB® TABLET also contains inactive ingredients: colloidal silicon dioxide, lactose, magnesium stearate, microcrystalline cellulose, pharmaceutical glaze, sodium starch glycolate, starch, talc, FD&C Blue #2, D&C Red #27.

Indications: For the temporary relief of nasal congestion associated with the common cold, sinusitis, hay fever or other upper respiratory allergies. Also helps loosen phlegm (mucus) and thin bronchial secretions to rid the bronchial passageways of bothersome mucus, drain bronchial tubes, and make coughs more productive.

Warnings: Do not exceed recommended dosage because at higher doses nervousness, dizziness or sleeplessness may occur. Do not use if you have high blood pressure, heart disease, diabetes, thyroid disease or a persistent chronic cough, except under the advice and supervision of a physician. Do not take this product for persistent or chronic cough such as occurs with smoking, asthma, chronic bronchitis, or emphysema, or where cough is accompanied by excessive phlegm (mucus) unless directed by a doctor. A persistent cough may be a sign of a serious condition. If cough persists for more than 1 week, tends to recur, or is accompanied by a fever, rash or persistent headache, consult a doctor.

Contraindications: Hypersensitivity to guaifenesin or sympathomimetic amines; marked hypertension, hyperthyroidism; or in patients receiving monoamine oxidase (MAO) inhibitors.

Adverse Reactions: Possible side effects include nausea, vomiting, nervousness, restlessness, rash (including urticaria), headache, or dry mouth.

Drug Interaction Precautions: Do not take this medication if you are presently taking a prescription antihypertensive or antidepressant drug containing a monoamine oxidase inhibitor except under the advice and supervision of a physician.

Geriatrics: Pseudoephedrine should be used with caution in the elderly because they may be more sensitive to the effect of the sympathomimetics.

Note: As with any drug, if you are pregnant or nursing a baby, seek the advice of a health professional before using this product.
In the case of accidental overdose, seek professional assistance or contact a Poison Control Center immediately.
Guaifenesin has been shown to produce a color interference with certain clinical laboratory determinations of 5-hydroxyindoleacetic acid (5-HIAA) and vanillylmandelic acid (VMA).

Directions: Guaitab® Tablets — Adults and Children 12 years of age and over: One Tablet every 4–6 hours, not to exceed four tablets in 24 hours. Children 6 to under 12 years of age: ½ the adult dosage (break tablet in half): ½ tablet every 4–6 hours, not to exceed two tablets in 24 hours.

How Supplied: Guaitab® Tablet is a purple layered Tablet in bottles of 100's. Each scored Tablet is coded "60/400" on one side and "Muro" on the other side. NDC 0451-4600-50.
Store at controlled room temperature between 15°C and 30°C (59°F and 86°F). Dispense in Child Resistant, tight and light resistant containers.

SALINEX® NASAL MIST AND DROPS
Buffered Isotonic Saline Solutions

Ingredients: Sodium Chloride 0.4%. Also contains edetate disodium, hydroxypropyl methylcellulose, sodium phosphate, polyethylene glycol, propylene glycol and purified water. Preservative used is benzalkonium chloride 0.01%.

Indications: Rhinitis Medicamentosa and Rhinitis Sicca. For relief of nasal congestion associated with overuse of nasal sprays, drops and inhalers.
To alleviate crusting due to nose bleeds; to compensate for nasal stuffiness and dryness due to lack of humidity.

Directions: Spray: Squeeze twice in each nostril as needed. Drops: Two drops in each nostril as needed or as directed by physician.

How Supplied: SPRAY: 50 ml plastic spray bottle. NDC 0451-4500-50. DROPS: 15 ml plastic dropper bottle. NDC 0451-4500-85.

Natren Inc.
3105 WILLOW LANE
WESTLAKE VILLAGE, CA 91361

BIFIDO FACTOR®
Bifidobacterium bifidum
Powder
Malyoth Strain

Ingredients: Active—Two billion viable *Bifidobacterium bifidum* strain Malyoth per gram with naturally occurring metabolic products retained in the supernatant. Potency guaranteed through expiration date. Inactive—Nonfat milk, whey.

Dosage: Low Frequency—¼ to ½ tsp. once daily. High Frequency—1 tsp. three times daily.

Precautions: Individuals sensitive to milk should not use this product.

How Supplied: Powder—
1.25 oz.   NDC-539830200-05
2.5 oz.   NDC-539830200-25
4.5 oz.   NDC-539830200-45

PRO-BIFIDONATE®
Bifidobacterium bifidum
Powder
Malyoth Strain

Ingredients: Active—Two billion viable *Bifidobacterium bifidum* strain Malyoth per gram with naturally occurring metabolic products retained in the supernatant. Potency guaranteed through expiration date. Inactive—Garbanzo bean (chick-pea) extract; powder also contains cellulose.

Dosage: Low Frequency—¼ to ½ tsp. once daily. High Frequency—1 tsp. three times daily.

Continued on next page

Natren—Cont.

How Supplied: Powder—
1.75 oz. NDC-539830700-15
3.0 oz. NDC-539830700-25

PRO-BIONATE®
Lactobacillus acidophilus
Powder and Capsules
NAS Strain

Ingredients: Active—Two billion viable *Lactobacillus acidophilus* strain NAS per capsule/gram with naturally occurring metabolic products retained in the supernatant. Potency guaranteed through expiration date. Inactive—Garbanzo bean (chick-pea) extract; powder also contains cellulose.

Dosage:
Capsule – Low Frequency—1 capsule per day. High Frequency—1 capsule three times per day.
Powder – Low Frequency—¼ to ½ tsp. once daily. High Frequency—1 tsp. three times daily.

How Supplied:
Powder—
1.75 oz. NDC-539830600-25
3.0 oz. NDC-539830600-35
Capsules—
30 count NDC-539830600-20
60 count NDC-539830600-15

SUPERDOPHILUS®
Lactobacillus acidophilus
POWDER
DDS-1 Strain

Ingredients: Active—Two billion viable *Lactobacillus acidophilus* strain DDS-1 per gram with naturally occurring metabolic products retained in the supernatant. Potency guaranteed through expiration date. Inactive—Non-fat milk, whey.

Dosage: Low Frequency—¼ to ½ tsp. once daily. High Frequency—1 tsp. three times daily.

Precautions: Individuals sensitive to milk should not use this product.

How Supplied: Powder—
1.25 oz. NDC-539830100-05
2.5 oz. NDC-539830100-15
4.5 oz. NDC-539830100-35

**IF YOU SUSPECT
AN INTERACTION...**
The 1,400-page
PDR Guide to Drug Interactions •
Side Effects • *Indications*
can help.
Use the order form
in the front of this book.

Nature's Bounty, Inc.
**90 ORVILLE DRIVE
BOHEMIA, NY 11716**

ENER–B®
**Vitamin B-12 Nasal Gel
Dietary Supplement**

Description: ENER-B™ is the first intra-nasal application for Vitamin B-12. Each delivery supplies 400 mcg. of Vitamin B-12. This method of delivery provides the highest Vitamin B-12 blood levels that can be obtained without a prescription. Clinical tests show that ENER-B produced 8.4 to 10 times more Vitamin B-12 in the blood than tablets.

Measured Vitamin B-12 Increase in Blood Levels

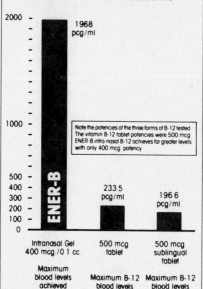

Clinical Tests results are available by writing Nature's Bounty.

Potency and Administration: Each nasal applicator delivers ¹⁄₁₀ cc of gel into the nose which adheres to the mucous membranes providing 400 mcg. of Vitamin B-12. Odorless and non-irritating to the nose.

Directions: As a dietary supplement, one unit every two to three days.

How Supplied: Packages of 12 unit doses. Supplies 400 mcg. of B-12 each.
*Shown in Product Identification
Guide, page 415*

UNKNOWN DRUG?
Consult the
Product Identification Guide
(Gray Pages)
for full-color photos of
leading over-the-counter
medications

Niché Pharmaceuticals, Inc.
**300 TROPHY CLUB DRIVE #400
ROANOKE, TX 76262**

MAGTAB® SR
[măg-tăb]
**(Magnesium L-lactate dihydrate)
Sustained-release Magnesium
Supplement**

Description: MagTab® SR is a sustained release oral magnesium supplement. Each pale yellow caplet contains 7mEq (84 Mg) magnesium as magnesium L-lactate dihydrate (835 Mg in a sustained release wax matrix formulation).

Indications/Uses: As a dietary supplement, MagTab® SR is indicated for patients with, or at risk for, magnesium deficiency. Hypomagnesemia and/or magnesium deficiency can result from inadequate nutritional intake or absorption, alcoholism, or magnesium depleting drugs such as diuretics.

Warnings/Side Effects: Patients with renal disease should not take magnesium supplements without the advice and direct supervision of a physician. Excessive dosage of magnesium can cause loose stools or diarrhea.

Dosage/How Supplied: As a dietary supplement, take 1 or 2 caplets b.i.d. or as directed by a physician. MagTab® SR is available for oral administration as uncoated yellow caplets, in bottles of 60 and 100.
U.S. Patent Number: 5,002,774

Ohm Laboratories, Inc.
**P. O. BOX 279
FRANKLIN PARK, NJ 08823**

CRAMP END
**Ibuprofen Tablets, USP, 200 mg
Menstrual Pain & Cramp Reliever**

WARNING: ASPIRIN-SENSITIVE PATIENTS: Do not take this product if you have had a severe allergic reaction to aspirin, e.g., asthma, swelling, shock or hives, because even though this product contains no aspirin or salicylates, cross-reactions may occur in patients allergic to aspirin.

Indications: For the temporary relief of painful menstrual cramps (Dysmenorrhea); also headaches, backaches and muscular aches and pains associated with Premenstrual Syndrome.

Directions: Adults: Take 1 tablet every 4 to 6 hours at the onset of menstrual symptoms and while pain persists. If pain does not respond to 1 tablet, 2 tablets may be used but do not exceed 6 tablets in 24 hours, unless directed by a doctor. The smallest effective dose should be used. Take with food or milk if occasional and mild heartburn, upset stomach, or stomach pain occurs with use. Consult a doctor if these symptoms are more than mild or if they persist.

Children: Do not give this product to children under 12 except under the advice and supervision of a doctor.

Warnings: Do not take for pain for more than 10 days unless directed by a doctor. If pain persists or gets worse, or if new symptoms occur, consult a doctor. These could be signs of serious illness. If you are under a doctor's care for any serious condition, consult a doctor before taking this product. As with aspirin and acetaminophen, if you have any condition which requires you to take prescription drugs or if you have had any problems or serious side effects from taking any non-prescription pain reliever, do not take this product without first discussing it with your doctor. If you experience any symptoms which are unusual or seem unrelated to the condition for which you took ibuprofen, consult a doctor before taking any more of it. Although ibuprofen is indicated for the same conditions as aspirin and acetaminophen, it should not be taken with them except under a doctor's direction. Do not combine this product with any other ibuprofen-containing product. As with any drug, if you are pregnant or nursing a baby, seek the advice of a health professional before using this product. IT IS **ESPECIALLY IMPORTANT NOT TO USE IBUPROFEN DURING THE LAST 3 MONTHS OF PREGNANCY UNLESS SPECIFICALLY DIRECTED TO DO SO BY A DOCTOR BECAUSE IT MAY CAUSE PROBLEMS IN THE UNBORN CHILD OR COMPLICATIONS DURING DELIVERY.** Keep this and all drugs out of the reach of children. In case of accidental overdose, seek professional assistance or contact a poison control center immediately.

How Supplied: Coated tablets in blister packs of 12's
Store at room temperature; avoid excessive heat 40°C (104°F).

Active Ingredient: Each tablet contains Ibuprofen 200 mg.
Manufactured by OHM LABORATORIES, INC, Franklin Park, NJ 08823

IBUPROHM®
Ibuprofen Tablets, USP
Ibuprofen Caplets, USP

Active Ingredient: Each tablet contains Ibuprofen USP, 200 mg.

Warning: ASPIRIN SENSITIVE PATIENTS: Do not take this product if you have had a severe allergic reaction to aspirin, e.g., asthma, swelling, shock or hives, because even though this product contains no aspirin or salicylates, cross-reactions may occur in patients allergic to aspirin.

Indications: For the temporary relief of minor aches and pains associated with

the common cold, headache, toothache, muscular aches, backache, for the minor pain of arthritis, for the pain of menstrual cramps, and for reduction of fever.

Directions: *Adults:* Take 1 tablet every 4 to 6 hours while symptoms persist. If pain or fever does not respond to 1 tablet, 2 tablets may be used but do not exceed 6 tablets in 24 hours, unless directed by a doctor. The smallest effective dose should be used. Take with food or milk if occasional and mild heartburn, upset stomach, or stomach pain occurs with use. Consult a doctor if these symptoms are more than mild or if they persist. Children: Do not give this product to children under 12 except under the advice and supervision of a doctor.

Warnings: Do not take for pain for more than 10 days or for fever for more than 3 days unless directed by a doctor. If pain or fever persists or gets worse, if new symptoms occur, or if the painful area is red or swollen, consult a doctor. These could be signs of serious illness. If you are under a doctor's care for any serious condition, consult a doctor before taking this product. As with aspirin and acetaminophen, if you have any condition which requires you to take prescription drugs or if you have had any problems or serious side effects from taking any nonprescription pain reliever, do not take this product without first discussing it with your doctor. If you experience any symptoms which are unusual or seem unrelated to the condition for which you took ibuprofen, consult a doctor before taking any more of it. Although ibuprofen is indicated for the same conditions as aspirin and acetaminophen, it should not be taken with them except under a doctor's direction. Do not combine the product with any other ibuprofen-containing product. As with any drug, if you are pregnant or nursing a baby, seek the advice of a health professional before using this product. IT IS ESPECIALLY IMPORTANT NOT TO USE IBUPROFEN DURING THE LAST 3 MONTHS OF PREGNANCY UNLESS SPECIFICALLY DIRECTED TO DO SO BY A DOCTOR BECAUSE IT MAY CAUSE PROBLEMS IN THE UNBORN CHILD OR COMPLICATIONS DURING DELIVERY. Keep this and all drugs out of the reach of children. In case of accidental overdose, seek professional assis-

tance or contact a poison control center immediately.

How Supplied: Coated tablets in bottles of 24, 50, 100, 165, 250, 500 and 1000. Coated caplets in bottles of 24, 50, 100 and 250.

Storage: Store at room temperature; avoid excessive heat 40° (104°F).

LOPERAMIDE HYDROCHLORIDE CAPLETS*
2 mg (Nonprescription Formula)
(Antidiarrheal)

Loperamide Hydrochloride Caplet relieves diarrhea for both adults and children 6 years of age and older, in many cases with just one dose. Each caplet contains loperamide hydrochloride, previously available only in a prescription product. This ingredient has been prescribed for millions of people, and has proven to be an exceptionally safe and effective antidiarrheal medication. Loperamide HCl caplets are small and easy to swallow.

Indication: Loperamide hydrochloride controls the symptoms of diarrhea.

Directions: Drink plenty of clear fluids to help prevent dehydration, which may accompany diarrhea.

Dosage and Administration:
[See table below.]

Warnings: DO NOT USE FOR MORE THAN TWO DAYS UNLESS DIRECTED BY A PHYSICIAN. Do not use if diarrhea is accompanied by high fever (greater than 101°F), or if blood is present in the stool, or if you have had a rash or other allergic reaction to loperamide HCl. If you are taking antibiotics or have a history of liver disease, consult a physician before using this product. As with any drug, if you are pregnant or nursing a baby, seek the advice of a health professional before using this product. Keep this and all drugs out of the reach of children. In case of accidental overdose, seek professional assistance or contact a poison control center immediately.

* Each Caplet (capsule-shaped tablet) contains 2 mg of Loperamide Hydrochloride.

Adults and Children 12 Years of Age and Older	Take 2 caplets after the first loose bowel movement and 1 caplet after each subsequent loose bowel movement but no more than 4 caplets a day for no more than two days.
Children 9–11 Years (60–95 lbs)	Take 1 caplet after the first loose bowel movement and ½ caplet after each subsequent loose bowel movement but no more than 3 caplets a day for no more than two days.
Children 6–8 Years (48–59 lbs)	Take 1 caplet after the first loose bowel movement and ½ caplet after each subsequent loose bowel movement but no more than 2 caplets a day for no more than two days.
Under 6 years old (up to 47 lbs):	**Consult a physician. Not intended for children under 6 years old.**

Continued on next page

Ohm—Cont.

Active Ingredient: Loperamide HCl 2 mg per caplet.

Inactive Ingredients: Croscarmellose sodium, Crospovidone, Hydrogenated vegetable oil, lactose, magnesium stearate, powdered cellulose, pregelatinized starch, FD&C Blue #1 and D&C Yellow #10.
See side panel for expiration date. Store at room temperature 15°–25°C (59°–77°F).

How Supplied: Green scored caplet with "122" engraved on the other side. The caplets in 6's, 10's, 12's, and 20's blister packaging which is tamper resistant and child resistant.

P & S Laboratories
**210 WEST 131st STREET
LOS ANGELES, CA 90061**

See Standard Homeopathic Company.

PRN Laboratories, Inc.
1275 BENNETT DRIVE

**SUITE 122
LONGWOOD, FLORIDA 32750
(407) 260 2225 local
(800) 881 2201 national watts
(800) 761 1210 fax**

PAIN FREE NATURAL AND PAIN FREE ALOE VERA GEL®

Composition: Aloe gel, carbopol 940, capsaicin (.025%), hydantoin, oleoresin of capsicum, DMDM, hydantoin, tetrasodium, germall 115, polysorbate, filtered water, triethanolamine.

Indications: For pain, relief of minor arthritis, backache, simple sprains, strains, fibromyalgia and pain associated with chronic fatigue and reflex sympathetic syndrome.

Actions: Although the precise mechanism of action is not fully understood, current scientific evidence suggests that capsaicin, a derivative from hot peppers, acts against pain by affecting a brain chemical known as substance P, thought to be a key to the tranmission of pain.

Warnings: FOR EXTERNAL USE ONLY. Keep out of reach of children. *Wash* hands thoroughly after application. Keep this and any analgesic products away from eyes, mouth and other mucous membranes.

Dosage and Administration: Apply a liberal amount (with Pain Free Natural), apply a dime-sized amount (with Pain Free Aloe Gel) to painful muscles and joints and gently massage until the Pain Free is absorbed in. Can be used before and after exercise. Repeat as needed for temporary relief of minor arthritis pain, bursitis pain, strains, sprains and cramps. Additional uses to help relieve pain from shingles and diabetic neuropathy have recently been discovered.

How Supplied:
1 oz. NDC 60459-0921-10 (aloe gel)
4 oz. NDC 60459-0921-40 (P.F. Natural)
4 oz. NDC 60459-0924-40 (P.F. Aloe)
Gallon NDC 60459-0922-80 (P.F. Aloe)

Parke-Davis
**Consumer Health Products Group
Division of Warner-Lambert
　　Company
201 TABOR ROAD
MORRIS PLAINS, NJ 07950
(See also Warner-Lambert)**

AGORAL® Raspberry
AGORAL® Marshmallow
[ă′gō-răl″]

Description: Each tablespoonful (15 mL) of Agoral Raspberry (pink) or of Agoral Marshmallow (white) contains 4.2 grams mineral oil and 0.2 gram phenolphthalein in a thoroughly homogenized emulsion.
Also contains acacia; agar; benzoic acid; egg albumin; flavors; glycerin; sodium benzoate; tragacanth; citric acid or sodium hydroxide to adjust pH; water. Agoral Raspberry Flavor also contains D&C Red No. 30 Lake and saccharin sodium.

Actions: Agoral, containing mineral oil, facilitates defecation by lubricating the fecal mass and softening the stool. More effective than nonemulsified oil in penetrating the feces, Agoral thereby greatly reduces the possibility of oil leakage at the anal sphincter. Phenolphthalein gently stimulates motor activity of the lower intestinal tract. Agoral's combined lubricating-softening and peristaltic actions can help to restore a normal pattern of evacuation.

Indications: Relief of occasional constipation. This product generally produces bowel movement in 6–8 hours.

Contraindication: Sensitivity to phenolphthalein.

Warning: Do not use laxative products when abdominal pain, nausea, or vomiting are present unless directed by a physician. If you have noticed a sudden change in bowel habits that persists over a period of 2 weeks, consult a physician before using a laxative. Laxative products should not be used for a period longer than 1 week unless directed by a physician. Rectal bleeding or failure to have a bowel movement after use of a laxative may indicate a serious condition. Discontinue use and consult your physician. Do not administer to children under 6 years of age, to pregnant women, to bedridden patients or to persons with difficulty swallowing. As with any drug, if you are nursing a baby, seek the advice of a health professional before using this product. Do not take with meals. If skin rash appears, do not use this product or any other preparation containing phenolphthalein. Keep this and all drugs out of the reach of children. In case of accidental overdose, seek professional assistance or contact a Poison Control Center immediately. Drug interaction precaution: Do not take this product if you are presently taking a stool softener laxative.

Dosage: Agoral Raspberry and Marshmallow—Adults—½ to 1 tablespoonful at bedtime only, unless other time is advised by physician. Children—Over 6 years, ½ to ¾ teaspoonfuls at bedtime only, unless other time is advised by physician. This product generally produces bowel movement in 6 to 8 hours.

Supplied: Agoral (raspberry flavor), plastic bottles of 16 fl oz. Agoral (marshmallow flavor), plastic bottles of 16 fl oz. **Store between 15°–30° C (59°–86° F). Keep this and all drugs out of the reach of children.**
In case of accidental overdose, seek professional assistance or contact a Poison Control Center immediately.

ANUSOL®
[ă′nū-sōl″]
Suppositories/Ointment

Description:
Anusol Suppositories: Active Ingredients: Phenylephrine HCl 0.25% and Hard Fat 88.7%. Also contains: Corn Starch, Methylparaben and Propylparaben.
Anusol Ointment: Active ingredients: Pramoxine HCl 1%, Mineral Oil 46.7% and Zinc Oxide 12.5%. Also contains: Benzyl Benzoate, Calcium Phosphate Dibasic, Cocoa Butter, Glyceryl Monooleate Glyceryl Monostearate, Kaolin, Peruvian Balsam and Polyethylene Wax.

Actions: Anusol Suppositories and Anusol Ointment help to relieve burning, itching and discomfort arising from irritated anorectal tissues. They have a soothing, lubricant action on mucous membranes. Pramoxine Hydrochloride in Anusol Ointment is a rapidly acting local anesthetic for the skin and mucous membranes of the anus and rectum. Pramoxine HCl is also chemically distinct from procaine, cocaine, and dibucaine and can often be used in the patient previously sensitized to other surface anesthetics. Surface analgesia lasts for several hours.

Indications: Anusol Ointment: Temporarily relieves the pain, soreness, and burning of hemorrhoids and other anorectal disorders while it forms a temporary protective coating over inflamed tissues. Anusol Suppositories: Temporarily shrinks the swelling associated with irritated hemorrhoidal tissues, and gives temporary relief from the itching, burning and discomfort of hemorrhoids and other anorectal disorders.

Contraindications: Anusol Suppositories and Anusol Ointment are contraindicated in those patients with a history of hypersensitivity to any of the components of the preparations.

Warnings: Anusol Ointment: Certain persons can develop allergic reactions to ingredients in this product. If the symptom being treated does not subside, if condition worsens or does not improve within 7 days, if redness, irritation, swelling, pain, or other symptoms develop or increase, discontinue use and consult a physician promptly. Do not exceed the recommended daily dosage unless directed by a physician. Do not put this product into the rectum by using fingers or any mechanical device or applicator. Keep this and all drugs out of the reach of children. In case of accidental ingestion seek professional advice or contact a Poison Control Center immediately. Anusol Suppositories: Do not exceed recommended daily dosage unless directed by a physician. Do not use this product if you have heart disease, high blood pressure, thyroid disease, diabetes, or difficulty in urination due to enlargement of the prostate gland unless directed by a physician. It condition worsens or does not improve within 7 days, consult a physician. In case of bleeding, consult a doctor. Keep this and all drugs out of the reach of children. In case of accidental ingestion seek professional advice or contact a Poison Control Center immediately. As with any drug, if you are pregnant or nursing a baby, seek the advice of a health professional before using this product.

Adverse Reactions: Upon application of Anusol Ointment, which contains Pramoxine HCl, a patient may occasionally experience burning, especially if the anoderm is not intact. Sensitivity reactions have been rare; discontinue medication if suspected. Certain persons can develop allergic reactions to ingredients in this product.

Drug Interaction Precaution: Anusol Suppositories: Do not use this product if you are presently taking a prescription drug for high blood pressure or depression without consulting a physician

Directions: Anusol Suppositories: Adults: When practical, cleanse the affected area with Tucks® Hemorrhoidal Pads or mild soap and warm water and rinse thoroughly. Gently dry by patting or blotting with toilet tissue or soft cloth before application of this product. Remove foil wrapper and insert suppository into the anus. Insert one suppository rectally up to four times daily: one in the morning, one in the evening, and one after each bowel movement. Children under 12 years of age: consult a physician. Anusol Ointment: Adults: When practical, cleanse the affected area with Tucks® Hemorrhoidal Pads or mild soap

and warm water and rinse thoroughly. Gently dry by patting or blotting with toilet tissue or soft cloth before application of this product. Apply ointment externally to the affected area up to five (5) times daily. To use dispensing cap, attach it to tube, lubricate well, then gently insert part way into the anus. Squeeze tube to deliver medication. Thoroughly cleanse dispensing cap after use. Children under 12 years of age: Consult a physician.
NOTE: If staining from either of the above products occurs, the stain may be removed from fabric by hand or machine washing with household detergent.

How Supplied: Anusol Suppositories— boxes of 12, 24 and 48; in silver foil strips. Anusol Ointment—1-oz tubes and 2-oz tubes with plastic applicator. Store between 15° and 30°C (59° and 86°F).
Shown in Product Identification Guide, page 415

ANUSOL HC-1

Active Ingredient: Hydrocortisone Acetate (equivalent to 1% Hydrocortisone).

Inactive Ingredients: Diazolidinyl Urea, Methylparaben, Microcrystalline Wax, Mineral Oil, Propylene Glycol, Propylparaben, Sorbitan Sesquioleate and White Petrolatum.

Indications: Temporarily relieves itch associated with external anal inflammation and irritation. Other uses of this product should be only under the advice and supervision of a physician.

Warnings: For external use only. Avoid contact with the eyes. If condition worsens, or if symptoms persist for more than 7 days or clear up and occur again within a few days, stop use of this product and do not begin use of any other hydrocortisone product unless you have consulted a physician. Do not exceed the recommended daily dosage unless directed by a physician. In case of bleeding, consult a physician promptly. Do not put this product into the rectum by using fingers or any mechanical device or applicator. Do not use for treatment of diaper rash. Consult a physician. Keep this and all drugs out of the reach of children. In case of accidental ingestion seek professional assistance or contact a Poison Control Center immediately.

Dosage and Administration: Adults: when practical cleanse affected area with mild soap and warm water. Rinse thoroughly. Gently dry by patting or blotting with tissue or soft cloth before application. Apply to affected area not more than 3 to 4 times daily. Children under 12 years: do not use, consult a physician.

How Supplied: Anusol HC-1 Ointment in 0.7 oz tube. Store at 59°–86°F.
Shown in Product Identification Guide, page 416

BENADRYL Children's Formula Itch Relief Cream
BENADRYL Itch Relief Cream Maximum Strength, 2%

Active Ingredients: Children's Formula contains Benadryl® (diphenhydramine hydrochloride USP) 1%; Maximum Strength contains Benadryl® (diphenhydramine hydrochloride USP) 2%.

Inactive Ingredients: Aloe Vera, Cetyl Alcohol, Diazolidinyl Urea, Methylparaben, Polyethylene Glycol Monostearate 1000, Propylene Glycol, Propylparaben, and Water Purified.

Indications: For the temporary relief of itching and pain associated with insect bites, allergic itches, minor skin irritations and rashes due to poison ivy, poison oak or poison sumac.

Actions: Benadryl is the most prescribed topical antihistamine available. It stops the itch at the source by blocking the action of histamine that causes the itch. Benadryl also provides local anesthetic action to stop the pain plus there is aloe to soothe the skin. Benadryl gives you the kind of itch and pain relief that you can't get from hydrocortisone. Benadryl cream is a soothing greaseless, vanishing cream.

Warnings: For external use only. Do not use on chicken pox, measles, blisters, or on extensive areas of skin except as directed by a physician. Avoid contact with the eyes. If condition worsens, or if symptoms persist for more than 7 days, or clear up and occur again within a few days, discontinue use of this product and consult a physician. Do not use any other drugs containing diphenhydramine while using this product. KEEP THIS AND ALL DRUGS OUT OF THE REACH OF CHILDREN. In case of accidental ingestion, seek professional assistance or contact a Poison Control Center immediately.

Dosage and Administration: Children's Formula For children 2 years of age and older: Apply to affected area not more than three to four times daily, or as directed by a physician. For children under 2 years of age: consult a physician. Maximum Strength 2%—For adults and children 12 years of age and older: Apply to affected area not more than three to four times daily, or as directed by a physician. For children under 12 years of age: consult a physician.

How Supplied: Benadryl Itch Relief Cream is available in ½ oz. Children's

Continued on next page

This product information was prepared in November 1993. On these and other Parke-Davis Products, detailed information may be obtained by addressing PARKE-DAVIS, Consumer Health Products Group, Division of Warner-Lambert Company, Morris Plains, NJ 07950.

Parke-Davis—Cont.

Formula and ½ oz. Maximum Strength tubes.

Shown in Product Identification Guide, page 416

BENADRYL®
[bĕ 'nă-drĭl]
Decongestant Elixir

Description: Each teaspoonful (5 mL) contains: Benadryl (diphenhydramine hydrochloride) 12.5 mg; pseudoephedrine hydrochloride 30 mg; alcohol 5%. Also contains: FD&C Yellow No. 6; glucose, liquid; glycerin, USP; flavors; menthol, USP; saccharin sodium, USP; sodium citrate, USP; sucrose, NF; water, purified, USP.

Indications: Temporarily relieves nasal congestion, runny nose, sneezing, itching of the nose or throat, itchy, watery eyes due to hay fever or other upper respiratory allergies, and runny nose, sneezing and nasal congestion of the common cold.

Warnings: Do not exceed recommended dosage because at higher doses nervousness, dizziness, or sleeplessness may occur. Do not take this product for more than 7 days. If symptoms do not improve or are accompanied by fever, consult a physician. Do not take this product if you have high blood pressure, heart disease, diabetes, thyroid disease, glaucoma, or difficulty in urination due to enlargement of the prostate gland, or breathing problems such as emphysema, or chronic pulmonary disease, unless directed by a physician. May cause excitability, especially in children. May cause marked drowsiness; alcohol, sedatives and tranquilizers may increase the drowsiness effect. Avoid driving a motor vehicle or operating machinery or drinking alcoholic beverages while taking this product. Do not take this product if you are taking sedatives or tranquilizers without first consulting your physician.

Do not use other products containing diphenhydramine while using this product. As with any drug, if you are pregnant or nursing a baby seek the advice of a health professional before using this product. Keep this and all drugs out of the reach of children. In case of accidental overdose, seek professional assistance or contact a Poison Control Center immediately.

Drug Interaction Precaution: Do not take this product if you are presently taking a prescription drug for high blood pressure or depression without first consulting your physician.

Directions: Follow dosage recommendations below, or as recommended by your doctor.
[See table below.]

How Supplied: Benadryl Decongestant Elixir is supplied in 4-oz bottles. Store below 30° C (86°F). Protect from freezing.

Shown in Product Identification Guide, page 416

BENADRYL® Decongestant
[bĕ 'nă-drĭl]
Decongestant Tablets

Active Ingredients: Each tablet contains: Benadryl® (diphenhydramine hydrochloride USP) 25 mg. and pseudoephedrine hydrochloride 60 mg.

Inactive Ingredients: Each tablet contains: Corn Starch, Croscarmellose Sodium, Dibasic Calcium Phosphate Dihydrate, FD&C Blue No. 1 Aluminum Lake, Hydroxypropyl Methylcellulose, Microcrystalline Cellulose, Polyethylene Glycol, Polysorbate 80, Stearic Acid, Titanium Dioxide and Zinc Stearate.

Indications: Temporarily relieves nasal congestion, runny nose, sneezing, itching of the nose or throat, itchy, watery eyes due to hay fever or other upper respiratory allergies, and runny nose, sneezing and nasal congestion of the common cold.

Warning: Do not exceed recommended dosage because at higher doses nervousness, dizziness, or sleeplessness may occur. Do not take this product for more than 7 days. If symptoms do not improve or are accompanied by fever, consult a physician. Do not take this product if you have high blood pressure, heart disease, diabetes, thyroid disease, asthma, glaucoma, or difficulty in urination due to enlargement of the prostate gland, or breathing problems such as emphysema, or chronic pulmonary disease, unless directed by a physician. May cause excitability, especially in children. May cause marked drowsiness; alcohol, sedatives and tranquilizers may increase the drowsiness effect. Avoid driving a motor vehicle or operating machinery or drinking alcoholic beverages while taking this product. Do not take this product if you are taking sedatives or tranquilizers without first consulting your physician. Do not use other products containing diphenhydramine while using this product. As with any drug, if you are pregnant or nursing a baby seek the advice of a health professional before using this product. Keep this and all drugs out of the reach of children. In case of accidental overdose, seek professional assistance or contact a Poison Control Center immediately.

Drug Interaction Precaution: Do not take this product if you are presently taking a prescription drug for high blood pressure or depression without first consulting your physician.

Directions: Adults and children over 12 years of age: 1 tablet every 4 to 6 hours not to exceed 4 tablets in 24 hours. Benadryl Decongestant is not recommended for children under 12 years of age, except under the advice of a physician.

How Supplied: Benadryl Decongestant Tablets are supplied in boxes of 24. Store at room temperature 15°–30° C (59°–86° F).
Protect from moisture.

Shown in Product Identification Guide, page 416

BENADRYL® Elixir

Active Ingredient: Each teaspoonful (5 mL) contains Benadryl (Diphenhydramine HCl) 12.5 mg.

Inactive Ingredients: Citric Acid, D&C Red No. 33, FD&C No. 40, Flavors, Glycerin, Poloxamer 407, Polysorbate 20, Sodium Benzoate, Sodium Citrate, Sodium Saccharin, Sugar, Water.

Indications: AS AN ANTIHISTAMINE: Benadryl relieves runny nose, sneezing, itching of the nose or throat and itchy, watery eyes due to hay fever or other upper respiratory allergies and runny nose and sneezing associated with the common cold.
AS AN ANTITUSSIVE: Benadryl provides relief of cough due to minor throat and bronchial irritations as may occur

BENADRYL DECONGESTANT ELIXIR

AGE	WEIGHT	DOSAGE
Under 2 years	Under 24 lbs	Consult a Physician
2 to 6 years*	24 to 47 lbs.	½ teaspoonful every 4 to 6 hours not to exceed 2 teaspoonfuls in 24 hours
6 to under 12 years	48 to 95 lbs.	1 teaspoonful every 4 to 6 hours not to exceed 4 teaspoonfuls in 24 hours
12 years & older	96 lbs & over	2 teaspoonfuls every 4 to 6 hours not to exceed 8 teaspoonfuls in 24 hours

*PROFESSIONAL LABELING ONLY

with common cold or with inhaled irritants.

Directions: Follow dosage recommendations below or use as recommended by your physician. [See table right.]

Warnings: Do not take this product, unless directed by a doctor, if you have persistent or chronic cough, breathing problems such as occurs with smoking, asthma, emphysema, chronic bronchitis, or if cough is accompanied by excessive phlegm (mucus), or if you have glaucoma or difficulty in urination due to enlargment of the prostate gland. A persistent cough may be a sign of a serious condition. If cough persists for more than one week, tends to recur, or is accompanied by fever, rash, or persistent headache, consult a physician. May cause excitability especially in children. May cause marked drowsiness; alcohol, sedative and tranquilizers may increase the drowsiness effect. Avoid driving a motor vehicle, operating machinery, or drinking alcoholic beverages while taking this product. Do not take this product if you are taking sedative or tranquilizers, without first consulting your doctor. Do not use any other products containing diphenhydramine while using this product. As with any drug, if you are pregnant or nursing a baby seek the advice of a health professional before using this product. KEEP THIS AND ALL DRUGS OUT OF THE REACH OF CHILDREN. In case of accidental overdose, seek professional assistance or contact a Poison Control Center immediately.

How Supplied: Benadryl Elixir is supplied in 4 and 8 fluid ounces bottles.

Shown in Product Identification Guide, page 416

BENADRYL® 25
[bĕ 'nă-drĭl]
Tablets and Kapseals®

Active Ingredient: Each tablet/kapseal contains: Benadryl (Diphenhydramine HCl) 25 mg.

Inactive Ingredients: Each tablet contains: Corn Starch, Croscarmellose Sodium, Dibasic Calcium Phosphate Dihydrate, D&C Red No. 27 Aluminum Lake, Hydroxypropyl Methylcellulose, Microcrystalline Cellulose, Polyethylene Glycol, Polysorbate 80, Stearic Acid, Titanium Dioxide and Zinc Stearate. Each Kapseal capsule contains: Lactose (hydrous) and Magnesium Stearate. The Kapseal capsule shell contains: Artificial Colors, Gelatin, Glyceryl Mono-oleate, PEG-200 Ricinoleate, and Titanium Dioxide.

Indications: AS AN ANTIHISTAMINE: Benadryl relieves runny nose, sneezing, itching of the nose or throat, itchy, watery eyes due to hay fever or other upper respiratory allergies and runny nose and sneezing associated with the common cold.

AGE	WEIGHT	ANTITUSSIVE DOSAGE	ANTIHISTAMINE DOSAGE
Under 2 years	Under 24 lbs	Consult a Physician	Consult a Physician
2 to under 6 years*	24 to 47 lbs.	6.25 mg (½ teaspoonful) every 4 hours not to exceed 3 teaspoonfuls in 24 hours	6.25 mg (½ teaspoonful) every 4 to 6 hours not to exceed 3 teaspoonfuls in 24 hours
6 to under 12 years	48 to 95 lbs.	12.5 mg (1 teaspoonful) every 4 hours not to exceed 6 teaspoonfuls in 24 hours	12.5 to 25 mg (1–2 teaspoonfuls) every 4 to 6 hours not to exceed 12 teaspoonfuls in 24 hours
12 years & older	96 lbs & over	25 mg (2 teaspoonfuls) every 4 hours not to exceed 12 teaspoonfuls in 24 hours	25 to 50 mg (2–4 teaspoonfuls) every 4 to 6 hours not to exceed 24 teaspoonfuls in 24 hours

*PROFESSIONAL LABELING ONLY

AS AN ANTITUSSIVE: Benadryl provides relief of cough due to minor throat and bronchial irritations as may occur with the common cold or with inhaled irritants.

Directions: ANTIHISTAMINE DOSAGE: Adult oral dosage is 25 to 50 mg (1 to 2 tablets/kapseals) every 4 to 6 hours not to exceed 12 tablets/kapseals in 24 hours, or as directed by a physician. Children 6 to under 12 years of age: oral dosage is 12.5 mg* to 25 mg (1 tablet/kapseal) every 4 to 6 hours, not to exceed 6 tablets/kapseals in 24 hours, or as directed by a physician. For children under 6 years of age your physician should be contacted for recommended dosage.
ANTITUSSIVE DOSAGE: Adult oral dose is 25 mg (1 tablet/kapseal) every 4 hours not to exceed 6 tablets/kapseals in 24 hours, or as directed by a physician. Children 6 to under 12 years of age: oral dose is 12.5 mg* every 4 hours not to exceed 3 tablets/kapseals in 24 hours. Children under 6 years of age consult a physician for recommended dosage.

How Supplied: Benadryl tablets and kapseals are supplied in boxes of 24 and 48.
Store at room temperature 15°–30° C (59°–86° F). Protect from moisture.

* This dosage is not available in this package. Do not attempt to break tablet/kapseal. This dosage is available in a pleasant tasting Benadryl Elixir.

Shown in Product Identification Guide, page 416

BENADRYL® Allergy Sinus Headache Formula

Active Ingredients: Each caplet contains Benadryl® (diphenhydramine HCl) 12.5 mg, pseudoephedrine HCl 30 mg and acetaminophen 500 mg.

Inactive Ingredients: Candelilla Wax, Carboxymethyl Cellulose, Corn Starch, Croscarmellose Sodium, D&C Yellow No. 10 Aluminum Lake, FD&C Blue No. 1 Aluminum Lake, FD&C Yellow No. 6 Aluminum Lake, Hydroxypropyl Cellulose, Hydroxypropyl Methylcellulose, Microcrystalline Cellulose, Polyethylene Glycol, Polysorbate 80, Stearic Acid, Titanium Dioxide, Zinc Stearate.

Indications: Temporarily relieves runny nose: sneezing; itching of the nose or throat; itchy, watery eyes; nasal congestion; sinus pain/pressure and headache due to hay fever or other upper respiratory allergies.

Action: BENADRYL ALLERGY/SINUS/HEADACHE is specially formulated to provide effective relief of your upper respiratory allergy symptoms complicated by sinus and headache problems. It combines the strength of BENADRYL to relieve your runny nose: sneezing; itchy water eyes; itchy nose or throat with a maximum strength NASAL DECONGESTANT to relieve nasal and sinus congestion and a maximum strength non-aspirin PAIN RELIEVER to relieve sinus pain and headache.

Warnings: Do not take this product for more than 7 days. Do not use any other drug containing diphenhydramine while using this product. Consult a physician promptly if symptoms do not improve or

Continued on next page

This product information was prepared in November 1993. On these and other Parke-Davis Products, detailed information may be obtained by addressing PARKE-DAVIS, Consumer Health Products Group, Division of Warner-Lambert Company, Morris Plains, NJ 07950.

Parke-Davis—Cont.

are accompanied by fever that lasts for more than 3 days or if new symptoms occur. Do not exceed recommended dosage because at higher doses nervousness, dizziness, or sleeplessness may occur. May cause marked drowsiness; alcohol, sedatives and tranquilizers may increase the drowsiness effect. Avoid driving a motor vehicle or operating machinery or drinking alcoholic beverages while taking this product. Do not take this product if you are presently taking sedatives or tranquilizers, without first consulting your physician. Do not take this product if you have high blood pressure, heart disease, diabetes, thyroid disease, glaucoma, or difficulty in urination due to enlargement of the prostate gland, or breathing problems such as emphysema or chronic pulmonary disease, unless directed by a physician. As with any drug, if you are pregnant or nursing a baby, seek the advice of a health professional before using this product. Keep this and all drugs out of the reach of children. In case of accidental overdose seek professional assistance or contact a Poison Control Center immediately.

Drug Interaction Precaution: Do not take this product if you are presently taking a prescription drug for high blood pressure or depression without first consulting your doctor.

Directions: Adults and children over 12 years of age: two (2) caplets every 6 hours, not to exceed 8 caplets in a 24 hour period. Benadryl Allergy Sinus Headache Formula is not recommended for children under 12 years of age.

How Supplied: Benadryl Allergy Sinus Headache Formula is available in boxes of 24. Store at room temperature, 15°–30°C (59°–86°F).

Shown in Product Identification Guide, page 416

BENADRYL® COLD/FLU
Tablets

Active Ingredients: Each tablet contains: Benadryl® (diphenhydramine hydrochloride USP) 12.5 mg., pseudoephedrine hydrochloride 30 mg., and acetaminophen 500 mg.

Inactive Ingredients: Each tablet contains: Carboxymethylcellulose, Croscarmellose Sodium, Hydroxypropyl Cellulose, Hydroxypropyl Methylcellulose, Magnesium Stearate, Microcrystalline Cellulose, Polyethylene Glycol, Propylene Glycol, Starch, Stearic Acid, Titanium Dioxide, and Zinc Stearate.

Indications: Benadryl Cold/Flu has been specially formulated to provide fast and effective relief of the symptoms of common colds and flu. Benadryl Cold/Flu tablets combine maximum strength ingredients for relief of nasal congestion, body aches and fever, with the trusted

relief of Benadryl for runny nose and sneezing.

Warnings: Do not take this product for more than 7 days. Consult a physician promptly for the following: (1) If symptoms do not improve or are accompanied by fever that lasts for more than 3 days or if new symptoms occur; (2) If sore throat is severe, persists for more than 2 days, is accompanied or followed by fever, headache, rash, nausea, or vomiting. Do not exceed recommended dosage because at higher doses nervousness, dizziness, or sleeplessness may occur. May cause excitability, especially in children. May cause marked drowsiness; alcohol, sedatives and tranquilizers may increase the drowsiness effect. Avoid driving a motor vehicle or operating heavy machinery, or drinking alcoholic beverages. Do not take this product if you are presently taking sedatives or tranquilizers without first consulting your physician. Do not use other products containing diphenhydramine while using this product. Do not take this product if you have high blood pressure, heart disease, diabetes, thyroid disease, glaucoma, or difficulty in urination due to enlargement of the prostate gland or breathing problems such as emphysema or chronic pulmonary disease, unless directed by a physician. As with any drug, if you are pregnant or nursing a baby, seek the advice of a health professional before using this product. Keep this and all drugs out of the reach of children. In case of accidental overdose seek professional assistance or contact a Poison Control Center immediately.

Drug Interaction Precaution: Do not take this product if you are presently taking a prescription drug for high blood pressure or depression without consulting your physician.

Directions: Adults (12 years and over): Two tablets every 6 hours, not to exceed 8 tablets in a 24-hour period. Benadryl Cold/Flu is not recommended for children under 12 years of age.

How Supplied: Benadryl Cold/Flu Tablets are supplied in boxes of 24. Store at room temperature 15°–30°C (59°–86°F). Protect from moisture.

Shown in Product Identification Guide, page 416

BENADRYL® Spray Children's Formula
BENADRYL® Spray Maximum Strength 2%

Active Ingredients: Children's Formula contains Benadryl® (diphenhydramine hydrochloride USP) 1%, Zinc Acetate 0.1%; Maximum Strength contains Benadryl® (diphenhydramine hydrochloride USP) 2%, Zinc Acetate 0.1%.

Inactive Ingredients: Alcohol, Aloe Vera, Glycerin, Povidone, Tromethamine, and Water, Purified.

Indications: For the temporary relief of itching and pain associated with insect bites, allergic itches, minor skin irritations and rashes due to poison ivy, poison oak, or poison sumac. Dries the oozing and weeping of poison ivy, poison oak, and poison sumac.

Actions: Benadryl Spray forms a clear, anti-itch "bandage" to protect and relieve affected areas. Benadryl stops the itch at the source by blocking the action of histamine that causes the itch. Benadryl also provides an anesthetic action to soothe the pain and aloe to soothe the skin. The spray feature allows soothing relief without touching or rubbing the affected area. Benadryl spray is clear, won't stain clothing and won't rinse off (can be easily removed with soap and water).

Warnings: FOR EXTERNAL USE ONLY. Do not use on chicken pox, measles, blisters, or extensive areas of skin except as directed by a physician. Avoid contact with the eyes. If condition worsens, or if symptoms persist for more than 7 days or clear up and occur again within a few days, discontinue use of this product and consult a physician. Do not use any other drugs containing diphenhydramine while using this product. KEEP THIS AND ALL DRUGS OUT OF THE REACH OF CHILDREN. In case of accidental ingestion, seek professional assistance or contact a Poison Control Center immediately. Flammable, keep away from fire or flame.

Dosage and Administration: Children's Formula—For children 2 years of age and older: Spray on affected area not more than three to four times daily, or as directed by a physician. For children under 2 years of age: consult a physician. **Maximum Strength 2%**—For adults and children 12 years of age or older: Spray on affected area not more than three to four times daily, or as directed by a physician. For children under 12 years of age: consult a physician.

How Supplied: Benadryl® Spray is available in a 2 oz. pump spray bottle.
Shown in Product Identification Guide, page 416

BENYLIN® Adult Formula
Cough Suppressant

Active Ingredient: Each teaspoonful (5 ml) contains: Dextromethorphan HBr 15 mg. Also contains: Caramel, Citric Acid, D&C Red No. 33, FD&C Red No. 40, Flavors, Glycerin, Poloxamer 407, Polysorbate 20, Sodium Benzoate, Sodium Carboxymethyl Cellulose, Sodium Citrate, Sodium Saccharin, Sorbitol Solution, and Water.

Warnings: A persistent cough may be a sign of a serious condition. If cough persists for more than one week, tends to recur, or is accompanied by fever, rash or persistent headache, consult a physician. Do not take this product for persistent or

Precaution: Keep this and all drugs out of the reach of children.

Symptoms and Treatment of Oral Overdosage: In case of accidental overdose, seek professional help or contact a Poison Control Center immediately.

Dosage and Administration: Adults 2 tablets or caplets every 6 hours, not to exceed 8 tablets or caplets in 24 hours or as directed by physician. Children under 12 should use only as directed by physician.

How Supplied: Sinutab® Sinus Medication, Maximum Strength Without Drowsiness Formula, Caplets are orange and coated. The Tablets are orange and uncoated. They are supplied in child-resistant blister packs in boxes of 24 tablets or caplets and in boxes of 48 caplets.
Shown in Product Identification Guide, page 417

TUCKS®
Pre-moistened Hemorrhoidal/Vaginal Pads

Indications: For prompt, temporary relief of minor external itching, burning and irritation associated with hemorrhoids.
—Soothe, cool, and comfort itching, burning, and irritation of sensitive rectal and outer vaginal areas.
—As a compress, to help relieve discomfort from rectal/vaginal surgical stitches.
—Effective hygienic wipe to cleanse rectal area of irritation-causing residue.

Directions: For external use only. *As a hemorrhoidal treatment* —Adults: When practical, cleanse the affected area with soap and warm water, and rinse thoroughly. Gently dry by patting or blotting with toilet tissue or soft cloth before each application of this product. Gently apply to affected area by patting and then discard. Can be used up to six times daily or after each bowel movement. Children under 12 years of age: consult a physician.
As a hygienic wipe —Use as a wipe instead of toilet tissue after bowel movement or after napkin or tampon change.
As a moist compress —For soothing relief, fold pad and place in contact with irritated tissue. Leave in place for 5 to 15 minutes. Repeat as needed.

Warnings: If condition worsens or does not improve within 7 days, consult a physician. Do not exceed recommended daily dosage unless directed by a physician. In case of bleeding, consult a physician promptly. Do not put this product in the rectum by using fingers or any mechanical device or applicator. Keep this and all drugs out of the reach of children. In case of accidental ingestion, seek professional assistance or contact a Poison Control Center immediately.

Contains: Soft pads pre-moistened with a solution containing 50%

Hamamelis Water (Witch Hazel). Also contains: Water, Glycerin, Alcohol 7%, Propylene Glycol, Sodium Citrate, Diazolidinyl, Urea, Citric Acid, Methylparaben, Aloe Vera Gel, Propylparaben.

How Supplied: Jars of 40 and 100. Also available as Tucks Take-Alongs®, individual, foil-wrapped, nonwoven wipes, 12 per box.
Shown in Product Identification Guide, page 417

The Parthenon Co., Inc.
3311 W. 2400 SOUTH
SALT LAKE CITY, UTAH 84119

DEVROM® CHEWABLE TABLETS

Description: DEVROM® is a safe and effective internal (oral) deodorant. Each tablet contains 200 mg of Bismuth Subgallate powder.

Indications: DEVROM® is indicated for the control of odors from ileostomies, colostomies and fecal incontinence.

Dosage: Take one or two tablets of DEVROM® three times a day with meals or as directed by physician. Chew or swallow whole if desired.

Note: The beneficial ingredient in DEVROM® may coat the tongue which may also darken in color. This condition is harmless and temporary. Darkening of the stool is also possible and equally harmless.

Warning: This product cannot be expected to be effective in the reduction of odor due to faulty personal hygiene. **KEEP THIS BOTTLE AND ALL MEDICATION OUT OF THE REACH OF CHILDREN.**

Inactive Ingredients: Mannitol, U.S.P., Lactose, N.F., Corn Starch, N.F., Confectioner's Sugar, N.F., Acacia Powder, N.F., Purified Water, U.S.P., Magnesium Stearate, N.F.
NO PHYSICIAN'S PRESCRIPTION IS NECESSARY

How Supplied: DEVROM® is supplied in bottles of 100 tablets.
DO NOT USE IF PRINTED OUTER SAFETY SEAL OR PRINTED INNER SAFETY SEAL IS BROKEN.
THE PARTHENON CO., INC./
3311 W. 2400 So./
Salt Lake City, Utah 84119

UNKNOWN DRUG?
Consult the
Product Identification Guide
(Gray Pages)
for full-color photos of
leading over-the-counter
medications

Pfizer Consumer Health Care Division
Division of Pfizer Inc.
100 JEFFERSON ROAD
PARSIPPANY, NJ 07054

BEN–GAY® External Analgesic Products

Description: Ben-Gay products contain menthol in an alcohol base gel, combinations of methyl salicylate and menthol in cream and ointment bases, as well as a combination of methyl salicylate, menthol and camphor in a non-greasy cream base; all suitable for topical application.
In addition to the Original Formula Pain Relieving Rub (methyl salicylate, 18.3%; menthol, 16%), Ben-Gay is offered as [Ben-Gay Greaseless/Stainless] (methyl salicylate, 15%; menthol, 10%), an Extra Strength Arthritis Rub (methyl salicylate, 30%; menthol, 8%), an Ultra Strength Pain Relieving Rub (methyl salicylate 30%; menthol 10%; camphor 4%), and Daytime Ben-Gay Pain Relieving Gel (2.5% menthol).

Action and Uses: Methyl salicylate, menthol and camphor are external analgesics which stimulate sensory receptors of warmth and/or cold. This produces a counter-irritant response which provides temporary relief of minor aches and pains of muscles and joints associated with simple backache, arthritis, strains, bruises and sprains.
Several double-blind clinical studies of Ben-Gay products containing menthol-methyl salicylate have shown the effectiveness of this combination in counteracting minor pain of skeletal muscle stress and arthritis.
Three studies involving a total of 102 normal subjects in which muscle soreness was experimentally induced showed statistically significant beneficial results from use of the active product vs. placebo for lowered Muscle Action Potential (spasms), greater rise in threshold of muscular pain and greater reduction in perceived muscular pain.
Six clinical studies of a total of 207 subjects suffering from minor pain due to osteoarthritis and rheumatoid arthritis showed the active product to give statistically significant beneficial results vs. placebo for greater relief of perceived pain, increased range of motion of the affected joints and increased digital dexterity. In two studies designed to measure the effect of topically applied Ben-Gay vs. Placebo on muscular endurance, discomfort, onset of exercise pain and fatigue, 30 subjects performed a submaximal three-hour run and another 30 subjects performed a maximal treadmill run. Ben-Gay was found to significantly decrease the discomfort during the submaximal and maximal runs, and increase the time before onset of fatigue during the maximal run.

Continued on next page

Pfizer Consumer—Cont.

Applied before workouts, Ben-Gay rubs relax tight muscles and increase circulation to make exercising more comfortable, longer.

To help reduce muscle ache and soreness after exercise, a Ben-Gay rub can be applied and allowed to work before taking a shower.

Directions: Apply generously and gently massage into painful area until Ben-Gay disappears. Repeat 3 to 4 times daily.

Warning: For external use only. Do not use with a heating pad. Keep away from children to avoid accidental poisoning. Do not bandage tightly. Do not swallow. If swallowed, induce vomiting and call a physician. Keep away from eyes, mucous membranes, broken or irritated skin. If skin redness or irritation develops, pain lasts for more than 10 days, or with arthritis—like conditions in children under 12, do not use and call a physician.

BONINE®
(meclizine hydrochloride)
Chewable Tablets

Action: BONINE (meclizine) is an H_1 histamine receptor blocker of the piperazine side chain group. It exhibits its action by an effect on the Central Nervous System (CNS), possibly by its ability to block muscarinic receptors in the brain.

Indications: BONINE is effective in the management of nausea, vomiting and dizziness associated with motion sickness.

Contraindications: Asthma, glaucoma, emphysema, chronic pulmonary disease, shortness of breath, difficulty in breathing, or difficulty in urination due to enlargement of the prostate gland unless directed by a doctor.

Warnings: May cause drowsiness; alcohol, sedatives and tranquilizers may increase the drowsiness effect. Avoid alcoholic beverages while taking this product. Do not take this product if you are taking sedatives or tranquilizers without first consulting your doctor. Do not drive or operate dangerous machinery while taking this medication.

Usage in Children: Clinical studies establishing safety and effectiveness in children have not been done; therefore, usage is not recommended in children under 12 years of age.

Usage in Pregnancy: As with any drug, if you are pregnant or nursing a baby, seek advice of a health care professional before taking this product.

Adverse Reactions: Drowsiness, dry mouth, and on rare occasions, blurred vision have been reported.

Dosage and Administration: For motion sickness, take one or two tablets of Bonine once daily, one hour before travel starts, for up to 24 hours of protection against motion sickness. The tablet can be chewed with or without water or swallowed whole with water. Thereafter, the dose may be repeated every 24 hours for the duration of the travel.

How Supplied: BONINE (meclizine hydrochloride) is available in convenient packets of 8 chewable tablets of 25 mg. meclizine hydrochloride. Store below 86°F (30°C)

Inactive Ingredients: FD&C Red No. 40, Lactose, Magnesium Stearate, Purified Siliceous Earth, Raspberry Flavor, Saccharin Sodium, Corn Starch, Talc.

DAILY CARE™ from DESITIN®
Diaper Rash Prevention Ointment
Skin Protectant (10% Zinc Oxide)

Description: Daily Care from DESITIN contains Zinc Oxide (10%) in a petrolatum base suitable for topical application. Also contains: cyclomethicone, dimethicone, fragrance, methylparaben, mineral oil, mineral wax, propylparaben, sodium borate, sorbitan sesquioleate, white wax and purified water.

Actions and Uses: Daily Care helps treat and prevent diaper rash. It helps seal out irritating wetness that can cause diaper rash by creating a protective wetness barrier at every diaper change. Daily Care has a pleasant formula that's easy to apply, easy to clean up and has a fresh scent.

Directions: Prevention—To help prevent diaper rash, change wet and soiled diaper promptly, cleanse the diaper area and allow to dry. Apply Daily Care ointment liberally as often as necessary with each diaper change—especially at bedtime or anytime when exposure to a wet diaper may be prolonged.

Treatment—At the first sign of redness or minor skin irritation, apply Daily Care liberally over the affected area and repeat as necessary. After the rash has cleared, continue to use Daily Care at every diaper change to help protect skin from future diaper rash.

Warnings: For external use only. Avoid contact with eyes. If condition worsens or does not improve within 7 days, consult your doctor. Keep out of reach of children. In case of accidental ingestion, seek professional assistance or contact a Poison Control Center immediately. Store between 2 and 30°C (36 and 86°F).

How Supplied: Daily Care Ointment is available in 2 oz. (57g) and 4 oz. (113g) tubes.

Shown in Product Identification Guide, page 417

DESITIN® OINTMENT

Description: Desitin Ointment combines Zinc Oxide (40%) with Cod Liver Oil in a petrolatum-lanolin base suitable for topical application. Also contains: BHA, fragrances, methylparaben, talc and water.

Actions and Uses: Desitin Ointment is designed to provide relief of diaper rash, superficial wounds and burns, and other minor skin irritations. It helps prevent incidents of diaper rash, protects against urine and other irritants, and soothes chafed skin.

Relief and protection is afforded by Zinc Oxide and Cod Liver Oil. These ingredients together with the petrolatum-lanolin base provide a physical barrier by forming a protective coating over skin or mucous membranes which serves to reduce further effects of irritants on the affected area and relieves burning, pain or itch produced by them.

Several studies have shown the effectiveness of Desitin Ointment in the relief and prevention of diaper rash.

Two clinical studies involving 90 infants demonstrated the effectiveness of Desitin Ointment in curing diaper rash. The diaper rash area was treated with Desitin Ointment at each diaper change for a period of 24 hours, while the untreated site served as controls. A significant reduction was noted in the severity and area of diaper dermatitis on the treated area.

Ninety-seven (97) babies participated in a 12-week study to show that Desitin Ointment helps prevent diaper rash. Approximately half of the infants (49) were treated with Desitin Ointment on a regular daily basis. The other half (48) received the ointment as necessary to treat any diaper rash which occurred. The incidence as well as the severity of diaper rash was significantly less among the babies using the ointment on a regular daily basis.

In a comparative study of the efficacy of Desitin Ointment vs. a baby powder, forty-five (45) babies were observed for a total of eight (8) weeks. Results support the conclusion that Desitin Ointment is a better prophylactic against diaper rash than the baby powder.

In another study, Desitin was found to be dramatically more effective in reducing the severity of medically diagnosed diaper rash than a commercially available diaper rash product in which only anhydrous lanolin and petrolatum were listed as ingredients. Fifty (50) infants participated in the study, half of whom were treated with Desitin and half with the other product. In the group (25) treated with Desitin, seventeen (17) infants showed significant improvement within 10 hours which increased to twenty-three improved infants within 24 hours. Of the group (25) treated with the other product, only three showed improvement at ten hours with a total of four improved within twenty-four hours. These results are statistically valid to conclude that Desitin Ointment reduces severity of diaper rash within ten hours.

Several other studies show that Desitin Ointment helps relieve other skin disorders, such as contact dermatitis.

Directions: Prevention: To prevent diaper rash, apply Desitin Ointment to the diaper area—especially at bedtime when exposure to wet diapers may be prolonged.

Treatment: If diaper rash is present, or at the first sign of redness, minor skin irritation or chafing, simply apply Desitin Ointment three or four times daily as needed. In superficial noninfected surface wounds and minor burns, apply a thin layer of Desitin Ointment, using a gauze dressing, if necessary. For external use only.

How Supplied: Desitin Ointment is available in 1 ounce (28g), 2 ounce (57g), and 4 ounce (114g) tubes, and 9 ounce (255g) and 1 lb. (454g) jars.

Shown in Product Identification Guide, page 417

RHEABAN® Maximum Strength FAST ACTING CAPLETS
[rē ´ăban]
(attapulgite)

Description: Maximum Strength Rheaban is an anti-diarrheal medication containing activated attapulgite and is offered in caplets form.

Each white Rheaban caplets contains 750 mg. of colloidal activated attapulgite. Rheaban provides the maximum level of medication when taken as directed. Rheaban contains no narcotics, opiates or other habit-forming drugs.

Actions and Uses: Rheaban is indicated for relief of diarrhea and the cramps and pains associated with it. Attapulgite, which has been activated by thermal treatment, is a highly sorptive substance which absorbs nutrients and digestive enzymes as well as noxious gases, irritants, toxins and some bacteria and viruses that are common causes of diarrhea.

In clinical studies to show the effectiveness in relieving diarrhea and its symptoms, 100 subjects suffering from acute gastroenteritis with diarrhea participated in a double-blind comparison of Rheaban to a placebo. Patients treated with the attapulgite product showed significantly improved relief of diarrhea and its symptoms vs. the placebo.

Dosage and Administration: CAPLETS

Adults—2 caplets after initial bowel movement, 2 caplets after each subsequent bowel movement. For a maximum of 12 caplets in 24 hours.

Children 6 to 12 years—1 caplet after initial bowel movement, 1 caplet after each subsequent bowel movement. For a maximum of 6 caplets in 24 hours, or as directed by a physician.

Warnings: Do not exceed 12 caplets in 24 hours. Swallow caplets with water, do not chew. Do not use for more than two days, or in the presence of high fever. Caplets should not be used for infants or children under 6 years of age unless directed by physician. If diarrhea persists consult a physician.

How Supplied:
Caplets—Boxes of 12 caplets.

Inactive Ingredients: Carnauba Wax, Croscarmellose Sodium, D&C Yellow No. 10 Aluminum Lake, FD&C Blue No. 1 Aluminum Lake, Hydroxypropyl Cellulose, Hydroxypropyl Methylcellulose, Methylparaben, Pectin, Pharmaceutical Glaze, Propylene Glycol, Propylparaben, Sucrose, Talc Titanium Dioxide, Zinc Stearate.

RID® Spray
Lice Control Spray

THIS PRODUCT IS NOT FOR USE ON HUMANS OR ANIMALS

Active Ingredient:
*Permethrin 0.50%
INERT INGREDIENTS 99.50%
100.00%
*(3-phenoxyphenyl) methyl ($\pm$) cis,trans 3-(2,2-dichloroethenyl) 2,2-dimethylcyclopropanecarboxylate. Cis, trans ratio: min. 35% ($\pm$) cis and max. 65% ($\pm$) trans

Actions: A highly active synthetic pyrethroid for the control of lice and louse eggs on garments, bedding, furniture and other inanimate objects.

Warnings: Harmful if swallowed. May be absorbed through skin. Avoid inhalation of spray mist. Avoid contact with skin, eyes or clothing. Wash thoroughly after handling and before smoking or eating. Avoid contamination of feed and foodstuffs. Remove pets and birds and cover fish aquaria before space spraying or surface applications. **This product is not for use on humans or animals.** If lice infestation should occur on humans, use Rid Lice Killing Shampoo. Vacate room after treatment and ventilate before reoccupying. Do not allow children or pets to contact treated areas until surfaces are dry. Do not overspray.

Physical and Chemical Hazards: Contents under pressure. Do not use or store near heat or open flame. Do not puncture or incinerate container. Exposure to temperatures above 130° F may cause bursting.
CAUTION: Avoid spraying in eyes. Avoid breathing spray mist. Use only in well ventilated areas. Avoid contact with skin. In case of contact wash immediately with soap and water. Vacate room after treatment and ventilate before reoccupying.
Statement of Practical Treatment: If inhaled: Remove affected person to fresh air. Apply artificial respiration if indicated.
If in eyes: Flush with plenty of water. Contact physician if irritation persists.
If on skin: Wash affected areas immediately with soap and water.

Direction For Use: It is a violation of Federal law to use this product in a manner inconsistent with its labeling.
Shake well before each use. Remove protective cap. Aim spray opening away from person. Push button to spray.
To kill lice and louse eggs: Spray in an inconspicuous area to test for possible staining or discoloration. Inspect again after drying, then proceed to spray entire area to be treated.
Hold container upright with nozzle away from you. Depress valve and spray from a distance of 8 to 10 inches.
Spray each square foot for 3 seconds. Spray only those garments, parts of bedding, including mattresses and furniture that cannot be either laundered or dry cleaned. Do not overspray.
Allow all sprayed articles to dry thoroughly before use. Repeat treatment as necessary.
Buyer assumes all risks of use, storage or handling of this material not in strict accordance with direction given herewith.
STORAGE AND DISPOSAL
Store in cool, dry area. Do not store below 32°F.
Wrap container in several layers of newspaper and dispose of in trash. Do not incinerate or puncture.

How Supplied: 5 oz. aerosol can.
Also available in combination with RID® Lice Treatment Kit as the RID® Lice Elimination System.

RID®
Lice Killing Shampoo

Description: Rid contains a liquid pediculicide whose active ingredients are: pyrethrins 0.33% and piperonyl butoxide, technical 4.00%, equivalent to min. 3.2% (butylcarbityl) (6-propylpiperonyl) ether and 0.8% related compounds. Inert ingredients include: C_{13}-C_{14} isoparaffin, Fragrance, Isopropyl Alcohol, PEG-25 Hydrogenated Castor Oil, Water, Xanthan Gum and totals 95.67%.

Actions: RID kills head lice (*Pediculus humanus capitis*), body lice (*Pediculus humanus humanus*), and pubic or crab lice (*Phthirus pubis*).
The pyrethrins act as a contact poison and affect the parasite's nervous system, resulting in paralysis and death. The efficacy of the pyrethrins is enhanced by the synergist, piperonyl butoxide. Rid rinses out completely after treatment.
The active ingredients in RID are poorly absorbed through the skin. Of the relatively minor amounts that are absorbed, they are rapidly metabolized to water-soluble compounds and eliminated from the body without ill-effects.

Indications: RID is indicated for the treatment of infestations of head lice, body lice and pubic (crab) lice, and their eggs.

Continued on next page

Pfizer Consumer—Cont.

Warning: RID should be used with caution by ragweed sensitized persons.

Precautions: This product is for external use only. It is harmful if swallowed. If accidentally swallowed, call a physician or Poison Control Center immediately. It should not be inhaled. It should be kept out of the eyes and contact with mucous membranes should be avoided. If accidental contact with eyes occur, flush eyes immediately with plenty of water and call a physician. In the case of infection or skin irritation, discontinue use immediately and consult a physician. Consult a physician before use if infestation of eyebrows or eyelashes occurs. Avoid contamination of feed or foodstuffs.

Storage and Disposal: Do not store below 32°F (0°C). Do not reuse empty container. Wrap in several layers of newspaper and discard in trash.

Dosage and Administration: (1) Shake well. Apply undiluted RID to dry hair and scalp or to any other infested area until entirely wet. Do not use on eyelashes or eyebrows. (2) Allow RID to remain on area for 10 minutes but no longer. (3) Wash thoroughly with warm water and soap or shampoo. (4) Dead lice and eggs should be removed with the special nit comb provided. (5) Repeat treatment in 7 to 10 days to kill any newly hatched lice. Do not exceed two consecutive applications within 24 hours.
Since lice infestations are spread by contact, each family member should be examined carefully. If infested, he or she should be treated promptly to avoid spread or reinfestation of previously treated individuals. Contaminated clothing and other articles, such as hats, etc. should be dry cleaned, boiled or otherwise treated until decontaminated to prevent reinfestation or spread.

How Supplied: In 2, 4 and 8 fl. oz. plastic bottles. Exclusive nit removal comb that removes nits and patient instruction booklet (English and Spanish) are included in each package of RID.
Also available in combination with RID Lice Control Spray as the RID Lice Elimination Kit.

MAXIMUM STRENGTH UNISOM SLEEPGELS
Nighttime Sleep Aid

Description: Maximum Strength Unisom SleepGels are liquid-filled, blue soft gelatin capsules.

Active Ingredient: Diphenhydramine Hydrochloride 50 mg.

Inactive Ingredients: FD&C Blue No. 1, Gelatin, Glycerin, Pharmaceutical Glaze, Polyethylene Glycol, Propylene Glycol, Purified Water, Sorbitol, Titanium Dioxide.

Indications: Helps to reduce difficulty falling asleep.

Action: Diphenhydramine Hydrochloride is an ethanolamine antihistamine with anticholinergic and sedative effects.

Administration and Dosage: Adults and children 12 years of age and over: Oral dosage is one softgel (50 mg.) at bedtime if needed, or as directed by a doctor.

Warnings: Do not take this product if you have asthma, glaucoma, emphysema, chronic pulmonary disease, shortness of breath, difficulty in breathing or difficulty in urination due to enlargement of the prostate gland unless directed by a doctor. Do not take this product if pregnant or nursing a baby.
• Do not give to children under 12 years of age.
• If sleeplessness persists continuously for more than two weeks, consult your doctor. Insomnia may be a symptom of serious underlying medical illness.
• Avoid alcoholic beverages while taking this product. Do not take this product if you are taking sedatives or tranquilizers, without first consulting your doctor.
• Keep this and all drugs out of the reach of children.
• In case of accidental overdose, seek professional assistance or contact a Poison Control Center immediately.

Drug Interaction: Monoamine oxidase (MAO) inhibitors prolong and intensify the anticholinergic effects of antihistamines. The CNS depressant effect is heightened by alcohol and other CNS depressant drugs.

Symptoms of Oral Overdosage: Antihistamine overdosage reactions may vary from central nervous system depression to stimulation.
Stimulation is particularly likely in children. Atropine-like signs and symptoms, such as dry mouth, fixed and dilated pupils, flushing, and gastrointestinal symptoms, may also occur.

Attention: Use only if softgel blister seals are unbroken.

How Supplied: Boxes of 16 liquid filled softgels in child resistant blisters and boxes of 8 with non-child resistant packaging.
Store between 15° and 30°C (59° and 86°F)

Shown in Product Identification Guide, page 417

UNISOM® NIGHTTIME SLEEP AID

Description: Unisom Nighttime Sleep Aid is a pale blue oval scored tablet.

Active Ingredient: Doxylamine succinate 25 mg.

Inactive Ingredients: FD&C Blue #1 Aluminum Lake, Microcrystalline Cellulose, Dibasic Calcium Phosphate Dihydrate, Sodium Starch Glycolate, Magnesium Stearate.

Indication: Helps to reduce difficulty falling asleep.

Action: An ethanolamine antihistamine that characteristically shows a high incidence of sedation.

Administration and Dosage: One tablet 30 minutes before retiring. Not for children under 12 years of age.

Side Effects: Occasional anticholinergic effects may be seen.

Precautions: Unisom® should be taken only at bedtime.

Contraindications: This product should not be taken by pregnant women, or those who are nursing a baby. This product is also contraindicated for asthma, glaucoma, enlargement of the prostate gland.

Warnings: Should be taken with caution if alcohol is being consumed. Product should not be taken if patient is concurrently on any other drug, without prior consultation with physician. Should not be taken for longer than two weeks unless approved by physician.

How Supplied: Boxes of 8, 32 and 48 tablets in child resistant blisters, and in boxes of 16 with non-child resistant packaging.

Shown in Product Identification Guide, page 417

UNISOM® WITH PAIN RELIEF
(formerly Unisom Dual Relief)
Nighttime Sleep Aid and
Pain Reliever

Description: Unisom® With Pain Relief is a pale blue, capsule-shaped, coated tablet.

Active Ingredients: 650 mg. acetaminophen and 50 mg. diphenhydramine HCl per tablet.

Inactive Ingredients: Corn starch, FD&C Blue #1 Aluminum Lake, FD&C Blue #2 Aluminum Lake, hydroxypropyl methylcellulose, magnesium stearate, polyethylene glycol, polysorbate 80, povidone, stearic acid, titanium dioxide.

Indications: Unisom With Pain Relief (diphenhydramine sleep aid formula) is indicated for the temporary relief of occasional headaches and minor aches and pains with accompanying sleeplessness. If there is difficulty in falling asleep, but pain is not being experienced at the same time, regular Unisom sleep aid is indicated which contains doxylamine succinate as its active ingredient.

Administration and Dosage: Adults and children 12 years of age and over: take one tablet 30 minutes before bedtime if needed, or as directed by a physician.

Warnings: Do not take this product if you have asthma, glaucoma, emphysema, chronic pulmonary disease, shortness of breath, difficulty in breathing, or difficulty in urination due to enlargement of the prostate gland unless directed by a doctor. Do not take this product for more than ten days unless directed by a doctor. If symptoms get worse, or if new symptoms occur, or if sleeplessness persists continuously for more than 2 weeks, consult a doctor because these could be signs of a serious underlying medical illness. Avoid alcoholic beverages while taking this product. Do not take this product if you are taking sedatives or tranquilizers without first consulting your doctor. As with any drug, if you are pregnant or nursing a baby, seek the advice of a health professional before using this product. Do not give to children under 12 years of age. Keep this and all medications out of the reach of children. In case of accidental overdose, seek professional assistance or contact a Poison Control center immediately. Prompt medical attention is critical for adults as well as for children even if you do not notice any signs of symptoms.

Drug Interaction: Monoamine oxidase (MAO) inhibitors prolong and intensify the anticholinergic effects of antihistamines. The CNS depressant effect is heightened by alcohol and other CNS depressant drugs.

Attention: Use only if tablet blister seals are unbroken. Child resistant packaging.

How Supplied: Boxes of 8 and 16 tablets in child resistant blisters.
Shown in Product Identification Guide, page 417

VISINE L. R.™ EYE DROPS
(oxymetazoline hydrochloride)

Description: Visine L. R. is a sterile, isotonic, buffered ophthalmic solution containing oxymetazoline hydrochloride 0.025%, boric acid, sodium borate, sodium chloride and water. It is preserved with benzalkonium chloride 0.01% and edetate disodium 0.1%.
Visine L. R. is produced by a process that assures sterility.

Indications: Visine L. R. is a decongestant ophthalmic solution designed for the relief of redness of the eye due to minor eye irritations. Visine L. R. is specially formulated to relieve redness of the eye in minutes with effective relief that lasts up to 6 hours.

Directions: *Adults and children 6 years of age and older*—Place 1 or 2 drops in the affected eye(s). This may be repeated as needed every 6 hours or as directed by a physician.

Warning: If you experience eye pain, changes in vision, continued redness or irritation of the eye, or if the condition worsens or persists for more than 72 hours, discontinue use and consult a physician. If you have glaucoma, do not use this product except under the advice and supervision of a physician. As with any medication, if you are pregnant seek the advice of a physician before using this product. Overuse of this product may

produce increased redness of the eye. If solution changes color or becomes cloudy, do not use. To avoid contamination of this product, do not touch tip of container to any surface. Replace cap after using. Remove contact lenses before using this product.

Parents: Before using with children under 6 years of age, consult your physician. Keep this and all other medications out of the reach of children. In case of accidental ingestion, seek professional assistance or contact a poison control center immediately.

Caution: Should not be used if Visine-imprinted neckband on bottle is broken or missing.

Storage: Store between 2° and 30°C (36° and 86°F).

How Supplied: In 0.5 fl. oz. and 1 fl. oz. plastic dispenser bottle.
Shown in Product Identification Guide, page 417

VISINE MAXIMUM STRENGTH ALLERGY RELIEF®
Astringent/Redness Reliever Eye Drops

Description: Visine with allergy relief is a sterile, isotonic, buffered ophthalmic solution containing tetrahydrozoline hydrochloride 0.05%, zinc sulfate 0.25%, boric acid, sodium chloride, sodium citrate and purified water. It is preserved with benzalkonium chloride 0.01% and edetate disodium 0.1%. Visine with allergy relief is an ophthalmic solution combining the effects of the vasoconstrictor tetrahydrozoline hydrochloride with the astringent effects of zinc sulfate. The vasoconstrictor provides symptomatic relief of conjunctival edema and hyperemia secondary to minor irritation due to conditions such as dust and airborne pollutants as well as so-called nonspecific or catarrhal conjunctivitis, while zinc sulfate provides relief from burning and itching, symptoms often associated with hay fever, allergies, etc. Beneficial effects include amelioration of burning, irritation, pruritis, and removal of mucus from the eye. Relief is afforded by both ingredients, tetrahydrozoline hydrochloride and zinc sulfate.
Tetrahydrozoline hydrochloride is a sympathomimetic agent, which brings about decongestion by vasoconstriction. Reddened eyes are rapidly whitened by this effective vasoconstrictor, which limits the local vascular response by constricting the small blood vessels. The onset of vasoconstriction becomes apparent within minutes. Zinc sulfate is an ocular astringent which, by precipitating protein, helps to clear mucus from the outer surface of the eye.
The effectiveness of Visine with allergy relief in relieving conjunctival hyperemia and associated symptoms induced by allergies has been clinically demonstrated. In one double-blind study allergy sufferers experienced acute episodes of

minor eye irritation. Visine with allergy relief produced statistically significant beneficial results versus a placebo of normal saline solution in relieving irritation of bulbar conjunctiva, irritation of palpebral conjunctiva, and mucous build-up. Treatment with Visine with allergy relief containing zinc sulfate also significantly improved burning and itching symptoms.

Indications: For temporary relief of discomfort and redness due to minor eye irritations.

Directions: Instill 1 to 2 drops in the affected eye(s) up to 4 times daily.

Warning: To avoid contamination, do not touch tip of container to any surface. Replace cap after using. If you experience eye pain, changes in vision, continued redness or irritation of the eye, or if the condition worsens or persists for more than 72 hours, discontinue use and consult a doctor. If you have glaucoma, do not use this product except under the advice and supervision of a doctor. Overuse of this product may produce increased redness of the eye. If solution changes color or becomes cloudy, do not use. Remove contact lenses before using.

Parents: Before using with children under 6 years of age, consult your physician. Keep this and all other drugs out of the reach of children. In case of accidental ingestion, seek professional assistance or contact a poison control center immediately.

How Supplied: In 0.5 fl. oz. and 1.0 fl. oz. plastic dispenser bottle.
Shown in Product Identification Guide, page 417

VISINE MOISTURIZING
Redness Reliever/Lubricant Eye Drops

Description: Visine Moisturizing is a sterile, isotonic, buffered ophthalmic solution containing tetrahydrozoline hydrochloride 0.05%, polyethylene glycol 400 1.0%, boric acid, sodium borate, sodium chloride and water. It is preserved with benzalkonium chloride 0.013% and edetate disodium 0.1%.
Visine Moisturizing is an ophthalmic solution combining the effects of the decongestant tetrahydrozoline hydrochloride with the demulcent effects of polyethylene glycol. It provides symptomatic relief of conjunctival edema and hyperemia secondary to ocular allergies, minor irritations and so-called nonspecific or catarrhal conjunctivitis. Tetrahydrozoline hydrochloride is a sympathomimetic agent, which brings about decongestion by vasoconstriction. Reddened eyes are rapidly whitened by this effective vasoconstrictor, which limits the local vascular response by constricting the small blood vessels. The onset of vasoconstriction becomes apparent within minutes. Additional effects include amelioration

Continued on next page

Pfizer Consumer—Cont.

of burning, irritation, pruritus, soreness, and excessive lacrimation. Relief is afforded by polyethylene glycol.

Polyethylene glycol is an ophthalmic demulcent which has been shown to be effective for the temporary relief of discomfort of minor irritations of the eye due to exposure to wind or sun. It is effective as a protectant and lubricant against further irritation or to relieve dryness of the eye.

The effectiveness of tetrahydrozoline hydrochloride in relieving conjunctival hyperemia and associated symptoms has been demonstrated by numerous clinicals, including several double-blind studies, involving more than 2000 subjects suffering from acute or chronic hyperemia induced by a variety of conditions. Visine Moisturizing is a product that combines the redness relieving effects of a vasoconstrictor and the soothing moisturizing and protective effects of a demulcent.

Indications: Relieves redness of the eye due to minor eye irritations. For use as a protectant against further irritation or to relieve dryness.

Directions: Instill 1 to 2 drops in the affected eye(s) up to 4 times daily.

Warning: To avoid contamination, do not touch tip of container to any surface. Replace cap after using. If you experience eye pain, changes in vision, continued redness or irritation of the eye, or if the condition worsens or persists for more than 72 hours, discontinue use and consult a doctor. If you have glaucoma, do not use this product except under the advice and supervision of a doctor. Overuse of this product may produce increased redness of the eye. If solution changes color or becomes cloudy, do not use. Remove contact lenses before using.

Parents: Before using with children under 6 years of age, consult your physician. Keep this and all other drugs out of the reach of children. In case of accidental ingestion, seek professional assistance or contact a poison control center immediately.

How Supplied: In 0.5 fl. oz. and 1.0 fl. oz. plastic dispenser bottle.

Shown in Product Identification Guide, page 417

VISINE® ORIGINAL
Tetrahydrozoline Hydrochloride Redness Reliever Eye Drops

Description: Visine is a sterile, isotonic, buffered ophthalmic solution containing tetrahydrozoline hydrochloride 0.05%, boric acid, sodium borate, sodium chloride and water. It is preserved with benzalkonium chloride 0.01% and edetate disodium 0.1%. Visine is a decongestant ophthalmic solution designed to provide symptomatic relief of conjunctival edema and hyperemia secondary to mi-

nor irritations, due to conditions such as smoke, dust, other airborne pollutants, swimming etc. and so-called nonspecific or catarrhal conjunctivitis. Relief is afforded by tetrahydrozoline hydrochloride, a sympathomimetic agent, which brings about decongestion by vasoconstriction. Reddened eyes are rapidly whitened by this effective vasoconstrictor, which limits the local vascular response by constricting the small blood vessels. The onset of vasoconstriction becomes apparent within minutes.

The effectiveness of Visine in relieving conjunctival hyperemia has been demonstrated by numerous clinicals, including several double-blind studies, involving more than 2,000 subjects suffering from acute or chronic hyperemia induced by a variety of conditions. Visine was found to be efficacious in providing relief from conjunctival hyperemia.

Indications: Relieves redness of the eye due to minor eye irritations.

Directions: Instill 1 to 2 drops in the affected eye(s) up to four times daily.

Warning: To avoid contamination, do not touch tip of container to any surface. Replace cap after using. If you experience eye pain, changes in vision, continued redness or irritation of the eye, or if the condition worsens or persists for more than 72 hours, discontinue use and consult a doctor. If you have glaucoma, do not use this product except under the advice and supervision of a doctor. Overuse of this product may produce increased redness of the eye. If solution changes color or becomes cloudy, do not use. Remove contact lenses before using.

Parents: Before using with children under 6 years of age, consult your physician. Keep this and all other drugs out of the reach of children. In case of accidental ingestion, seek professional assistance or contact a poison control center immediately.

How Supplied: In 0.5 fl. oz., 0.75 fl. oz., and 1.0 fl. oz. plastic dispenser bottle and 0.5 fl. oz. plastic bottle with dropper.

Shown in Product Identification Guide, page 417

WART–OFF®
Liquid

Active Ingredient: Salicylic Acid 17% w/w.

Inactive Ingredients: Alcohol, 26.35% w/w, Flexible Collodion, Propylene Glycol Dipelargonate.

Indications: For the removal of common warts and plantar warts on the bottom of the foot. The common wart is easily recognized by the rough "cauliflower-like" appearance of the surface. The plantar wart is recognized by its location only on the bottom of the foot, its tenderness, and the interruption of the footprint pattern.

Warnings: For external use only. Keep this and all medications out of the reach

of children to avoid accidental poisoning. In case of accidental ingestion, contact a physician or a Poison Control Center immediately. Do not use this product on irritated skin, on any area that is infected or reddened, if you are a diabetic, or if you have poor blood circulation. Do not use on moles, birthmarks, warts with hair growing from them, genital warts, or warts on the face or mucous membranes. If product gets into the eye, flush with water for 15 minutes. Avoid inhaling vapors. If discomfort persists, see your doctor.

Extremely Flammable—Keep away from fire or flame. Cap bottle tightly and store at room temperature away from heat (59°–86°F).

Instructions For Use: Read warnings and enclosed instructional brochure. Wash affected area. Dry area thoroughly. Using the special pinpoint applicator, apply one drop at a time to sufficiently cover each wart. Apply Wart-Off to warts only—not to surrounding skin. Let dry. Repeat this procedure once or twice daily as needed (until wart is removed) for up to 12 weeks. Replace cap tightly to prevent evaporation.

How Supplied: 0.5 fluid ounce bottle with special pinpoint plastic applicator and instructional brochure.

Pharma-Singer AG
WINDEGGSTRASSE 1
NIEDERURNEN
GLARUS 8867
SWITZERLAND

PERSKINDOL® Liniment
PERSKINDOL® Spray
PERSKINDOL® Gel

Active Ingredient: Menthol 1.5%.

Other Ingredients: Pine Needle Oil, Orange Oil, Wintergreen Oil, Lemon Oil, Bergamot Oil (free of furocumarin), Rosemary Oil, Lavender Oil, Terpineol, Terpenyl Acetate, Benzyl Benzoate, Ethyl Acetate, Isopropyl Alcohol and Water. In addition, Perskindol Gel include Miglyol 812, Methylparaben, Propylparaben, Carbomer 934 P and Ammonium Hydroxide. Perskindol Spray include as propellant propane/butane.

Description: A unique formulation with menthol and essential oils providing fast and effective relief of muscles aches and pain.

Indications: For the temporary relief of minor aches and pains of muscles and joints associated with arthritis, simple backache, strains, cramps, bruises, sprains and sports injuries.

Directions: Adults and children 6 years of age and older:
Gently massage into affected area not more than 3 to 4 times daily.
Children under 6 years of age: Consult a physician.

Warnings: KEEP OUT OF REACH OF CHILDREN. FOR EXTERNAL USE ONLY. Avoid contact with eyes and mucous membranes. **Do not Use With Heating Pads Or Heating Devices.** If condition worsens, skin redness or irritation develops or if symptoms persist for more than 7 days, discontinue use of this product and consult a doctor. Do not apply to wounds or damaged skin. Do not bandage tightly. If you have sensitive skin, consult a doctor **before** use. If skin irritation develops, discontinue use and consult a doctor. As with any drug, if you are pregnant or nursing a baby, seek the advice of a health professional before using this product. Do not use, pour, spill or store near heat or open flame.

How Supplied:
NDC 57219-107-15 Perskindol Liniment 9 fl. oz.
NDC 57219-107-25 Perskindol Spray 6 fl. oz.
NDC 57219-107-35 Perskindol Gel 3.5 oz.

Pharmavite Corp.
15451 SAN FERNANDO MISSION BLVD. MISSION HILLS, CA 91345

NATURE MADE® ANTIOXIDANT FORMULA
(Vitamins C, E, & Beta Carotene)

Description: Nature Made® Antioxidant Formula contains high levels of Vitamin C, Vitamin E and Beta Carotene which are "free radical fighters". This product is manufactured to contain no artificial colors, no artificial flavors, no preservatives, no chemical solvents, no yeast, no sugar, no sodium and no starch.

Each tablet contains: For adults percentage of U.S. Recommended Daily Allowance (U.S. RDA):

Vitamin A (from Beta Carotene)	6 mg (10,000 I.U.)	200%
Vitamin C	250 mg	417%
Vitamin E	200 I.U.	667%

Active Ingredients: Ascorbic Acid, dl-Alpha Tocopheryl Acetate and Beta Carotene.

Inactive Ingredients: Cottonseed Oil, Gelatin, Glycerin, Water, Partially Hydrogenated Cottonseed and Soybean Oils.

Indications: Supplementation to diet as only one in ten Americans consume the recommended 5 servings of fruits and vegetables daily. Antioxidant vitamins (Vitamin C, Vitamin E and Beta Carotene) may help protect cells against the damaging effects of free radicals. Free radicals are highly reactive oxygen molecules created by environmental factors such as ultraviolet light, pollution, X-rays and alcohol, as well as by normal body processes.

Recommended Intake: Take one softgel daily, with a meal. Nature Made

Suggested use: As a dietary supplement, take one tablet daily.

Each tablet contains:

	Quantity	%U.S.* RDA
Vitamin A (As Acetate and Beta Carotene)	5000 I.U.	100
Vitamin E (From d-Alpha Tocopheryl Succinate)	**40 I.U.**	**133**
Vitamin C (With Rose Hips)	**120 mg**	**200**
Folic Acid	400 mcg	100
Vitamin B1 (As Thiamine Mononitrate)	1.5 mg	100
Vitamin B2 (Riboflavin)	1.7 mg	100
Niacin (From Niacinamide Ascorbate)	20 mg	100
Vitamin B6 (From Pyridoxine Hydrochloride)	2 mg	100
Vitamin B12 (Cyanocobalamin)	6 mcg	100
Vitamin D	400 I.U.	100
Biotin	30 mcg	10
Pantothenic Acid (From d-Calcium Pantothenate)	10 mg	100
Vitamin K (As Phylloquinone)	25 mcg	**
Calcium (From Dibasic Calcium Phosphate)	100 mg	10
Phosphorus (From Dibasic Calcium Phosphate)	77 mg	8
Iodine (From Kelp and Potassium Iodide)	150 mcg	100
Iron (From Ferrous Fumarate)	18 mg	100
Magnesium (From Magnesium Oxide)	100 mg	25
Copper (From Cupric Oxide)	2 mg	100
Zinc (From Zinc Oxide)	15 mg	100
Manganese (From Manganese Sulfate)	2.5 mg	**
Potassium (From Potassium Chloride)	40 mg	**
Chloride (From Potassium Chloride)	36.3 mg	**
Chromium (From Chromium Chloride)	25 mcg	**
Molybdenum (From Sodium Molybdate)	25 mcg	**
Selenium (From Sodium Selenate)	25 mcg	**
Nickel (From Nickelous Sulfate)	5 mcg	**
Tin (From Stannous Chloride)	10 mcg	**
Silicon (From Sodium Metasilicate & Silicon Dioxide)	2 mg	**
Vanadium (From Sodium Metavanadate)	10 mcg	**
Boron (As Borates)	150 mcg	**

In a base containing Rose Hips-50 mg, Lemon Bioflavonoid Complex-2.5 mg, Rutin-2.5 mg, Hesperidin Complex-2.5 mg.

* Percentage of the U.S. Recommended Daily Allowance for Adults.
** No U.S. RDA has been established for this nutrient.

Antioxidant Formula can be taken by itself or with a multiple vitamin.

Warnings: Keep out of the reach of children.

How Supplied: Softgels, bottle of 60. Store at room temperature.
Shown in Product Identification Guide, page 417

NATURE MADE® ESSENTIAL BALANCE®
Complete High Potency Multivitamin-Multimineral Formula

Description: Nature Made® Essential Balance® offers a complete and more natural multivitamin/multimineral with higher levels of antioxidant vitamins C and Natural E than the leading multivitamin brand. This product is manufactured to contain no artificial colors, no artificial flavors, no preservatives, no yeast and no gluten.

Each tablet contains: For adults percentage of U.S. Recommended Daily Allowance (U.S.RDA):
[See table above.]

Inactive Ingredients: Cellulose, Glycerides of Fatty Acids, Croscarmellose Sodium, Stearic Acid, Sugar, Magnesium Stearate, Hydroxypropyl Methylcellulose, Corn Starch, Silicon Dioxide, Acety-

lated Monoglycerides, Ethylcellulose, Polyethylene Glycol, Carnauba Wax, Lactose.

Recommended Intake: Take one tablet daily, with a meal.

Warnings: Keep out of the reach of children.

How Supplied: Oval shaped scored tablet, bottles of 100 plus 30. Store at room temperature.
Shown in Product Identification Guide, page 417

IF YOU SUSPECT AN INTERACTION...
The 1,400-page
*PDR Guide to Drug Interactions •
Side Effects • Indications*
can help.
Use the order form
in the front of this book.

PolyMedica Pharmaceuticals (U.S.A.), Inc.
2 CONSTITUTION WAY
WOBURN, MA 01801

ALCONEFRIN®
Phenylephrine hydrochloride
Nasal Decongestant

How Supplied:
Drops 1 oz., 0.16%, 0.25%, 0.50%
Spray 1 oz., 0.25%

AZO-STANDARD™
Phenazopyridine hydrochloride
Urinary Tract Analgesic Tablets

Description: Each tablet contains phenazopyridine hydrochloride 95mg.

Indication: An analgesic for use as an aid for the prompt temporary relief of minor pain, urgency, frequency and burning of urination.

Directions: Adults: 2 tablets 3 times a day after meals. Use is only recommended for up to 2 days. For children under 12, consult a physician.

Warnings: Do not administer to children under 12 unless directed by a physician. Individuals with any hepatic or renal trouble should not use this product unless directed by a physician. Do not use for more than two days without consulting a physician. If you are pregnant or nursing a baby, seek the advice of a physician before using this product. Keep out of the reach of children. If symptoms persist, consult a physician.
Store at room temperature.

How Supplied: Cartons of 30 tablets.

NEOPAP®
Acetaminophen, 125mg
Analgesic

How Supplied: Pediatric Suppositories, 12's

EDUCATIONAL MATERIAL

An educational brochure is available
Title: "What Every Woman Needs to Know about Urinary Discomfort"
Subject: Urinary discomfort

Description: Educational brochure discussing the causes, symptoms, and possible prevention of urinary discomfort
Size: Height = 8.5 inches, Length = 3.5 inches, 6 panels
Quantity Available: 25 brochures per store; includes one counter top holder
Available to: physicians, pharmacists, consumers
Brochures carry no charge (from requests sent to our office)
No samples available

Premier, Inc.
GREENWICH OFFICE PARK ONE
GREENWICH, CT 06831

EXACT™
[Ex-act]
Benzoyl Peroxide Acne Medication Tinted Cream

Active Ingredient: Benzoyl Peroxide 5.0% in a flesh toned, odorless, and greaseless cream base containing water, acrylates co-polymer, glycerin, titanium dioxide, sorbitol, cetyl alcohol, glyceryl dilaurate, stearyl alcohol, sodium, lauryl sulfate, magnesium aluminum silicate, sodium citrate, silica, iron oxides, citric acid, methylparaben, xanthan gum and propylparaben.

Indications: For the topical treatment of acne vulgaris.

Actions: Exact cream contains 5% benzoyl peroxide. The product clears existing pimples and helps prevent new pimples from forming.

Additional Benefits: Exact utilizes a patented Microsponge® system to provide prolonged release of benzoyl peroxide to the skin. This special Microsponge formula was designed for low irritancy and to provide 50% higher oil absorbancy than other benzoyl peroxide medications. Exact tinted is flesh toned so it hides acne pimples while it treats them.

Warning: For external use only. Using other topical acne medications at the same time or immediately following use of this product may increase dryness or irritation of the skin. If this occurs, only one medication should be used unless directed by a doctor. Do not use this medication if you have very sensitive skin or if you are sensitive to benzoyl peroxide. This product may cause irritation, characterized by redness, burning, itching, peeling, or possibly swelling. Mild irritation may be reduced by using the product less frequently or in a lower concentration. If irritation becomes severe, discontinue use; if irritation still continues, consult a doctor. Keep away from eyes, lips, and mouth. This product may bleach hair or dyed fabrics. Store at room temperature. Keep away from flame, fire and heat.
KEEP THIS AND ALL DRUGS OUT OF REACH OF CHILDREN.

Symptoms and Treatment of Ingestion: These symptoms are based upon medical judgement, not on actual experience. Theoretically, ingestion of very large amounts may cause nausea, vomiting, abdominal discomfort and diarrhea. Treatment is symptomatic, with bed rest and observation.

Direction for Use: Cleanse the skin thoroughly before applying medication. Cover the entire affected area with a thin layer one to three times daily. Because excessive drying of the skin may occur, start with one application daily, then gradually increase to two or three times daily if needed or as directed by a doctor. If bothersome dryness or peeling occurs, reduce application to once a day or every other day.

How Supplied: .65 oz. plastic squeeze tubes.

EXACT™
[Ex-áct]
Benzoyl Peroxide Acne Medication Vanishing Cream

Active Ingredient: Benzoyl Peroxide 5.0% in a colorless, odorless, and greaseless cream base containing water, acrylates co-polymer, glycerin, sorbitol, cetyl alcohol, glyceryl dilaurate, stearyl alcohol, sodium lauryl sulfate, magnesium aluminum silicates, sodium citrate, silica, citric acid, methylparaben, xanthan gum and propylparaben.

Indications: For the topical treatment of acne vulgaris.

Actions: Exact cream contains 5% benzoyl peroxide. The product clears existing pimples and helps prevent new pimples from forming.

Additional Benefits: Exact utilizes a patented Microsponge® system to provide prolonged release of benzoyl peroxide to the skin. This special Microsponge formula was designed for low irritancy and to provide 50% higher oil absorbancy than other benzoyl peroxide medications.

Warning: For external use only. Using other topical acne medications at the same time or immediately following use of this product may increase dryness or irritation of the skin. If this occurs, only one medication should be used unless directed by a doctor. Do not use this medication if you have very sensitive skin or if you are sensitive to benzoyl peroxide. This product may cause irritation, characterized by redness, burning, itching, peeling, or possibly swelling. Mild irritation may be reduced by using the product less frequently or in a lower concentration. If irritation becomes severe, discontinue use; if irritation still continues, consult a doctor. Keep away from eyes, lips, and mouth. This product may bleach hair or dyed fabrics. Store at room temperature. Keep away from flame, fire and heat.
KEEP THIS AND ALL DRUGS OUT OF REACH OF CHILDREN.

Symptoms and Treatment of Ingestion: These symptoms are based upon medical judgement, not on actual experience. Theoretically, ingestion of very large amounts may cause nausea, vomiting, abdominal discomfort and diarrhea. Treatment is symptomatic, with bed rest and observation.

Directions for Use: Cleanse the skin thoroughly before applying medication. Cover the entire affected area with a thin layer one to three times daily. Because excessive drying of the skin may occur, start with one application daily, then gradually increase to two or three times daily if needed or as directed by a doctor. If bothersome dryness or peeling occurs, reduce application to once a day or every other day.

How Supplied: .65 oz. plastic squeeze tubes.

Procter & Gamble
P. O. BOX 5516
CINCINNATI, OH 45201

CHILDREN'S CHLORASEPTIC®
SORE THROAT LOZENGES
Benzocaine/Oral Anesthetic
(Grape Flavor)

Active Ingredient: Benzocaine 5 mg per lozenge.

Inactive Ingredients: Corn syrup, FD&C Blue No. 1, FD&C Red No. 40, flavor, and sucrose.

Indications: For temporary relief of occasional minor mouth irritation and pain, sore mouth and sore throat. Also for pain associated with canker sores.

Directions: Adults and children 2 years of age and older: Allow 1 lozenge to dissolve slowly in mouth. May be repeated every 2 hours as needed or as directed by a physician or dentist. Children under 2 years of age: Consult a physician or a dentist.

WARNINGS: If sore throat is severe, or is accompanied by difficulty in breathing, or persists for more than two days, do not use, and consult a doctor promptly. If sore throat is accompanied or followed by fever, headache, rash, swelling, nausea, or vomiting, consult a doctor promptly. If sore mouth symptoms do not improve in 7 days, or if irritation, pain, or redness persists or worsens, see your doctor promptly. Do not use this product if you have a history of allergy to local anesthetics such as procaine, butacaine, benzocaine, or other "caine" anesthetics. **Keep this and all drugs out of the reach of children.** In case of accidental overdose seek professional assistance or contact a poison control center immediately. As with any drug, if you are pregnant or nursing a baby, seek the advice of a health professional before using this product.

How Supplied: Cartons of 18.

VICKS® CHILDREN'S CHLORASEPTIC®
SORE THROAT SPRAY
Phenol/Oral
Anesthetic/Antiseptic

Children's Chloraseptic is specially formulated with a reduced concentration of phenol, the active ingredient in Advanced Formula Chloraseptic, to provide fast, effective relief in a great-tasting grape flavor your child will like.

Active Ingredient: Phenol 0.5%

Inactive Ingredients: FD&C Blue No. 1, FD&C Red No. 40, flavor, glycerin, purified water, saccharin sodium, and sorbitol.

Indications: For temporary relief of occasional minor sore throat pain and sore mouth. Also, for temporary relief of pain due to canker sores, minor irritation or injury of the mouth and gums, minor dental procedures, or appliances.

Directions—Children 2 Years of Age and Older: Spray 5 times directly into throat or affected area and swallow. Repeat every two hours or as directed by a physician or dentist. Children under 12 years of age should be supervised in product use.
Children Under 2 Years of Age: Consult a physician or dentist.

WARNINGS: If sore throat is severe, or is accompanied by difficulty in breathing, or persists for more than 2 days, do not use, and consult a doctor promptly. If sore throat is accompanied or followed by fever, headache, rash, swelling, nausea or vomiting, consult a doctor promptly. If sore mouth symptoms do not improve in 7 days, or if irritation, pain, or redness persists or worsens, see your doctor promptly. **Keep this and all drugs out of the reach of children.** In case of accidental overdose, seek professional assistance or contact a poison control center immediately. As with any drug, if you are pregnant or nursing a baby, seek the advice of a health professional before using this product.

How Supplied: Available in 6 FL. OZ. (177 mL) plastic bottles with sprayer.

CHLORASEPTIC®
SORE THROAT LOZENGES
Cherry, Menthol, and Cool Mint
Flavor
Menthol/Benzocaine
Oral Anesthetic

Active Ingredients: Benzocaine 6 mg, Menthol 10 mg

Inactive Ingredients:
Menthol Lozenges: Corn syrup, D&C Yellow No. 10, FD&C Blue No. 1, FD&C Yellow No. 6, flavor and sucrose.
Cherry Lozenges: Corn syrup, FD&C Blue No. 1, FD&C Red No. 40, flavor and sucrose.
Cool Mint Lozenges: Corn syrup, FD&C Blue No. 1, flavor and sucrose.

Indications: For temporary relief of occasional minor mouth pain and irritation, sore mouth and sore throat. Also, for pain associated with canker sores.

Directions:
Adults and children 2 years of age and older: Allow 1 lozenge to dissolve slowly in mouth. May be repeated every 2 hours as needed or as directed by a physician or dentist. Children under 2 years of age: Consult a physician or a dentist.

WARNINGS: If sore throat is severe, or is accompanied by difficulty in breathing, or persists for more than 2 days, do not use, and consult a doctor promptly. If sore throat is accompanied or followed by fever, headache, rash, swelling, nausea, or vomiting, consult a doctor promptly. If sore mouth symptoms do not improve in 7 days, see your doctor promptly. Do not use this product if you have a history of allergy to local anesthetics such as procaine, butacaine, or other "caine" anesthetics. **Keep this and all drugs out of the reach of children.** In case of accidental overdose seek professional assistance or contact a poison control center immediately. As with any drug if you are pregnant or nursing a baby, seek the advice of a health professional before using this product.

How Supplied: Available in Cool Mint, Cherry, and Menthol lozenges in packages of 18.

CHLORASEPTIC®
SORE THROAT SPRAY & GARGLE
Phenol/oral anesthetic/antiseptic
Cherry, Menthol and Cool Mint
Flavors

Active Ingredient: Gargle and Spray—Phenol 1.4%.

Inactive Ingredients: Original Menthol Liquid: D&C Green No. 5, D&C Yellow No. 10, FD&C Green No. 3, flavor, glycerin, purified water, saccharin sodium.
Cherry Liquid: FD&C Red No. 40, flavor, glycerin, purified water, saccharin sodium.
Cool Mint Liquid: FD&C Blue No. 1, flavor, glycerin, purified water, saccharin sodium.

Indications: For temporary relief of occasional minor sore throat pain and sore mouth. Also for the temporary relief of pain due to canker sores, minor irritation or injury of the mouth and gums, minor dental procedures, dentures or orthodontic appliances.

Administration and Dosage: Chloraseptic Spray (Pump): Spray 5 times directly into throat or affected area and swallow. Children 2–12 years of age, spray 3 times and swallow. Repeat every 2 hours or as directed by a physician or dentist. Children under 12 years of age should be supervised in product use. Children under 2 years: consult a physician or dentist.
Chloraseptic Gargle: Adults and children 12 years of age and older: Gargle or swish around the mouth for at least 15 seconds and then spit out. Use every 2 hours or as directed by a physician or dentist. Children 6 to under 12 years: Gargle or swish around in mouth 2 teaspoonsful for at least 15 seconds and then spit out. Use every 2 hours or as directed by a physician or dentist. Children under 12 years should be supervised in product

Continued on next page

Procter & Gamble—Cont.

use. Children under 6 years: Consult a physician or dentist.

WARNINGS: If sore throat is severe, or is accompanied by difficulty in breathing, or persists for more than 2 days, do not use, and consult a doctor promptly. If sore throat is accompanied or followed by fever, headache, rash, swelling, nausea, or vomiting, consult a doctor promptly. If sore mouth symptoms do not improve in 7 days, or if irritation, pain, or redness persists or worsens, consult your doctor promptly. **Keep this and all drugs out of the reach of children.** In case of accidental overdose, seek professional assistance or contact a poison control center immediately. As with any drug, if you are pregnant or nursing a baby, seek the advice of a health professional before using this product.

How Supplied: Available in Original Menthol, Cherry, and Cool Mint flavors in 6 FL. OZ. (177 mL) plastic bottles with sprayer. Menthol Flavor is also available in 12 FL. OZ. (355 mL) gargle.

HEAD & SHOULDERS® INTENSIVE TREATMENT DANDRUFF SHAMPOO

Head & Shoulders Intensive Treatment Dandruff Shampoo offers effective control of persistent dandruff, and beautiful hair from a pleasant-to-use formula. Double-blind and expert-graded testing have proven that Intensive Treatment Dandruff Shampoo reduces persistent dandruff. It is also gentle enough to use every day for clean, manageable hair.

Active Ingredient: 1% selenium sulfide suspended in a mild surfactant base. Shampoo also includes mild conditioning agents.

Indications: For effective control of seborrheic dermatitis and dandruff of the scalp.

Actions: Selenium sulfide is substantive to the scalp and remains after rinsing. Its mechanism is believed to be antiproliferative, and to also control the microorganisms associated with persistent dandruff flaking and itching.

WARNINGS: For external use only. Avoid contact with eyes—if this happens, rinse thoroughly with water. If scalp condition worsens, or does not improve, consult a doctor. Keep out of reach of children.

Caution: If used on light, gray, or chemically treated hair, rinse **(VIGOROUSLY)** for 5 minutes.

Dosage and Administration: For best results in controlling persistent dandruff, Head & Shoulders Intensive Treatment Dandruff Shampoo should be used regularly. It is gentle enough to use for every shampoo.

Composition:
Lotion—Intensive Treatment Regular Formula: Ingredients: Selenium sulfide in a shampoo base of water, ammonium laureth sulfate, ammonium lauryl sulfate, cocamide MEA, glycol distearate, ammonium xylenesulfonate, dimethicone, fragrance, tricetylmonium chloride, cetyl alcohol, DMDM hydantoin, sodium chloride, stearyl alcohol, hydroxypropyl methylcellulose, FD&C Red no. 4.
Lotion—Intensive Treatment 2-in-1 (Persistent Dandruff Shampoo plus Conditioner in One) Formula: Selenium sulfide in a shampoo base of water, ammonium laureth sulfate, ammonium lauryl sulfate, cocamide MEA, glycol distearate, dimethicone, ammonium xylenesulfonate, fragrance, tricetylmonium chloride, cetyl alcohol, DMDM hydantoin, sodium chloride, stearyl alcohol, hydroxypropyl methylcellulose, FD&C Red no. 4.

How Supplied: Intensive Treatment Regular Lotion is available in 7.0 and 11.0 fl. oz. unbreakable plastic bottles. Intensive Treatment 2-in-1 is available in 6.0 and 8.9 fl. oz. unbreakable plastic bottles.

METAMUCIL®

[met 'uh-mū 'sil]
(psyllium hydrophilic mucilloid)

Description: Metamucil is a bulk-forming natural therapeutic fiber for restoring and maintaining regularity as recommended by a physician. It contains hydrophilic mucilloid, a highly efficient dietary fiber derived from the husk of the psyllium seed (*Plantago ovata*). Metamucil contains no chemical stimulants and does not disrupt normal bowel function. Each dose contains approximately 3.4 grams of psyllium hydrophilic mucilloid. Inactive ingredients, sodium, potassium, calories, carbohydrate, fat and phenylalanine content are shown in Table 1 for all forms and flavors. NutraSweet®* brand sweetener (aspartame) is used in flavored sugar-free Metamucil powdered products. Phenylketonurics should be aware that phenylalanine is present in Metamucil products that contain Nutrasweet. Metamucil Sugar-Free Regular Flavor contains no sugar and no artificial sweeteners.
Metamucil in powdered forms is gluten-free. Wafers contain gluten: Apple Crisp contains 0.7 g/dose, Cinnamon Spice contains 0.5 g/dose.

Actions: The active ingredient in Metamucil is psyllium, a natural fiber which promotes elimination due to its bulking effect in the colon. This bulking effect is due to both the water-holding capacity of undigested fiber and the increased bacterial mass following partial fiber digestion. These actions result in enlargement

---

*NutraSweet® is a registered trademark of the NutraSweet Company.

of the lumen of the colon, and softer stool, thereby decreasing intraluminal pressure and straining, and speeding colonic transit in constipated patients.

Indications: Metamucil is indicated in the management of chronic constipation, in irritable bowel syndrome, as adjunctive therapy in the constipation of diverticular disease, in the bowel management of patients with hemorrhoids, for constipation associated with convalescence and senility and for occasional constipation during pregnancy when under the care of a physician. Pregnancy: Category B.

Contraindications: Intestinal obstruction, fecal impaction. Known allergy to any component.

Warnings: Patients are advised they should not use the product without consulting a doctor when abdominal pain, nausea, or vomiting are present or if they have noticed a sudden change in bowel habits that persists over a period of 2 weeks, or rectal bleeding. Patients are advised to consult a physician if constipation persists for longer than one week, as this may be a sign of a serious medical condition. **PATIENTS ARE CAUTIONED THAT TAKING THIS PRODUCT WITHOUT ADEQUATE FLUID MAY CAUSE IT TO SWELL AND BLOCK THE THROAT OR ESOPHAGUS AND MAY CAUSE CHOKING. THEY SHOULD NOT TAKE THE PRODUCT IF THEY HAVE DIFFICULTY IN SWALLOWING. IF THEY EXPERIENCE CHEST PAIN, VOMITING, OR DIFFICULTY IN SWALLOWING OR BREATHING AFTER TAKING THIS PRODUCT, THEY ARE ADVISED TO SEEK IMMEDIATE MEDICAL ATTENTION.** Psyllium products may cause allergic reaction in people sensitive to inhaled or ingested psyllium. Keep this and all medications out of the reach of children.

Precaution: *Notice to Health Care Professionals:* To minimize the potential for allergic reaction, health care professionals who frequently dispense powdered psyllium products should avoid inhaling airborne dust while dispensing these products. *Handling and Dispensing:* To minimize generating airborne dust, spoon product from the canister into a glass according to label directions.

Dosage and Administration: The usual adult dosage is 1 rounded teaspoonful or 1 rounded tablespoonful depending on product form. Generally the sugar-free products are dosed by the teaspoonful, sucrose-containing products by the tablespoonful. Some forms are available in packets. The appropriate dose should be mixed with 8 oz. of liquid (e.g. cool water, fruit juice, milk) following the labeled instructions. Metamucil wafers should be consumed with 8 oz. of liquid. **THE PRODUCT (CHILD OR ADULT DOSE) SHOULD BE TAKEN WITH AT LEAST 8 OZ (A FULL GLASS) OF WATER OR OTHER FLUID. TAKING**

TABLE 1

Forms/ Flavors	Inactive Ingredients	Sodium mg/ Dose	Potas- sium mg/ Dose	Calo- ries per Dose	Carbo- hy- drate g/ Dose	Fat g/ Dose	Phenyl- alanine mg/Dose	Dosage 1–3 Times Daily. Each Dose Contains 3.4 g Psyllium Hydrophilic Mucilloid	How Supplied
Smooth Texture Orange Flavor **METAMUCIL** Powder	Citric acid, D&C Yellow No. 10, FD&C Yellow No. 6, Flavoring, Sucrose	< 5	30	35	12	—	—	1 rounded tablespoonful 12 g	Canisters: 13, 20.3, and 30.4 ozs. (Doses: 30, 48 and 72); Cartons: 30 single-dose packets (OTC)
Smooth Texture Sugar-Free Orange Flavor **METAMUCIL** Powder	Aspartame, Citric acid, D&C Yellow No. 10, FD&C Yellow No. 6, Flavoring, Maltodextrin	< 5	30	10	5	—	25	1 rounded teaspoonful 5.8 g	Canisters: 10, 15 and 23.3 ozs. (Doses: 48, 72 and 114); Cartons: 30 single-dose packets (OTC), 100 single-dose packets (Institutional)
Smooth Texture Citrus Flavor **METAMUCIL** Powder	Citric acid, D&C Yellow No. 10, FD&C Yellow No. 6, Flavoring, Sucrose	< 5	40	35	12	—	—	1 rounded tablespoonful 12 g	Canisters: 13, 20.3 and 30.4 ozs. (Doses: 30, 48 and 72); Cartons: 30 single-dose packets (OTC) 100 single-dose packets (Institutional)
Smooth Texture Sugar-Free Citrus Flavor **METAMUCIL** Powder	Aspartame, Citric acid, D&C Yellow No. 10, FD&C Yellow No. 6, Flavoring, Maltodextrin	< 5	30	10	5	—	25	1 rounded teaspoonful 5.8 g	Canisters: 10, 15 and 23.3 ozs. (Doses: 48, 72 and 114); Cartons: 30 single-dose packets (OTC)
Smooth Texture Sugar-Free Regular Flavor **METAMUCIL** Powder	Citric acid (less than 1%), Magnesium sulfate**, Maltodextrin	< 5	30	10	5	—	—	1 rounded teaspoonful 5.8 g	Canisters: 10, 15 and 23.3 ozs. (Doses: 48, 72 and 114)
Regular Flavor **METAMUCIL** Powder	Dextrose	< 5	30	14	6	—	—	1 rounded teaspoonful 7 g	Canisters: 13, 19 and 29 ozs. (Doses: 48, 72 and 114)
Orange Flavor **METAMUCIL** Powder	Citric acid, FD&C Yellow No. 6, Flavoring, Sucrose	< 5	35	30	10	—	—	1 rounded tablespoonful 11 g	Canisters: 13, 19 and 29 ozs. (Doses: 30, 48 and 72)
Sugar-Free Lemon-Lime Flavor **METAMUCIL** Effervescent Powder	Aspartame, Calcium carbonate, Citric acid, Flavoring, Potassium bicarbonate, Silicon dioxide, Sodium bicarbonate	10	280	6	4	—	30	1 packet 5.4 g	Cartons: 30 single-dose packets (OTC), 100 single-dose packets (Institutional)
Sugar-Free Orange-Flavor **METAMUCIL** Effervescent Powder	Aspartame, Citric acid, FD&C Yellow No. 6, Flavoring, Potassium bicarbonate, Silicon dioxide, Sodium bicarbonate	5	280	6	4	—	28	1 packet 5.2 g	Cartons: 30 single-dose packets (OTC)

Continued on next page

Procter & Gamble—Cont.

TABLE 1 (continued)

Forms/ FLavors	Inactive Ingredients	Sodium mg/ Dose	Potas- sium mg/ Dose	Calo- ries per Dose	Carbo- hy- drate g/ Dose	Fat g/ Dose	Phenyl- alanine mg/Dose	Dosage 1–3 Times Daily. Each Dose Contains 3.4 g Psyllium Hydrophilic Mucilloid	How Supplied
Apple Crisp **METAMUCIL** Wafers	Ascorbic acid, Brown sugar, Cinnamon, Corn oil, Flavors, Fructose, Lecithin, Modified food starch, Molasses, Oat hull fiber, Sodium bicarbonate, Sucrose, Water, Wheat flour	20	50	100	19	5	—	2 wafers 25 g	Cartons: 12 doses; 24 doses
Cinnamon Spice **METAMUCIL** Wafers	Ascorbic acid, Cinnamon, Corn oil, Flavors, Fructose, Lecithin, Modified food starch, Molasses, Nutmeg, Oat hull fiber, Oats, Sodium bicarbonate, Sucrose, Water Wheat flour	15	45	100	18	5	—	2 wafers 25 g	Cartons: 12 doses; 24 doses

**Metamucil Sugar-Free Regular Flavor contains 26 mg of magnesium per dose.

THIS PRODUCT WITHOUT ENOUGH LIQUID MAY CAUSE CHOKING (SEE WARNINGS). Metamucil can be taken orally one to three times a day, depending on the need and response. It may require continued use for 2 to 3 days to provide optimal benefit. For children (6 to 12 years old), use ½ the adult dose in/with 8 oz. of liquid, 1 to 3 times daily.

New Users: (Label statement)
Your doctor can recommend the right dosage of Metamucil to best meet your needs. In general, start by taking one dose each day. Gradually increase to three doses per day, if needed or recommended by your doctor. If minor gas or bloating occurs when you increase doses, try slightly reducing the amount you are taking.

How Supplied: Powder: canisters (OTC) and cartons of single-dose packets (OTC and Institutional). Wafers: cartons of single-dose packets (OTC). (See Table 1).
[See table on preceding page]
[See table above.]

OIL OF OLAY®—Daily UV Protectant SPF 15 Beauty Fluid—Original & Fragrance Free Versions (Olay Co., Inc.)

Oil of Olay Daily UV Protectant Beauty Fluid is a light, greaseless lotion that is specially formulated to provide effective moisturization and SPF 15 protection with minimal migration to reduce the likelihood of eye sting. Oil of Olay Daily UV Protectant is PABA free. It is non-comedogenic and is suitable for daily use under facial make-up.

Active Ingredients: Octyl Methoxycinnamate, Phenylbenzimidazole Sulfonic Acid

Inactive Ingredients: Water, Isohexadecane, Butylene Glycol, Triethanolamine, Glycerin, Stearic Acid, Cetyl Alcohol, Cetyl Palmitate, DEA-Cetyl Phosphate, Aluminum Starch Octenylsuccinate, Titanium Dioxide, Imidazolidinyl Urea, Methylparaben, Propylparaben, Carbomer, Acrylates/C10–30 Alkyl Acrylate Crosspolymer, PEG-10 Soya Sterol, Disodium EDTA, Castor Oil, Fragrance, FD&C Red No. 4, FD&C Yellow No. 5.
Available in both lightly scented original version and a 100% color free and fragrance free version.

Indications: Filters out the sun's harmful rays to help prevent skin damage. Provides SPF 15 protection in a light, greaseless moisturizer. Regular use over the years may reduce the chance of skin damage, some types of skin cancer, and other harmful effects due to the sun.

Directions: Adults and children 6 months of age and over: Apply liberally as often as necessary. Children under 6 months of age: Consult a doctor.

Warnings: For external use only, not to be swallowed. Avoid contact with eyes. If contact occurs, rinse eyes thoroughly with water. Discontinue use if signs of irritation or rash appear. If irritation or rash persists, consult a doctor. **KEEP OUT OF REACH OF CHILDREN.**

How Supplied: Available in 3.5 fl. oz. and 5.25 fl. oz. plastic bottles.

PEPTO-BISMOL® ORIGINAL LIQUID AND ORIGINAL AND CHERRY TABLETS
For diarrhea, heartburn, indigestion, upset stomach and nausea.

Multi-symptom Pepto-Bismol contains bismuth subsalicylate and is the only leading OTC stomach remedy clinically proven effective for both upper and lower GI symptoms. Pepto-Bismol is in more households than any other stomach remedy, making it a convenient recommendation with a name your patients will know. It has been clinically-proven in double-blind placebo-controlled trials for relief of upset stomach symptoms and diarrhea.

Description: Each Pepto-Bismol Tablet contains 262 mg bismuth subsalicylate and each tablespoonful (15ml) of Pepto-Bismol Liquid contains 262 mg bismuth subsalicylate. Each tablet contains 102 mg salicylate (99 mg salicylate for Cherry) and each tablespoonful of liquid contains 130 mg salicylate. Liquid and tablets contain no sugar. Tablets are very low in sodium (less than 2 mg/tablet) and Liquid is low in sodium (less than 3 mg/tablespoonful). Inactive ingredients include (Tablets): adipic acid (in Cherry only), calcium carbonate, D&C Red No. 27, FD&C Red No. 40 (in Cherry only), flavors, magnesium stearate, mannitol, povidone, saccharin sodium and talc; (Liquid): benzoic acid, D&C Red No. 22, D&C Red No. 28, flavor, magnesium aluminum silicate, methylcellulose, saccharin sodium, salicylic acid, sodium salicylate, sorbic acid and water.

Indications: Pepto-Bismol controls diarrhea within 24 hours, relieving associated abdominal cramps; soothes heartburn and indigestion without constipating; and relieves nausea and upset stomach.

Actions: For upset stomach symptoms (i.e. heartburn, indigestion, nausea and fullness caused by over-indulgence), the active ingredient is believed to work via a topical effect on the stomach mucosa. For diarrhea, it is believed to work by several mechanisms in the gastro-intestinal tract, including: 1) by normalizing fluid movement via an antisecretory mechanism and 2) by binding bacterial toxins and antimicrobial activity.

Warnings: Children and teenagers who have or are recovering from chicken pox or flu should not use this medicine to treat nausea or vomiting. If nausea or vomiting is present, patients are advised to consult a doctor because this could be an early sign of Reye Syndrome, a rare but serious illness.
This product contains salicylates. If taken with aspirin and ringing in the ears occurs, discontinue use. This product does not contain aspirin, but should not be administered to those patients who have a known allergy to aspirin or salicylates. Caution is advised in the administration to patients taking medication for anticoagulation, diabetes and gout.
If diarrhea is accompanied by a high fever or continues more than 2 days, patients are advised to consult a physician. As with any drug, caution is advised in the administration to pregnant or nursing women.

Note: This medication may cause a temporary and harmless darkening of the tongue and/or stool. Stool darkening should not be confused with melena.

Overdosage: In case of overdose, patients are advised to contact a physician or Poison Control Center. Emesis induced by ipecac syrup is indicated in large ingestions provided ipecac can be administered within one hour of ingestion. Activated charcoal should be administered after gastric emptying. Patients should be evaluated for signs and symptoms of salicylate toxicity.

Dosage and Administration
Tablets:
Adults—Two tablets
Children (according to age)—

9–12 yrs.	1 tablet
6–9 yrs.	2/3 tablet
3–6 yrs.	1/3 tablet

Chew or dissolve in mouth. Repeat every 1/2 to 1 hour as needed, to a maximum of 8 doses in a 24-hour period. Drink plenty of clear fluids to help prevent dehydration, which may accompany diarrhea.

Liquid: Shake well before using.
Adults—2 tablespoonsful (1 dose cup)
Children (according to age)—

9–12 yrs.	1 tablespoonful (1/2 dose cup)
6–9 yrs.	2 teaspoonsful (1/3 dose cup)
3–6 yrs.	1 teaspoonful (1/6 dose cup)

Repeat dosage every 1/2 to 1 hour, if needed, to a maximum of 8 doses in a 24-hour period. Drink plenty of clear fluids to help prevent dehydration which may accompany diarrhea.
For children under 3 years of age, consult physician.

How Supplied: Pepto-Bismol Liquid is available in: 4 fl. oz. bottle, 8 fl. oz. bottle, 12 fl. oz. bottle, 16 fl. oz. bottle. Pepto-Bismol Tablets are pink, round, chewable, tablets imprinted with "Pepto-Bismol" on one side. Tablets are available in: box of 30, box of 48, and roll pack of 12 (cherry only).

PEPTO-BISMOL®MAXIMUM STRENGTH LIQUID
For diarrhea, heartburn, indigestion, upset stomach and nausea.

Multi-symptom Pepto-Bismol contains bismuth subsalicylate and is the only leading OTC stomach remedy clinically proven effective for both upper and lower GI symptoms. Pepto-Bismol is in more households than any other stomach remedy, making it a convenient recommendation with a name your patients will know. It has been clinically-proven in double-blind placebo-controlled trials for relief of upset stomach symptoms and diarrhea.

Description: Each tablespoonful (15ml) of Maximum Strength Pepto-Bismol Liquid contains 525 mg bismuth subsalicylate (236 mg salicylate). Maximum Strength Pepto-Bismol Liquid contains no sugar and is low in sodium (less than 3 mg/tablespoonful). Inactive ingredients include: benzoic acid, D&C Red No. 22, D&C Red No. 28, flavor, magnesium aluminum silicate, methylcellulose, saccharin sodium, salicylic acid, sodium salicylate, sorbic acid, and water.

Indications: Maximum Strength Pepto-Bismol controls diarrhea within 24 hours, relieving associated abdominal cramps; soothes heartburn and indigestion without constipating; and relieves nausea and upset stomach.

Actions: For upset stomach symptoms (i.e. heartburn, indigestion, nausea and fullness caused by over-indulgence), the active ingredient is believed to work via a topical effect on the stomach mucosa. For diarrhea, it is believed to work by several mechanisms in the gastro-intestinal tract, including: 1) by normalizing fluid movement via an antisecretory mechanism and 2) by binding bacterial toxins and antimicrobial activity.

Warnings: Children and teenagers who have or are recovering from chicken pox or flu should NOT use this medicine to treat nausea or vomiting. If nausea or vomiting is present, patients are advised to consult a doctor because this could be an early sign of Reye Syndrome, a rare but serious illness.
This product contains salicylates. If taken with aspirin and ringing in the ears occurs, discontinue use. This product does not contain aspirin, but should not be administered to those patients who have a known allergy to aspirin or salicylates. Caution is advised in the administration to patients taking medication for anticoagulation, diabetes and gout.
If diarrhea is accompanied by a high fever or continues more than 2 days, patients are advised to consult a physician. As with any drug, caution is advised in the administration to pregnant or nursing women.

Note: This medication may cause a temporary and harmless darkening of the tongue and/or stool. Stool darkening should not be confused with melena.

Overdosage: In case of overdose, patients are advised to contact a physician or Poison Control Center. Emesis induced by ipecac syrup is indicated in large ingestions provided ipecac can be administered within one hour of ingestion. Activated charcoal should be administered after gastric emptying. Patients should be evaluated for signs and symptoms of salicylate toxicity.

Dosage and Administration: Shake well before using.

Adults—2 tablespoonfuls (1 dose cup)
Children (according to age)—

9–12 yrs.	1 tablespoonful (1/2 dose cup)
6–9 yrs.	2 teaspoonfuls (1/3 dose cup)
3–6 yrs.	1 teaspoonful (1/6 dose cup)

Repeat dosage every hour, if needed, to a maximum of 4 doses in a 24-hour period. Drink plenty of clear fluids to help prevent dehydration, which may accompany diarrhea.

How Supplied: Maximum Strength Pepto-Bismol is available in:
4 fl. oz. bottle
8 fl. oz. bottle
12 fl. oz. bottle

PEPTO DIARRHEA CONTROL®
Loperamide Hydrochloride Oral Solution & Caplets

Description: Each 5 ml (teaspoon) of Pepto Diarrhea Control liquid contains Loperamide Hydrochloride 1 mg. Pepto Diarrhea Control is a non-chalky, cherry flavored, clear liquid. Each caplet of Pepto Diarrhea Control contains 2 mg of Loperamide Hydrochloride and is scored and colored white.

Actions: Pepto Diarrhea Control contains a clinically proven antidiarrheal medication, Loperamide Hydrochloride, that works in many cases with just one dose. Loperamide Hydrochloride acts by

Continued on next page

Procter & Gamble—Cont.

slowing intestinal motility and by affecting water and electrolyte movement through the bowel.

Indication: Pepto Diarrhea Control controls the symptoms of diarrhea.

Directions: A dose cup is provided to accurately measure liquid doses as noted below. Drink plenty of clear fluids to help prevent dehydration, which may accompany diarrhea.

Usual Dosage: Adults and children 12 years of age and older: Take four teaspoonfuls or two caplets after first loose bowel movement followed by two teaspoonfuls or one caplet after each subsequent loose bowel movement but not more than eight teaspoonfuls or four caplets a day for no more than two days.
Children 9–11 years old (60–95 lbs.): Two teaspoonfuls or one caplet after first loose bowel movement, followed by one teaspoonful or one-half caplet after each subsequent loose bowel movement. Do not exceed six teaspoonfuls or three caplets a day for no more than two days.
Children 6–8 years old (48–59 lbs.): Two teaspoonfuls or one caplet after first loose bowel movement, followed by one teaspoonful or one-half caplet after each subsequent loose bowel movement. Do not exceed four teaspoonfuls or two caplets a day for no more than two days.
Professional Dosage Schedule for children 2–5 years old (24–47 lbs.): One teaspoon after first loose bowel movement, followed by one after each subsequent loose bowel movement. Do not exceed three teaspoonfuls a day.

Warnings: DO NOT USE FOR MORE THAN TWO DAYS UNLESS DIRECTED BY A PHYSICIAN. Do not use if diarrhea is accompanied by high fever (greater than 101°F), or if blood is present in the stool, or if you have had a rash or other allergic reaction to Loperamide Hydrochloride. If you are taking antibiotics or have a history of liver disease, consult a physician before using this product. As with any drug, if you are pregnant or nursing a baby, seek the advice of a health professional before using this product. Keep this and all drugs out of the reach of children. In case of accidental overdose, seek professional assistance or contact a poison control center immediately. Store at room temperature.

Overdosage: Overdosage of Loperamide Hydrochloride in man may result in constipation, CNS depression and nausea. A slurry of activated charcoal administered promptly after ingestion of Loperamide Hydrochloride can reduce the amount of drug which is absorbed. If vomiting occurs spontaneously upon ingestion, a slurry of 100 grams of activated charcoal should be administered orally as soon as fluids can be retained. If vomiting has not occurred, and CNS depression is evident, gastric lavage should be performed followed by administration of 100 gms of the activated charcoal

slurry through the gastric tube. In the event of overdosage, patients should be monitored for signs of CNS depression for at least 24 hours. Children may be more sensitive to central nervous system effects than adults. If CNS depression is observed, naloxone may be administered. If responsive to naloxone, vital signs must be monitored carefully for recurrence of symptoms of drug overdose for at least 24 hours after the last dose of naloxone.

Inactive Ingredients: Liquid: Alcohol (5.25%), citric acid, flavors, glycerin, methylparaben, propylparaben and purified water.
Caplets: Corn starch, lactose, magnesium stearate, microcrystalline cellulose.

How Supplied: Cherry flavored liquid (clear) 2 fl. oz. and 4 fl. oz. tamper resistant bottles with child resistant safety caps and special dosage cups. White scored caplets in 6's, 12's and 18's blister packaging which is tamper resistant and child resistant.

PERCOGESIC®
[pěr·kō-jē 'zĭk]
Analgesic Tablets
Pain Reliever/Fever Reducer

Active Ingredients: Each tablet contains:
Acetaminophen .... 325 mg
Phenyltoloxamine citrate .... 30 mg

Inactive Ingredients: Cellulose, FD&C Yellow No. 6, Flavor, Hydroxypropyl Methylcellulose, Magnesium Stearate, Polyethylene Glycol, Povidone, Silica Gel, Starch, Stearic Acid, Sucrose.

Indications: For temporary relief of minor aches and pains associated with headaches, muscular aches, backaches, premenstrual and menstrual periods, colds, the flu, toothaches, as well as for minor pain from arthritis, and to reduce fever.

Dosage and Administration: Adults (12 years and over)—1 or 2 tablets every four hours. Maximum daily dose—8 tablets.
Children (6 to under 12 years)—1 tablet every 4 hours. Maximum daily dose—4 tablets.
Children under 6 years of age: consult a doctor.

Warnings: Do not take this product for pain for more than 10 days (adults) or 5 days (children), and do not take for fever for more than 3 days unless directed by a doctor. If pain or fever persists or worsens, new symptoms occur or redness or swelling is present, consult a doctor as these could be signs of a serious condition. Do not give to children for arthritis pain unless directed by a doctor. May cause excitability especially in children. Do not take this product if you have asthma, glaucoma, emphysema, chronic pulmonary disease, shortness of breath, or difficulty in breathing unless directed by a doctor. May cause drowsiness; alco-

hol, sedatives, and tranquilizers may increase the drowsiness effect. Avoid alcoholic beverages while taking this product. Do not take this product if you are taking sedatives or tranquilizers without first consulting your doctor. Use caution when driving a motor vehicle or operating machinery. **KEEP THIS AND ALL DRUGS OUT OF THE REACH OF CHILDREN.** In case of accidental overdose, seek professional assistance or contact a poison control center immediately. Prompt medical attention is critical for adults as well as for children even if you do not notice any signs or symptoms. As with any drug, if you are pregnant or nursing a baby, seek the advice of a health professional before using this product.

How Supplied: Light orange tablets engraved with "Percogesic". Child-resistant bottles of 24 and 90 tablets, and non-child-resistant bottles of 50 tablets.

VICKS® CHILDREN'S NYQUIL®
NIGHTTIME COLD/COUGH
MEDICINE
Antihistamine/Nasal Decongestant/
Cough Suppressant

Children's NyQuil was specially formulated with three effective ingredients to relieve nighttime cough, nasal congestion, and runny nose so children can rest. Children's NyQuil is alcohol free and analgesic free and has a pleasant cherry flavor.

Active Ingredients: Per ½ FL. OZ. dose (1 TBSP.): Chlorpheniramine Maleate 2 mg, Pseudoephedrine HCl 30 mg, Dextromethorphan Hydrobromide 15 mg.

Inactive Ingredients: Citric Acid, FD&C Red No. 40, Flavor, Potassium Sorbate, Propylene Glycol, Purified Water, Sodium Citrate, Sucrose.

Indications: For temporary relief of nasal congestion, runny nose, sneezing, and coughing due to a cold, so your child can rest.

Directions: Take at bedtime as directed. Use medicine cup provided.
If cold symptoms keep your child at home, 4 doses may be given per day, each 6 hours apart, or use as directed by a doctor.

Age	Weight	Dose
Under 6 yrs	Under 48 lbs.	Consult physician*
6–11 yrs	48–95 lbs.	½ FL. OZ. 1 TABLESPOON (TBSP.)
12 yrs and over	96 lbs. and over	1 FL. OZ. 2 TABLESPOONS (TBSP.)

***Professional Labeling:** Children under 6 years of age: Use only as directed by a physician.

Suggested doses for children under 6 years of age:

Age	Weight	Dose
*6–11 mo.	17–21 lbs.	1 teaspoon (tsp.) (5 mL)
*12–23 mo.	22–27 lbs.	1¼ teaspoon (tsp.) (6.25 mL)
2–5 yrs.	28–47 lbs.	½ TABLE-SPOON (TBSP.) (7.5 mL)

Repeat every 6 hours, not to exceed 4 doses in 24 hours, or as directed by doctor.

* Based on extrapolation from studies on the safety and efficacy of active ingredients conducted among older children and adults. Use caution in treating children under 2 years of age who were born prematurely.

WARNINGS: Do not exceed recommended dosage because at higher doses nervousness, dizziness, or sleeplessness may occur. Do not take this product for more than 7 days. If symptoms do not improve or are accompanied by fever, consult a doctor. Do not take this product if you have heart disease, high blood pressure, thyroid disease, diabetes, glaucoma, or difficulty in urination due to enlargement of the prostate gland unless directed by a doctor. *Drug Interaction Precaution:* Do not take this product if you are presently taking a prescription drug for high blood pressure or depression, without first consulting your doctor. May cause excitability especially in children. Do not take this product, unless directed by a doctor, if you have a breathing problem such as emphysema or chronic bronchitis. May cause marked drowsiness; alcohol, sedatives, and tranquilizers may increase the drowsiness effect. Avoid alcoholic beverages while taking this product. Do not take this product if you are taking sedatives or tranquilizers, without first consulting your doctor. Use caution when driving a motor vehicle or operating machinery. A persistent cough may be a sign of a serious condition. If cough persists for more than 1 week, tends to recur, or is accompanied by fever, rash, or persistent headache, consult a doctor. Do not take this product for persistent or chronic cough such as occurs with smoking, asthma, emphysema, or if cough is accompanied by excessive phlegm (mucus) unless directed by a doctor. **Keep this and all drugs out of the reach of children.** In case of accidental overdose, seek professional assistance or contact a poison control center immediately. As with any drug, if you are pregnant or nursing a baby, seek the advice of a health professional before using this product.

How Supplied: Available in 4 FL. OZ. (118 mL) bottles with child-resistant, tamper-evident cap and a calibrated medicine cup.

VICKS® COUGH DROPS
Menthol Cough Suppressant/Oral Anesthetic

Flavors: Available in two popular flavors: Menthol and Cherry.

Active Ingredient: Menthol.

Inactive Ingredients:
Menthol Flavor: Benzyl Alcohol, Camphor, Caramel, Corn Syrup, Eucalyptus Oil, Flavor, Sucrose, Tolu Balsam, Thymol.
Cherry Flavor: Citric Acid, Corn Syrup, FD&C Blue No. 1, FD&C Red No. 40, Flavor, Sucrose.

Indications: Temporarily relieves sore throat and coughs due to colds or inhaled irritants.

Directions: **Adults and children 3 to 12 years:** Allow drop to dissolve slowly in mouth. **Cough:** may be repeated every hour as needed or as directed by a doctor. **Sore Throat:** may be repeated every 2 hours—as needed or as directed by a doctor. **Children under 3 years of age:** consult a doctor.

WARNINGS: A persistent cough may be a sign of a serious condition. If cough persists for more than 1 week, tends to recur, or is accompanied by fever, rash, or persistent headache, consult a doctor. Do not take this product for persistent or chronic cough such as occurs with smoking, asthma, emphysema, or if cough is accompanied by excessive phlegm (mucus), unless directed by a doctor. If sore throat is severe, or is accompanied by difficulty in breathing, or persists for more than 2 days, do not use, and consult a doctor promptly. If sore throat is accompanied or followed by fever, headache, rash, swelling, nausea, or vomiting, consult a doctor promptly. **Keep this and all drugs out of the reach of children.** As with any drug, if you are pregnant or nursing a baby, seek the advice of a health professional before using this product.

How Supplied: Vicks Cough Drops are available in boxes of 14 drops each and bags of 30 drops.

EXTRA STRENGTH VICKS® COUGH DROPS
Menthol Cough Suppressant/Oral Anesthetic

Flavors: Available in Cherry, Menthol, Honey Lemon and Peppermint flavors.

Active Ingredient: Menthol Flavor: Menthol 8.4 mg. Cherry: Menthol 10 mg, Honey Lemon: Menthol 10 mg, Peppermint: Menthol 10 mg.

Inactive Ingredients:
Menthol Flavor: Corn Syrup, FD&C Blue No. 1, Flavor, Sucrose, Cherry Flavor: Corn Syrup, FD&C Blue No. 2, FD&C Red No. 40, Flavor, Sucrose Honey Lemon: Citric Acid, Corn Syrup, D&C Yellow No. 10, FD&C Yellow No. 6, Flavor, Sucrose, Peppermint: Corn Syrup, Flavor, Peppermint Oil, Sucrose.

Indications: Temporarily relieves sore throat and coughs due to colds or inhaled irritants.

Directions: **Adults and children 3 to 12 years:** Allow drop to dissolve slowly in mouth. **Cough:** may be repeated every hour as needed or as directed by a doctor. **Sore Throat:** may be repeated every 2 hours as needed or as directed by a doctor. **Children under 3 years of age:** consult a doctor.

WARNINGS: A persistent cough may be a sign of a serious condition. If cough persists for more than 1 week, tends to recur, or is accompanied by fever, rash, or persistent headache, consult a doctor. Do not take this product for persistent or chronic cough such as occurs with smoking, asthma, emphysema, or if cough is accompanied by excessive phlegm (mucus), unless directed by a doctor. If sore throat is severe, or is accompanied by difficulty in breathing, or persists for more than 2 days, do not use, and consult a doctor promptly. If sore throat is accompanied or followed by fever, headache, rash, swelling, nausea, or vomiting, consult a doctor promptly. **Keep this and all drugs out of the reach of children.** As with any drug, if you are pregnant or nursing a baby, seek the advice of a health professional before using this product.

How Supplied: Extra Strength Vicks Cough Drops are available in single sticks of 9 drops each and bags of 30 drops.

VICKS® DAYQUIL® ALLERGY RELIEF 4 HOUR TABLETS
Nasal Decongestant/Antihistamine

Active Ingredients: Each Tablet Contains:
25 mg Phenylpropanolamine Hydrochloride, 4 mg Brompheniramine Maleate

Inactive Ingredients: D&C Yellow No. 10 Aluminum Lake, FD&C Yellow No. 6 Aluminum Lake, Magnesium Stearate, Microcrystalline Cellulose, Starch.

Action: Nasal Decongestant and Antihistamine. The anytime stuffy nose, sneezing, runny nose, itchy, watery eyes, so you can face your allergy season medicine.™

Directions: Adults and children 12 years of age and older: One tablet every 4 hours. Do not exceed 1 tablet every 4 hours or 6 tablets in a 24-hour period. Children under 12 years of age: consult a doctor.

Warnings: Do not exceed recommended dosage because at higher doses nervous-

Continued on next page

Procter & Gamble—Cont.

ness, dizziness, or sleeplessness may occur. Do not take this product for more than 7 days. If symptoms do not improve or are accompanied by fever, consult a doctor. Do not take this product if you have heart disease, high blood pressure, thyroid disease, diabetes, glaucoma, or difficulty in urination due to enlargement of the prostate gland unless directed by a doctor. *Drug Interaction Precaution:* Do not take this product if you are presently taking a prescription drug for high blood pressure or depression without first consulting your doctor. May cause excitability especially in children. Do not take this product, unless directed by a doctor, if you have a breathing problem such as emphysema or chronic bronchitis. May cause drowsiness; alcohol, sedatives and tranquilizers may increase the drowsiness effect. Avoid alcoholic beverages while taking this product. Do not take this product if you are taking sedatives or tranquilizers without first consulting your doctor. Use caution when driving a motor vehicle or operating machinery. **Keep this and all drugs out of the reach of children.** In case of accidental overdose, seek professional assistance or contact a poison control center immediately. As with any drug, if you are pregnant or nursing a baby, seek the advice of a health professional before using this product.

How Supplied: Available in 24 count blister package. Each yellow tablet is imprinted with the letter A inside the vicks shield

---

VICKS® DAYQUIL® ALLERGY RELIEF 12 HOUR EXTENDED RELEASE TABLETS
Nasal Decongestant/Antihistamine

Active Ingredients: Each Extended Release Tablet Contains:
75 mg Phenylpropanolamine Hydrochloride, 12 mg Brompheniramine Maleate

Inactive Ingredients: Dimethyl Polysiloxane Oil, FD&C Blue No. 1 Aluminum Lake, Hydroxypropyl Methylcellulose, Lactose, Magnesium Stearate, Polyethylene Glycol. Talc, Titanium Dioxide.

Indications: For the temporary relief of nasal congestion due to the common cold, hay fever or other upper respiratory allergies, or associated with sinusitis; temporarily relieves runny nose, sneezing, and itchy and watery eyes as may occur in allergic rhinitis (such as hay fever). Temporarily restores freer breathing through the nose.

Action: Nasal Decongestant and Antihistamine. The anytime stuffy nose, sneezing, runny nose, itchy, watery eyes, so you can face your allergy season medicine.™

Directions: Adults and children 12 years of age and older: One tablet every 12 hours. DO NOT EXCEED 1 TABLET EVERY 12 HOURS, OR 2 TABLETS IN A 24-HOUR PERIOD. Children under 12 years of age: consult a doctor.

Warnings: This product may cause excitability, especially in children. Do not take this product if you have heart disease, high blood pressure, thyroid disease, diabetes, glaucoma, or difficulty in urination due to enlargement of the prostate gland, except under the advice and supervision of a doctor. Do not take this product, unless directed by a doctor, if you have a breathing problem such as emphysema or chronic bronchitis. Do not give this product to children under 12 years, except under the advice and supervision of a doctor. May cause drowsiness. Do not exceed recommended dosage because at higher doses nervousness, dizziness, or sleeplessness may occur. If symptoms do not improve within 7 days or are accompanied by fever, consult a doctor before continuing use. Do not take if hypersensitive to any of the ingredients. As with any drug, if you are pregnant or nursing a baby, seek the advice of a health professional before using this product. **CAUTION:** Avoid driving a motor vehicle or operating machinery and avoid alcoholic beverages while taking this product. **DRUG INTERACTION PRECAUTION:** Do not take this product if you are presently taking a prescription antihypertensive or antidepressant drug containing a monoamine oxidase inhibitor, except under the advice and supervision of a doctor. KEEP THIS AND ALL DRUGS OUT OF THE REACH OF CHILDREN. IN CASE OF ACCIDENTAL OVERDOSE, SEEK PROFESSIONAL ASSISTANCE OR CONTACT A POISON CONTROL CENTER IMMEDIATELY.

How Supplied: Available in 12 and 24 count blister packages. Each blue tablet is imprinted with the letter A inside the Vicks shield.

CHILDREN'S VICKS® DAYQUIL® ALLERGY RELIEF
Antihistamine/Nasal Decongestant

Children's Vicks DayQuil Allergy Relief was specially formulated with two effective ingredients to relieve allergy symptoms and head colds without coughs.

Active Ingredients per ½ FL. OZ., Dose (1 TBSP): Chlorpheniramine Maleate 2 mg, Pseudoephedrine HCl 30 mg

Inactive Ingredients: Citric Acid, FD&C Blue No. 1, FD&C Red No. 40, Flavor, Methylparaben, Potassium Sorbate, Propylene Glycol, Purified Water, Sodium Citrate, Sorbitol and Sucrose.

Indications: For temporary relief of nasal and sinus congestion, sneezing, runny nose, and itchy, watery eyes due to hay fever or other upper respiratory allergies.

Directions: Take as directed. Use medicine cup provided. If symptoms keep your child at home, 4 doses may be given per day, each 6 hours apart, or use as directed by a doctor.

Age	Weight	Dose
Under 6 yrs	Under 48 lbs.	Consult physician*
6–11 yrs	48–95 lbs.	1 TABLESPOON (TBSP.)
12 yrs and over	96 lbs. and over	2 TABLESPOONS (TBSP.)

*Professional Labeling: Children under 6 years of age: Use only as directed by a physician. Suggested doses for children under 6 years of age:

Age	Weight	Dose
*6–11 mo.	17–21 lbs.	1 teaspoon (tsp.) (5 mL)
*12–23 mo.	22–27 lbs.	1¼ teaspoon (tsp.) (6.25 mL)
2–5 yrs.	28–47 lbs.	½ TABLESPOON (TBSP.) (7.5 mL)

Repeat every 6 hours, not to exceed 4 doses in 24 hours, or as directed by doctor.
*Based on extrapolation from studies on the safety and efficacy of active ingredients conducted among older children and adults. Use caution in treating children under 2 years of age who were born prematurely.

Warnings: Do not exceed recommended dosage, because at higher doses nervousness, dizziness or sleeplessness may occur. Do not take this product for more than 7 days. If symptoms do not improve or are accompanied by fever, consult a doctor. Do not take this product if you have heart disease, high blood pressure, thyroid disease, diabetes, glaucoma, or difficulty in urination due to enlargement of the prostate gland unless directed by a doctor.
Drug Interaction Precaution: Do not take this product if you are presently taking a prescription drug for high blood pressure or depression, without first consulting your doctor. May cause excitability especially in children. Do not take this product, unless directed by a doctor, if you have a breathing problem such as emphysema or chronic bronchitis. May cause drowsiness; alcohol, sedatives, and tranquilizers may increase the drowsiness effect. Avoid alcoholic beverages while taking this product. Do not take this product if you are taking sedatives or tranquilizers, without first consulting your doctor. Use caution when driving a motor vehicle or operating machinery. **Keep this and all drugs out of the reach of children.** In case of accidental overdose, seek professional assistance or contact a poison control center immediately. As with any drug, if you are pregnant or nursing a baby, seek the advice of

a health professional before using this product.

How Supplied: Available in 4 FL. OZ. (118 mL) plastic bottles with child-resistant, tamper-evident cap and a calibrated medicine cup.

VICKS® DAYQUIL® LIQUID
VICKS® DAYQUIL® LIQUICAPS®
Multi-Symptom Cold/Flu Relief
Nasal Decongestant/Expectorant/
Pain Reliever/Cough
Suppressant/Fever Reducer

Active Ingredients: LIQUID—per fluid ounce (2 TBSP.) or LIQUI-CAPS—per two softgels, contains Pseudoephedrine Hydrochloride 60 mg, Guaifenesin 200 mg, Acetaminophen 650 mg (Liquid) or 500 mg (softgels), Dextromethorphan Hydrobromide 20 mg.

Inactive Ingredients: Liquid: Citric Acid, FD&C Yellow No. 6, Flavor, Glycerin, Polyethylene Glycol, Propylene Glycol, Purified Water, Saccharin Sodium, Sodium Citrate, Sucrose.
Softgels: FD&C Red No. 40, FD&C Yellow No. 6, Gelatin, Glycerin, Polyethylene Glycol, Povidone, Propylene Glycol, Purified Water. May contain Sorbitol.

Indications: For the temporary relief of minor aches, pains, headache, muscular aches, sore throat pain, and fever associated with a cold or flu. Temporarily relieves nasal congestion and coughing due to a cold. Helps loosen phlegm (mucus) and thin secretions to drain bronchial tubes and make coughs more productive.

Directions: Take as directed.
Adults 12 years and over: one FL. OZ. in medicine cup (2 tablespoons), or swallow 2 softgels with water.
Children 6 to under 12 years of age: ½ FL. OZ in medicine cup (1 tablespoon), or swallow 1 softgel with water.
Children under 6 years of age: Consult a doctor.
Repeat every 4 hours, not to exceed 4 doses per day, or as directed by a doctor.

Warnings: Do not exceed recommended dosage because at higher doses nervousness, dizziness, or sleeplessness may occur. Do not take this product if you have heart disease, high blood pressure, thyroid disease, diabetes, or difficulty in urination due to enlargement of the prostate gland unless directed by a doctor. *Drug Interaction Precaution:* Do not take this product if you are presently taking a prescription drug for high blood pressure or depression, without first consulting your doctor. Do not take this product for persistent or chronic cough such as occurs with smoking, asthma, chronic bronchitis, emphysema, or if cough is accompanied by excessive phlegm (mucus) unless directed by a doctor. Do not take this product for more than 7 days (for adults) or 5 days (for children). A persistent cough may be a sign

of serious condition. If cough persists for more than 7 days, tends to recur, or is accompanied by rash, or persistent headache, consult a doctor. If symptoms do not improve or are accompanied by fever that lasts for more than 3 days, or if new symptoms occur, consult a doctor. If sore throat is severe, persists for more than 2 days, is accompanied or followed by fever, headache, rash, nausea, or vomiting, consult a doctor promptly. **Keep this and all drugs out of the reach of children.** In case of accidental overdose, seek professional assistance or contact a poison control center immediately. Prompt medical attention is critical for adults as well as for children even if you do not notice any signs or symptoms. As with any drug, if you are pregnant or nursing a baby, seek the advice of a health professional before using this product.

How Supplied: Available in: **LIQUID** 6 FL. OZ. (177 mL) plastic bottles with child-resistant, tamper-evident cap and a calibrated medicine cup.
LIQUICAP in 12 count child-resistant packages and 20-count non-child resistant packages. Each softgel is imprinted: DayQuil

---

VICKS® DAYQUIL® SINUS
PRESSURE & CONGESTION RELIEF
Nasal Decongestant/Expectorant

Active Ingredients: (per caplet)
Guaifenesin 200 mg
Phyenylpropanolamine Hydrochloride 25 mg

Inactive Ingredients: Colloidal Silicone Dioxide, Crospovidone, FD&C Yellow No. 6 Aluminum Lake, Hydroxypropyl Methylcellulose, Microcrystalline Cellulose, Polyethylene Glycol, Polysorbate 80, Povidone, Stearic Acid, Titanium Dioxide.

Indications: For the temporary relief of nasal/sinus congestion and pressure associated with sinusitis, hay fever, upper respiratory allergies or the common cold. Also helps to loosen phlegm and thin bronchial secretions to relieve chest congestion.

Action: DayQuil® SINUS Pressure & CONGESTION Relief is available without a prescription to relieve congestion and pressure so you can breathe easier without drowsiness.

Directions: Adults and Children 12 years and over: 1 caplet every 4 hours. Maximum: 6 caplets per day.
Not recommended for children under 12 years of age.

Warnings: Do not exceed recommended dosage because at higher doses nervousness, dizziness, or sleeplessness may occur. Do not take this product for more than 7 days. If symptoms do not improve or are accompanied by fever, consult a doctor. Do not take this product if you have heart disease, high blood pressure, thyroid disease, diabetes, or difficulty in urination due to enlargement of

the prostate gland unless directed by a doctor. *Drug Interaction Precaution:* Do not take this product if you are presently taking a prescription drug for high blood pressure or depression without first consulting your doctor. Do not take this product for persistent or chronic cough such as occurs with smoking, asthma, chronic bronchitis, or emphysema, or where cough is accompanied by excessive phlegm (mucus) unless directed by a doctor. A persistent cough may be a sign of a serious condition. If cough persists for more than 1 week, tends to recur, or is accompanied by fever, rash, or persistent headache, consult a doctor. **Keep this and all drugs out of the reach of children.** In case of accidental overdose, seek professional assistance or contact a poison control center immediately. As with any drug, if you are pregnant or nursing a baby, seek the advice of a health professional before using this product.

How Supplied: Available in 12 and 24 caplet blister packages. Each caplet is imprinted DQ SC.

VICKS® DAYQUIL® SINUS
PRESSURE & PAIN RELIEF
Nasal Decongestant/Pain Reliever

Active Ingredients: (per caplet)
Acetaminophen 500 mg
Pseudoephedrine Hydrochloride 30 mg

Inactive Ingredients: Colloidal Silicon Dioxide, Croscarmellose Sodium, D&C Red No. 27 Aluminum Lake, D&C Yellow No. 10 Aluminum Lake, FD&C Blue No. 1 Aluminum Lake, Hydrogenated Vegetable Oil, Hydroxypropyl Cellulose, Hydroxypropyl Methylcellulose, Magnesium Stearate, Polyethylene Glycol, Polysorbate 80, Starch, Titanium Dioxide.

Indications: For the temporary relief of nasal/sinus congestion and pressure, sinus headache pain associated with sinusitis, hay fever, upper respiratory allergies, or the common cold.

Action: DayQuil® SINUS Pressure & PAIN Relief eases congestion and pressure so you can breathe easier without drowsiness.

Directions: Adults and Children 12 years and over: 2 caplets every 6 hours. Maximum: 8 caplets per day.
Children under 12 years of age: consult a doctor.

Warnings: Do not exceed recommended dosage because at higher doses nervousness, dizziness, or sleeplessness may occur. Do not take this product for more than 10 days. If symptoms do not improve or are accompanied by fever that lasts for more than 3 days, or if new symptoms occur, consult a doctor. Do not take this product if you have heart disease, high blood pressure, thyroid disease, diabetes, or difficulty in urination due to enlargement of the prostate gland

Continued on next page

Procter & Gamble—Cont.

unless directed by a doctor. *Drug Interaction Precaution:* Do not take this product if you are presently taking a prescription drug for high blood pressure or depression without first consulting your doctor. **Keep this and all drugs out of the reach of children.** In case of accidental overdose, seek professional assistance or contact a poison control center immediately. Prompt medical attention is critical for adults as well as for children even if you do not notice any signs or symptoms. As with any drug, if you are pregnant or nursing a baby, seek the advice of a health professional before using this product.

How Supplied: Available in 24 caplet, child-resistant, tamper-evident blister packages. Each caplet is imprinted DQ SP.

**VICKS® FORMULA 44®
MAXIMUM STRENGTH COUGH**
Dextromethorphan HBr/
Cough Suppressant

Active Ingredient per 2 tsp. (10 mL.): Dextromethorphan Hydrobromide 30 mg

Inactive Ingredients: Alcohol 10%, Caramel, Carboxymethylcellulose Sodium, Citric Acid, FD&C Red No. 40, Flavor, Invert Sugar, Propylene Glycol, Purified Water, Sodium Citrate.

Indications: VICKS® FORMULA 44® provides temporary relief of coughs due to minor throat and bronchial irritation associated with a cold.

Actions: VICKS® FORMULA 44® COUGH MEDICINE is a cough suppressant.

Directions:
Adults and Children 12 years of age and over: 2 teaspoons

Children under 12 years of age: consult a doctor.
Repeat every 6–8 hours. No more than 4 doses per day or as directed by doctor.

WARNINGS: A persistent cough may be a sign of a serious condition. If cough persists for more than 1 week, tends to recur, or is accompanied by fever, rash, or persistent headache, consult a doctor. Do not take this product for persistent or chronic cough such as occurs with smoking, asthma, emphysema, or if cough is accompanied by excessive phlegm (mucus) unless directed by a doctor. **Keep this and all drugs out of the reach of children.** In case of accidental overdose, seek professional assistance or contact a poison control center immediately. As with any drug, if you are pregnant or nursing a baby, seek the advice of a health professional before using this product.

How Supplied: Available in 4 FL. OZ. (118 mL) and 8 FL. OZ. (236 mL) squeeze

bottles with Vicks AccuTip® Dispenser for accurate, easy dosing.

**VICKS® FORMULA 44®
NON-DROWSY COLD & COUGH
LIQUICAPS®**
Cough Suppressant/Nasal Decongestant

Active Ingredient (per softgel): Dextromethorphan Hydrobromide 30 mg, Pseudoephedrine Hydrochloride 60 mg.

Inactive Ingredients: D&C Red No. 33, FD&C Blue No. 1, FD&C Red No. 40, Gelatin, Glycerin, Polyethylene Glycol, Povidone, Purified Water, Sorbitol. Edible Ink.

Indications: Formula 44 Non-Drowsy Cold & Cough LiquiCaps provide temporary relief of coughs and nasal congestion due to the common cold.

Directions: **Adults and Children 12 years and over:** Swallow 1 softgel with water. Do not chew. Repeat every 6 hours, not to exceed 4 softgels per day. Not recommended for children under 12.

Warnings: A persistent cough may be a sign of a serious condition. If cough persists for more than 1 week, tends to recur, or is accompanied by fever, rash, or persistent headache, consult a doctor. Do not take this product for persistent or chronic cough such as occurs with smoking, asthma, emphysema, or if cough is accompanied by excessive phlegm (mucus) unless directed by a doctor. Do not exceed recommended dosage because at higher doses nervousness, dizziness, or sleeplessness may occur. Do not take this product for more than 7 days. If symptoms do not improve or are accompanied by fever, consult a doctor. Do not take this product if you have heart disease, high blood pressures, thyroid disease, diabetes, or difficulty in urination due to enlargement of the prostate gland unless directed by a doctor. *Drug Interaction Precaution:* Do not take this product if you are presently taking a prescription drug for high blood pressure or depression without first consulting your doctor. **Keep this and all drugs out of the reach of children.** In case of accidental overdose, seek professional assistance or contact a poison control center immediately. As with any drug, if you are pregnant or nursing a baby, seek the advice of a health professional before using this product.

How Supplied: Available in 10 count blister packages. Each red liquicap is imprinted 44.

**VICKS® FORMULA 44D®
COUGH & HEAD CONGESTION**
Cough Suppressant/
Nasal Decongestant

Active Ingredients per 3 tsp. (15 mL): Dextromethorphan Hydrobromide 30 mg, Pseudoephedrine Hydrochloride 60 mg.

Inactive Ingredients: Alcohol 10%, Citric Acid, FD&C Red No. 40, Flavor, Glycerin, Propylene Glycol, Purified Water, Saccharin Sodium, Sodium Citrate, Sucrose.

Indications: VICKS® FORMULA 44D® provides temporary relief of coughs and nasal congestion due to a common cold.

Actions: VICKS® FORMULA 44D® is a cough suppressant and a nasal decongestant.

Dosage Directions:
Adults and children 12 years of age and over: 3 teaspoons

Children under 12 years of age, consult a doctor.
Repeat every 6 hours. No more than 4 doses per day or as directed by a doctor.

WARNINGS: A persistent cough may be a sign of a serious condition. If cough persists for more than 1 week, tends to recur, or is accompanied by fever, rash, or persistent headache, consult a doctor. Do not take this product for persistent or chronic cough such as occurs with smoking, asthma, emphysema, or if cough is accompanied by excessive phlegm (mucus) unless directed by a doctor. Do not exceed recommended dosage because at higher doses nervousness, dizziness, or sleeplessness may occur. Do not take this product for more than 7 days. If symptoms do not improve or are accompanied by fever, consult a doctor. Do not take this product if you have heart disease, high blood pressure, thyroid disease, diabetes, or difficulty in urination due to enlargement of the prostate gland unless directed by a doctor. *Drug Interaction Precaution:* Do not take this product if you are presently taking a prescription drug for high blood pressure or depression, without first consulting your doctor. **Keep this and all drugs out of the reach of children.** In case of accidental overdose, seek professional assistance or contact a poison control center immediately. As with any drug, if you are pregnant or nursing a baby, seek the advice of a health professional before using this product.

How Supplied: Available in 4 FL. OZ.(118 mL) and 8 FL. OZ. (236 mL) squeeze bottles with Vicks AccuTip® Dispenser for accurate, easy dosing.

VICKS® FORMULA 44E®
Cough & Chest Congestion
Cough Suppressant/Expectorant

Active Ingredients per 3 teaspoons (15mL): Dextromethorphan Hydrobromide 20 mg, Guaifenesin 200 mg

Inactive Ingredients: Alcohol 10%, Citric Acid, FD&C Blue No. 1, FD&C Red No. 40, Flavor, Glycerin, Propylene Glycol, Purified Water, Saccharin Sodium, Sodium Citrate, Sucrose.

Indications: VICKS® FORMULA 44E® provides temporary relief of coughs due to the common cold and helps loosen phlegm to make coughs more productive.

Actions: VICKS® FORMULA 44E® is a cough suppressant and expectorant.

Directions:

Adults and Children 12 years of age and over: 3 teaspoons.

Children under 12 years of age: consult a doctor.

Repeat every 4 hours. No more than 6 doses per day, or as directed by a doctor.

WARNINGS: A persistent cough may be a sign of a serious condition. If cough persists for more than 1 week, tends to recur, or is accompanied by fever, rash, or persistent headache, consult a doctor. Do not take this product for persistent or chronic cough such as occurs with smoking, asthma, chronic bronchitis, or emphysema, or if cough is accompanied by excessive phlegm (mucus) unless directed by a doctor. **Keep this and all drugs out of the reach of children.** In case of accidental overdose, seek professional assistance or contact a poison control center immediately. As with any drug, if you are pregnant or nursing a baby, seek the advice of a health professional before using this product.

How Supplied: Available in 4 FL. OZ. (118 mL) and 8 FL. OZ. (236 mL) squeeze bottles with Vicks AccuTip® Dispenser for accurate, easy dosing.

VICKS® FORMULA 44M® COLD, FLU & COUGH LIQUICAPS®
Cough Suppressant • Nasal Decongestant
•Antihistamine • Pain Reliever/Fever Reducer

Active Ingredients (per softgel): Dextromethorphan Hydrobromide 10 mg, Pseudoephedrine Hydrochloride 30 mg, Chlorpheniramine Maleate 2 mg, Acetaminophen 250 mg.

Inactive Ingredients: D&C Red No. 33 Lake, FD&C Blue No. 1 Lake, Gelatin, Glycerin, Polyethylene Glycol, Povidone, Propylene Glycol, Purified Water. Edible Ink.

Indications: Vicks Formula 44 Cold, Flu & Cough LiquiCaps provide temporary relief of coughing, nasal congestion, runny nose and sneezing due to a cold. Also for temporary relief of headache, fever, muscular aches and sore throat pain due to a cold or flu.

Directions: Adults and 12 years and over): Swallow 2 softgels with water. **Children (6 to under 12 years):** Swallow 1 softgel with water. Do not chew. Repeat every 4 hours not to exceed 4 doses per day. Not recommended for children under 6 years.

Warnings: Do not take this product for persistent or chronic cough such as occurs with smoking, asthma, emphysema, or if cough is accompanied by excessive phlegm (mucus) unless directed by a doctor. Do not exceed recommended dosage because at higher doses nervousness, dizziness, or sleeplessness may occur. Do not take this product if you have heart disease, high blood pressure, thyroid disease, diabetes, glaucoma, or difficulty in urination due to enlargement of the prostate gland unless directed by a doctor. *Drug Interaction Precaution:* Do not take this product if you are presently taking a prescription drug for high blood pressure or depression without first consulting your doctor. May cause excitability especially in children. Do not take this product, unless directed by a doctor, if you have a breathing problem such as emphysema or chronic bronchitis. May cause marked drowsiness: alcohol, sedatives and tranquilizers may increase the drowsiness effect. Avoid alcoholic beverages while taking this product. Do not take this product if you are taking sedatives or tranquilizers without first consulting your doctor. Use caution when driving a motor vehicle or operating machinery. Do not take this product for more than 7 days (for adults) or 5 days (for children). A persistent cough may be a sign of a serious condition. If cough persists for more than 7 days, tends to recur, or is accompanied by rash, persistent headache, fever that lasts for more than 3 days, or if new symptoms occur, consult a doctor. If symptoms do not improve or are accompanied by fever that lasts for more than 3 days, or if new symptoms occur, consult a doctor. If sore throat is severe, persists for more than 2 days, is accompanied or followed by fever, headache, rash, nausea or vomiting, consult a doctor promptly. **Keep this and all drugs out of the reach of children.** In case of accidental overdose, seek professional assistance or contact a poison control center immediately. Prompt medical attention is critical for adults as well as for children even if you do not notice any signs or symptoms. As with any drug, if you are pregnant or nursing a baby, seek the advice of a health professional before using this product.

How Supplied: Available in 12 count blister packages. Each blue liquicap is imprinted 44.

VICKS® FORMULA 44M®
COUGH, COLD & FLU
Cough Suppressant/Nasal Decongestant/Antihistamine/ Pain Reliever–Fever Reducer

Active Ingredients: per 4 tsp. (20 mL): Dextromethorphan Hydrobromide 30 mg, Pseudoephedrine Hydrochloride 60 mg, Chlorpheniramine Maleate 4 mg, Acetaminophen 650 mg

Inactive Ingredients: Alcohol 10%, Citric Acid, FD&C Blue No. 1, FD&C Red No. 40, Flavor, Glycerin, Purified Water, Saccharin Sodium, Sodium Benzoate, Sodium Citrate, Sorbitol, and Sucrose.

Indications: VICKS® FORMULA 44M® provides temporary relief of coughing, nasal congestion, runny nose, and sneezing due to a cold. Also for temporary relief of headache, fever, muscular aches and sore throat due to a cold or flu.

Actions: VICKS® FORMULA 44M® is a cough suppressant, nasal decongestant, antihistamine and analgesic.

Directions: Adults and children 12 years of age and over: fill cup to top line or 4 teaspoons
Repeat every 6 hours. No more than 4 doses per day or as directed by a doctor. Children under 12 years of age: consult a doctor

Warnings: Do not take this product for persistent or chronic cough such as occurs with smoking, asthma, or emphysema, or if cough is accompanied by excessive phlegm (mucus) unless directed by a doctor. Do not exceed recommended dosage because at higher doses nervousness, dizziness, or sleeplessness may occur. Do not take this product if you have heart disease, high blood pressure, thyroid disease, diabetes, glaucoma, or difficulty in urination due to enlargement of the prostate gland unless directed by a doctor. *Drug Interaction Precaution:* Do not take this product if you are presently taking a prescription drug for high blood pressure or depression, without first consulting a doctor. May cause excitability especially in children. Do not take this product, unless directed by a doctor, if you have a breathing problem such as emphysema or chronic bronchitis. May cause marked drowsiness; alcohol, sedatives, and tranquilizers may increase the drowsiness effect. Avoid alcoholic beverages while taking this product. Do not take this product if you are taking sedatives or tranquilizers, without first consulting your doctor. Use caution when driving a motor vehicle or operating machinery. Do not take this product for more than 7 days. A persistent cough may be a sign of a serious condition. If cough persists for more than 7 days, tends to recur, or is accompanied by rash, persistent headache, fever that lasts for more than 3 days, or if new symptoms occur, consult a doctor. If symptoms do not improve or are accompanied by fever that lasts for more than 3 days, or if new symptoms occur, consult a doctor. If sore throat is severe, persists for more than 2 days, is accompanied or followed by fever, headache, rash, nausea or vomiting, consult a doctor. **Keep this and all drugs out of the reach of children.** In case of accidental overdose, seek professional assistance or contact a poison control center immediately. Prompt medical attention is critical for adults as well as for children, even if you do not notice any signs or symptoms. As with any drug, if you are pregnant or nursing a baby, seek the advice of a health professional before using this product.

Continued on next page

Procter & Gamble—Cont.

How Supplied: Available in 4 FL. OZ. (118 mL) and 8 FL. OZ. (236 mL) squeeze bottles with Vicks AccuTip® Dispenser for accurate, easy dosing. A calibrated dose cup accompanies each bottle.

VICKS® NYQUIL® HOT THERAPY™
ADULT NIGHTTIME COLD/FLU HOT LIQUID MEDICINE
Honey Lemon Hot Liquid Drink
Nasal Decongestant/Antihistamine/
Cough Suppressant
Pain Reliever• Fever Reducer

Active Ingredients: (per packet) Acetaminophen 1000, Pseudoephedrine Hydrochloride 60 mg, Dextromethorphan Hydrobromide 30 mg, Doxylamine Succinate 12.5 mg.

Inactive Ingredients: Citric Acid, Flavor, and Sucrose.

Indications: For the temporary relief of minor aches, pains, headache, muscular aches, sore throat pain, and fever associated with a cold or flu. Temporarily relieves nasal congestion, cough due to minor throat and bronchial irritations, runny nose and sneezing associated with the common cold.

Actions: The nighttime sniffling, sneezing, coughing, aching, stuffy head, fever, so you can rest HOT LIQUID medicine.™

Directions: Adults and Children 12 years and over: Take one dose at bedtime. DISSOLVE ONE PACKET IN 6 OZ. CUP OF HOT WATER. SIP WHILE HOT. If your cold or flu symptoms keep you confined to be or at home, a total of 4 doses may be taken per day, each 6 hours apart, or as directed by a doctor. **MICROWAVE HEATING INSTRUCTIONS:** Add contents of packet and 6 ounces of cool water to a microwave safe cup and stir briskly. Microwave on high 1½ minutes or until hot. **DO NOT BOIL.** Sweeten to taste if desired.

Warnings: Do not exceed recommended dosage because at higher doses nervousness, dizziness, or sleeplessness may occur. Do not take this product if you have heart disease, high blood pressure, thyroid disease, diabetes, glaucoma, or difficulty in urination due to enlargement of the prostate gland unless directed by a doctor. *Drug Interaction Precaution:* Do not take this product if you are presently taking a prescription drug for high blood pressure or depression without first consulting your doctor. Do not take this product for persistent or chronic cough such as occurs with smoking, asthma, emphysema, or if cough is accompanied by excessive phlegm (mucus) unless directed by a doctor. May cause excitability especially in children. Do not take this product, unless directed by a doctor, if you have a breathing prob-

lem such as emphysema or chronic bronchitis. May cause marked drowsiness; alcohol, sedatives and tranquilizers may increase the drowsiness effect. Avoid alcoholic beverages while taking this product. Do not take this product if you are taking sedatives or tranquilizers without first consulting your doctor. Use caution when driving a motor vehicle or operating machinery. Do not take this product for more than 7 days. A persistent cough may be a sign of a serious condition. If cough persists for more than 7 days, tends to recur, or is accompanied by rash, or persistent headache, consult a doctor. If symptoms do not improve or are accompanied by fever that lasts for more than 3 days, or if new symptoms occur, consult a doctor. If sore throat is severe, persists for more than 2 days, is accompanied or followed by fever, headache, rash, nausea or vomiting, consult a doctor promptly. **Keep this and all drugs out of the reach of children.** In case of accidental overdose, seek professional assistance or contact a poison control center immediately. Prompt medical attention is critical for adults as well as for children even if you do not notice any signs or symptoms. As with any drug, if you are pregnant or nursing a baby, seek the advice of a health professional before using this product.

How Supplied: Available in child-resistant packages of 6 and 10 individual dose pouches.

VICKS® NYQUIL® LIQUICAPS®
VICKS® NYQUIL® LIQUID
(Original and Cherry)
Adult Nighttime Cold/Flu Medicine
Nasal Decongestant/Antihistamine/
Cough Suppressant/Pain
Reliever–Fever Reducer

Active Ingredients (per softgel): Acetaminophen 250 mg, Pseudoephedrine HCl 30 mg, Dextromethorphan HBr 10 mg, Doxylamine Succinate 6.25 mg

(per fluid oz) (2 TBSP): Acetaminophen 1000 mg, Dextromethorphan HBr 30 mg, Pseudoephedrine HCl 60 mg, Doxylamine succinate 12.5 mg

Inactive Ingredients: (per softgel): D&C Yellow No. 10, FD&C Blue No. 1, Gelatin, Glycerin, Polyethylene Glycol, Povidone, Propylene Glycol and Purified Water. May contain Edible Ink. Contains no alcohol.
(Liquid): Alcohol 10%, Citric Acid, Flavor, Glycerin, Polyethylene Glycol, Purified Water, Saccharin Sodium, Sodium Citrate, Sucrose.
Original flavor also has D&C Yellow No. 10, FD&C Green No. 3, FD&C Yellow No. 6.
Cherry flavor also has FD&C Blue No. 1, FD&C Red No. 40.

Indications: For the temporary relief of minor aches, pains, headache, muscular aches, sore throat pain, and fever associated with a cold or flu. Temporarily relieves nasal congestion, cough due to

minor throat and bronchial irritations, runny nose and sneezing associated with the common cold.

Actions: The nighttime sniffling, sneezing, coughing, aching, stuffy head, fever, so you can rest medicine.®

Directions: (LiquiCaps) ADULTS (12 years and older): Swallow two softgels. If your cold or flu symptoms keep you confined to bed or at home a <u>total</u> of <u>4 doses</u> may be taken <u>per day</u>, each 4 hours apart, or as directed by a doctor.
(liquid) Take one fluid ounce (2 tablespoons) at bedtime in medicine cup provided. If your cold or flu symptoms keep you confined to bed or at home, a <u>total</u> of <u>4 doses</u> may be taken per day, each 6 hours apart, or as directed by a doctor. **NOT RECOMMENDED FOR CHILDREN.**

Warnings: Do not exceed recommended dosage because at higher doses nervousness, dizziness or sleeplessness may occur. Do not take this product if you have heart disease, high blood pressure, thyroid disease, diabetes, glaucoma, or difficulty in urination due to enlargement of the prostate gland unless directed by a doctor. *Drug Interaction Precaution:* Do not take this product if you are presently taking a prescription drug for high blood pressure or depression, without first consulting your doctor. Do not take this product for persistent or chronic cough such as occurs with smoking, asthma, emphysema, or if cough is accompanied by excessive phlegm (mucus) unless directed by a doctor. May cause excitability especially in children. Do not take this product, unless directed by a doctor, if you have a breathing problem such as emphysema or chronic bronchitis. May cause marked drowsiness; alcohol, sedatives, and tranquilizers may increase the drowsiness effect. Avoid alcoholic beverages while taking this product. Do not take this product if you are taking sedatives or tranquilizers, without first consulting your doctor. Use caution when driving a motor vehicle or operating machinery. Do not take this product for more than 7 days. A persistent cough may be a sign of a serious condition. If cough persists for more than 7 days, tends to recur, or is accompanied by rash, persistent headache, consult a doctor. If symptoms do not improve or are accompanied by fever that lasts for more than 3 days, or if new symptoms occur, consult a doctor. If sore throat is severe, persists for more than 2 days, is accompanied or followed by fever, headache, rash, nausea, or vomiting, consult a doctor promptly. **Keep this and all drugs out of the reach of children.** In case of accidental overdose, seek professional assistance or contact a poison control center immediately. Prompt medical attention is critical for adults as well as for children even if you do not notice any signs or symptoms. As with any drug, if you are pregnant or nursing a baby, seek the advice of a health professional before using this product.

How Supplied: **(LiquiCaps)** Available in 12-count child-resistant blister packages and 20-count non-child resistant blister packages. Each softgel is imprinted NyQuil.

(Liquid) Available in 6, 10, and 14 fl. oz (177, 295, and 414 mL, respectively) plastic bottles with child-resistant, tamper-evident cap and calibrated medicine cup.

VICKS® PEDIATRIC FORMULA 44®
COUGH MEDICINE
Dextromethorphan HBr/Cough Suppressant

Active Ingredient per 1 Tablespoon (15 mL): Dextromethorphan Hydrobromide 15 mg
CONTAINS NO ALCOHOL

Inactive Ingredients: Carboxymethylcellulose Sodium, Cellulose, Citric Acid, FD&C Red No. 40, Flavor, Glycerin, Polysorbate 80, Potassium Sorbate, Propylene Glycol, Purified Water, Sodium Citrate, Sorbitol, Sucrose.

Indications: For the temporary relief of coughs due to the common cold.

Actions: VICKS® PEDIATRIC FORMULA 44® is an alcohol-free cough suppressant.

Administration and Dosage:
Directions: SHAKE WELL BEFORE USING
Squeeze bottle to accurately dispense medicine into dosage cup provided. 1 TBSP. ½ TBSP.

Dosage:

Age	Weight	Dose
Under 2 yrs	Under 28 lbs.	Consult physician*
2–5 yrs	28–47 lbs.	Fill cup to ½ TABLESPOON (TBSP.)
6–11 yrs	48–95 lbs.	Fill cup to 1 TABLESPOON (TBSP.)
12 yrs. and over	96 lbs. and over	2 TABLESPOONS (TBSP.) or Try one of the Adult Formula 44® Medicines

Repeat every 6–8 hours, no more than 4 doses in 24 hours, or as directed by a doctor.

Professional Dosage:

*Physicians: Suggested doses for children under 2 years of age.

Age	Weight	Dose
* 6–11 mo.	17–21 lbs.	1 teaspoon (tsp.) (5 mL)
*12–23 mo.	22–27 lbs.	1¼ teaspoon (tsp.) (6.25 mL)

Repeat every 6–8 hours, no more than 4 doses in 24 hours or as directed by doctor.

*Based on extrapolation from studies on the safety and efficacy of active ingredients conducted among older children and adults. Use caution in treating children under 2 years of age who were born prematurely.

WARNINGS: A persistent cough may be a sign of a serious condition. If cough persists for more than 1 week, tends to recur, or is accompanied by fever, rash, or persistent headache, consult a doctor. Do not take this product for persistent or chronic cough such as occurs with smoking, asthma, emphysema, or if cough is accompanied by excessive phlegm (mucus) unless directed by a doctor. **Keep this and all drugs out of the reach of children.** In case of accidental overdose, seek professional assistance or contact a poison control center immediately. As with any drug, if you are pregnant or nursing a baby, seek the advice of a health professional before using this product.

How Supplied: 4 FL. OZ. squeeze bottles with Vicks® AccuTip® Dispenser for accurate, easy dosing. Calibrated dose cup accompanies each bottle.

VICKS® PEDIATRIC FORMULA 44d®
COUGH & HEAD CONGESTION

Active Ingredients Per 1 Tablespoon (TBSP.) (15 mL): Dextromethorphan Hydrobromide 15 mg, Pseudoephedrine Hydrochloride 30 mg

CONTAINS NO ALCOHOL

Inactive Ingredients: Carboxymethylcellulose Sodium, Cellulose, Citric Acid, FD&C Red No. 40, Flavor, Glycerin, Polysorbate 80, Potassium Sorbate, Propylene Glycol, Purified Water, Sodium Citrate, Sorbitol, Sucrose.

Indications: For the temporary relief of coughs and nasal congestion due to the common cold.

Actions: VICKS® PEDIATRIC FORMULA 44d® is an alcohol-free cough suppressant and nasal decongestant.

Administration and Dosage:
Directions: SHAKE WELL BEFORE USING
Squeeze bottle to accurately dispense medicine into dosage cup provided. 1 TBSP. ½ TBSP.

Dosage:

Age	Weight	Dose
Under 2 yrs	Under 28 lbs.	Consult physician*
2–5 yrs	28–47 lbs.	Fill cup to ½ TABLESPOON (TBSP.)
6–11 yrs	48–95 lbs.	Fill cup to 1 TABLESPOON (TBSP.)
12 yrs. and over	96 lbs. and over	2 TABLESPOONS (TBSP.) or Try one of the Adult Formula 44® Medicines

Repeat every 6 hours, no more than 4 doses in 24 hours, or as directed by a doctor.

*Professional Dosage:
Physicians: Suggested doses for children under 2 years of age.

Age	Weight	Dose
* 6–11 mo.	17–21 lbs.	1 teaspoon (tsp.) (5 mL)
*12–23 mo.	22–27 lbs.	1¼ teaspoon (tsp.) (6.25 mL)

Repeat every 6 hours. No more than 4 doses in 24 hours, or as directed by doctor.

*Based on extrapolation from studies on the safety and efficacy of active ingredients conducted among older children and adults. Use caution in treating children under 2 years who were born prematurely.

WARNINGS: A persistent cough may be a sign of a serious condition. If cough persists for more than 1 week, tends to recur, or is accompanied by fever, rash, or persistent headache, consult a doctor. Do not take this product for persistent or chronic cough such as occurs with smoking, asthma, emphysema, or if cough is accompanied by excessive phlegm (mucus) unless directed by a doctor. Do not exceed recommended dosage because at higher doses nervousness, dizziness, or sleeplessness may occur. Do not take this product for more than 7 days. If symptoms do not improve or are accompanied by fever, consult a doctor. Do not take this product if you have heart disease, high blood pressure, thyroid disease, diabetes, or difficulty in urination due to enlargement of the prostate gland unless directed by a doctor. *Drug Interaction Precaution:* Do not take this product if you are presently taking a prescription drug for high blood pressure or depression, without first consulting your doctor. **Keep this and all drugs out of the reach of children.** In case of accidental overdose, seek professional assistance or contact a poison control center immediately. As with any drug, if you are pregnant or nursing a baby, seek the advice of a health professional before using this product.

How Supplied: 4 FL. OZ. (118 mL) squeeze bottles with Vicks® AccuTip® Dispenser for accurate, easy dosing. A calibrated dose cup accompanies each bottle.

Continued on next page

Procter & Gamble—Cont.

VICKS® PEDIATRIC FORMULA 44e®
Cough & Chest Congestion

Active Ingredients per 1 tablespoon (TBSP.) (15 mL):
Dextromethorphan Hydrobromide 10 mg,
Guaifenesin 100 mg

CONTAINS NO ALCOHOL

Inactive Ingredients: Carboxymethylcellulose Sodium, Cellulose, Citric Acid, FD&C Red No. 40, Flavor, Glycerin, Polysorbate 80, Potassium Sorbate, Propylene Glycol, Purified Water, Sodium Citrate, Sorbitol, Sucrose.

Indications: For the temporary relief of coughs due to the common cold and helps loosen phlegm to make coughs more productive.

Actions: VICKS® PEDIATRIC 44e® is an alcohol-free cough suppressant and expectorant.

Administration and Dosage:
Directions: (SHAKE WELL BEFORE USING) Squeeze bottle to accurately dispense medicine into dosage cup provided. 1 TBSP. ½ TBSP.

Dosage:

Age	Weight	Dose
Under 2 yrs	Under 28 lbs.	Consult physician*
2–5 yrs	28–47 lbs.	Fill cup to ½ TABLESPOON (TBSP.)
6–11 yrs	48–95 lbs.	Fill cup to 1 TABLESPOON (TBSP.)
12 yrs and over	96 lbs. and over	2 TABLESPOONS (TBSP.) or Try one of the Adult Formula 44® Medicines

Repeat every 4 hours. No more than 6 doses in 24 hours, or as directed by a doctor.

*Professional Dosage:

Physicians: Suggested doses for children under 2 years of age.

Age	Weight	Dose
* 6–11 mo.	17–21 lbs.	1 teaspoon (tsp.)(5 mL)
*12–23 mo.	22–27 lbs.	1¼ teaspoon (tsp.) (6.25 mL)

Repeat every 4 hours. No more than 6 doses in 24 hours, or as directed by a doctor.

* Based on extrapolation from studies on the safety and efficacy of active ingredients conducted among older children and adults. Use caution in treating children under 2 years who were born prematurely.

WARNINGS: A persistent cough may be a sign of a serious condition. If cough persists for more than 1 week, tends to recur, or is accompanied by fever, rash, or persistent headache, consult a doctor. Do not take this product for persistent or chronic cough such as occurs with smoking, asthma, chronic bronchitis, emphysema, or if cough is accompanied by excessive phlegm (mucus) unless directed by a doctor. **Keep this and all drugs out of the reach of children.** In case of accidental overdose, seek professional assistance or contact a poison control center immediately. As with any drug, if you are pregnant or nursing a baby, seek the advice of a health professional before using this product.
How Supplied: 4 FL. OZ. (118 mL) squeeze bottles with Vicks® AccuTip® Dispenser for accurate, easy dosing. A calibrated dose cup accompanies each bottle.

VICKS® PEDIATRIC FORMULA 44m®
COUGH & COLD
Cough Suppressant/Nasal Decongestant/Antihistamine

Active Ingredients Per 1 tablespoon (TBSP.) (15 mL): Dextromethorphan Hydrobromide 15 mg, Pseudoephedrine Hydrochloride 30 mg, Chlorpheniramine Maleate 2 mg

CONTAINS NO ALCOHOL

Inactive Ingredients: Carboxymethylcellulose Sodium, Cellulose, Citric Acid, FD&C Red No. 40, Flavor, Glycerin, Polysorbate 80, Potassium Sorbate, Propylene Glycol, Purified Water, Sodium Citrate, Sorbitol, Sucrose.

Indications: For the temporary relief of coughs, nasal congestion, runny nose and sneezing due to the common cold.

Actions: VICKS® PEDIATRIC FORMULA 44m® is an alcohol-free cough suppressant, nasal decongestant and antihistamine.

Administration and Dosage:
Directions: SHAKE WELL BEFORE USING Squeeze bottle to accurately dispense medicine into dosage cup provided. 1 TBSP. ½ TBSP.

Dosage:

Age	Weight	Dose
Under 6 yrs	Under 48 lbs.	Consult Physician*
6–11 yrs	48–95 lbs.	Fill cup to 1 TABLESPOON (TBSP.)
12 yrs and over	96 lbs. and over	2 TABLESPOON (TBSP.) or try one of the Adult Formula 44® Medicines

Repeat every 6 hours. No more than 4 doses in 24 hours, or as directed by a doctor.

Professional Dosage:
*Physicians: Suggested doses for children under 6 years of age.

Age	Weight	Dose
* 6–11 mo.	17–21 lbs.	1 teaspoon (tsp.) (5 mL)
*12–23 mo.	22–27 lbs.	1¼ teaspoon (tsp.) (6.25 mL)
2–5 yrs.	28–47 lbs.	½ TABLESPOON (TBSP.) (7.5 mL)

Repeat every 6 hours, no more than 4 doses in 24 hours, or as directed by doctor.

*Based on extrapolation from studies on the safety and efficacy of active ingredients conducted among older children and adults. Use caution in treating children under 2 years of age who were born prematurely.

WARNINGS: A persistent cough may be a sign of a serious condition. If cough persists for more than 1 week, tends to recur, or is accompanied by fever, rash, or persistent headache, consult a doctor. Do not take this product for persistent or chronic cough such as occurs with smoking, asthma, emphysema, or if cough is accompanied by excessive phlegm (mucus) unless directed by a doctor. Do not exceed recommended dosage because at higher doses nervousness, dizziness, or sleeplessness may occur. Do not take this product for more than 7 days. If symptoms do not improve or are accompanied by fever, consult a doctor. Do not take this product if you have heart disease, high blood pressure, thyroid disease, diabetes, glaucoma, or difficulty in urination due to enlargement of the prostate gland unless directed by a doctor. *Drug Interaction Precaution:* Do not take this product if you are presently taking a prescription drug for high blood pressure or depression, without first consulting your doctor. May cause excitability especially in children. Do not take this product, unless directed by a doctor, if you have a breathing problem such as emphysema or chronic bronchitis. May cause marked drowsiness; alcohol, sedatives, and tranquilizers may increase the drowsiness effect. Avoid alcoholic beverages while taking this product. Do not take this product if you are taking sedatives or tranquilizers, without first consulting your doctor. Use caution when driving a motor vehicle or operating machinery. **Keep this and all drugs out of the reach of children.** In case of accidental overdose, seek professional assistance or contact a poison control center immediately. As with any drug, if you are pregnant or nursing a baby, seek the advice of a health professional before using this product.

How Supplied: 4 FL OZ (118 mL) squeeze bottles with Vicks® AccuTip® Dispenser for accurate easy dosing. A calibrated dose cup accompanies each bottle.

VICKS® SINEX® REGULAR
[sĭ 'nĕx]
Decongestant Nasal Spray and Ultra Fine Mist

Active Ingredient: Phenylephrine Hydrochloride 0.5%.

Inactive Ingredients: Aromatic Vapors (Camphor, Eucalyptol, Menthol), Citric Acid, Purified Water, Tyloxapol. Preservatives: Benzalkonium Chloride, Chlorhexidine Gluconate, Disodium EDTA.

Indications: For temporary relief of nasal congestion due to colds, hay fever, upper respiratory allergies or sinusitis.

Actions: Provides fast decongestant relief.

Dosage and Administration: Keep head and dispenser upright. May be used every 4 hours as needed.
Ultra Fine Mist: Remove protective cap. Before using for the first time, prime the pump by firmly depressing its rim several times. Hold container with thumb at base and nozzle between first and second fingers. Without tilting your head, insert nozzle into nostril. Fully depress rim with a firm even stroke and inhale deeply.
Adults and Children—age 12 and over: 2 or 3 sprays in each nostril not more often than every 4 hours. Do not give to children under 12 years of age unless directed by a doctor.
Squeeze Bottle: Adults and Children— age 12 and over: 2 or 3 sprays in each nostril not more often than every 4 hours. Do not give to children under 12 years of age unless directed by a doctor.

WARNINGS: Do not exceed recommended dosage because burning, stinging, sneezing, or increase of nasal discharge may occur. The use of this container by more than one person may spread infection. Do not use this product for more than 3 days. If symptoms persist, consult a doctor. Do not use this product if you have heart disease, high blood pressure, thyroid disease, diabetes, or difficulty in urination due to enlargement of the prostate gland unless directed by a doctor.
Keep this and all drugs out of the reach of children. In case of accidental ingestion, seek professional assistance or contact a poison control center immediately.

How Supplied: Available in ½ FL. OZ. (14 mL) and 1 FL. OZ. (29 mL) plastic squeeze bottles and ½ FL. OZ. (14 mL) measured dose Ultra Fine mist pump.

VICKS® SINEX® LONG-ACTING
[sĭ 'nĕx]
12-hour Formula Decongestant Nasal Spray and Ultra Fine Mist

Active Ingredient: Oxymetazoline Hydrochloride 0.05%.

Inactive Ingredients: Aromatic Vapors (Camphor, Eucalyptol, Menthol), Potassium Phosphate, Purified Water, Sodium Chloride, Sodium Phosphate, Tyloxapol. Preservatives: Benzalkonium Chloride, Chlorhexidine Gluconate, Disodium EDTA.

Indications: For temporary relief of nasal congestion due to colds, hay fever, upper respiratory allergies or sinusitis.

Actions: Provides fast relief of head and nasal congestion and lasts up to 12 hours.

Dosage and Administration: Keep head and dispenser upright. May be used twice daily (morning and evening) or as directed by a physician.
Ultra Fine Mist: Remove protective cap. Before using for the first time, prime the pump by firmly depressing its rim several times. Hold container with thumb at base and nozzle between first and second fingers. Without tilting head, insert nozzle into nostril. Fully depress rim with a firm even stroke and inhale deeply.
Adults and children 6 years of age and over (with adult supervision): 2 or 3 sprays in each nostril not more often than every 10 to 12 hours. Do not exceed 2 applications in any 24-hour period. Children under 6 years of age: consult a doctor.
Squeeze Bottle: Adults and children 6 years of age and over (with adult supervision): 2 or 3 sprays in each nostril not more often than every 10 to 12 hours. Do not exceed 2 applications in any 24-hour period. Children under 6 years of age: consult a doctor.

WARNINGS: Do not exceed recommended dosage because burning, stinging, sneezing or increase of nasal discharge may occur. The use of this container by more than one person may spread infection. Do not use this product for more than 3 days. If symptoms persist, consult a doctor. Do not use this product if you have heart disease, high blood pressure, thyroid disease, diabetes, or difficulty in urination due to enlargement of the prostate gland unless directed by a doctor.
Keep this and all drugs out of the reach of children. In case of accidental ingestion, seek professional assistance or contact a poison control center immediately.

How Supplied: Available in ½ FL. OZ. (14 mL) and 1 FL. OZ. (29 mL) plastic squeeze bottles and ½ FL. OZ. (14 mL) measured-dose Ultra Fine mist pump.

VICKS® VAPOR INHALER
with decongestant action
***l* -Desoxyephedrine/Nasal Decongestant**

Active Ingredient per inhaler: *l* -Desoxyephedrine 50 mg.

Inactive Ingredients: Special Vicks Vapors (bornyl acetate, camphor, lavender oil, menthol).

Indications: For the temporary relief of nasal congestion due to the common cold, hay fever, upper respiratory allergies or sinusitis.

Actions: Fast relief from nasal congestion due to colds, hay fever, upper respiratory allergies or sinusitis.

Directions: Adults: 2 inhalations in each nostril not more often than every 2 hours.
Children 6 to under 12 years of age (with adult supervision): 1 inhalation in each nostril not more often than every 2 hours. Children under 6 years of age: consult a doctor.

WARNINGS: Do not exceed recommended dosage because burning, stinging, sneezing, or increase of nasal discharge may occur. The use of this container by more than one person may spread infection. Do not use this product for more than 7 days. If symptoms persist, consult a doctor. **Keep this and all drugs out of the reach of children.** In case of accidental ingestion, seek professional assistance or contact a poison control center immediately.

VICKS VAPOR INHALER is effective for a minimum of 3 months after first use. Keep tightly closed.

How Supplied: Available as a cylindrical plastic nasal inhaler
Net weight: 0.007 OZ (198 mg)

VICKS® VAPORUB®
VICKS® VAPORUB® CREAM
[vā 'pō-rub]
Nasal Decongestant/Cough Suppressant

Active Ingredients: Camphor 4.7%, Menthol 2.6%, Eucalyptus Oil 1.2%.

Inactive Ingredients: (ointment) Cedarleaf Oil, Mineral Oil, Nutmeg Oil, Petrolatum, Spirits of Turpentine, Thymol.
(cream) Carbomer, Cedarleaf Oil, Cetyl Alcohol, Cetyl Palmitate, Cyclomethicone and Dimethicone Copolyol, Dimethicone, EDTA, Glycerin, Imidazolidinyl Urea, Isopropyl Palmitate, Methylparaben, Nutmeg Oil, PEG-100, Stearate, Propylparaben, Purified Water, Sodium Hydroxide, Spirits of Turpentine, Stearic Acid, Stearyl Alcohol, Thymol, Titanium Dioxide.

Indications: For the temporary relief of nasal congestion and coughs associated with a cold.

Continued on next page

Procter & Gamble—Cont.

Actions: VICKS VAPORUB has antitussive and nasal decongestant effects.

Directions: Adults and children 2 years of age and over: Rub a thick layer of Vicks VapoRub on chest and throat. If desired, cover with a dry, soft cloth, but keep clothing loose to let vapors rise to the nose and mouth. Repeat up to three times daily, especially at bedtime, or as directed by a doctor. Children under two years of age, consult a doctor.
Do not heat. Never expose VapoRub to flame, microwave, or place in any container in which you are heating water. [Such improper use may cause the mixture to splatter. (VapoRub Ointment, only)]

Warnings: For external use only. Do not take by mouth or place in nostrils. A persistent cough may be a sign of a serious condition. If cough persists for more than 1 week, tends to recur, or is accompanied by fever, rash, or persistent headache, consult a doctor. Do not use this product for persistent or chronic cough such as occurs with smoking, asthma, emphysema, or if cough is accompanied by excessive phlegm (mucus) unless directed by a doctor. **Keep this and all drugs out of the reach of children.** In case of accidental ingestion, seek professional assistance or contact a poison control center immediately.

How Supplied: (ointment) Available in 1.5 OZ. (42.5 g), 3.0 OZ. (85 g) and 6.0 OZ. plastic jars.
(cream) 2.0 oz. (56.7 g)

VICKS® VAPOSTEAM®
[vā ′pō ″stēm]
**Liquid Medication for
Hot Steam Vaporizers.
Nasal Decongestant/Cough
Suppressant**

Active Ingredients: Camphor 6.2%, Menthol 3.2%, Eucalyptus Oil 1.5%.

Inactive Ingredients: Alcohol 74%, Cedarleaf Oil, Nutmeg Oil, Poloxamer 124, Polyoxyethylene Dodecanol, Silicone.

Indications: For temporary relief of nasal congestion due to colds, hay fever or other upper respiratory allergies. Temporarily relieves cough occurring with a cold.

Actions: VAPOSTEAM increases the action of steam to relieve cold symptoms in the following ways: relieves coughs of colds, eases nasal congestion, and moistens dry, irritated breathing passages.

Directions:
Adults and children 2 years of age and older: Use VAPOSTEAM only in hot/warm steam vaporizers, as described below. Follow directions for use carefully. Breathe in medicated vapors. May

be repeated up to 3 times daily or as directed by a doctor.
Children under 2 years of age: consult a doctor.
In Hot/Warm Steam Vaporizers: VAPOSTEAM is formulated to be added directly to the water in your hot/warm steam vaporizer. Add one tablespoon of VAPOSTEAM with each quart of water added to the vaporizer. Do not direct steam from vaporizer close to face. For best performance, vaporizer should be thoroughly cleaned after each use according to manufacturer's instructions. To promote steaming, follow directions of vaporizer manufacturer.
Never expose VAPOSTEAM to flame, microwave, or place in any container in which you are heating water except for a hot-warm steam vaporizer. Never use VAPOSTEAM in any bowl or washbasin with hot water. Improper use may cause the mixture to splatter and cause burns.

Warnings: For hot/warm steam vaporizers only. Do not use in cold steam vaporizers or humidifiers. **Not to be taken by mouth.** A persistent cough may be a sign of a serious condition. If cough persists for more than one week, tends to recur or is accompanied by fever, rash, or persistent headache, consult a doctor. Do not use this product for persistent or chronic cough such as occurs with smoking, asthma, emphysema, or if cough is accompanied by excessive phlegm (mucus) unless directed by a doctor. **Keep this and all drugs out of the reach of children.**

Accidental Ingestion: In case of accidental ingestion, seek professional assistance or contact a poison control center immediately.

How Supplied: Available in 4 FL. OZ. (118 mL) and 8 FL. OZ. (236 mL) bottles.

VICKS® VATRONOL®
[vātrōnōl]
**Ephedrine Sulfate/Nasal
Decongestant
Nose Drops**

Active Ingredient: Ephedrine Sulfate 0.5%.

Inactive Ingredients: Camphor, Cedarleaf Oil, Eucalyptol, Menthol, Nutmeg Oil, Potassium Phosphate, Purified Water, Sodium Chloride, Sodium Phosphate, Tyloxapol.
Preservative: Thimerosal 0.001%.

Indications: For temporary relief of nasal congestion due to a cold, hay fever, or other upper respiratory allergies, or associated with sinusitis.

Actions: VICKS VATRONOL helps restore freer breathing by relieving nasal stuffiness. Relieves sinus pressure.

Dosage: Adults: Fill dropper to upper mark. Children 6 to under 12 years of age (with adult supervision): Fill dropper to lower mark. Children under 6 years of age: consult a doctor.

Apply in each nostril, not more often than every four hours.

WARNINGS: Do not exceed recommended dosage because burning, stinging, sneezing, or increase of nasal discharge may occur. The use of this container by more than one person may spread infection. Do not use this product for more than 3 days. If symptoms persist, consult a doctor. Do not use this product if you have heart disease, high blood pressure, thyroid disease, diabetes, or difficulty in urination due to enlargement of the prostate gland unless directed by a doctor. **KEEP THIS AND ALL DRUGS OUT OF THE REACH OF CHILDREN.** In case of accidental ingestion, seek professional assistance or contact a poison control center immediately.

How Supplied: Available in 1 FL. OZ. dropper bottles.

| **EDUCATIONAL MATERIAL** |

Journal Reprints for Physicians
Reprints of published journal articles illustrating the effectiveness of bismuth subsalicylate (Pepto-Bismol) for the treatment of diarrhea.

Reed & Carnrick
Division of Block Drug Company, Inc.
**257 CORNELISON AVENUE
JERSEY CITY, NJ 07302**

PHAZYME® and PHAZYME®-95
[fay-zime]
Tablets

Description: Contains simethicone, an antiflatulent to alleviate or relieve the symptoms of gas. It has no known side effects or drug interactions.

Actions: Simethicone minimizes gas formation and relieves gas entrapment in both the stomach and the lower G.I. tract. This action combats the distress due to gastrointestinal gas.

Indication: To alleviate or relieve the symptoms of gas. May also be used for postoperative gas pain.

Warnings: Keep this and all drugs out of the reach of children. If condition persists, consult your physician.

Store at controlled room temperature 59°–86°F (15°–30°C).

PHAZYME®

Active Ingredient: Each tablet contains simethicone 60 mg.

Inactive Ingredients: Acacia, calcium sulfate, carnauba wax, crospovidone, D&C red No. 7 calcium lake, FD&C blue No. 1 aluminum lake, gelatin, lactose, methylparaben, microcrystalline cellulose, polyoxyl-40 stearate, povidone, pregelatinized starch, propylparaben, rice starch, sodium benzoate, sucrose, talc, titanium dioxide, white wax.

Dosage: One tablet four times a day after meals and at bedtime. Do not exceed 8 tablets a day unless directed by a physician.

How Supplied: Pink coated tablet imprinted "Phazyme" in bottles of 100, NDC #0021-1400-01

PHAZYME® 95

Active Ingredient: Each tablet contains simethicone 95 mg.

Inactive Ingredients: Acacia, carnauba wax, compressible sugar, crosscarmellose sodium, FD&C red No. 40 aluminum lake, FD&C yellow No. 6 aluminum lake, hydroxypropyl methylcellulose, microcrystalline cellulose, polyoxyl 40 stearate, povidone, sodium benzoate, sucrose, talc, titanium dioxide, white wax.

Dosage: One tablet four times a day after meals and at bedtime. Do not exceed 5 tablets per day unless directed by a physician.

How Supplied: Red coated tablet imprinted "Phazyme 95" in
10 pack, NDC #0021-1420-02
50's   NDC #0021-1420-50
100's,   NDC #0021-1420-01
Shown in Product Identification Guide, page 417

PHAZYME® DROPS
[*fay-zime*]

Description: Contains simethicone, an antiflatulent to alleviate or relieve the symptoms of gas. It has no known side effects or drug interactions.

Active Ingredients: Each 0.6 mL contains simethicone, 40 mg.
Inactive Ingredients: Carbomer 934 P, citric acid, flavor (natural orange), hydroxypropyl methylcellulose, PEG-8 stearate, potassium sorbate, sodium citrate, sodium saccharin, water.

Actions: Simethicone minimizes gas formation and relieves gas entrapment in both the stomach and the lower G.I. tract. This action combats the distress due to gastrointestinal gas.

Indication: To alleviate or relieve the symptoms of gas. May also be used for postoperative gas pain or endoscopic examination.

Warnings: Keep this and all drugs out of the reach of children. If condition persists, consult your physician.

Store at controlled room temperature 59°–86°F (15°–30°C).

Dosage/Administration: Shake well before using.
Infants (under 2 years):
0.3 ml four times daily after meals and at bedtime or as directed by a physician. Can also be mixed with liquids for easier administration.

Children (2 to 12 years):
0.6 ml four times daily after meals and at bedtime or as directed by a physician.
Adults: 1.2 ml (take two 0.6 ml doses) four times daily after meals and at bedtime. Do not take more than six times per day unless directed by a physician.

How Supplied: Dropper bottles of 15 mL (0.5 fl oz) and 30 mL (1 fl oz).
15 mL NDC-0021-4300-33
30 mL NDC-0021-4300-17
Shown in Product Identification Guide, page 418

Maximum Strength
PHAZYME–125 Chewable Tablets
[*fayzime*]

Description: Phazyme Chewables contain the highest dose of simethicone available in a single clean, fresh mint tasting chewable tablet. It has no known side effects or drug interactions.

Active Ingredient: Each tablet contains simethicone 125 mg.

Inactive Ingredients: Citric acid, D&C Yellow #10, dextrates, FD&C Blue #1, peppermint flavor, sorbitol, starch, sucrose, talc, tribasic calcium phosphate.

Actions: Simethicone minimizes gas formation and relieves gas entrapment in both the stomach and the lower G.I. tract. This action combats the distress due to gastrointestinal gas.

Indication: To alleviate or relieve the symptoms of gas. May also be used for postoperative gas pain.

Warnings: Keep this and all drugs out of the reach of children. If condition persists, consult your physician.

Store at controlled room temperature 59°–89°F (15°–30°C).

Dosage: One tablet, chewed thoroughly, four times a day after meals and at bedtime. Do not exceed 4 chewable tablets per day unless directed by a physician.

How Supplied: White, bevel-edged tablets with green speckles and imprinted with "Phazyme 125" in 10 pack NDC #0021-4450-15; 50's NDC #0021-4450-31.
Shown in Product Identification Guide, page 418

Maximum Strength
PHAZYME®–125 Softgel Capsules
[*fayzime*]

Description: A red softgel containing the highest dose of simethicone available in a single capsule. It has no known side effects or drug interactions.
Active Ingredient: Each capsule contains simethicone, 125 mg.
Inactive Ingredients: FD&C red No. 40, gelatin, glycerin, hydrogenated soybean oil, lecithin, methylparaben, polysorbate 80, propylparaben, soybean oil,

titanium dioxide, vegetable shortening, yellow wax.

Actions: Simethicone minimizes gas formation and relieves gas entrapment in both the stomach and the lower G.I. tract. This action combats the distress due to gastrointestinal gas.

Indication: To alleviate or relieve the symptoms of gas. May also be used for postoperative gas pain.

Warnings: Keep this and all drugs out of the reach of children. If condition persists, consult your physician.

Store at controlled room temperature 59°–86°F (15°–30°C).

Dosage: One softgel capsule four times a day after meals and at bedtime. Do not exceed 4 softgel capsules per day unless directed by a physician.

How Supplied: Red capsule imprinted rc 125 in bottles of 50, NDC #0021-0450-50 and 10 pack, NDC #0021-0450-02.
Shown in Product Identification Guide, page 417 and 418

The Reese Chemical Co.
**10617 FRANK AVENUE
CLEVELAND, OHIO 44106**

RE-AZO
RE-AZO TABLETS

Active Ingredients: Each tablet contains: Phenazopyridine HCl 1½ gr.

Indications: For the temporary relief of the discomfort of urinary tract irritations, pain, burning, urgency and frequency of voiding.

Warnings: Do not administer to children under 12 years of age. If symptoms persist or if abdominal cramps, diarrhea, dizziness or nausea develops, discontinue use and consult a physician. If you are pregnant, nursing a baby, or kidney disease is present, do not use this product without consulting a physician. Keep this and all medication out of reach of children. In case of accidental overdose, seek professional assistance or contact a poison control center immediately.

Dosage and Administration: Adults: two tablets three times a day after meals. Children under 12 years of age, consult a physician.

How Supplied: Cartons of 32 tablets.

RECAPSIN™ CREME
[*Rĕ "căp'sin Crēme*]
CAPSAICIN

Active Ingredient: Capsaicin 0.025% in a cream base.

Indications: For the temporary relief of minor aches and pains of muscles and joints associated with simple backache, arthritis, strains, bruises, and sprains.

Continued on next page

Reese Chemical—Cont.

Actions: Capsaicin is classified as a counterirritant and appears to affect Substance P by decreasing it from the sensory neurons associated with pain relating to the skin. Local application of Capsaicin results in the depletion of Substance P.

Warnings: For external use only. Avoid contact with the eyes, mouth, and other mucous membranes. Do not apply to wounds or damaged skin. Keep this and all drugs out of the reach of children. In case of accidental ingestion, seek professional assistance or contact a poison control center immediately.

Directions: Apply only the smallest amount of Recapsin™ Creme needed to cover the skin surrounding the affected joint. Massage directly into the skin on all sides of the affected joint repeating application 3–4 times daily. A burning sensation may or may not occur following use.

How Supplied: Available in a 1.5 oz. (45gms) tube
Shown in Product Identification Guide, page 418

REDACON DX PEDIATRIC DROPS

Active Ingredients: Each ml contains Phenylpropanolamine HCl 6.25 mg. Guaifenesin 50 mg. Dextromethorphan HBr 5 mg.

Indications: For the temporary relief of nasal congestion due to the common cold, hay fever or other respiratory allergies. Helps loosen phlegm and thin bronchial secretions and temporarily quiet cough.

Warnings: Do not exceed recommended dosage because at higher doses nervousness, dizziness, or sleeplessness may occur. Do not give to children who have heart disease, high blood pressure, thyroid disease, or diabetes unless directed by a physician.

Warnings: If cough persists for more than one week, tends to recur or is accompanied by fever, rash or persistent headache, consult a physician. Keep this and all drugs out of the reach of children. In case of accidental overdose, seek professional assistance or contact a Poison Control Center immediately.

Dosage and Administration: Children 2 to 6 years of age; oral dosage is 1 ml every 4 hours, not to exceed 6 doses in 24 hours, or as directed by a physician. Children under 2 years of age; consult a physician.

Professional Labeling: Children under 2 years of age: Dosage should be adjusted to age or weight and be administered every 4 hours as shown in the dosage table, not to exceed 6 doses in 24 hours.

Age	Weight	Dosage
1–3 months	8–12 lb	¼ mL
4–6 months	13–17 lb	½ mL
7–9 months	18–20 lb	¾ mL
10–24 months	21 + lb	1.0 mL

How Supplied: Available in 30 ml (1 fl. oz) plastic bottle with child-resistant cap and graduated dropper.

REESE'S PINWORM MEDICINE
Pyrantel Pamoate

Active Ingredient: Oral suspension—Pyrantel pamoate, 144 mg/cc (the equivalent of 50 mg Pyrantel base per cc). Caplets—Pyrantel pamoate, 180 mg (the equivalent of 62.5 mg Pyrantel pamate base).

Indications: For the treatment of enterobiasis (pinworm infection).

Warnings: Keep this and all drugs out of the reach of children. In case of accidental overdose, seek professional assistance or contact a poison control center immediately.

Precaution: If you are pregnant or have liver disease, do not take this product unless directed by a doctor.

Dosage and Administration: Adults, children 12 years of age and over, and children 2 years to under 12 years of age —Oral dosage is a single dose of 5 mg of pyrantel pamoate base per pound of body weight, not to exceed 1 gram.
Read package insert before taking this medicine. Do not administer to children under 2 years of age.

How Supplied: Reese's Pinworm Medicine is available in one-ounce bottles as a pleasant-tasting suspension which contains the equivalent of 50 mg Pyrantel pamoate base per cc. Also available in bottles of 24 caplets. It is supplied with English and Spanish label copy and directions.

Requa, Inc.
BOX 4008
1 SENECA PLACE
GREENWICH, CT 06830

CHARCOAID
Poison Adsorbent, liquid has sweet, pleasant taste and feel.

Active Ingredient: Activated vegetable charcoal U.S.P., 30 g per bottle, suspended in 70% sorbitol solution U.S.P., 110 g.

Indication: For the emergency treatment of acute ingested poison.

Action: Adsorbent

Warnings: Before using call a poison control center, emergency room, or a physician for advice. If the patient has been given Ipecac Syrup, do not give activated charcoal until after patient has vomited. Do not use in a semi-conscious or unconscious person.

Precaution: May cause laxation. Careful attention to fluids and electrolytes is important, especially with young children. Not recommended for multiple dose therapy.

Dosage and Administration: Adults: Shake well and drink entire contents (add water if too sweet). To insure a full dose, rinse bottle with water and drink. For children, refer to Poison Control Center.

Professional Labeling: Some dilution may be necessary for administration via lavage tube. Add a small amount of water to bottle and shake.

How Supplied: 5 fl. oz. unit dose bottle, 30 g activated charcoal U.S.P., suspended in 70% sorbitol solution U.S.P., 110 g.
U.S. Patent #4,122,169

CharcoAid 2000
Emergency Poison Adsorbent with super activated charcoal.

Active Ingredient: Super Activated Charcoal U.S.P., 50g

Indication: For the emergency treatment of acute ingested poison.

Action: Adsorbent

Warnings: See Charcoaid

Dosage and Administration: Shake bottle vigorously for at least 15 seconds. Drink entire contents, or for children use as directed by a health professional.

How Supplied: 240 ml bottle contains 50g charcoal in water suspension

---

CHARCOCAPS®
Digestive Aid Activated Charcoal Capsules and Caplets

Active Ingredient: Activated vegetable charcoal U.S.P., 260 mg per capsule.

Indications: Relief of intestinal gas or gastrointestinal distress. Also to aid in the prevention of non-specific pruritus associated with kidney dialysis treatment.

Actions: Adsorbent, detoxicant, soothing agent. Reduces the volume of intestinal gas and allays related discomfort.

Warnings: If symptoms of distress persist, stop this medication and consult your physician. Consults a physician if taking other drugs as this medication may interfere with their effectiveness.

Drug Interaction: Activated Charcoal USP can adsorb medication while they are in the digestive tract.

Precaution: General Guidelines— Take two hours before or one hour after medication including oral contraceptives.

Symptoms and Treatment of Oral Overdosage: Overdosage has not been encountered. Medical evidence indicates that high dosage or prolonged use does not cause side effect or harm the nutritional state of the patient.

Dosage and Administration: Two capsules after meals or at first sign of discomfort. Repeat as needed up to eight doses (16 capsules) per day.

Professional Labeling: None.

How Supplied: Bottles of 8, 36, 100 capsules

EDUCATIONAL MATERIAL

Questions & Answers
Brochure with questions and answers about the use of activated charcoal.
Trial Size
Free professional samples of Charcocaps, which includes coupon for regular size for the patient.

Rhône-Poulenc Rorer Pharmaceuticals Inc.
Consumer Pharmaceutical Products
500 ARCOLA ROAD
P.O. BOX 1200
COLLEGEVILLE, PA 19426-0107

Regular Strength
ASCRIPTIN®
[ă"skrĭp'tin]
Analgesic
Aspirin buffered with Maalox® for stomach comfort

Active Ingredients: Each tablet contains Aspirin (325 mg), buffered with Maalox® (Alumina-Magnesia) and Calcium Carbonate.

Inactive Ingredients: Hydroxypropyl Methylcellulose, Magnesium Stearate, Microcrystalline Cellulose, Starch, Talc, Titanium Dioxide, and other ingredients.

Description: Ascriptin is an excellent analgesic, antipyretic, and anti-inflammatory agent for general use, particularly where there is concern over aspirin-induced gastric distress. Coated tablets make swallowing easy.

Indications: As an analgesic for the temporary relief of minor pain in such conditions as headache, neuralgia, minor injuries, and dysmenorrhea. As an analgesic and antipyretic in adult colds. As an analgesic and anti-inflammatory agent for the minor aches and pains of arthritis and other rheumatic diseases. As an inhibitor of platelet aggregation, see MI's and TIA's indications.

Usual Adult Dose: Two tablets with water every 4 hours while symptoms persist; do not exceed 12 tablets in 24 hours. For children under twelve, consult a doctor.
WARNINGS: Children and teenagers should not use this medicine for

chicken pox or flu symptoms before a doctor is consulted about Reye syndrome, a rare but serious illness reported to be associated with aspirin. Keep this and all medicines out of children's reach. If pain persists more than 10 days, redness or swelling is present, fever persists more than 3 days, or symptoms worsen, consult a doctor immediately. If you are under medical care or have a history of stomach, kidney, or bleeding disorders or asthma, consult a doctor before using. Do not use if allergic to aspirin. As with any drug, if you are pregnant or nursing a baby, consult a doctor before using. **IT IS ESPECIALLY IMPORTANT NOT TO USE ASPIRIN DURING THE LAST 3 MONTHS OF PREGNANCY UNLESS SPECIFICALLY DIRECTED TO DO SO BY A DOCTOR BECAUSE IT MAY CAUSE PROBLEMS IN THE UNBORN CHILD OR COMPLICATIONS DURING DELIVERY.** If ringing in the ears or loss of hearing occurs, consult a doctor before taking any more of this product. **In case of accidental overdose, contact a doctor immediately.**
Drug Interaction Precaution: Do not use if taking a prescription drug for anticoagulation (blood thinning), diabetes, gout or arthritis, or a tetracycline antibiotic unless directed by a doctor.

Professional Labeling
ASCRIPTIN FOR MYOCARDIAL INFARCTION

Indication: Aspirin is indicated to reduce the risk of death and/or non-fatal myocardial infarction in patients with a previous infarction or unstable angina pectoris.

Clinical Trials: The indication is supported by the results of six, large, randomized multicenter, placebo-controlled studies[1–7] involving 10,816, predominantly male, post-myocardial infarction (MI) patients and one randomized placebo-controlled study of 1,266 men with unstable angina. Therapy with aspirin was begun at intervals after the onset of acute MI varying from less than 3 days to more than 5 years and continued for periods of from less than one year to four years. In the unstable angina study, treatment was started within 1 month after the onset of unstable angina and continued for 12 weeks and complicating conditions such as congestive heart failure were not included in the study.
Aspirin therapy in MI patients was associated with about a 20 percent reduction in the risk of subsequent death and/or nonfatal reinfarction, a median absolute decrease of 3 percent from the 12 to 22 percent event rates in the placebo groups. In the aspirin-treated unstable angina patients the reduction in risk was about 50 percent, a reduction in the event rate of 5% from the 10% rate in the placebo group over the 12 weeks of the study.
Daily dosage of aspirin in the post-myocardial infarction studies was 300 mg. in one study and 900 and 1500 mg. in five

studies. A dose of 325 mg. was used in the study of unstable angina.

Adverse Reactions: Gastrointestinal Reactions: Doses of 1000 mg. per day of aspirin caused gastrointestinal symptoms and bleeding that in some cases were clinically significant. In the largest post-infarction study (The Aspirin Myocardial Infaration Study (AMIS) with 4,500 people), the percentage incidences of gastrointestinal symptoms for the aspirin (1000 mg. of a standard, solid-tablet formulation) and placebo-treated subjects, respectively, were: stomach pain (14.5%; 4.4%); heartburn (11.9%; 4.8%); nausea and/or vomiting (7.6%; 2.1%); hospitalization for gastrointestinal disorder (4.8%; 3.5%). In the AMIS and other trials, aspirin treated patients had increased rates of gross gastrointestinal bleeding. Symptoms and signs of gastrointestinal irritation were not significantly increased in subjects treated for unstable angina with buffered aspirin in solution.

Cardiovascular and Biochemical:
In the AMIS trial, the dosage of 1000 mg. per day of aspirin was associated with small increases in systolic blood pressure (BP) (average 1.5 to 2.1 mm) and diastolic BP (0.5 to 0.6 mm), depending upon whether maximal or last available readings were used. Blood urea nitrogen and uric acid levels were also increased, but by less than 1.0 mg%.
Subjects with marked hypertension or renal insufficiency had been excluded from the trial so that the clinical importance of these observations for such subjects or for any subjects treated over more prolonged periods is not known. It is recommended that patients placed on long-term aspirin treatment, even at doses of 300 mg. per day, be seen at regular intervals to assess changes in these measurements.

Dosage and Administration: Although most of the studies used dosages exceeding 300 mg, two trials used only 300 mg, and pharmacologic data indicate that this dose inhibits platelet function fully. Therefore, 300 mg or a conventional 325-mg aspirin dose is a reasonable, routine dose that would minimize gastrointestinal adverse reactions. This use of aspirin applies to both solid, oral dosage forms (buffered and plain aspirin), and buffered aspirin in solution.

References: 1. Elwood P.C., et al., "A Randomized Controlled Trial of Acetylsalicylic Acid in the Secondary Prevention of Mortality from Myocardial Infarction," *British Medical Journal*, 1:436–440, 1974. 2. The Coronary Drug Project Research Group, "Aspirin in Coronary Heart Disease," *Journal of Chronic Disease*, 29:625–642, 1976. 3. Breddin K. et al., "Secondary Prevention of Myocardial Infarction; Comparison of Acetylsalicylic Acid Phenprocoumon and Placebo," *Thromb, Haemost.*, 41:225–236. 1979. 4. Aspirin Myocardial Infarction Study Research Group, "A Randomized.

Continued on next page

Rhône-Poulenc Rorer—Cont.

Controlled Trial of Aspirin in Persons Recovered from Myocardial Infarction." *Journal American Medical Association,* 243:661–669, 1980. 5. Elwood P.C., and Sweetnam, P.M., "Aspirin and Secondary Mortality after Myocardial Infartion," *Lancet,* pp. 1313–1315, December 22–29, 1979. 6. The Persantine-Aspirin Reinfarction Study Research Group "Persantine and Aspirin in Coronary Heart Disease," *Circulation* 62;449–460. 1980. 7. Lewis H.D., et al., "Protective Effects of Aspirin Against Acute Myocardial Infarction and Death in Men with Unstable Angina, Results of a Veterans Administration Cooperative Study." *New England Journal of Medicine,* 309;396–403, 1983.

ASCRIPTIN FOR RECURRENT TIA's IN MEN

Clinical Trials: The indication is supported by the results of a Canadian study (1) in which 585 patients with threatened stroke were followed in a randomized clinical trial for an average of 26 months to determine whether aspirin or sulfinpyrazone, singly or in combination was superior to placebo in preventing transient ischemic attacks, stroke, or death. The study showed that, although sulfinpyrazone had no statistically significant effect, aspirin reduced the risk of continuing transient ischemic attacks, stroke, or death by 19 percent and reduced the risk of stroke or death by 31 percent. Another aspirin study carried out in the United States with 178 patients, showed a statistically significant number of "favorable outcomes" including reduced transient ischemic attacks, stroke, and death (2).

Indications: For reducing the risk of recurrent transient ischemic attacks (TIA's) or stroke in men who have had transient ischemia of the brain due to fibrin platelet emboli. There is inadequate evidence that aspirin or buffered aspirin is effective in reducing TIA's in women at the recommended dosage. There is no evidence that aspirin or buffered aspirin is of benefit in the treatment of completed strokes in men or women.

Precautions: (1) Patients presenting with signs and symptoms of TIA's should have a complete medical and neurologic evaluation. Consideration should be given to other disorders which resemble TIA's. (2) Attention should be given to risk factors; it is important to evaluate and treat, if appropriate, other diseases associated with TIA's and stroke such as hypertension and diabetes. (3) Concurrent administration of absorbable antacids at therapeutic doses may increase the clearance of salicylates in some individuals. The concurrent administration of nonabsorbable antacids may alter the rate of absorption of aspirin, thereby resulting in a decreased acetylsalicylic acid/salicylate ratio in plasma. The clinical significance on TIA's of

these decreases in available aspirin is unknown.
Aspirin at dosages of 1,000 milligrams per day has been associated with small increases in blood pressure, blood urea nitrogen, and serum uric acid levels. It is recommended that patients placed on long-term aspirin treatment be seen at regular intervals to assess changes in these measurements.

Adverse Reactions: At dosages of 1,000 milligrams or higher of aspirin per day, gastrointestinal side effects include stomach pain, heartburn, nausea and/or vomiting, as well as increased rates of gross gastrointestinal bleeding.

Dosage: Adults dosage for men is 1300 mg a day, in divided doses of 650 mg twice a day or 325 mg four times a day.

References: (1) The Canadian Cooperative Study Group. "A Randomized Trial of Aspirin and Sulfinpyrazone in Threatened Stroke," *New England Journal of Medicine,*299:53–59, 1978.
(2) Fields, W.S., et al., "Controlled Trial of Aspirin in Cerebral Ischemia," *Stroke* 8:301–316, 1977.

How Supplied: Bottles of 60 tablets (0067-0145-60), 100 tablets (0067-0145-68), 160 (0067-0145-30) and 225 tablets (0067-0145-77).
Bottles of 500 tablets (0067-0145-74) without child-resistant closures (for arthritic patients).

Shown in Product Identification Guide, page 418

Maximum Strength ASCRIPTIN®
Analgesic
Aspirin Buffered with Maalox®
for Stomach Comfort

Active Ingredients: Each coated caplet contains Aspirin (500 mg), buffered with Maalox®(Alumina-Magnesia) and Calcium Carbonate.

Inactive Ingredients: Hydroxypropyl Methylcellulose, Magnesium Stearate, Microcrystalline Cellulose, Starch, Talc, Titanium Dioxide, and other ingredients.

Description: Maximum Strength Ascriptin contains the maximum dose of aspirin for fast, effective pain relief, and is buffered with Maalox for stomach comfort. Coated caplets make swallowing easy.

Indications: Use Maximum Strength Ascriptin for temporary relief of minor pain in headache, neuralgia, minor injuries, dysmenorrhea, discomfort and fever of ordinary colds. Also provides relief from the minor aches and pains of arthritis and rheumatism.

Usual Adult Dose: Two caplets with water every 6 hours while symptoms persist, not to exceed 8 caplets in 24 hours. For children under 12, consult a doctor.
**WARNINGS: Children and teenagers should not use this medicine for chicken pox or flu symptoms before a doctor is consulted about Reye syn-

drome, a rate but serious illness reported to be associated with aspirin. Keep this and all medicines out of children's reach. If pain persists more than 10 days, redness or swelling is present, fever persists more than 3 days, or symptoms worsen, consult a doctor immediately.** If you are under medical care or have a history of stomach, kidney, or bleeding disorders or asthma, consult a doctor before using. Do not use if allergic to aspirin. As with any drug, if you are pregnant or nursing a baby, consult a doctor before using.
IT IS ESPECIALLY IMPORTANT NOT TO USE ASPIRIN DURING THE LAST 3 MONTHS OF PREGNANCY UNLESS SPECIFICALLY DIRECTED TO DO SO BY A DOCTOR BECAUSE IT MAY CAUSE PROBLEMS IN THE UNBORN CHILD OR COMPLICATIONS DURING DELIVERY. If ringing in the ears or loss of hearing occurs, consult a doctor before taking any more of this product. **In case of accidental overdose, contact a doctor immediately.** *Drug interaction precaution:* Do not use if taking a prescription drug for anticoagulation (blood thinning), diabetes, gout or arthritis, or a tetracycline antibiotic unless directed by a doctor.

Professional Labeling see detail under Regular Strength Ascriptin®

How Supplied: Bottles of 60 tablets (0067-0145-60), 100 tablets (0067-0145-68), 160 (0067-0145-30) and 225 tablets (0067-0145-77).
Bottles of 500 tablets (0067-0145-74) without child-resistant closures (for arthritic patients).

Shown in Product Identification Guide, page 418

ARTHRITIS PAIN ASCRIPTIN®
Analgesic
Aspirin buffered with extra Maalox®
for extra stomach comfort

Active Ingredients: Each caplet contains Aspirin (325 mg), buffered with Maalox® (Alumina-Magnesia) and Calcium Carbonate.

Inactive Ingredients: Hydroxypropyl Methylcellulose, Magnesium Stearate, Microcrystalline Cellulose, Starch, Talc, Titanium Dioxide, and other ingredients.

Description: Arthritis Pain Ascriptin is a highly buffered analgesic, anti-inflammatory, and antipyretic agent which relieves the minor pain associated with rheumatoid arthritis, osteoarthritis, and other arthritic conditions. It is formulated with more Maalox® than Regular Strength Ascriptin to provide increased neutralization of gastric acid, thus reducing the likelihood of GI disturbance. Coated caplets make swallowing easy.

Indications: As an analgesic, anti-inflammatory, and antipyretic agent to relieve the minor pain associated with rheumatoid arthritis, osteoarthritis, and other arthritic conditions.

Usual Adult Dose: Two caplets with water, four times daily, or as directed by the physician for arthritis therapy. For children under twelve, consult a doctor. **WARNINGS: Children and teenagers should not use this medicine for chicken pox or flu symptoms before a doctor is consulted about Reye syndrome, a rare but serious illness reported to be associated with aspirin. Keep this and all medicines out of children's reach. If pain persists more than 10 days, redness or swelling is present, fever persists more than 3 days, or symptoms worsen, consult a doctor immediately.** If you are under medical care or have a history of stomach, kidney, or bleeding disorders or asthma, consult a doctor before using. Do not use if allergic to aspirin. As with any drug, if you are pregnant or nursing a baby, consult a doctor before using. **IT IS ESPECIALLY IMPORTANT NOT TO USE ASPIRIN DURING THE LAST 3 MONTHS OF PREGNANCY UNLESS SPECIFICALLY DIRECTED TO DO SO BY A DOCTOR BECAUSE IT MAY CAUSE PROBLEMS IN THE UNBORN CHILD OR COMPLICATIONS DURING DELIVERY.** If ringing in the ears or loss of hearing occurs, consult a doctor before taking any more of this product. **In case of accidental overdose, contact a doctor immediately.**
Drug Interaction Precaution: Do not use if taking a prescription drug for anticoagulation (blood thinning), diabetes, gout or arthritis, or a tetracycline antibiotic unless directed by a doctor.

Professional Labeling see detail under Regular Strength Ascriptin®

How Supplied: Bottles of 60 tablets (0067-0145-60), 100 tablets (0067-0145-68), 160 (0067-0145-30) and 225 tablets (0067-0145-77).
Bottles of 500 tablets (0067-0145-74) without child-resistant closures (for arthritic patients).

Shown in Product Identification Guide, page 418

MAALOX® Antacid Caplets
Antacid

Description: New, Maalox® antacid caplets provide fast, effective relief of acid indigestion, heartburn, and sour stomach. Because they are easy-to-swallow caplets, there is no chalky aftertaste.

Active Ingredients: Each caplet contains 1000 mg calcium carbonate.

Inactive Ingredients: Corn starch, croscarmellose, magnesium stearate and sodium lauryl sulfate. Contains not more than 0.4 mEq sodium per caplet.
[See chart top of next column]

Indications: For the relief of acid indigestion, heartburn, sour stomach and upset stomach associated with these symptoms.

Directions for Use: Take 1 caplet as needed or as directed by physician.

Minimum Recommended Dosage: Maalox Antacid Caplets Per caplet	
Acid neutralizing capacity	NLT 20.0 mEq/ caplet
Sodium content	NMT 5 mg/ caplet

CAPLETS SHOULD NOT BE CHEWED.

Patient Warnings: Do not take more than 8 caplets in a 24-hour period or use the maximum dosage for more than 2 weeks except under the advice and supervision of a physician. If you have a history of calcium stones or decreased renal function, consult a physician before use. Keep this and all drugs out of the reach of children.

Drug Interaction Precaution: Calcium antacid salts can decrease absorption of beta-adrenergic blockers and Dilantin. Thiazide diuretics can cause hypercalcemia by decreasing renal excretion of calcium antacids. The milk-alkali syndrome can occur with prolonged sodium bicarbonate use and/or homogenized milk containing Vitamin D.

Drug Interaction Precaution: Antacids may interact with certain prescription drugs. If you are presently taking a prescription drug, do not take this product without checking with your physician or other health professional.

Professional Labeling: Indicated for the symptomatic relief of hyperacidity associated with the diagnosis of peptic ulcer, gastritis, peptic esophagitis, gastric hyperacidity, and hiatal hernia.

How Supplied: Maalox Antacid Caplets are available in blister packs of 24 caplets (0067-0183-24) and plastic bottle of 50 caplets (0067-0183-50).

Storage: Store at room temperature. Protect from moisture.
Shown in Product Identification Guide, page 418

MAALOX™ ANTI-DIARRHEAL
Loperamide Hydrochloride
Caplets, 2mg

Description: Maalox™ Anti-Diarrheal relieves diarrhea for both adults and children 6 years of age and older, in many cases with just one dose. Maalox Anti-Diarrheal contains Loperamide Hydrochloride, previously available only in a leading prescription product. Loperamide Hydrochloride has been prescribed for millions of people, and has proven to be an exceptionally safe and effective anti-diarrheal medication.

Actions: Maalox Anti-Diarrheal contains loperamide hydrochloride which has been clinically proven to slow intestinal motility. It also affects water and electrolyte movement through the bowel.

Indications: Maalox Anti-Diarrheal controls the symptoms of diarrhea.

Active Ingredient: Loperamide Hydrochloride 2 mg per caplet.

Inactive Ingredients: Corn starch, lactose, magnesium stearate, microcrystalline cellulose, FD&C Blue #1 and D&C Yellow #10.

Directions for Use: Follow specific dosing information below, and drink plenty of clear fluids to help prevent dehydration, which may accompany diarrhea.
Adults and children 12 years of age and older—
Take 2 caplets after the first loose bowel movement and 1 caplet after each subsequent loose bowel movement, but no more than 4 caplets a day for no more than 2 days.
Children 9–11 years (60–95 lbs.)—Take 1 caplet after the first loose bowel movements and ½ caplet after each subsequent loose bowel movement, but no more than 3 caplets a day for no more than 2 days.
Children 6–8 years (48–59 lbs.)—Take 1 caplet after the first loose bowel movement and ½ caplet after each subsequent loose bowel movement, but no more than 2 caplets a day for no more than 2 days.
Children under 6 years (up to 47 lbs.)—Consult a physician. Not intended for use in children under 6 years old.

Warnings: DO NOT USE FOR MORE THAN TWO DAYS UNLESS DIRECTED BY A PHYSICIAN. Do not use if diarrhea is accompanied by high fever (greater than 101°), or if blood is present in the stool, or if you have had a rash or other allergic reaction to Loperamide Hydrochloride. If you are taking antibiotics or have a history of liver disease, consult a physician before using this product. As with any drug, if you are pregnant or nursing a baby, seek the advice of a health professional before using this product. In case of accidental overdose, seek professional assistance or contact poison control center immediately.

Overdosage: Overdosage of loperamide HCl in man may result in constipation, CNS depression and nausea. A slurry of activated charcoal administered promptly after ingestion of loperamide hydrochloride can reduce the amount of drug which is absorbed. If vomiting occurs spontaneously upon ingestion, a slurry of 100 grams of activated charcoal should be administered orally as soon as fluids can be retained. If vomiting has not occurred, and CNS depression is evident, gastric lavage should be performed followed by administration to 100 grams of the activated charcoal slurry through the gastric tube. In the event of overdosage, patients should be monitored for signs of CNS depression for at least 24 hours. Children may be more sensitive to central nervous system

Continued on next page

Rhône-Poulenc Rorer—Cont.

effects than adults. If CNS depression is observed, naloxone may be administered. If responsive to naloxone, vital signs must be monitored carefully for recurrence of symptoms of drug overdose for at least 24 hours after the last dose of naloxone.

How Supplied: Cartons of 6 and 12 caplets.

Shown in Product Identification Guide, page 418

MAALOX™ ANTI-DIARRHEAL
(Loperamide Hydrochloride)
Oral Solution

Description: Maalox™ Anti-Diarrheal relieves diarrhea for both adults and children 6 years of age and older, in many cases with just one dose. Maalox Anti-Diarrheal contains Loperamide Hydrochloride, previously available only in a leading prescription product. Loperamide Hydrochloride has been prescribed for millions of people, and has proven to be an exceptionally safe and effective anti-diarrheal medication.
Maalox Anti-Diarrheal is a non-chalky, cherry flavored, clear liquid.

Actions: Maalox Anti-Diarrheal contains Loperamide Hydrochloride which has been clinically proven to slow intestinal motility. It also affects water and electrolyte movement through the bowel.

Indications: Maalox Anti-Diarrheal controls the symptoms of diarrhea.

Active Ingredient: Loperamide Hydrochloride 1 mg per teaspoonful (5 ml).

Inactive Ingredients: Alcohol 5.25%, citric acid, flavors, glycerin, methylparaben and purified water. May contain sodium hydroxide to adjust pH.

Directions for use: A dose cup is provided to accurately measure doses as noted below. Drink plenty of clear fluids to help prevent dehydration, which may accompany diarrhea.
Adults and children 12 years of age and older —
Take 4 teaspoonfuls (1 dosage cup) after the first loose bowel movement and 2 teaspoonfuls after each subsequent loose bowel movement, but no more than 8 teaspoonfuls per day for no more than 2 days.
Children 9–11 years (60–95 lbs.) —
Take 2 teaspoonfuls (½ dosage cup) after the first loose bowel movement and 1 teaspoonful after each subsequent loose bowel movement. Do not exceed 6 teaspoonfuls per day.
Children 6–8 years (48–59 lbs.) —
Take 2 teaspoonfuls (½ dosage cup) after the first loose bowel movement and 1 teaspoonful after each subsequent loose bowel movement. Do not exceed 4 teaspoonfuls per day.
Children under 6 years (up to 47 lbs.) —
Consult a physician. Not intended for use in children 6 years old.

Warnings: DO NOT USE FOR MORE THAN TWO DAYS UNLESS DIRECTED BY A PHYSICIAN. Do not use if diarrhea is accompanied by high fever (greater than 101°), or if blood is present in the stool, or if you have had a rash or other allergic reaction to Loperamide Hydrochloride. If you are taking antibiotics or have a history of liver disease, consult a physician before using this product. As with any drug, if you are pregnant or nursing a baby, seek the advice of a health professional before using this product. In case of accidental overdose, seek professional assistance or contact poison control center immediately.

Overdosage: Overdosage of loperamide HCl in man may result in constipation, CNS depression and nausea. A slurry of activated charcoal administered promptly after ingestion of loperamide hydrochloride can reduce the amount of drug which is absorbed. If vomiting occurs spontaneously upon ingestion, a slurry of 100 grams of activated charcoal should be administered orally as soon as fluids can be retained. If vomiting has not occurred, and CNS depression is evident, gastric lavage should be performed followed by administration to 100 grams of the activated charcoal slurry through the gastric tube. In the event of overdosage, patients should be monitored for signs of CNS depression for at least 24 hours. Children may be more sensitive to central nervous system effects than adults. If CNS depression is observed, naloxone may be administered. If responsive to naloxone, vital signs must be monitored carefully for recurrence of symptoms of drug overdose for at least 24 hours after the last dose of naloxone.

How Supplied: Cherry flavored liquid (2 fl oz and 4 fl oz) in tamper resistant bottles and child resistant safety caps and dosage cup.

Shown in Product Identification Guide, page 418

MAALOX™ ANTI-GAS
(Simethicone)
Tablets (Regular Strength)

Description: Maalox Anti-Gas relieves painful gas, bloating, and pressure quickly and effectively. It is formulated with the active ingredient that diffuses the excess gas in the stomach and digestive tract.

Active Ingredient: Simethicone (80 mg per tablet)

Inactive Ingredients: Corn starch, D&C Red No. 27, aluminum lake, flavor, gelatin, mannitol, sucrose, and tribasic calcium phosphate.

Indications: For relief of painful symptoms of excess gas in the digestive tract. Such gas is frequently caused by excessive swallowing of air or by eating foods that disagree.
Maalox™ Anti-Gas acts in the stomach and intestines to change the surface tension of gas bubbles enabling them to co-

alesce: thus, the gas is freed and is eliminated more easily by belching or passing flatus.

Directions for Use: Chew 1 tablet thoroughly 4 times daily after meals and at bedtime or as directed by a physician. May also be taken as needed, up to 6 tablets daily.
If symptoms persist, contact your physician.

Warnings: Keep this and all drugs out of the reach of children.

How Supplied: Cartons of 12 and 48 tablets.

Shown in Product Identification Guide, page 418

EXTRA STRENGTH MAALOX™ ANTI-GAS
(Simethicone) Tablets

Description: Maalox Anti-Gas relieves painful gas, bloating, and pressure quickly and effectively. It is formulated with the active ingredient that diffuses the excess gas in the stomach and digestive tract.

Active Ingredient: Simethicone (150 mg per tablet)

Inactive Ingredients: Corn starch, D&C red No. 27, aluminum lake, flavor, gelatin, mannitol, sucrose and tribasic calcium phosphate.

Indications: For relief of painful symptoms of excess gas in the digestive tract. Such gas is frequently caused by excessive swallowing of air or by eating foods that disagree.
Maalox™ Anti-Gas acts in the stomach and intestines to change the surface tension of gas bubbles enabling them to coalesce: thus, the gas is freed and is eliminated more easily by belching or passing flatus.

Directions for Use: Chew 1 tablet thoroughly. Use after meals or at bedtime, or as directed by a physician. May also be taken as needed, up to 3 tablets daily. If symptoms persist, contact your physician.

Warnings: Keep this and all drugs out of the reach of children.

How Supplied: Cartons of 10 tablets.

Shown in Product Identification Guide, page 418

MAALOX™ DAILY FIBER THERAPY
(psyllium hydrophilic mucilloid)

Description: Maalox™ Daily Fiber Therapy is a bulk-producing, natural psyllium fiber encouraging normal elimination naturally, without chemical stimulants. It contains hydrophilic mucilloid fiber which is derived from the husk of the psyllium seed. It is a finely ground, ultra-smooth powder that mixes easily. It provides a daily source of soluble fiber that is effective in restoring and maintaining regularity.

Actions: Maalox Daily Fiber Therapy promotes natural elimination due to its

Forms	Inactive Ingredients	Dosage	How Supplied	Per Dose Information
Maalox™ Daily Fiber Therapy Orange Flavor Powder	Citric Acid, D&C Yellow No. 10, FD&C Yellow No. 6, Flavoring, Sucrose	One rounded tablespoonful (12g) in 8 ounces of liquid up to 3 times per day	Canisters: 13 Ounce/30 Doses 20.3 Ounce/48 Doses Packettes: Cartons of Three Single Dose Packets	Calories: 35 Sodium: Carbohydrates: 8g Fat: 100 mg Phenylaline: 0mg
Maalox™ Daily Fiber Therapy Citrus Flavor Powder	Citric Acid, D&C Yellow No. 10, Flavoring, Sucrose	One rounded tablespoonful (12g) in 8 ounces of liquid up to 3 times per day	Canisters: 13 Ounce/30 Doses 20.3 Ounce/48 Doses	Calories: 35 Sodium: Carbohydrates: 8g Fat: 100mg Phenylaline: 0mg
Maalox™ Daily Fiber Therapy Orange Flavor Sugar Free Powder	Aspartame, Citric Acid, D&C Yellow No. 10, FD&C Yellow No. 6, Flavoring, Maltodextrin	One rounded teaspoonful (5.8g) in 8 ounces of liquid up to 3 times per day	Canisters: 10 Ounce/48 Doses Packettes: Cartons of Three Single Dose Packets	Calories: 9 Sodium: Carbohydrates: 2g Fat: 100mg Phenylaline: 21mg
Maalox™ Daily Fiber Therapy Citrus Flavor Sugar Free Powder	Aspartame, Citric Acid, D&C Yellow No. 10, Flavoring, Maltodextrin	One rounded teaspoonful (5.8g) in 8 ounces of liquid up to 3 times per day	Canisters: 10 Ounce/48 Dose	Calories: 9 Sodium: Carboyhdrates: 2g Fat: 100mg Phenylaline: 21mg

bulking effect in the colon. The bulking effect is due to both the water-holding capacity of undigested fiber and the increased bacterial mass following partial fiber digestion. This results in enlargement of the lumen of the colon, thereby decreasing intraluminal pressure and speeding colonic transit in constipated patients.

Indications: Maalox Daily Fiber Therapy is indicated in the management of chronic constipation, in irritable bowel syndrome, as adjunctive therapy in constipation of diverticular disease, in the bowel management of patients with hemorrhoids, and for constipation during pregnancy, convalescence, and senility.

Contraindications: Intestinal obstruction, fecal impaction.

Warnings: TAKING THIS PRODUCT WITHOUT ADEQUATE FLUID MAY CAUSE IT TO SWELL AND BLOCK YOUR THROAT OR ESOPHAGUS AND MAY CAUSE CHOKING. DO NOT TAKE THIS PRODUCT IF YOU HAVE DIFFICULTY IN SWALLOWING. IF YOU EXPERIENCE CHEST PAIN, VOMITING, OR DIFFICULTY IN SWALLOWING OR BREATHING AFTER TAKING THIS PRODUCT, SEEK IMMEDIATE MEDICAL ATTENTION. Patients are advised they should not use the product without consulting a doctor when abdominal pain, nausea, or vomiting are present, if they have noticed a sudden change in bowel habits that persists over a period of 2 weeks, or rectal bleeding, or if they have been diagnosed with esophageal narrowing or have difficulty in swallowing.
Patients are advised to consult a physician if constipation persists for longer than 1 week, as this may be a sign of serious medical condition.

Psyllium products may cause allergic reaction in people sensitive to inhaled or ingested psyllium. Keep this and all medications out of the reach of children.

Precaution: *Notice to Health Care Professionals:* To minimize the potential for allergic reaction, health care professionals who frequently dispense powdered psyllium products should avoid inhaling airborne dust while dispensing these products. *Handling and Dispensing:* To minimize generating airborne dust, spoon product from the canister into a glass according to label directions.

Dosage & Administration: MIX THIS PRODUCT (CHILD OR ADULT DOSE) WITH AT LEAST 8 OUNCES (A FULL GLASS) OF WATER OR OTHER FLUID. MIXING THIS PRODUCT WITHOUT ENOUGH LIQUID MAY CAUSE CHOKING. SEE WARNINGS. Recommended dosage is for sugar-free product 1 rounded teaspoonful or for sucrose product 1 rounded tablespoonful. The appropriate dose should be mixed with 8 ounces of water or your favorite cool beverage. Drinking another glass of liquid is helpful.
Children (6–12 years of age) should take ½ the adult dose with 8 ounces of liquid up to 3 times daily.

New Users: Start by taking 1 dose each day. Gradually increase to 3 doses per day if needed or recommended by your doctor. If minor gas or bloating occurs, reduce the amount you take until your system adjusts. Also useful in the treatment of disorders other than constipation, when recommended by a physician.

How Supplied: See chart above

Shown in Product Identification Guide, page 419

MAALOX® HEARTBURN RELIEF
Heartburn Relief™ Antacid Tablets

Description: Maalox® Heartburn Relief tablets are specially formulated to provide fast, effective relief of heartburn, acid indigestion, and sour stomach. Each tablet contains aluminum hydroxide-magnesium carbonate codried gel 180 mg and magnesium carbonate 160 mg. It is formulated in a pleasant, cool mint flavor.

Inactive Ingredients: Compressible sugar, corn starch, D&C Yellow No. 10, FD&C Blue No. 2, flavors, magnesium alginate, magnesium stearate, potassium bicarbonate.

Minimum Recommended Dosage: Maalox Heartburn Relief Antacid Tablets	Per 2 tablets
Acid neutralizing Capacity	NLT 14.7 mEq
Sodium	NMT 6mg

Directions for Use: Chew 2–4 tablets thoroughly, after meals and at bedtime, or as directed by physician. For best results, follow with a half glass (4 fl. oz.) of water or other cool liquid.

Patient Warnings: Do not take more than 16 tablets in a 24-hour period or use the maximum dosage for more than 2 weeks or use if you have kidney disease except under the advice and supervision of a physician.

Continued on next page

Rhône-Poulenc Rorer—Cont.

Drug Interaction Precaution: Antacids may interact with certain prescription drugs. If you are presently taking a prescription drug, do not take this product without checking with your physician or other health professional.

Professional Labeling:

Warnings: Prolonged use of aluminum-containing antacids in patients with renal failure may result in or worsen dialysis osteomalacia. Elevated tissue aluminum levels contribute to the development of the dialysis encephalopathy and osteomalacia syndromes. Small amounts of aluminum are absorbed from the gastrointestinal tract and renal excretion of aluminum is impaired in renal failure. Aluminum is not well removed by dialysis because it is bound to albumin and transferrin, which do not cross dialysis membranes. As a result, aluminum is deposited in bone and dialysis osteomalacia may develop when large amounts of aluminum are ingested orally by patients with impaired renal function. Aluminum forms insoluble complexes with phosphate in the gastrointestinal tract, thus decreasing phosphate absorption. Prolonged use of antacids containing aluminum by normophosphatemic patients may result in hypophosphatemia if phosphate intake is not adequate. In its more severe forms, hypophosphatemia can lead to anorexia, malaise, muscle weakness, and osteomalacia.

How Supplied: Maalox HRF antacid tablets are available in plastic bottles of 30 tablets (0067-0353-30), 60 tablets (0067-0353-60) and blister packs of 12 tablets (0067-0353-12).

Shown in Product Identification Guide, page 418

MAALOX® HEARTBURN RELIEF Suspension (Antacid)

Description: Maalox® Heartburn Relief provides symptomatic relief of heartburn, acid indigestion and/or sour stomach. Each 10 ml (2 teaspoonfuls) contains aluminum hydroxide-magnesium carbonate codried gel 280 mg and magnesium carbonate USP 350 mg. It is formulated in a pleasant, cool mint flavor to help provide a cooling and soothing sensation as it goes down the esophagus.

Inactive Ingredients: Calcium carbonate, calcium saccharin, FD&C Blue No. 1, FD&C Yellow No. 5 (tartrazine) as a color additive, flavors, magnesium alginate, methyl and propyl parabens, potassium bicarbonate, purified water, sorbitol and other ingredients.

[See table top of next column]

Directions for Use: Two to four teaspoonfuls 4 times a day, taken 20 min to 1 hour after meals and at bedtime, or as directed by a physician.

Patient Warnings: Do not take more than 16 teaspoonfuls in a 24-hour period

Minimum Recommended Dosage: Maalox Heartburn Relief Suspension	
	Per 2 tsp. (10 mL)
Acid neutralizing capacity	NLT 17 mEq
Sodium content	NMT 5 mg

or use the maximum dosage for more than 2 weeks or use if you have kidney disease except under the advice and supervision of a physician. Keep this and all drugs out of the reach of children.

Drug Interaction Precaution: Antacids may interact with certain prescription drugs. If you are presently taking a prescription drug, do not take this product without checking with your physician or other health professional.

Professional Labeling:

Warnings:
Prolonged use of aluminum-containing antacids in patients with renal failure may result in or worsen dialysis osteomalacia. Elevated tissue aluminum levels contribute to the development of the dialysis encephalopathy and osteomalacia syndromes. Small amounts of aluminum are absorbed from the gastrointestinal tract and renal excretion of aluminum is impaired in renal failure. Aluminum is not well removed by dialysis because it is bound to albumin and transferrin, which do not cross dialysis membranes. As a result, aluminum is deposited in bone, and dialysis osteomalacia may develop when large amounts of aluminum are ingested orally by patients with impaired renal function.
Aluminum forms insoluble complexes with phosphate in the gastrointestinal tract, thus decreasing phosphate absorption. Prolonged use of antacids containing aluminum by normophosphatemic patients may result in hypophosphatemia if phosphate intake is not adequate. In its more severe forms, hypophosphatemia can lead to anorexia, malaise, muscle weakness, and osteomalacia.

How Supplied: Maalox® Heartburn Relief is available in a 10 fl oz plastic bottle (0067-0350-71).

Shown in Product Identification Guide, page 418

MAALOX®
Magnesia and Alumina
Oral Suspension
Antacid

Liquids
Mint Flavored
Cherry Creme

Description: Maalox® is used for the relief of acid indigestion, heartburn, sour stomach and upset stomach associated with these symptoms.

Active Ingredients	Maalox Suspension 5 mL teaspoon
Magnesium Hydroxide	200 mg.
Aluminum Hydroxide (equivalent to dried gel, USP)	225 mg.

Inactive Ingredients: Flavors, methylparaben, propylparaben, saccharin, sorbitol, purified water and other ingredients. May also contain citric acid.

Minimum Recommended Dosage: Maalox Suspension	
	Per 2 Tsp. (10 mL)
Acid neutralizing capacity	NLT 26.6 mEq
Sodium content	NMT 2 mg

Indications: As an antacid for symptomatic relief of hyperacidity associated with the diagnosis of peptic ulcer, gastritis, peptic esophagitis, gastric hyperacidity, heartburn, or hiatal hernia.

Professional Labeling

Warnings: (i) Prolonged use of aluminum-containing antacids in patients with renal failure may result in or worsen dialysis osteomalacia. Elevated tissue aluminum levels contribute to the development of the dialysis encephalopathy and osteomalacia syndromes. Small amounts of aluminum are absorbed from the gastrointestinal tract and renal excretion of aluminum is impaired in renal failure. Aluminum is not well removed by dialysis because it is bound to albumin and trensferrin, which do not cross dialysis membranes. As a result, aluminum is deposited in bone, and dialysis osteomalacia may develop when large amounts of aluminum are ingested orally by patients with impaired renal function. (ii) Aluminum forms insoluble complexes with phosphate in the gastrointestinal tract, thus decreasing phosphate absorption. Prolonged use of aluminum-containing antacids by normophosphatemic patients may result in hypophosphatemia if phosphate intake is not adequate. In its more severe forms, hypophosphatemia can lead to anorexia, malaise, muscle weakness, and osteomalacia.

Directions for Use. Two to four teaspoonfuls, four times a day, taken 20 minutes to 1 hour after meals and at bedtime, or as directed by a physician.

Patient Warnings: Do not take more than 16 teaspoonfuls in a 24-hour period or use the maximum dosage for more than 2 weeks or use if you have kidney disease except under the advice and supervision of a physician. Keep this and all drugs out of the reach of children.

Drug Interaction Precaution: Antacids may interact with certain prescription drugs. If you are presently taking a prescription drug, do not take this product without checking with your physician or other health professional.

How Supplied:
Maalox Mint Flavored Suspension is available in plastic bottles of 12 oz (0067-0330-71) and 26 oz (0067-0330-44).
Maalox Cherry Creme Flavored Suspension is available in plastic bottles of 12 oz (0067-0331-71) and 26 oz (0067-0331-44).

Shown in Product Identification Guide, page 418

MAALOX® Plus
Alumina, Magnesia and Simethicone Tablets,
Rhône-Poulenc Rorer
Antacid/Anti-Gas

Tablets
   Lemon Creme
   Cherry Creme, Mint Creme
☐ Physician-proven Maalox® formula for antacid effectiveness.
☐ Simethicone, at a recognized clinical dose, for antiflatulent action.

Description: Maalox® Plus, a balanced combination of magnesium and aluminum hydroxides plus simethicone, is a non-constipating antacid/anti-gas which comes in pleasant tasting flavors.

Composition: To provide symptomatic relief of hyperacidity plus alleviation of gas symptoms, each tablet contains:

Active Ingredients	Maalox® Plus Per Tablet
Magnesium Hydroxide	200 mg
Aluminum Hydroxide (equivalent to dried gel, USP)	200 mg
Simethicone	25 mg

Inactive Ingredients: Maalox® Plus Tablets: Citric acid, confectioners' sugar, D&C Red No. 30, D&C Yellow No. 10, dextrose, flavors, glycerin, magnesium stearate, mannitol, saccharin sodium, sorbitol, starch, talc.
To aid in establishing proper dosage schedules, the following information is provided:
[See table top of next column]

Directions for Use: Chew 1 to 4 tablets 4 times a day, 20 minutes to 1 hour after meals and at bedtime, or as directed by a physician.

Patient Warnings: Do not take more than 16 tablets in a 24-hour period or use the maximum dosage for more than 2 weeks or use if you have kidney disease

Minimum Recommended Dosage:	
	Per Tablet
Acid neutralizing capacity	NLT 10.65 mEq
Sodium content*	NMT <1 mg
Sugar content	0.57 g
Lactose content	None

*Dietetically insignificant.

except under the advice and supervision of a physician. Keep this and all drugs out of the reach of children.

Drug Interaction Precaution: Antacids may interact with certain prescription drugs. If you are presently taking a prescription drug, do not take this product without checking with your physician or other health professional.

Professional Labeling

Indications: As an antacid for symptomatic relief of hyperacidity associated with the diagnosis of peptic ulcer, gastritis, peptic esophagitis, gastric hyperacidity, heartburn, or hiatal hernia. As an antiflatulent to alleviate the symptoms of gas, including postoperative gas pain.

Warnings: Prolonged use of aluminum-containing antacids in patients with renal failure may result in or worsen dialysis osteomalacia. Elevated tissue aluminum levels contribute to the development of the dialysis encephalopathy and osteomalacia syndromes. Small amounts of aluminum are absorbed from the gastrointestinal tract and renal excretion of aluminum is impaired in renal failure. Aluminum is not well removed by dialysis because it is bound to albumin and transferrin, which do not cross dialysis membranes. As a result, aluminum is deposited in bone, and dialysis osteomalacia may develop when large amounts of aluminum are ingested orally by patients with impaired renal function.
Aluminum forms insoluble complexes with phosphate in the gastrointestinal tract, thus decreasing phosphate absorption. Prolonged use of aluminum-containing antacids by normophosphatemic patients may result in hypophosphatemia if phosphate intake is not adequate. In its more severe forms, hypophosphatemia can lead to anorexia, malaise, muscle weakness, and osteomalacia.

Advantages: Maalox® Plus Tablets are uniquely palatable—an important feature which encourages patients to follow your dosage directions. Maalox® Plus Tablets have the time-proven, non-constipating, sodium-free* Maalox® formula—useful for those patients suffering from the problems associated with hyperacidity. Additionally, Maalox® Plus Tablets contain simethicone to alleviate discomfort associated with entrapped gas.

How Supplied: Maalox® Plus Lemon Creme Tablets are available in plastic bottles of 50 tablets (0067-0339-50) and 100 tablets (0067-0339-67), convenience packs of 12 tablets (0067-0339-19), tray of 12 rolls (0067-0339-23), and 3 roll packs of 36 tablets (0067-0339-33).
Maalox Plus Cherry Creme Tablets are available in plastic bottles of 50 tablets (0067-0341-50) and 100 tablets (0067-0341-68), tray of 12 rolls (0067-0341-23) and 3 roll packs of 36 tablets (0067-0341-33).

Shown in Product Identification Guide, page 418

EXTRA STRENGTH MAALOX® ANTACID PLUS ANTI-GAS
Alumina, Magnesia and Simethicone
Oral Suspension
and Tablets, Antacid/Anti-Gas

Liquids   **Tablets**
☐ Lemon Creme   Mint Creme
   Cherry Creme
   Mint Creme
☐ Physician-proven Maalox® formula for antacid effectiveness.
☐ Simethicone, at a recognized clinical dose, for antiflatulent action.

Description: Extra Strength Maalox® Antacid Plus Anti-Gas, a balanced combination of magnesium and aluminum hydroxides plus simethicone, is a non-constipating antacid/anti-gas product to provide symptomatic relief of hyperacidity plus alleviation of gas symptoms. Available in liquid form in Cherry Creme, Mint Creme or Lemon Creme flavors, and in tablet form in the Mint Creme flavor.

Composition: To provide symptomatic relief of hyperacidity plus alleviation of gas symptoms, each teaspoonful/tablet contains:

Active Ingredients	Extra Strength Maalox® Antacid Plus Per Tsp. (5 mL)	Extra Strength Maalox® Anti-Gas Per Tablet
Magnesium Hydroxide	450 mg	350 mg
Aluminum Hydroxide (equivalent to dried gel, USP)	500 mg	350 mg
Simethicone	40 mg	30 mg

Inactive Ingredients: FD&C Red No. 40, flavors, methylparaben, propylparaben, purified water, saccharin, sorbitol, and other ingredients. May also contain citric acid.
Extra Strength Maalox® Plus Tablets: Citric acid, confectioners' sugar, D&C Yellow No. 10, dextrose, FD&C Blue

Continued on next page

Rhône-Poulenc Rorer—Cont.

No. 1, flavors, glycerin, hydrogenated vegetable oil, magnesium stearate, mannitol, saccharin sodium, sorbitol, starch, talc.

To aid in establishing proper dosage schedules, the following information is provided:

Minimum Recommended Dosage: Extra Strength Maalox® Antacid Plus Anti-Gas		
	Per 2 Tsp. (10 mL)	Per Tablet
Acid neutralizing capacity	58.1 mEq	18.6 mEq
Sodium content*	<2 mg	<1.7 mg
Sugar content	None	0.72 g
Lactose content	None	None

*Dietetically insignificant.

Professional Labeling

Indications: As an antacid for symptomatic relief of hyperacidity associated with the diagnosis of peptic ulcer, gastritis, peptic esophagitis, gastric hyperacidity, heartburn, or hiatal hernia. As an antiflatulent to alleviate the symptoms of gas, including postoperative gas pain.

Advantages: Among antacids, Extra Strength Maalox® Plus Suspension and Extra Strength Maalox® Plus Tablets are uniquely palatable—an important feature which encourages patients to follow your dosage directions. Extra Strength Maalox® Plus Suspension and Extra Strength Maalox® Plus Tablets have the time-proven, nonconstipating, sodium-free* Maalox® formula—useful for those patients suffering from the problems associated with hyperacidity. Additionally, Extra Strength Maalox® Plus Suspension and Extra Strength Maalox® Plus Tablets contain simethicone to alleviate discomfort associated with entrapped gas.

Warnings:
(i) Prolonged use of aluminum-containing antacids in patients with renal failure may result in or worsen dialysis osteomalacia. Elevated tissue aluminum levels contribute to the development of the dialysis encephalopathy and osteomalacia syndromes. Small amounts of aluminum are absorbed from the gastrointestinal tract and renal excretion of aluminum is impaired in renal failure. Aluminum is not well removed by dialysis because it is bound to albumin and transferrin, which do not cross dialysis membranes. As a result, aluminum is deposited in bone, and dialysis osteomalacia may develop when large amounts of aluminum are ingested orally by patients with impaired renal function.

(ii) Aluminum forms insoluble complexes with phosphate in the gastrointestinal tract, thus decreasing phosphate absorption. Prolonged use of aluminum-containing antacids by normophosphatemic patients may result in hypophosphatemia if phosphate intake is not adequate. In its more severe forms, hypophosphatemia can lead to anorexia, malaise, muscle weakness, and osteomalacia.

Extra Strength Maalox® Antacid Plus Anti-Gas Suspension

Directions for Use: Two to four teaspoonfuls, taken twenty minutes to one hour after meals and at bedtime, or as directed by a physician.

Patient Warnings: Do not take more than 12 teaspoonfuls in a 24-hour period or use the maximum dosage for more than 2 weeks or use if you have kidney disease except under the advice and supervision of a physician. Keep this and all drugs out of the reach of children.

Extra Strength Maalox® Antacid Plus Anti-Gas Tablets

Directions for Use: Chew one to three tablets twenty minutes to one hour after meals and at bedtime, or as directed by a physician.

Patient Warnings: Do not take more than 12 tablets in a 24-hour period or use the maximum dosage for more than two weeks or use if you have kidney disease except under the advice and supervision of a physician. Keep this and all drugs out of the reach of children.

Drug Interaction Precaution: Antacids may interact with certain prescription drugs. If you are presently taking a prescription drug, do not take this product without checking with your physician or other health professional.

How Supplied:
Extra Strength Maalox® Plus Suspension
Available in Lemon Creme in the following sizes: 5 fl. oz. (148 mL) (0067-0333-62), 12 fl. oz. (355 mL) (0067-0333-71), and 26 fl. oz. (769 mL) (0067-0333-44).
Cherry Creme is available in plastic bottles of 5 fl. oz. (148 mL) (0067-0336-62, 12 fl. oz. (355 mL) (0067-0336-71), and 26 fl. oz. (769 mL) (0067-0336-44).
Mint Creme is available in plastic bottles of 5 fl. oz. (148 mL) (0067-0338-62), 12 fl. oz. (355 mL) (0067-0338-71) and 26 fl. oz. (769 mL) (0067-0338-44).
Extra Strength Maalox® Antacid Plus Anti-Gas Mint Creme Tablets are available in flip-top bottles of 38 tablets (0067-0345-38) and 75 tablets (0067-0345-75).

Shown in Product Identification Guide, page 418

PERDIEM®
[pĕr″dē′ŭm]

Indication: For relief of constipation. Perdiem®, with its 100% natural, gentle action provides comfortable relief from constipation. Perdiem® is a unique combination of bulk-forming fiber and natural stimulant. The vegetable mucilages of Perdiem® soften the stool and provide pain-free evacuation of the bowel with no chemical stimulants. Perdiem® is also effective as an aid to elimination for the hemorrhoid or fissure patient prior to and following surgery.

Composition: Perdiem® contains as its active ingredients, 82% psyllium (Plantago Hydrocolloid) a natural grain and 18% senna (Cassia Pod Concentrate), a natural vegetable derivative. Each rounded teaspoonful (6.0 g) contains approximately 3.25 g psyllium, 0.74 g senna, 1.8 mg of sodium, 35.5 mg of potassium, and only 4 calories. Perdiem® is "Dye-Free" and contains no artificial sweeteners.

Inactive Ingredients: Acacia, iron oxides, natural flavors, paraffin, sucrose, talc.

Directions for Use: TAKE THIS PRODUCT (CHILD OR ADULT DOSE) WITH AT LEAST 8 OUNCES (A FULL GLASS) OF COOL WATER OR OTHER FLUID. TAKING THIS PRODUCT WITHOUT ENOUGH LIQUID MAY CAUSE CHOKING. SEE WARNINGS.

Adults and Children 12 years and older: In the evening and/or before breakfast, 1 to 2 rounded teaspoonfuls of Perdiem (in full or partial doses) should be placed in the mouth and swallowed with at least 8 ounces of cool liquid. Perdiem should not be chewed.

Children 7 to 11 years: One (1) rounded teaspoon one to two times daily with at least 8 ounces of cool liquid.

For Severe Cases of Constipation: Perdiem may be taken more frequently, up to 2 rounded teaspoonfuls every 6 hours not to exceed 5 teaspoonfuls in a 24-hour period. Perdiem generally takes effect within 12 hours; in severe cases, 24 to 72 hours may be required for optimal relief.

Warnings: TAKING THIS PRODUCT WITHOUT ADEQUATE ADEQUATE FLUID MAY CAUSE IT TO SWELL AND BLOCK YOUR THROAT OR ESOPHAGUS AND MAY CAUSE CHOKING. DO NOT TAKE THIS PRODUCT IF YOU HAVE DIFFICULTY IN SWALLOWING. IF YOU EXPERIENCE CHEST PAIN, VOMITING, OR DIFFICULTY IN SWALLOWING OR BREATHING AFTER TAKING THIS PRODUCT, SEEK IMMEDIATE MEDICAL ATTENTION.

Frequent or prolonged use without the direction of a doctor is not recommended. If use of this product for one week has produced no effect, discontinue use and consult a doctor.

If you have noticed a sudden change in bowel habits that persists over a two week period, consult a doctor before using any laxative product.

Do not use in patients with a history of psyllium allergy. Psyllium allergy is rare but can be severe. If an allergic reaction occurs, discontinue use and consult a doctor immediately.

Consult a physician before using any laxative or bulk fiber product in the presence of rectal bleeding or undiagnosed abdominal pain.

Keep this and all drugs out of the reach of children. In case of accidental overdose, seek professional assistance or contact a poison control center immediately. If you are pregnant or nursing a baby, seek the advice of a health professional before using this product and consider using Perdiem Fiber.

For Patients Habituated to Strong Purgatives: Two rounded teaspoonfuls of Perdiem® in the morning and evening may be required along with half the usual dose of the purgative being used. The purgative should be discontinued as soon as possible and the dosage of Perdiem® granules reduced when and if bowel tone shows lessened laxative dependence.

For Colostomy Patients: To ensure formed stools, give one to two rounded teaspoonfuls of Perdiem® in the evening.

For Clinical Regulation: For patients confined to bed, for those of inactive habits, and in the presence of cardiovascular disease where straining must be avoided, one rounded teaspoonful of Perdiem® taken once or twice daily will provide regular bowel habits.

How Supplied: Granules: 250-gram (8.8 oz) (0067-0690-70) plastic container, 6 single serving packets 6 gm (0067-0690-16) and 20 single serving packets 6 gm (0067-0690-17).
Shown in Product Identification Guide, page 419

PERDIEM® FIBER
[pĕr "dē 'ŭm]

Indications: Perdiem® Fiber provides gentle relief from simple, chronic, and spastic constipation. In addition, it relieves constipation associated with convalescence, pregnancy, and advanced age. Perdiem® Fiber is also indicated for use in special diets lacking in residue fiber to aid regularity and in the management of constipation associated with irritable bowel syndrome, diverticular disease, hemorrhoids, and anal fissures.

Perdiem® Fiber is a 100% natural bulk-forming fiber that gently helps maintain regularity and prevents constipation. Perdiem® Fiber's unique form is easy to swallow and requires no mixing but must be followed by at least 8 ounces (a full glass) of water or other cool liquid. Perdiem® Fiber contains no chemical stimulants and may be used daily by those who may lack sufficient dietary fiber. When recommended by a doctor, Perdiem® Fiber is also useful for the treatment of bowel disorders other than constipation.

Composition: Perdiem® Fiber contains as its active ingredient 100% psyllium (Plantago Hydrocolloid), a natural grain with no chemical stimulants. Each rounded teaspoonful (6.0 g) contains approximately 4 g of psyllium, 1.8 mg of sodium, 36.1 mg of potassium, and only 4 calories. Perdiem® Fiber is "Dye-Free" and contains no artificial sweeteners.

Inactive Ingredients: Acacia, iron oxides, natural flavors, paraffin, sucrose, talc, titanium dioxide.

Directions for Use: TAKE THIS PRODUCT (CHILD OR ADULT DOSE) WITH AT LEAST 8 OUNCES (A FULL GLASS) OF COOL WATER OR OTHER FLUID. TAKING THIS PRODUCT WITHOUT ENOUGH LIQUID MAY CAUSE CHOKING. SEE WARNINGS.

Adults and children 12 years and older: In the evening and/or before breakfast, 1 to 2 rounded teaspoonfuls of Perdiem® Fiber (in full or partial doses) should be placed in the mouth and swallowed with at least 8 ounces of cool liquid. Perdiem® Fiber should not be chewed.

Children 7 to 11 years: One (1) rounded teaspoonful one to two times daily with at least 8 ounces of cool liquid.

For Severe Cases of Constipation: Perdiem® Fiber may be taken more frequently, up to 2 rounded teaspoonfuls every 6 hours not to exceed 5 teaspoonfuls in a 24-hour period. Perdiem® Fiber generally takes effect within 12 hours; in severe cases, 24 to 72 hours may be required to provide optimal relief.

During Pregnancy: Because of its natural ingredients and bulking action, Perdiem® Fiber is effective for expectant mothers—follow directions.

Warnings: TAKING THIS PRODUCT WITHOUT ADEQUATE FLUID MAY CAUSE IT TO SWELL AND BLOCK YOUR THROAT OR ESOPHAGUS AND MAY CAUSE CHOKING. DO NOT TAKE THIS PRODUCT IF YOU HAVE DIFFICULTY IN SWALLOWING. IF YOU EXPERIENCE CHEST PAIN, VOMITING, OR DIFFICULTY IN SWALLOWING OR BREATHING AFTER TAKING THIS PRODUCT, SEEK IMMEDIATE MEDICAL ATTENTION.

Frequent or prolonged use without the direction of a doctor is not recommended. If use of this product for one week has produced no effect, discontinue use and consult a doctor.

If you have noticed a sudden change in bowel habits that persists over a two week period, consult a doctor before using any laxative product.

Do not use in patients with a history of psyllium allergy. Psyllium allergy is rare but can be severe. If an allergic reaction occurs, discontinue use and consult a doctor immediately.

Consult a physician before using any laxative or bulk fiber product in the pres-

ence of rectal bleeding or undiagnosed abdominal pain.

Keep this and all drugs out of the reach of children. In case of accidental overdose, seek professional assistance or contact a poison control center immediately.

After Rectal Surgery: The vegetable mucilages of Perdiem® Fiber soften the stool and provide pain-free evacuation of the bowel. Perdiem® Fiber is effective as an aid to elimination for the hemorrhoid or fissure patient prior to and following surgery.

For Clinical Regulation: For patients confined to bed—after an operation for example—and for those of inactive habits, 1 rounded teaspoonful of Perdiem® Fiber taken 1–2 times daily will ensure regular bowel habits.

How Supplied: Granules: 250-gram (8.8 oz) (0067-0795-70) plastic container, 6 single serving packets 6 gm (0067-0795-09) and 20 single serving packets 6 gm (0067-0795-10).
Shown in Product Identification Guide, page 419

Richardson-Vicks Inc.
(See Procter & Gamble.)

Roberts Pharmaceutical Corporation
4 INDUSTRIAL WAY WEST EATONTOWN, NJ 07724

CHERACOL® Nasal Spray Pump Cherry Scented

Description: CHERACOL® NASAL SPRAY PUMP is a cherry scented long acting topical nasal decongestant. One application lasts up to 12 hours.

Indications: For the temporary relief of a nasal congestion associated with colds ("flu"), hay fever, and sinusitis.

Active Ingredients: Oxymetazoline hydrochloride USP 0.05% (0.5 mg/ml).

Inactive Ingredients: Benzalkonium chloride, glycine, sodium hydroxide, phenylmercuric acetate (0.02 mg/ml), sorbitol, artificial cherry flavor, and purified water.

Dosage and Administration: CHERACOL Nasal Spray has a long duration of action lasting up to 12 hours with each topical application. One application mornings and at bedtime is usually sufficient for round-the-clock action. For adults and children 6 years of age and over: Two or three sprays in each nostril twice daily—morning and bedtime. Remove protective cap. Hold bottle with thumb at base and nozzle between first and second fingers. With head upright, insert metered pump spray nozzle in nostril. Depress pump 2 or 3 times all the way down with a firm even stroke and

Continued on next page

Roberts—Cont.

sniff deeply. Repeat in other nostril. Do not tilt head backward while spraying. Wipe tip clean after each use. Before using the first time, remove the protective cap from the tip and prime the metered pump by depressing pump firmly several times.

Warning: Do not give this product to children under 6 years of age except under the advice and supervision of a physician. Do not exceed recommended dosage because symptoms may occur such as burning, stinging, sneezing or increase of nasal discharge. Do not use this product for more than 3 days. If symptoms persist, consult a physician. The use of this dispenser by more than one person may spread infection. Store at room temperature. Keep this and all medicines out of children's reach.

Overdose: In case of accidental overdose contact a physician or regional poison control center immediately.

How Supplied: Available in 1 fluid ounce bottles fitted with a metered pump (NDC 54092-880-30).

CHERACOL® SINUS
12 Hour Formula

Description: Cheracol® SINUS sustained-action tablets combine a nasal decongestant with an antihistamine in a special continuous-acting timed-release tablet to provide temporary relief of nasal congestion due to the common cold, and associated with sinusitis. Also alleviates running nose and sneezing due to hay fever.

Each Cheracol® SINUS Sustained-Action Tablet Contains: 6 mg of dex-brompheniramine maleate and 120 mg of pseudoephedrine sulfate. Half of the medication is released after the tablet is swallowed and the remaining amount of medication is sustained-release, providing continuous long-lasting relief for 12 hours.

Indications: For temporary relief of nasal congestion due to the common cold, hay fever, or other upper respiratory allergies, and associated with sinusitis. Helps decongest sinus openings, sinus passages. Reduces swelling of nasal passages; shrinks swollen membranes; and temporarily restores freer breathing through the nose. Alleviates running nose, sneezing, itching of the nose or throat, and itchy and watery eyes as may occur in allergic rhinitis (such as hay fever).

Directions: Adults and Children 12 Years and Over—one tablet every 12 hours. Do not exceed two tablets in 24 hours.

Warnings: If symptoms do not improve within 7 days or are accompanied by high fever, consult a physician before continuing use. May

cause drowsiness; alcohol may increase the drowsiness effect. Avoid alcoholic beverages while taking this product. Use caution when driving a motor vehicle or operating machinery. May cause excitability especially in children. Do not exceed recommended dosage, because at higher doses nervousness, dizziness, or sleeplessness may occur. Do not give this product to children under 12 years, except under the advice and supervision of a physician. Do not take this product if you have emphysema, chronic pulmonary disease, shortness of breath, and difficulty in breathing, asthma, glaucoma, difficulty in urination due to enlargement of the prostate gland, high blood pressure, heart disease, diabetes, or thyroid disease except under the advice and supervision of a physician. As with any drug, if you are pregnant or nursing a baby, seek the advice of a health professional before using this product. Keep this and all drugs out of the reach of children. In case of accidental overdose, seek professional assistance or contact a Poison Control Center immediately.

Drug Interaction Precaution: Do not take this product if you are presently taking a prescription drug for high blood pressure or depression, without first consulting your doctor.

Active Ingredients: Dexbrompheniramine Meleate 6 mg, Pseudoephedrine Sulfate 120 mg.

Also Contains: Acacia, Calcium Carbonate, Carnauba Wax, Confectioner's Sugar, D&C Yellow #10, FD&C Blue #1, FD&C Yellow #6, Gelatin, Hydrogenated Castor Oil, Magnesium Stearate, Methylparaben, Povidone, Propylparaben, Shellac, Sodium Benzoate, Sucrose, Talc, Titanium Dioxide.
Use by expiration date printed on package.
Store between 2° and 30°C (36° and 86°F). Protect from excessive moisture.

How Supplied: 10 sustained-action release tablets. NDC 54092-045-10
Manufactured for:
Roberts Laboratories Inc., a subsidiary of
ROBERTS PHARMACEUTICAL CORPORATION
Eatontown, NJ 07724, USA

CHERACOL® Sore Throat Spray
Anesthetic/Antiseptic Liquid

Description: A pleasant tasting cherry flavored liquid spray with anesthetic and antiseptic properties.

Indications: For the temporary relief of occasional minor sore throat pain and irritation. Also for temporary relief of pain associated with sore mouth, canker sores, tonsillitis, pharyngitis and throat infections.

Active Ingredients: Phenol 1.4%.

Inactive Ingredients: Alcohol 12.5%, citric acid, FD&C Red No. 40, flavor, glycerin, propylene glycol, sodium citrate, sodium saccharin, sorbitol and purified water.

Directions For Use: Mouthwash and gargle: Irritated throat: Spray 5 times (children 3–12 years of age, 3 times) and swallow. May be used as a gargle. Repeat every 2 hours or as directed by physician or dentist. Children under 12 years of age should be supervised in the use of this product.

Warning: If sore throat is severe, persists for more than 2 days, is accompanied or followed by fever, headache, rash, nausea or vomiting, consult a doctor promptly. If sore mouth symptoms do not improve in 7 days, see your doctor or dentist promptly. As with any drug, if you are pregnant or nursing a baby, seek the advice of a health professional before using this product. Do not administer to children under 2 years unless directed by a physician or dentist. Keep this and all medicines out of the reach of children.

Overdose: In case of accidental overdose contact a physician or a poison control center immediately.

How Supplied: Available in 6 fluid ounce spray pump bottle (NDC 54092-340-06).

CHERACOL–D® Cough Formula
Maximum Strength Cough Formula

Description: CHERACOL-D® is a non-narcotic cough formula which combines two important medicines in one safe, fast-acting pleasant tasting liquid:
● The highest level of cough suppressant available without prescription.
● A clinically proven expectorant to help loosen phlegm and drain bronchial tubes.

Indications: CHERACOL-D® cough formula helps quiet dry, hacking coughs, and helps loosen phlegm and mucus. Recommended for adults and children 2 years of age and older.

Active Ingredients: Each teaspoonful (5 ml) contains dextromethorphan hydrobromide, 10 mg; guaifenesin, 100 mg; alcohol, 4.75%. Also contains benzoic acid, FD&C Red #40, flavors, fragrances, fructose, glycerin, propylene glycol, sodium chloride, sucrose, and purified water.

Dosage and Administration: Adults and children 12 years of age and over: 2 teaspoonfuls. Children 6 to 12 years: 1 teaspoonful. Children 2 to 6 years: ½ teaspoonful. May be repeated every 4 hours if necessary. Children under 2 years, consult a physician.

Warnings: Keep this and all drugs out of the reach of children. Do not give this product to children under 2 years of age except under the advice and supervision of a physician. Do not use this product for persistent or chronic cough such as occurs with smoking, asthma, or emphysema or where cough is accompanied by excessive secretions except under the advice and supervision of a physician. As with any drug, if you are pregnant or nursing a baby, seek the advice of a health professional before using this product.

Caution: A persistent cough may be a sign of a serious condition. If cough persists for more than 1 week, tends to recur or is accompanied by high fever, rash or persistent headache, consult a physician.

Overdose: In case of accidental overdose contact a physician or a poison control center immediately.

How Supplied: Available in 2 oz bottle (NDC 54092-400-60), 4 oz bottle (NDC 54092-400-04), and 6 oz bottle (NDC 54092-400-06).

Shown in Product Identification Guide, page 419

CHERACOL PLUS® Cough Syrup
Multisymptom cough/cold formula

Description: CHERACOL PLUS® Cough Syrup is a pleasant tasting 3-ingredient non-narcotic liquid formulation.

Indications: Cheracol Plus syrup is an effective 3-ingredient, maximum strength formula for the temporary relief of head cold symptoms and cough (without narcotic side effects).

Active Ingredients: Each tablespoonful (15ml) contains phenylpropanolamine HCl, 25 mg; dextromethorphan hydrobromide, 20 mg; chlorpheniramine maleate, 4 mg; and alcohol, 8%.

Inactive Ingredients: Flavors, glycerin, methylparaben, propylene glycol, propylparaben, FD&C Red No. 40, sodium chloride, sorbitol solution, and purified water.

Dosage and Administration: Adults and children over 12 years of age: 1 tablespoonful (15ml) every 4 hours or as directed by a physician. Do not take more than 6 tablespoonfuls in a 24 hour period. Do not administer to children under 12 years of age.

Uses: Cheracol Plus® multisymptom head cold/cough formula provides cough suppressant and decongestant activity and controls runny nose associated with the common cold ("flu").

Warnings: Do not take this product for persistent or chronic cough such as occurs with smoking, asthma, or emphysema or where cough is accompanied by excessive secretions or if you have high blood pressure, heart or thyroid disease, diabetes, asthma, glaucoma, or difficulty in urination due to enlargement of the prostate gland except under the advice and supervision of a physician. If symptoms do not improve within 7 days or are accompanied by high fever, consult a

physician before continuing use. May cause excitability, especially in children. Do not give this product to children under 12 years except under the advice and supervision of a physician. As with any drug, if you are pregnant or nursing a baby consult a health professional before using this product. Keep out of reach of children.

Drug Interaction Precaution: Do not take this product if you are presently taking antihypertensive or antidepressant medication containing a monoamine oxidase inhibitor except under the advice and supervision of a physician.

Overdose: In case of accidental overdose contact a physician or a poison control center immediately.

How Supplied: Available in 4 oz bottle (NDC 54092-401-04), 6 oz bottle (54092-401-06).

CITROCARBONATE® Antacid

Active Ingredients: When dissolved, each 4.1 grams (1 teaspoonful) contains approximately: sodium bicarbonate, 0.78 gram and sodium citrate, 1.82 grams. **As derived from (per teaspoonful):** sodium bicarbonate, 2.34 gram; citric acid anhydrous, 1.19 gram; sodium citrate hydrous, 254 mg; calcium lactate pentahydrate, 151 mg; sodium chloride, 79 mg; monobasic sodium phosphate anhydrous, 44 mg; and magnesium sulfate dried, 42 mg. Each 3.9 grams (teaspoonful) contains 30.46 mEq (700.6 mg) of sodium.

Indications: For the relief of heartburn, acid indigestion, and sour stomach; and upset stomach associated with these symptoms.

Dosage and Administration: Adults: 1 to 2 teaspoonfuls (not to exceed 5 level teaspoonfuls per day) in a glass of cold water after meals. Persons 60 years or older: ½ to 1 teaspoonful after meals. Children 6 to 12 years: ¼ to ½ teaspoonful. For children under 6 years: Consult physician.

How Supplied: Available in 5 oz (NDC 54092-900-05) and 10 oz (NDC 54092-900-10) bottles.

CLOCREAM®
Skin Protectant Cream

Description: CLOCREAM® skin protectant cream contains Vitamins A and D in a greaseless vanishing cream base that leaves no residue. Also contains cetylpalmitate, cottonseed oil, glycerin, glyceryl monostearate, fragrance, methylparaben, mineral oil, potassium stearate, propylparaben, sodium citrate, Vitamin A palmitate and purified oil. Each ounce of CLOCREAM® contains Vitamins A and D equivalent to 1 ounce of cod liver oil.

Indications: CLOCREAM® is indicated for the temporary relief of chapped skin, diaper rash, wind burn, sunburn

and minor non-infected skin irritations. CLOCREAM® promotes epitheliazation.

Uses: CLOCREAM® may be particularly useful for health care personnel or others who frequently wash their hands and for general patient care to reduce dermal excoriation and breakdown from prolonged bed rest, bedwetting and abrasions. The vanishing action of CLOCREAM skin protectant cream makes it cosmetically acceptable when the skin treated is on an exposed part of the body such as the hands or arms.

Warnings: CLOCREAM® skin protectant cream is for external use only. Avoid contact with the eyes. If condition worsens or if symptoms persist for more than 7 days, discontinue use of this product and consult a physician. Keep this and all medications out of the reach of children. In case of accidental ingestion seek professional assistance or contact a poison control center immediately.

Dosage and Administration: Gently massage or apply liberally to unbroken skin or abraded skin where promotion of epitheliazation is denied. Use as often as desired.

How Supplied: Available in 1 ounce tubes (NDC 54092-300-30).

COLACE®
[kōlās]
docusate sodium,
capsules • syrup • liquid (drops)

Description: Colace (docusate sodium) is a stool softener.
Colace Capsules, 50 mg, contain the following inactive ingredients: citric acid, D&C Red No. 33, FD&C Red No. 40, nonporcine gelatin, edible ink, polyethylene glycol, propylene glycol, and purified water.
Colace Capsules, 100 mg, contain the following inactive ingredients: citric acid, D&C Red No. 33, FD&C Red No. 40, FD&C Yellow No. 6, nonporcine gelatin, edible ink, polyethylene glycol, propylene glycol, titanium dioxide, and purified water.
Colace Liquid, 1%, contains the following inactive ingredients: citric acid, D&C Red No. 33, methylparaben, poloxamer, polyethylene glycol, propylene glycol, propylparaben, sodium citrate, vanillin, and purified water.
Colace Syrup, 20 mg/5 mL, contains the following inactive ingredients: alcohol (not more than 1%), citric acid, D&C Red No. 33, FD&C Red No. 40, flavor (natural), menthol, methylparaben, peppermint oil, poloxamer, polyethylene glycol, propylparaben, sodium citrate, sucrose, and purified water.

Actions and Uses: Colace, a surface-active agent, helps to keep stools soft for easy, natural passage and is not a laxative, thus, not habit forming. Useful in constipation due to hard stools, in pain-

Continued on next page

Roberts—Cont.

ful anorectal conditions, in cardiac and other conditions in which maximum ease of passage is desirable to avoid difficult or painful defecation, and when peristaltic stimulants are contraindicated. *Note:* When peristaltic stimulation is needed due to inadequate bowel motility, see Peri-Colace® (laxative and stool softener).

Contraindications: There are no known contraindications to Colace.

Warning: As with any drug, if you are pregnant or nursing a baby, seek the advice of a health professional before using this product.

Side Effects: The incidence of side effects—none of a serious nature—is exceedingly small. Bitter taste, throat irritation, and nausea (primarily associated with the use of the syrup and liquid) are the main side effects reported. Rash has occurred.

Administration and Dosage: *Orally*—Suggested daily Dosage: *Adults and older children:* 50 to 200 mg *Children 6 to 12:* 40 to 120 mg *Children 3 to 6:* 20 to 60 mg. *Infants and children under 3:* 10 to 40 mg. The higher doses are recommended for initial therapy. Dosage should be adjusted to individual response. The effect on stools is usually apparent 1 to 3 days after the first dose. Give Colace liquid in half a glass of milk or fruit juice or in infant formula, to mask bitter taste. *In enemas*—Add 50 to 100 mg Colace (5 to 10 mL Colace liquid) to a retention or flushing enema.

How Supplied: Colace capsules, 50 mg
NDC 54092-052-30 Bottles of 30
NDC 54092-052-60 Bottles of 60
NDC 54092-052-02 Bottles of 250
NDC 54092-052-52 Cartons of 100
single unit packs
Colace capsules, 100 mg
NDC 54092-053-30 Bottles of 30
NDC 54092-053-02 Bottles of 250
NDC 54092-053-52 Cartons of 100
single unit packs
Note: Colace capsules should be stored at controlled room temperature (59°–86°F or 15°–30°C)
Colace liquid, 1% solution; 10 mg/mL (with calibrated dropper)
NDC 54092-414-16 Bottles of 16 fl oz
NDC 54092-414-30 Bottles of 30 mL
Colace syrup, 20 mg/5-mL teaspoon; contains not more than 1% alcohol
NDC 54092-415-08 Bottles of 8 fl oz
NDC 54092-415-16 Bottles of 16 fl oz
Shown in Product Identification Guide, page 419

HALTRAN® Tablets
Ibuprofen/Analgesic
MENSTRUAL CRAMP RELIEVER
WARNING: ASPIRIN SENSITIVE PATIENTS. Do not take this product if you have had a severe allergic reaction to aspirin, eg—asthma, swelling, shock or hives, because even though this product contains no aspirin or salicylates cross-reactions may occur in patients allergic to aspirin.

Indications: For the pain of menstrual cramps and also the temporary relief of minor aches and pains associated with the common cold, headache, toothache, muscular aches, backache, for the minor pain of arthritis and for reduction of fever.

Directions: *Adults:* Take 1 tablet every 4 to 6 hours while symptoms persist. If pain or fever does not respond to 1 tablet, 2 tablets may be used, but do not exceed 6 tablets in 24 hours, unless directed by a doctor. The smallest effective dose should be used. Take with food or milk if occasional and mild heartburn, upset stomach, or stomach pain occurs with use. Consult a doctor if these symptoms are more than mild or if they persist. *Children:* Do not give this product to children under 12 except under the advice and supervision of a doctor.

Warnings: Do not take for pain for more than 10 days or for fever for more than 3 days unless directed by a doctor. If pain or fever persists or gets worse, if new symptoms occur, or if the painful area is red or swollen, consult a doctor. These could be signs of serious illness. If you are under a doctor's care for any serious condition, consult a doctor before taking this product. As with aspirin and acetaminophen, if you have any condition which requires you to take prescription drugs or if you have had any problems or serious side effects from taking any non-prescription pain reliever, do not take HALTRAN Tablets (ibuprofen) without first discussing it with your doctor. If you experience any symptoms which are unusual or seem unrelated to the condition for which you took ibuprofen, consult a doctor before taking any more of it. Although ibuprofen is indicated for the same conditions as aspirin and acetaminophen, it should not be taken with them except under a doctor's direction. Before using any drug, including HALTRAN, you should seek the advice of a health professional if you are pregnant or nursing a baby. IT IS ESPECIALLY IMPORTANT NOT TO USE IBUPROFEN DURING THE LAST 3 MONTHS OF PREGNANCY UNLESS SPECIFICALLY DIRECTED TO DO SO BY A DOCTOR BECAUSE IT MAY CAUSE PROBLEMS IN THE UNBORN CHILD OR COMPLICATIONS DURING DELIVERY. Keep this and all drugs out of the reach of children. In case of accidental overdose, seek professional assistance or contact a poison control center immediately.

Active Ingredient: Each tablet contains ibuprofen USP 200 mg.

Other Ingredients: Carnauba wax, cornstarch, hydroxypropyl methylcellulose, propylene glycol, silicon dioxide, pregelatinized starch, stearic acid, and titanium dioxide.

Store at room temperature. Avoid excessive heat 40°C (104°F).

How Supplied: Available in bottles of 30 (NDC 54092-020-30).
Shown in Product Identification Guide, page 419

ORTHOXICOL® Cough Syrup
Multisymptom cough/cold formula

Description: ORTHOXICOL® Cough Syrup is a pleasant tasting 3-ingredient non-narcotic liquid formulation.

Indications: Orthoxicol syrup is an effective 3-ingredient, maximum strength formula for the temporary relief of head cold symptoms and cough (without narcotic side effects).

Active Ingredients: Each tablespoonful (15 ml) contains phenylpropanolamine, HCl 25 mg; dextromethorphan hydrobromide, 20 mg; chlorpheniramine maleate, 4 mg; and alcohol, 8%.

Inactive Ingredients: Flavors, glycerin, methylparaben, propylene glycol, propylparaben, FD&C Red No. 40, sodium chloride, sorbitol solution, and purified water.

Dosage and Administration: Adults and children over 12 years of age: 1 tablespoonful (15 ml) every 4 hours or as directed by a physician. Do not take more than 6 tablespoonfuls in a 24 hour period. Do not administer to children under 12 years of age.

Uses: Orthoxicol multisymptom head cold/cough formula provides cough suppressant and decongestant activity and controls runny nose associated with the common cold ("flu").

Warnings: Do not take this product for persistent or chronic cough such as occurs with smoking, asthma, or emphysema or where cough is accompanied by excessive secretions or if you have high blood pressure, heart or thyroid disease, diabetes, asthma, glaucoma, or difficulty in urination due to enlargement of the prostate gland except under the advice and supervision of a physician. If symptoms do not improve within 7 days or are accompanied by high fever, consult a physician before continuing use. May cause excitability, especially in children. Do not give this product to children under 12 years except under the advice and supervision of a physician. As with any drug, if you are pregnant or nursing a baby consult a health professional before using this product. Keep this and all other drugs out of the reach of children.

Drug Interaction Precaution: Do not take this product if you are presently taking antihypertensive or antidepressant medication containing a monoamine oxidase inhibitor except under the advice and supervision of a physician.

Overdose: In case of accidental overdose contact a physician or a poison control center immediately.

How Supplied: Available in 2 oz bottle (NDC 54092-410-60), 4 oz bottle (NDC 54092-410-04), 16 oz bottle (NDC 54092-410-16).

PERI-COLACE® capsules • syrup
(casanthranol and docusate sodium)

Description: Peri-Colace is a combination of the mild stimulant laxative casanthranol, and the stool-softener Colace® (docusate sodium). Each capsule contains 30 mg of casanthranol and 100 mg of Colace; the syrup contains 30 mg of casanthranol and 60 mg of Colace per 15-mL tablespoon (10 mg of casanthranol and 20 mg of Colace per 5-mL teaspoon) and 10% alcohol.
Peri-Colace Capsules contain the following inactive ingredients: D&C Red No. 33, FD&C Red No. 40, nonporcine gelatin, edible ink, polyethylene glycol, propylene glycol, titanium dioxide, and purified water.
Peri-Colace Syrup contains the following inactive ingredients: alcohol (10% v/v), citric acid, flavors, methyl salicylate, methylparaben, poloxamer, polyethylene glycol, propylparaben, sodium citrate, sorbitol solution, sucrose, and purified water.

Action and Uses: Peri-Colace provides gentle peristaltic stimulation and helps to keep stools soft for easier passage. Bowel movement is induced gently—usually overnight or in 8 to 12 hours. Nausea, griping, abnormally loose stools, and constipation rebound are minimized. Useful in management of chronic or temporary constipation.
Note: To prevent hard stools when laxative stimulation is not needed or undesirable, see Colace (stool softener).

Warnings: Do not use when abdominal pain, nausea, or vomiting are present. Frequent or prolonged use of this preparation may result in dependence on laxatives.
As with any drug, if you are pregnant or nursing a baby, seek the advice of a health professional before using this product.

Side Effects: The incidence of side effects—none of a serious nature—is exceedingly small. Nausea, abdominal cramping or discomfort, diarrhea, and rash are the main side effects reported.

Administration and Dosage:
Adults —1 or 2 capsules, or 1 or 2 tablespoons syrup at bedtime, or as indicated. In severe cases, dosage may be increased to 2 capsules or 2 tablespoons twice daily, or 3 capsules at bedtime. *Children* —1 to 3 teaspoons of syrup at bedtime, or as indicated.

Overdosage: In addition to symptomatic treatment, gastric lavage, if timely, is recommended in cases of large overdosage.

How Supplied: Peri-Colace® Capsules
NDC 54092-054-30 Bottles of 30
NDC 54092-054-10 Bottles of 1000
NDC 54092-054-52 Cartons of 100 single unit packs
Note: Peri-Colace capsules should be stored at controlled room temperatures (59°–86°F or 15°–30°C).
Peri-Colace® Syrup
NDC 54092-418-08 Bottles of 8 fl oz
NDC 54092-418-16 Bottles of 16 fl oz
Shown in Product Identification Guide, page 419

PYRROXATE® Caplets
Extra Strength Decongestant/ Antihistamine/ Analgesic Caplets

Description: *Pyrroxate®* provides single-caplet, multisymptom relief for colds, allergies, nasal/sinus congestion, runny nose, sneezing, and watery eyes. Because it contains the non-aspirin analgesic **acetaminophen,** *Pyrroxate* gives temporary relief of occasional minor aches, pains, headache, and helps in the reduction of fever. *Pyrroxate* is caffeine and aspirin-free.

Active Ingredients: Each *Pyrroxate* Caplet contains: chlorpheniramine maleate, 4 mg; phenylpropanolamine HCl, 25 mg; acetaminophen, 650 mg.

Inactive Ingredients: Cellulose, Croscarmalose sodium, stearic acid, magnesium stearate, hydroxypropyl methylcellulose, titatium dioxide, polyethylene glycol, dicalcium phosphate, FD&C yellow Lake No. 6, D&C yellow Lake No. 10, D&C yellow No. 10.

Indications: *Pyrroxate* Caplets are for the temporary relief of runny nose, sneezing, itching of the nose or throat; for the temporary relief of nasal congestion due to the common cold, allergies (hay fever), sinus congestion and for the temporary relief of occasional minor aches, pains, headache, and for the reduction of fever.

Actions: Chlorpheniramine maleate is an antihistamine effective in controlling runny nose, sneezing, watery eyes, and itching of the nose and throat. Phenylpropanolamine HCl is an oral nasal decongestant effective in relieving nasal/sinus congestion due to the common cold or allergies (hay fever). Acetaminophen is a clinically effective analgesic and antipyretic without aspirin side effects.

Warnings: Do not take this product for more than 7 days. If symptoms persist, do not improve, or new ones occur, or if fever persists for more than 3 days, discontinue use and consult your physician. Do not take this product if you have asthma, glaucoma, difficulty in urination due to the enlargement of the prostate gland, high blood pressure, diabetes, thyroid disease, or if you are presently taking a prescription antihypertensive or antidepressant drug containing a monamine oxidase inhibitor, except under the advice and supervision of a physician. As with any drug, if you are pregnant or nursing a baby, seek the advice of a health professional before using this product. Do not exceed recommended dosage because severe liver damage may occur and at higher doses, nervousness, dizziness or sleeplessness may occur. Do not take other medications containing acetaminophen simultaneously, to avoid the risk of overdosage. Do not take this product for the treatment of arthritis except under the advice and supervision of a physician.

Cautions: Avoid alcoholic beverages, driving a motor vehicle, or operating heavy machinery while taking this product. This product may cause drowsiness or excitability, especially in children. Keep this and all drugs out of the reach of children. In case of accidental overdose, seek professional assistance or contact a poison control center immediately.

Dosage and Administration: Take 1 caplet every 4 hours or as directed by a physician. Do not take more than 6 caplets in a 24-hour period. Do not administer to children under 12 years of age.

How Supplied: Yellow caplets available in bottles of 24 (NDC 54092-041-24) and 500 (NDC 54092-041-05).
Shown in Product Identification Guide, page 419

SIGTAB® Tablets
High Potency Vitamin Supplement

Each Tablet Contains:		% U.S. RDA*
Vitamin A	5000 IU	100
Vitamin D	400 IU	100
Vitamin E	15 IU	50
Vitamin C	333 mg	555
Folic Acid	0.4 mg	100
Thiamine	10.3 mg	687
Riboflavin	10 mg	588
Niacin	100 mg	500
Vitamin B$_6$	6 mg	300
Vitamin B$_{12}$	18 mcg	300
Pantothenic Acid	20 mg	200

*Percentage of U.S. Recommended Daily Allowance.

Recommended Dosage: For adults, 1 tablet daily

Ingredient List: Sucrose, Ascorbic acid (Vit. C), Calcium Sulfate, Niacinamide, Vitamin E Acetate, Calcium Pantothenate, Vitamin A Acetate, Thiamine Mononitrate (B-1), Riboflavin (B-2), Gelatin, Pyridoxine HCl (B-6), Povidone, Lacca, Magnesium Stearate, Silica, Artificial Color, Sodium Benzoate, Folic Acid, Polyethylene Glycol, Cholecalciferol (Vit. D), Carnauba Wax, Cyanocobalamin (B-12), Medical Antifoam, Sesame Seed Oil and Titanium Dioxide.

How Supplied: Available in bottles of 90 (NDC 54092-033-90) and 500 (NDC 54092-033-05).

Continued on next page

Roberts—Cont.

SIGTAB®-M Tablets

[See table below.]

How Supplied: Bottle of 100 tablets.
NDC 54092-038-01

Recommended dosage for adults: 1 tablet daily.

Warning: Keep out of the reach of children.

Keep container tightly closed. Store at room temperature.
Do not use if seal under cap is broken.
Manufactured for:
Roberts Laboratories Inc., a subsidiary of
ROBERTS PHARMACEUTICAL CORPORATION
Eatontown, NJ 077244, USA
Shown in Product Identification Guide, page 419

ZYMACAP® Capsules
High Potency Vitamin Supplement

Description: Dietary multivitamin supplement providing 150% of the RDA for Vitamin B and Vitamin C plus 100% of the RDA for Vitamins A and D.

Each Capsule Contains:

		% US RDA*
Vitamin A	5,000 IU	100
Vitamin D	400 IU	100
Vitamin E	15 IU	50
Vitamin C	90 mg	150
Folic Acid	400 mcg	100
Thiamine	2.25 mg	150
Riboflavin	2.6 mg	150
Niacin	30 mg	150
Vitamin B-6	3 mg	150
Vitamin B-12	9 mcg	150
Pantothenic Acid	15 mg	150

*Percentage of U.S. recommended daily allowance.

Recommended Dosage: 1 Capsule daily.

Ingredient List: Soybean oil, ascorbic acid (Vitamin C), gelatin, glycerin, niacinamide, calcium pantothenate, Vitamin E acetate, lecithin, pyridoxine hydrochloride (Vitamin B-6), yellow wax, thiamine mononitrate (Vitamin B-1), riboflavin (Vitamin B-2), Vitamin A palmitate, corn oil, FD&C Red No. 40, folic acid, titanium dioxide, ethyl vanillin, vanilla enhancer, cholecalciferol (Vitamin D), cyanocobalamin (Vitamin B-12).

How Supplied: Available in bottles of 90 capsules (NDC 54092-030-90).

SIGTAB®-M Tablets
Each Tablet Contains:

Active Ingredients:

		% U.S. RDA*
Vitamin A (From Vit. A & Beta Carotene)	6000 Intl. Units	120
Vitamin D3	400 Intl. Units	100
Vitamin E (DL-Alpha Tocopherol Acetate)	45 Intl. Units	150
Vitamin C (Ascorbic Acid)	100 mg	166
Niacinamide	25 mg	125
Thiamine Mononitrate	5 mg	333
Riboflavin	5 mg	294
Pyridoxine (Pyridoxine HCl)	3 mg	150
Folic Acid	400 mcg	100
Pantothenic Acid (D-Calcium Pant.)	15 mg	150
Vitamin B12	18 mcg	300
Vitamin K1	25 mcg	8
Biotin	45 mcg	15
Calcium	200 mg	20
Phosphorus (Dicalcium Phosphate)	150 mg	15
Iron (Ferrous Fumarate)	18 mg	100
Magnesium (Magnesium Oxide)	100 mg	25
Copper (Copper Oxide)	2 mg	100
Zinc (Zinc Oxide)	15 mg	100
Iodine (Potassium Iodide)	150 mcg	100
Manganese (Manganese Sulfate)	5 mg	**
Potassium (Potassium Chloride)	40 mg	**
Chloride	36.3 mg	**
Selenium (Sodium Selenate)	25 mcg	**
Molybdenum (Sodium Molybdate)	25 mcg	**
Chromium (Chromium Chloride)	25 mcg	**
Nickel	5 mcg	**
Tin	10 mcg	**
Vanadium	10 mcg	**
Silicon	2 mcg	**
Boron	150 mcg	**

Inactive Ingredients:
Microcrystalline Cellulose NF, Stearic Acid NF, Croscarmellose Sodium NF, Magnesium Stearate NF, Hydroxypropyl Methylcellulose NF, Propylene Glycol, USP, FD&C Yellow #6

*Percentage of U.S. Recommended Daily Allowances
**These beneficial minerals are in addition to the Recommended Daily Allowances of the vitamins.

A. H. Robins Consumer Products Division
American Home Products Corporation
FIVE GIRALDA FARMS
MADISON, NJ 07940-0871

DIMETAPP® Cold & Allergy
[di 'mĕ-tap]
Chewable Tablets

Description: Each chewable tablet contains:
Brompheniramine Maleate, USP .... 1 mg
Phenylpropanolamine Hydrochloride, USP .... 6.25 mg

Inactive Ingredients: Aspartame, Citric Acid, Crospovidone, D&C Red 30 Aluminum Lake, D&C Red 7 Calcium Lake, FD&C Blue 1 Aluminum Lake, Flavor, Glycine, Magnesium Stearate, Mannitol, Microcrystalline Cellulose, Pregelatinized Starch, Silicon Dioxide, Sorbitol, Stearic Acid.

Indications: For temporary relief of nasal congestion due to the common cold, hay fever, or other upper respiratory allergies or associated with sinusitis. Temporarily relieves runny nose, sneezing, and itchy, watery eyes due to allergic rhinitis (hay fever). Temporarily restores freer breathing through the nose.

Warnings: Parents are warned not to give this product to children with the following conditions, unless directed by a physician: a breathing problem such as chronic bronchitis, glaucoma, high blood pressure, heart disease, diabetes, or thyroid disease. This product may cause drowsiness, or in some cases, excitability. Sedatives and tranquilizers may increase the drowsiness effect. Parents are warned not to give this product to children who are taking sedatives or tranquilizers without first consulting the child's physician.

Parents are warned not to exceed the recommended dosage, because at higher doses, nervousness, dizziness, or sleeplessness may occur. They are also warned not to give this product to children for more than 7 days. If their child's symptoms do not improve, or are accompanied by a fever, parents are instructed to consult a physician. Children should not be given this product if they are hypersensitive to any of the ingredients. As with any drug, if the person taking the drug is pregnant or nursing a baby, she should seek the advice of a health professional before using this product.

Drug Interaction Precaution: Concomitant administration of phenylpropanolamine with other sympathomimetic agents may produce additive effects and increased toxicity; with monoamine oxidase inhibitors (MAOIs) may produce a hypertensive crisis; with certain antihypertensive agents may diminish their antihypertensive effect.

This and all drugs should be kept out of the reach of children. In case of acciden-

tal overdose, professional assistance should be sought, or a poison control center contacted immediately.
Phenylketonurics are advised that this product contains 8 mg of phenylalanine per tablet.

Directions: Children 6 to under 12 years of age: 2 chewable tablets every 4 hours. Children under 6: consult a physician. DO NOT EXCEED 6 DOSES IN A 24-HOUR PERIOD.

Professional Labeling: The suggested dosage for children age 2 to under 6 years, only when the child is under the care of a physician, is 1 tablet every 4 hours, not to exceed 6 doses in a 24-hour period.

How Supplied: Purple tablet scored on one side and engraved with AHR 2290 on the other in bottles of 24 tablets (NDC 0031–2290–54).
Store at Controlled Room Temperature, Between 15°C and 30°C (59°F and 86°F).

DIMETAPP® Elixir
[dī´ mĕ-tap]

Description: Each 5 mL (1 teaspoonful) contains:
Brompheniramine
    Maleate, USP ....2 mg
Phenylpropanolamine
    Hydrochloride, USP ....12.5 mg

Inactive Ingredients: Citric Acid, FD&C Blue 1, FD&C Red 40, Flavors, Glycerin, Saccharin Sodium, Sodium Benzoate, Sorbitol, Water.

Indications: For temporary relief of nasal congestion due to the common cold, hay fever or other upper respiratory allergies or associated with sinusitis; temporarily relieves runny nose, sneezing, and itchy and watery eyes due to allergic rhinitis (hay fever). Temporarily restores freer breathing through the nose.

Warnings: Patients with the following conditions are warned not to take this product, unless directed by a physician: a breathing problem such as emphysema or chronic bronchitis, high blood pressure, heart disease, diabetes, thyroid disease, glaucoma, or difficulty in urination due to enlargement of the prostate gland. This product may cause drowsiness; alcohol, sedatives and tranquilizers may increase the drowsiness effect. Patients are told to avoid alcoholic beverages while taking this product and not to take it if they are taking sedatives or tranquilizers without first consulting their physician. Caution should be used when driving a motor vehicle or operating machinery. May cause excitability, especially in children.
Patients are warned not to exceed the recommended dosage because at higher doses, nervousness, dizziness or sleeplessness may occur. They also are told not to take this product for more than 7 days. If symptoms do not improve, or are accompanied by fever, patients should consult a physician.

Patients should not take this product if they are hypersensitive to any of the ingredients. As with any drug, women who are pregnant or nursing a baby should seek the advice of a health professional before using this product.
Patients are also warned to keep this and all drugs out of the reach of children, and that in case of accidental overdose, to seek professional assistance or contact a poison control center immediately.

Drug Interaction Precaution: Concomitant administration of phenylpropanolamine with other sympathomimetic agents may produce additive effects and increased toxicity; with monamine oxidase inhibitors (MAOIs) may produce a hypertensive crisis; with certain antihypertensive agents may diminish their antihypertensive effect.

Directions: Adults and children 12 years of age and over: 2 teaspoonfuls every 4 hours; children 6 to under 12 years: 1 teaspoonful every 4 hours; DO NOT EXCEED 6 DOSES IN A 24-HOUR PERIOD. Children under 6 years: use only as directed by a physician.

Professional Labeling: The suggested dosage for children age 2 to under 6 years, only when the child is under the care of a physician, is ½ teaspoonful every 4 hours, not to exceed 6 doses in a 24-hour period. The dosage for children under 2 years should be determined by the physician on the basis of the patients' weight, physical condition, or other appropriate consideration. Dimetapp Elixir is contraindicated in neonates (children under the age of one month).

How Supplied: Purple, grape-flavored liquid in bottles of 4 fl. oz. (NDC 0031-2230-12), 8 fl. oz. (NDC 0031-2230-18), 12 fl. oz. (NDC 0031-2230-22), pints (NDC 0031-2230-25), gallons (NDC 0031-2230-29), and 5 mL Dis-Co® Unit Dose Packs (10 × 10s) (NDC 0031-2230-23).
Store at Controlled Room Temperature, between 15°C and 30°C (59°F and 86°F). Not a USP elixir.
Shown in Product Identification Guide, page 419

DIMETAPP® DM ELIXIR
[dī´mĕ-tap]

Description: Each 5 mL (1 teaspoonful) contains:
Brompheniramine
    Maleate, USP .... 2 mg
Phenylpropanolamine
    Hydrochloride, USP .... 12.5 mg
Dextromethorphan
    Hydrobromide, USP .... 10.0 mg

Inactive Ingredients: Citric Acid, FD&C Blue 1, FD&C Red 40, Flavors, Glycerin, Propylene Glycol, Saccharin Sodium, Sodium Benzoate, Sorbitol, Water.

Indications: Temporarily relieves cough due to minor throat and bronchial irritation as may occur with a cold. For temporary relief of nasal congestion due to the

common cold, hay fever or other upper respiratory allergies or associated with sinusitis; temporarily relieves runny nose, sneezing, and itchy and watery eyes due to allergic rhinitis (hay fever). Temporarily restores freer breathing through the nose.

Warnings: Patients with the following conditions are warned not to take this product, unless directed by a physician: a breathing problem such as emphysema or chronic bronchitis or other persistent or chronic cough such as occurs with smoking or asthma, or cough that is accompanied by excessive phlegm (mucus). Likewise, patients with high blood pressure, heart disease, diabetes, thyroid disease, glaucoma, or difficulty in urination due to enlargement of the prostate gland are warned not to take this product unless directed by a physician.
This product may cause marked drowsiness; alcohol, sedatives and tranquilizers may increase the drowsiness effect. Patients are instructed to avoid alcoholic beverages while taking this product and not to take it if they are taking sedatives or tranquilizers without first consulting their physician. Caution should be used when driving a motor vehicle or operating machinery. May cause excitability, especially in children.
Patients are warned not to exceed the recommended dosage because at higher doses, nervousness, dizziness or sleeplessness may occur. They also are told not to take the product for more than 7 days. A persistent cough may be a sign of a serious condition. If cough or other symptoms persist for more than one week, tend to recur, or are accompanied by fever, rash or persistent headache, patients should consult a physician.
Patients should not take this product if they are hypersensitive to any of the ingredients. As with any drug, women who are pregnant or nursing a baby should seek the advice of a health professional before using this product.
Patients are also warned to keep this and all drugs out of the reach of children, and that in case of accidental overdose, to seek professional assistance or contact a poison control center immediately.

Drug Interaction Precautions: Concomitant administration of phenylpropanolamine with other sympathomimetic agents may produce additive effects and increased toxicity; with monamine oxidase inhibitors (MAOIs) may produce a hypertensive crisis; with certain antihypertensive agents may diminish their antihypertensive effect. Serious toxicity

Continued on next page

Prescribing information on A. H. Robins products listed here is based on official labeling in effect November 1, 1993, with Indications, Contraindications, Warnings, Precautions, Adverse Reactions, and Dosage stated in full.

A. H. Robins—Cont.

may result if dextromethorphan is used with MAOIs.

Directions: Adults and children 12 years of age and over: Two teaspoonfuls every 4 hours; children 6 to under 12 years: one teaspoonful every 4 hours. DO NOT EXCEED 6 DOSES IN A 24-HOUR PERIOD. Children under 6 years: use only as directed by a physician.

Overdose: Symptoms that may be associated with dextromethorphan overdose include ataxia, respiratory depression and convulsions in children, whereas adults may exhibit altered sensory perception, ataxia, slurred speech and dysphoria.

Professional Labeling: The suggested dosage for children age 2 to under 6 years, only when the child is under the care of a physician, is ½ teaspoonful every 4 hours, not to exceed 6 doses in a 24-hour period. The dosage for children under 2 years should be determined by the physician on the basis of the patients' weight, physical condition, or other appropriate consideration. Dimetapp DM Elixir is contraindicated in neonates (children under the age of one month).

How Supplied: Red, grape-flavored liquid in bottles of 4 fl. oz. (NDC 0031-2240-12), 8 fl. oz. (NDC 0031-2240-18), and 12 fl. oz. (NDC 0031-2240-22).
Store at Room Temperature.
Not a USP elixir.

DIMETAPP® Extentabs®
[dī' mě-tap]

Description: Each **Dimetapp Extentabs**® Tablet contains:
Brompheniramine Maleate,
    USP .... 12 mg
Phenylpropanolamine
    Hydrochloride, USP .... 75 mg

Inactive Ingredients: Acacia, Acetylated Monoglycerides, Calcium Sulfate, Carnauba Wax, Castor Wax or Oil, Citric Acid, Edible Ink, FD&C Blue 1, FD&C Blue 2 Aluminum Lake, Gelatin, Magnesium Stearate, Magnesium Trisilicate, Pharmaceutical Glaze, Polysorbates, Povidone, Silicon Dioxide, Stearyl Alcohol, Sucrose, Titanium Dioxide, Wheat Flour, White Wax. May contain FD&C Red 40 and FD&C Yellow 6 Aluminum Lakes.

Indications: For temporary relief of nasal congestion due to the common cold, hay fever or other upper respiratory allergies or associated with sinusitis; temporarily relieves runny nose, sneezing, and itchy and watery eyes due to allergic rhinitis (hay fever). Temporarily restores freer breathing through the nose.

Warnings: Patients with the following conditions are warned not to take this product, unless directed by a physician: a breathing problem such as emphysema or chronic bronchitis, or high blood pressure, heart disease, diabetes, thyroid dis-

ease, glaucoma, or difficulty in urination due to enlargement of the prostate gland. This product may cause drowsiness; alcohol, sedatives and tranquilizers may increase the drowsiness effect. Patients are told to avoid alcoholic beverages while taking this product and not to take it if they are taking sedatives or tranquilizers without first consulting their physician. Caution should be used when driving a motor vehicle or operating machinery. May cause excitability, especially in children.
Patients are warned not to exceed the recommended dosage because at higher doses, nervousness, dizziness or sleeplessness may occur. They also are told not to take this product for more than 7 days. If symptoms do not improve, or are accompanied by fever, patients should consult a physician.
Dimetapp Extentabs should not be given to children under 12 years, except under the advice and supervision of a physician. Patients should not take this product if they are hypersensitive to any of the ingredients. As with any drug, women who are pregnant or nursing a baby should seek the advice of a health professional before using this product. Patients are also warned to keep this and all drugs out of the reach of children, and that in case of accidental overdose, to seek professional assistance or contact a poison control center immediately.

Drug Interaction Precaution: Concomitant administration of phenylpropanolamine with other sympathomimetic agents may produce additive effects and increased toxicity; with monoamine oxidase inhibitors (MAOIs) may produce a hypertensive crisis; with certain antihypertensive agents may diminish their antihypertensive effect.

Directions: Adults and children 12 years of age and over: one tablet every 12 hours. DO NOT EXCEED 1 TABLET EVERY 12 HOURS OR 2 TABLETS IN A 24-HOUR PERIOD.

How Supplied: Pale blue sugar-coated tablets monogrammed DIMETAPP AHR in bottles of 100 (NDC 0031-2277-63), 500 (NDC 0031-2277-70); Dis-Co® Unit Dose Packs of 100 (NDC 0031-2277-64); and consumer packages of 12 tablets (NDC 0031-2277-46), 24 tablets (NDC 0031-2277-54) and 48 tablets (NDC 0031-2277-59) (individually packaged).
Store at Controlled Room Temperature, between 15°C and 30°C (59°F and 86°F).
Dimetapp Extentabs® Tablets are the A. H. Robins Company's uniquely constructed extended action tablets.

Shown in Product Identification Guide, page 419

DIMETAPP® Sinus Caplets*
[di 'mě-tap]
*Oval-Shaped tablets

Description: Each Dimetapp Caplet contains:
Ibuprofen .... 200 mg
Pseudoephedrine HCl .... 30 mg

Inactive Ingredients: Carnauba or Equivalent Wax, Croscarmellose Sodium, Iron Oxide, Methylparaben, Microcrystalline Cellulose, Propylparaben, Silicon Dioxide, Sodium Benzoate, Sodium Lauryl Sulfate, Starch, Stearic Acid, Sucrose, Titanium Dioxide.

Indications: For temporary relief of symptoms associated with the common cold, sinusitis or flu including nasal congestion, headache, fever, body aches, and pains.

Warnings: Aspirin sensitive patients are warned not to take this product if they have had a severe allergic reaction to aspirin, e.g. - asthma, swelling, shock, or hives because, even though this product contains no aspirin or salicylates, cross-reactions may occur in patients allergic to aspirin.
Patients are warned not to take this product for colds for more than 7 days or for fever for more than 3 days unless directed by a doctor. If the cold or fever persists or gets worse or if new symptoms occur patients are directed to consult a physician because these could be signs of a serious illness. Patients are directed that as with aspirin and acetaminophen, if they have any condition which requires them to take prescription drugs or if they have had any problems or serious side effects from taking any non-prescription pain reliever, not to take this product without first discussing it with their physician. They are also directed to consult their physician IF THEY EXPERIENCE ANY SYMPTOMS WHICH ARE UNUSUAL OR SEEM UNRELATED TO THE CONDITION FOR WHICH THEY TOOK THIS PRODUCT BEFORE TAKING ANY MORE OF IT, and to consult a physician if they are under a physician's care for any serious condition. Patients are warned not to exceed the recommended dosage because at higher doses nervousness, dizziness or sleeplessness may occur. Patients with the following conditions are warned not to take this product unless directed by a physician: high blood pressure, heart disease, diabetes, thyroid disease or difficulty in urination due to enlargement of the prostate gland. As with any drug, women who are pregnant or nursing a baby should seek the advice of a health professional before using this product. Women are warned that IT IS ESPECIALLY IMPORTANT NOT TO USE THIS PRODUCT DURING THE LAST 3 MONTHS OF PREGNANCY UNLESS SPECIFICALLY DIRECTED TO DO SO BY A DOCTOR BECAUSE IT MAY CAUSE PROBLEMS IN THE UNBORN CHILD OR COMPLICATIONS DURING DELIVERY. Patients are warned to keep this and all drugs out of the reach of children and that in case of accidental overdose to seek professional assistance or contact a poison control center immediately.

Drug Interaction Precaution: Concomitant administration of pseudoephedrine with other sympathomimetic amines may produce additive effects and increased toxicity; with monoamine oxidase inhibitors (MAOIs) may produce a hypertensive crisis; with certain antihypertensive agents may diminish their antihypertensive effect. Because of these effects patients are advised not to take this product if they are presently taking a prescription drug for high blood pressure or depression without first consulting their doctor. Patients are also instructed not to combine this product with other non-prescription pain relievers or with any other ibuprofen-containing product.

Directions: Adults: 1 caplet every 4 to 6 hours while symptoms persist. If symptoms do not respond to 1 caplet, 2 caplets may be used but do not exceed 6 caplets in 24 hours, unless directed by a physician. The smallest effective dose should be used. Take with food or milk if occasional and mild heartburn, upset stomach, or stomach pain occurs with use. Consult a physician if these symptoms are more than mild or if they persist. Children: Do not give this product to children under 12 years of age except under the advice and supervision of a doctor.

How Supplied: White coated caplet monogrammed DIMETAPP SINUS in packages of 20 tablets (NDC 0031–2260–52), and bottles of 40 tablets (NDC 0031–2260–56).
Store at room temperture; avoid excessive heat (40°C, 104°F).

DIMETAPP® Tablets and Liqui-Gels®
[dī' mĕ-tap]

Description: Each **Dimetapp** Tablet or Liquigel® contains:
Brompheniramine
  Maleate, USP .... 4 mg
Phenylpropanolamine
  Hydrochloride, USP .... 25 mg

Inactive Ingredients: Tablets: Corn Starch, FD&C Blue 1 Aluminum Lake, Magnesium Stearate, Microcrystalline Cellulose. Liqui-Gels: D&C Red 33, FD&C Blue 1, Gelatin, Glycerin, Mannitol, Pharmaceutical Glaze, Polyethylene Glycol, Povidone, Propylene Glycol, Sorbitan, Sorbitol, Titanium Dioxide, Water.

Indications: For temporary relief of nasal congestion due to the common cold, hay fever or other upper respiratory allergies or associated with sinusitis; temporarily relieves runny nose, sneezing, and itchy and watery eyes due to allergic rhinitis (hay fever). Temporarily restores freer breathing through the nose.

Warnings: Patients with the following conditions are warned not to take this product, unless directed by a physician: a breathing problem such as emphysema or chronic bronchitis, or high blood pressure, heart disease, diabetes, thyroid disease, glaucoma, or difficulty in urination due to enlargement of the prostate gland. This product may cause drowsiness; alcohol, sedatives and tranquilizers may increase the drowsiness effect. Patients are told to avoid alcoholic beverages while taking this product and not to take it if they are taking sedatives or tranquilizers without first consulting their physician. Caution should be used when driving a motor vehicle or operating machinery. May cause excitability, especially in children. Patients are warned not to exceed the recommended dosage because at higher doses, nervousness, dizziness or sleeplessness may occur. They also are told not to take this product for more than 7 days. If symptoms do not improve, or are accompanied by fever, patients should consult a physician.
Patients should not take this product if they are hypersensitive to any of the ingredients. As with any drug, women who are pregnant or nursing a baby should seek the advice of a health professional before using this product.
Patients are also warned to keep this and all drugs out of the reach of children, and that in case of accidental overdose, to seek professional assistance or contact a poison control center immediately.

Drug Interaction Precaution: Concomitant administration of phenylpropanolamine with other sympathomimetic agents may produce additive effects and increased toxicity; with monoamine oxidase inhibitors (MAOIs) may produce a hypertensive crisis; with certain antihypertensive agents may diminish their antihypertensive effect.

Directions: Tablets: Adults and children 12 years of age and over: one tablet every 4 hours. Children 6 to under 12 years: one-half tablet every 4 hours. DO NOT EXCEED 6 DOSES IN A 24-HOUR PERIOD. Children under 6 years: Use only as directed by a physician. Liqui-Gels: Adults and children 12 years of age and over: one Liquigel® every 4 hours. Children under 12, consult a physician. DO NOT EXCEED 6 Liqui-Gels in a 24-hour period.

How Supplied: Tablets: Blue, scored compressed tablets engraved AHR and 2254 in consumer packages of 24 (NDC 0031-2254-54) (individually packaged). Liqui-Gels: Purple Liquigel imprinted AHR and 2255 in consumer packages of 12 (NDC 0031-2255-46) and 24 (NDC 0031-2255-54) (individually packaged). Tablets and Liqui-Gels: Store at Controlled Room Temperature, between 15°C and 30°C (59°F and 86°F).
Liqui-Gels and Liquigel are registered trademarks of R.P. Scherer International Corporation.

ROBITUSSIN® COLD & COUGH LIQUI-GELS®
[ro "bĭ-tuss 'ĭn]

Description: Each Robitussin Cold & Cough Liquigel® contains:

Guaifenesin, USP .... 200 mg
Dextromethorphan Hydrobromide,
  USP .... 10 mg
Pseudoephedrine Hydrochloride,
  USP .... 30 mg

Inactive Ingredients: FD&C Blue 1, FD&C Red 40, Gelatin, Glycerin, Mannitol, Pharmaceutical Glaze, Polyethylene Glycol, Povidone, Propylene Glycol, Sorbitan, Sorbitol, Titanium Dioxide, Water.

Indications: Temporarily relieves coughs due to minor throat and bronchial irritation and nasal congestion as may occur with a cold. Expectorant action to help loosen phlegm and thin bronchial secretions to make coughs more productive.

Warnings: Patients with the following conditions are warned not to take this product, unless directed by a physician: persistent or chronic cough such as occurs with smoking, asthma, chronic bronchitis, emphysema, or if cough is accompanied by excessive phlegm (mucus). Likewise, patients with heart disease, high blood pressure, thyroid disease, diabetes, or difficulty in urination due to enlargement of the prostate gland are warned not to take this product unless directed by a physician.
Patients are warned not to exceed the recommended dosage because at higher doses, nervousness, dizziness or sleeplessness may occur. They are also told not to take this product for more than 7 days. A persistent cough may be a sign of a serious condition. If cough or other symptoms persist for more than one week without improvement, tend to recur, or are accompanied by fever, rash, or persistent headache, patients should consult a physician.
Patients should not take this product if they are hypersensitive to any of the ingredients. As with any drug, women who are pregnant or nursing a baby should seek the advice of a health professional before using this product.
Patients are also warned to keep this and all drugs out of reach of children and that in case of accidental overdose, to seek professional assistance or contact a poison control center immediately.

Overdose: Symptoms that may be associated with dextromethorphan overdose include ataxia, respiratory depres-

Continued on next page

Prescribing information on A. H. Robins products listed here is based on official labeling in effect November 1, 1993, with Indications, Contraindications, Warnings, Precautions, Adverse Reactions, and Dosage stated in full.

A. H. Robins—Cont.

sion and convulsions in children, whereas adults may exhibit altered sensory perception, ataxia, slurred speech and dysphoria.

Note: Guaifenesin had been shown to produce a color interference with certain clinical laboratory determinations of 5-hydroxyindoleacetic acid (5-HIAA) and vanillylmandelic acid (VMA).

Drug Interaction Precaution: Concomitant administration of pseudoephedrine with other sympathomimetic agents may produce additive effects and increased toxicity; with monoamine oxidase inhibitors (MAOIs) may produce a hypertensive crisis; with certain antihypertensive agents may diminish their antihypertensive effect. Serious toxicity may result if dextromethorphan is used with MAOIs.

Directions: Adults and children 12 years of age and over: swallow two Liqui-Gels every 4 hours. Children 6 to under 12 years: swallow one Liquigel every 4 hours. DO NOT EXCEED 4 DOSES IN A 24-HOUR PERIOD. Children under 6, consult a physician.

How Supplied: Red Liquigel imprinted AHR and 8600 in consumer packages of 12 (NDC 0031-8600-46) and 20 (NDC 0031-8600-52) (individually packaged).
Store at controlled room temperature, between 15°C and 30°C (59°F and 86°F)
Liqui-Gels and Liquigel are registered trademarks of R.P. Scherer International Corporation.
Shown in Product Identification Guide, page 419

ROBITUSSIN® SEVERE CONGESTION LIQUI-GELS®
[ro "bĭ-tuss 'ĭn]

Description: Each Robitussin Severe Congestion Liquigel® contains:

Guaifenesin, USP .... 200 mg
Pseudoephedrine Hydrochloride,
USP .... 30 mg

Inactive Ingredients: FD&C Green 3, Gelatin, Glycerin, Mannitol, Pharmaceutical Glaze, Polyethylene Glycol, Povidone, Propylene Glycol, Sorbitan, Sorbitol, Titanium Dioxide, Water.

Indications: Temporarily relieves nasal congestion as may occur with a cold. Expectorant action to help loosen phlegm and thin bronchial secretions to make coughs more productive.

Warnings: Patients with the following conditions are warned not to take this product, unless directed by a physician: persistent or chronic cough such as occurs with smoking, asthma, chronic bronchitis, emphysema, or if cough is accompanied by excessive phlegm (mucus). Likewise, patients with heart disease, high blood pressure, thyroid disease, diabetes, or difficulty in urination due to

enlargement of the prostate gland are warned not to take this product unless directed by a physician.
Patients are warned not to exceed the recommended dosage because at higher doses, nervousness, dizziness or sleeplessness may occur. They are also told not to take this product for more than 7 days. A persistent cough may be a sign of a serious condition. If cough or other symptoms persist for more than one week without improvement, tend to recur, or are accompanied by fever, rash, or persistent headache, patients should consult a physician.
Patients should not take this product if they are hypersensitive to any of the ingredients. As with any drug, women who are pregnant or nursing a baby should seek the advice of a health professional before using this product.
Patients are also warned to keep this and all drugs out of reach of children and that in case of accidental overdose, to seek professional assistance or contact a poison control center immediately.

Note: Guaifenesin has been shown to produce a color interference with certain clinical laboratory determinations of 5-hydroxyindoleacetic acid (5-HIAA) and vanillylmandelic acid (VMA).

Drug Interaction Precaution: Concomitant administration of pseudoephedrine with other sympathomimetic agents may produce additive effects and increased toxicity; with monoamine oxidase inhibitors (MAOIs) may produce a hypertensive crisis; with certain antihypertensive agents may diminish their antihypertensive effect.

Directions: Adults and children 12 years of age and over: swallow two Liqui-Gels every 4 hours. Children 6 to under 12 years: swallow one Liquigel every 4 hours. DO NOT EXCEED 4 DOSES IN A 24-HOUR PERIOD. Children under 6, consult a physician.

How Supplied: Aqua Liquigel imprinted AHR and 8501 in consumer packages of 12 (NDC 0031-8601-46) and 20 (NDC 0031-8601-52) (individually packaged).
Store at controlled room temperature, between 15°C and 30°C (59°F and 86°F).
Liqui-Gels and Liquigel are registered trademarks of R.P. Scherer International Corporation.
Shown in Product Identification Section, page 419

ROBITUSSIN®
[ro "bĭ-tuss 'ĭn](Guaifenesin Syrup, USP)

Active Ingredients: Each teaspoonful (5 mL) contains:
Guaifenesin, USP .... 100 mg
in a pleasant tasting syrup.

Inactive Ingredients: Alcohol 3.5%, Caramel, Citric Acid, FD&C Red 40, Flavors, Glucose, Glycerin, High Fructose Corn Syrup, Saccharin Sodium, Sodium Benzoate, Water.

Indications: Expectorant action to help loosen phlegm and thin bronchial

secretions to make coughs more productive.

Professional Labeling: Helps loosen phlegm and thin bronchial secretions in patients with stable chronic bronchitis.

Warnings: Patients with the following conditions are warned not to take this product, unless directed by a physician: persistent or chronic cough such as occurs with smoking, asthma, chronic bronchitis, emphysema or where cough is accompanied by excessive phlegm (mucus).
A persistent cough may be a sign of a serious condition. If cough persists for more than one week, tends to recur, or is accompanied by fever, rash, or persistent headache, patients should consult a physician.
Patients should not take this product if they are hypersensitive to any of the ingredients. As with any drug, women who are pregnant or nursing a baby should seek the advice of a health professional before using this product.

Note: Guaifenesin has been shown to produce a color interference with certain clinical laboratory determinations of 5-hydroxyindoleacetic acid (5-HIAA) and vanillylmandelic acid (VMA).

Directions: Adults and children 12 years and over: 2–4 teaspoonfuls every 4 hours; children 6 years to under 12 years: 1–2 teaspoonfuls every 4 hours. Children 2 years to under 6 years: ½–1 teaspoonful every 4 hours; children under 2 years—consult your doctor. DO NOT EXCEED RECOMMENDED DOSAGE.

How Supplied: Robitussin (wine-colored) in bottles of 4 fl. oz. (NDC 0031-8624-12), 8 fl. oz. (NDC 0031-8624-18), pint (NDC 0031-8624-25) and gallon (NDC 0031-8624-29).
Robitussin also available in 1 fl. oz. bottles (4 × 25's) (NDC 0031-8624-02) and Dis-Co® Unit Dose Packs of 10 × 10's in 5 mL (NDC 0031-8624-23), 10 mL (NDC 0031-8624-26) and 15 mL (NDC 0031-8624-28).
Store at Controlled Room Temperature, between 15°C and 30°C (59°F and 86°F).
Shown in Product Identification Guide, page 419

ROBITUSSIN®-CF
[ro "bĭ-tuss 'ĭn]

Active Ingredients: Each teaspoonful (5 mL) contains:
Guaifenesin, USP .... 100 mg
Phenylpropanolamine HCl,
USP .... 12.5 mg
Dextromethorphan HBr, USP ... 10 mg
in a pleasant tasting syrup.

Inactive Ingredients: Alcohol 4.75%, Citric Acid, FD&C Red 40, Flavors, Glycerin, Propylene Glycol, Saccharin Sodium, Sodium Benzoate, Sorbitol, Water.

Indications: Temporarily relieves coughs due to minor throat and bronchial irritation and nasal congestion as may occur with a cold. Expectorant action to help loosen phlegm and thin bronchial secretions to make coughs more productive.

Warnings: Patients with the following conditions are warned not to take this product, unless directed by a physician: persistent or chronic cough such as occurs with smoking, asthma, chronic bronchitis, emphysema, or if cough is accompanied by excessive phlegm (mucus). Likewise, patients with heart disease, high blood pressure, thyroid disease, diabetes, or difficulty in urination due to enlargement of the prostate gland are warned not to take this product unless directed by a physician.

Patients are warned not to exceed the recommended dosage because at higher doses, nervousness, dizziness or sleeplessness may occur. They also are told not to take this product for more than 7 days. A persistent cough may be a sign of a serious condition. If cough or other symptoms persist for more than one week, tend to recur, or are accompanied by fever, rash, or persistent headache, patients should consult a physician.

Patients should not take this product if they are hypersensitive to any of the ingredients. As with any drug, women who are pregnant or nursing a baby should seek the advice of a health professional before using this product.

Patients are also warned to keep this and all drugs out of the reach of children, and that in case of accidental overdose, to seek professional assistance or contact a poison control center immediately.

Overdose: Symptoms that may be associated with dextromethorphan overdose include ataxia, respiratory depression and convulsions in children, whereas adults may exhibit altered sensory perception, ataxia, slurred speech and dysphoria.

Note: Guaifenesin has been shown to produce a color interference with certain clinical laboratory determinations of 5-hydroxyindoleacetic acid (5-HIAA) and vanillylmandelic acid (VMA).

Drug Interaction Precautions: Concomitant administration of phenylpropanolamine with other sympathomimetic agents may produce additive effects and increased toxicity; with MAOIs may produce a hypertensive crisis; with certain antihypertensive agents may diminish their antihypertensive effect. Serious toxicity may result if dextromethorphan is used with MAOIs.

Directions: Adults and children 12 years and over, 2 teaspoonfuls every 4 hours; children 6 years to under 12 years, 1 teaspoonful every 4 hours; children 2 years to under 6 years, ½ teaspoonful every 4 hours; children under 2 years —as directed by a physician. DO NOT EXCEED 6 DOSES IN A 24-HOUR PERIOD.

How Supplied: Robitussin-CF (red-colored) in bottles of 4 fl. oz. (NDC 0031-8677-12), 8 fl. oz. (NDC 0031-8677-18), 12

fl. oz. (NDC 0031-8677-22), and one pint (NDC 0031-8677-25).

Store at Controlled Room Temperature, between 15°C and 30°C (59°F and 86°F).

Shown in Product Identification Guide, page 419

ROBITUSSIN®-DM
[ro "bĭ-tuss 'ĭn]

Active Ingredients: Each teaspoonful (5 mL) contains:
Guaifenesin, USP .... 100 mg
Dextromethorphan HBr,
  USP .... 10 mg
in a pleasant tasting syrup.

Inactive Ingredients: Citric Acid, FD&C Red 40, Flavors, Glucose, Glycerin, High Fructose Corn Syrup, Saccharin Sodium, Sodium Benzoate, Water.

Indications: Temporarily relieves coughs due to minor throat and bronchial irritation as may occur with a cold. Expectorant action to help loosen phlegm and thin bronchial secretions to make coughs more productive.

Warnings: Patients with the following conditions are warned not to take this product, unless directed by a physician: persistent or chronic cough such as occurs with smoking, asthma, chronic bronchitis, emphysema, or if cough is accompanied by excessive phlegm (mucus). A persistent cough may be a sign of a serious condition. If cough persists for more than one week, tends to recur, or is accompanied by a fever, rash, or persistent headache, patients should consult a physician.

Patients should not take this product if they are hypersensitive to any of the ingredients. As with any drug, women who are pregnant or nursing a baby should seek the advice of a health professional before using this product.

Patients are also warned to keep this and all drugs out of the reach of children, and that in case of accidental overdose, to seek professional assistance or contact a poison control center immediately.

Overdose: Symptoms may include ataxia, respiratory depression and convulsions in children, whereas adults may exhibit altered sensory perception, ataxia, slurred speech and dysphoria.

Note: Guaifenesin has been shown to produce a color interference with certain clinical laboratory determinations of 5-hydroxyindoleacetic acid (5-HIAA) and vanillylmandelic acid (VMA).

Drug Interaction Precaution: Serious toxicity may result if dextromethorphan is used with MAOIs.

Directions: Adults and children 12 years and over, 2 teaspoonfuls every 4 hours; children 6 years to under 12 years, 1 teaspoonful every 4 hours; children 2 years to under 6 years, ½ teaspoonful every 4 hours; children under 2 years— consult your doctor. DO NOT EXCEED 6 DOSES IN A 24-HOUR PERIOD.

How Supplied: Robitussin-DM (cherry-colored) in bottles of 4 fl. oz. (NDC 0031-8685-12), 8 fl. oz. (NDC 0031-8685-18), 12 fl. oz. (NDC 0031-8685-22), single doses: 6 premeasured doses—⅓ fl. oz. each (NDC 0031-8685-06), pint (NDC 0031-8685-25), and gallon (NDC 0031-8685-29).

Robitussin-DM also available in Dis-Co® Unit Dose Packs of 10 × 10's in 5 mL (NDC 0031-8685-23) and 10 mL (NDC 0031-8685-26).

Store at Controlled Room Temperature, between 15°C and 30°C (59°F and 86°F).

Shown in Product Identification Guide, page 419

ROBITUSSIN®-PE
[ro "bĭ-tuss 'ĭn]

Active Ingredients: Each teaspoonful (5 mL) contains:
Guaifenesin, USP .... 100 mg
Pseudoephedrine HCl, USP ...... 30 mg
in a pleasant tasting syrup.

Inactive Ingredients: Alcohol 1.4%, Citric Acid, FD&C Red 40, Flavors, Glucose, Glycerin, High Fructose Corn Syrup, Saccharin Sodium, Sodium Benzoate, Water.

Indications: Temporarily relieves nasal congestion as may occur with a cold. Expectorant action to help loosen phlegm and thin bronchial secretions to make coughs more productive.

Warnings: Patients with the following conditions are warned not to take this product, unless directed by a physician: persistent or chronic cough such as occurs with smoking, asthma, chronic bronchitis, emphysema, or if cough is accompanied by excessive phlegm (mucus). Likewise, patients with heart disease, high blood pressure, thyroid disease, diabetes, or difficulty in urination due to enlargement of the prostate gland are warned not to take this product unless directed by a physician.

Patients are warned not to exceed the recommended dosage because at higher doses, nervousness, dizziness or sleeplessness may occur. They also are told not to take this product for more than 7 days. A persistent cough may be a sign of a serious condition. If cough or other symptoms persist for more than one week, tend to recur, or are accompanied by fever, rash, or persistent headache, patients should consult a physician.

Patients should not take this product if they are hypersensitive to any of the ingredients. As with any drug, women who are pregnant or nursing a baby should

Continued on next page

Prescribing information on A. H. Robins products listed here is based on official labeling in effect November 1, 1993, with Indications, Contraindications, Warnings, Precautions, Adverse Reactions, and Dosage stated in full.

A. H. Robins—Cont.

seek the advice of a health professional before using this product.

Patients are also warned to keep this and all drugs out of the reach of children, and that in case of accidental overdose, to seek professional assistance or contact a poison control center immediately.

Note: Guaifenesin has been shown to produce a color interference with certain clinical laboratory determinations of 5-hydroxyindoleacetic acid (5-HIAA) and vanillylmandelic acid (VMA).

Drug Interaction Precautions: Concomitant administration of pseudoephedrine with other sympathomimetic agents may produce additive effects and increased toxicity; with MAOIs may produce a hypertensive crisis; with certain antihypertensive agents may diminish their antihypertensive effect.

Directions: Adults and children 12 years and over, 2 teaspoonfuls every 4 hours; children 6 years to under 12 years, 1 teaspoonful every 4 hours; children 2 years to under 6 years, ½ teaspoonful every 4 hours; children under 2 years —as directed by physician. DO NOT EXCEED 4 DOSES IN A 24-HOUR PERIOD.

How Supplied: Robitussin-PE (orange-red) in bottles of 4 fl. oz. (NDC 0031-8695-12), 8 fl. oz. (NDC 0031-8695-18) and pint (NDC 0031-8695-25).

Store at Controlled Room Temperature, between 15°C and 30°C (59°F and 86°F).

Shown in Product Identification Guide, page 419

ROBITUSSIN® MAXIMUM STRENGTH COUGH SUPPRESSANT
[ro "bĭ-tuss 'ĭn]

Description: Each 5 mL (1 teaspoonful) contains:
Dextromethorphan
  Hydrobromide, USP .... 15 mg
in a pleasant tasting liquid.

Inactive Ingredients: Alcohol 1.4%, Citric Acid, FD&C Red 40, Flavors, Glucose, Glycerin, High Fructose Corn Syrup, Saccharin Sodium, Sodium Benzoate, Water.

Indications: Temporarily relieves coughs due to minor throat and bronchial irritation as may occur with a cold.

Warnings: Patients with the following conditions are warned not to take this product unless directed by a physician: persistent or chronic cough such as occurs with smoking, asthma, emphysema, or if cough is accompanied by excessive phlegm (mucus).

A persistent cough may be a sign of a serious condition. If cough persists for more than one week, tends to recur, or is accompanied by fever, rash, or persistent headache, patients should consult a physician.

Patients should not take this product if they are hypersensitive to any of the ingredients. As with any drug, women who are pregnant or nursing a baby should seek the advice of a health professional before using this product.

Patients are also warned to keep this and all drugs out of the reach of children, and that in case of accidental overdose, to seek professional assistance or contact a poison control center immediately.

Overdose: Symptoms may include ataxia, respiratory depression and convulsions in children, whereas adults may exhibit altered sensory perception, ataxia, slurred speech and dysphoria.

Drug Interaction Precaution: Serious toxicity may result if dextromethorphan is used with MAOIs.

Directions: Adults and children 12 years and over: 2 teaspoonfuls every 6–8 hours in medicine cup. Do not exceed 4 doses in a 24-hour period.

Professional Labeling: Children 6 years to under 12 years, 1 teaspoonful every 6–8 hours; children 2 years to under 6 years, ½ teaspoonful every 6–8 hours. Do not exceed 4 doses in a 24-hour period.

How Supplied: Robitussin Maximum Strength (dark red-colored) in bottles of 4 fl. oz. (NDC 0031-8670-12) and 8 fl. oz. (NDC 0031-8670-18).

Store at Controlled Room Temperature, between 15°C and 30°C (59°F and 86°F).

ROBITUSSIN® MAXIMUM STRENGTH COUGH & COLD
[ro "bĭ-tuss 'ĭn]

Description: Each teaspoonful (5 mL) contains:
Dextromethorphan HBr, USP ... 15 mg
Pseudoephedrine HCl, USP .... 30 mg

Inactive Ingredients: Alcohol 1.4%, Citric Acid, FD&C Red 40, Flavors, Glycerin, Glucose, High Fructose Corn Syrup, Saccharin Sodium, Sodium Benzoate, Water.

Indications: Temporarily relieves coughs due to minor throat and bronchial irritation and nasal congestion as may occur with a cold.

Warnings: Patients with the following conditions are warned not to take this product unless directed by a physician: persistent or chronic cough such as occurs with smoking, asthma, emphysema, or if cough is accompanied by excessive phlegm (mucus). Likewise patients with heart disease, high blood pressure, thyroid disease, diabetes, or difficulty in urination due to enlargement of the prostate gland are warned not to take this product unless directed by a physician. Patients are warned not to exceed the recommended dosage because at higher doses nervousness, dizziness or sleeplessness may occur. They are also told not to take this product for more than 7 days. A persistent cough may be a sign of a seri-

ous condition. If cough or other symptoms persist for more than one week without improvement, tend to recur, or are accompanied by fever, rash, or persistent headache, patients should consult a physician.

Patients should not take this product if they are hypersensitive to any of the ingredients. As with any drug, women who are pregnant or nursing a baby should seek the advice of a health professional before using this product.

Patients are also warned to keep this and all drugs out of the reach of children, and that in case of accidental overdose, to seek professional assistance or contact a poison control center immediately.

Overdose: Symptoms that may be associated with dextromethorphan overdose include ataxia, respiratory depression and convulsions in children, whereas adults may exhibit altered sensory perception, ataxia, slurred speech and dysphoria.

Drug Interaction Precaution: Concomitant administration of pseudoephedrine with other sympathomimetic amines may produce additive effects and increased toxicity; with monoamine oxidase inhibitors (MAOIs) may produce a hypertensive crisis; with certain antihypertensive agents may diminish their antihypertensive effect. Serious toxicity may result if dextromethorphan is used with MAOIs.

Directions: Adults and children 12 years and over: 2 teaspoonfuls every 6 hours, in medicine cup. Children under 12: consult a physician. Do not exceed 4 doses in a 24 hour period.

How Supplied: Red syrup in bottles of 4 fl. oz. (NDC 0031-8671-12) and 8 fl. oz. (NDC-0031-8671-18).

Store at Controlled Room Temperature, Between 15°C and 30°C (59°F and 86°F).

ROBITUSSIN® PEDIATRIC COUGH & COLD FORMULA
[ro "bĭ-tuss 'ĭn]

Description: Each 5 mL (1 teaspoonful) contains:
Dextromethorphan
  Hydrobromide, USP .... 7.5 mg
Pseudoephedrine
  Hydrochloride .... 15 mg
in a pleasant tasting alcohol-free syrup.

Inactive Ingredients: Citric Acid, FD&C Red 40, Flavors, Glycerin, Propylene Glycol, Saccharin Sodium, Sodium Benzoate, Sorbitol, Water.

Indications: Temporarily relieves coughs due to minor throat and bronchial irritation and nasal congestion as may occur with a cold.

Warnings: Patients with the following conditions are warned not to take this product unless directed by a physician: persistent or chronic cough such as occurs with smoking, asthma, or emphysema, or if cough is accompanied by excessive phlegm (mucus). Likewise, pa-

Age	Weight	Dose
Under 2 yrs.	Under 24 lbs.	As directed by physician.
2 to under 6 yrs.	24–47 lbs.	1 Teaspoonful
6 to under 12 yrs.	48–95 lbs.	2 Teaspoonfuls
12 yrs. and older	96 lbs. and over	4 Teaspoonfuls

tients with heart disease, high blood pressure, thyroid disease, diabetes, or difficulty in urination due to enlargement of the prostate gland are warned not to take this product unless directed by a physician.

Patients are warned not to exceed the recommended dosage because at higher doses, nervousness, dizziness or sleeplessness may occur. They also are told not to take this product for more than 7 days. A persistent cough may be a sign of a serious condition. If cough or other symptoms persist for more than one week, tend to recur, or are accompanied by fever, rash, or persistent headache, patients should consult a physician.

Patients should not take this product if they are hypersensitive to any of the ingredients. As with any drug, women who are pregnant or nursing a baby should seek the advice of a health professional before using this product.

Patients are also warned to keep this and all drugs out of the reach of children, and that in case of accidental overdose, to seek professional assistance or contact a poison control center immediately.

Drug Interaction Precautions: Concomitant administration of pseudoephedrine with other sympathomimetic agents may produce additive effects and increased toxicity; with monoamine oxidase inhibitors (MAOIs) may produce a hypertensive crisis; with certain antihypertensive agents may diminish their antihypertensive effect. Serious toxicity may result if dextromethorphan is used with MAOIs.

Overdose: Symptoms that may be associated with dextromethorphan overdose include ataxia, respiratory depression and convulsions in children, whereas adults may exhibit altered sensory perception, ataxia, slurred speech and dysphoria.

Directions: Patients are instructed to follow recommendations on the bottle or carton (see below) or to use as directed by a physician. Doses may be repeated every 6–8 hours, not to exceed 4 doses in a 24-hour period. Dosage should be chosen by weight, if known; if weight is not known, choose by age.
[See table above.]

How Supplied: Robitussin Pediatric Cough & Cold formula (bright red) in bottles of 4 fl. oz. (NDC 0031-8609-12) and 8 fl. oz. (NDC 0031-8609-18).
Store at Controlled Room Temperature, between 15°C and 30°C (59°F and 86°F).

Age	Weight	Dose
Under 2 yrs.	Under 24 lbs.	As directed by physician.
2 to under 6 yrs.	24–47 lbs.	1 Teaspoonful
6 to under 12 yrs.	48–95 lbs.	2 Teaspoonfuls
12 yrs. and older	96 lbs. and over	4 Teaspoonfuls

ROBITUSSIN® PEDIATRIC COUGH SUPPRESSANT
[ro "bĭ-tuss 'ĭn]

Description: Each 5 mL (1 teaspoonful) contains:
Dextromethorphan
  Hydrobromide, USP .... 7.5 mg
in a pleasant tasting alcohol-free syrup.

Inactive Ingredients: Citric Acid, FD&C Red 40, Flavors, Glycerin, Propylene Glycol, Saccharin Sodium, Sodium Benzoate, Sorbitol, Water.

Indications: Temporarily relieves coughs due to minor throat and bronchial irritation as may occur with a cold.

Warnings: Patients with the following conditions are warned not to take this product unless directed by a physician: persistent or chronic cough such as occurs with smoking, asthma, or emphysema, or if cough is accompanied by excessive phlegm (mucus).
A persistent cough may be a sign of a serious condition. If cough persists for more than one week, tends to recur, or is accompanied by fever, rash, or persistent headache, patients should consult a physician.
Patients should not take this product if they are hypersensitive to any of the ingredients. As with any drug, women who are pregnant or nursing a baby should seek the advice of a health professional before using this product.
Patients are also warned to keep this and all drugs out of the reach of children, and that in case of accidental overdose, to seek professional assistance or contact a poison control center immediately.

Overdose: Symptoms may include ataxia, respiratory depression and convulsions in children, whereas adults may exhibit altered sensory perception, ataxia, slurred speech and dysphoria.

Drug Interaction Precaution: Serious toxicity may result if dextromethorphan is used with MAOIs.

Directions: Patients are instructed to follow recommendations on the bottle or carton (see below) or to use as directed by a physician. Doses may be repeated every 6–8 hours, not to exceed 4 doses in a 24-hour period. Dosage should be chosen by weight, if known; if weight is not known, choose by age.
[See table below.]

How Supplied: Robitussin Pediatric (cherry-colored) in bottles of 4 fl. oz.

(NDC 0031-8610-12) and 8 fl. oz. (NDC 0031-8610-18).
Store at Controlled Room Temperature, between 15°C and 30°C (59°F and 86°F).

Ross Products Division
Abbott Laboratories
COLUMBUS, OHIO 43215-1724

PEDIATRIC NUTRITIONAL PRODUCTS

Alimentum® Protein Hydrolysate Formula With Iron

Isomil® Soy Formula With Iron

Isomil® DF Soy Formula For Diarrhea

Isomil® SF Sucrose-Free Soy Formula With Iron

PediaSure® Complete Liquid Nutrition

PediaSure® With Fiber Complete Liquid Nutrition

RCF® Ross Carbohydrate Free Low-Iron Soy Formula Base

Similac® Low-Iron Infant Formula

Similac® PM 60/40 Low-Iron Infant Formula

Similac® Special Care® With Iron 24 Premature Infant Formula

Similac® With Iron Infant Formula

For most current information, refer to product labels.

CLEAR EYES®
[klēr īz]
Lubricating Eye Redness Reliever

Description: Clear Eyes is a sterile, isotonic buffered solution containing the active ingredients naphazoline hydrochloride (0.012%) and glycerin (0.2%). It also contains boric acid, purified water and sodium borate. Edetate disodium and benzalkonium chloride are added as preservatives. Clear Eyes is a lubricating, decongestant ophthalmic solution specially designed for temporary relief of redness and drying due to minor eye irritation caused by dust, smoke, smog, sun glare, wearing contact lenses, allergies or swimming. Clear Eyes contains laboratory-tested and scientifically blended ingredients, including an effective vasoconstrictor which narrows swollen blood vessels and rapidly whitens reddened eyes

Continued on next page

If desired, additional information on any Ross product will be provided upon request to Ross Products Division, Abbott Laboratories, Columbus, Ohio 43215-1724.

Ross—Cont.

in a formulation which also contains a lubricant and produces a refreshing, soothing effect. Clear Eyes is a sterile, isotonic solution compatible with the natural fluids of the eye.

Indications: For the temporary relief of redness due to minor eye irritation AND for protection against further irritation or dryness of the eye.

Warnings: To avoid contamination, do not touch tip of container to any surface. Replace cap after using. If you experience eye pain, changes in vision, continued redness or irritation of the eye, or if the condition worsens or persists for more than 72 hours, discontinue use and consult a doctor. If you have glaucoma, do not use this product except under the advice and supervision of a doctor. Overuse of this product may produce increased redness of the eye. If solution changes color or becomes cloudy, do not use. Keep this and all drugs out of the reach of children.

Directions: Instill 1 or 2 drops in the affected eye(s), up to four times daily.

How Supplied: In 0.5-fl-oz and 1.0-fl-oz plastic dropper bottles.
(FAN 2348)

Shown in Product Identification Guide, page 419

CLEAR EYES® ACR
[klēr īz]
Astringent/Lubricating Eye Redness Reliever Drops

Description: Clear Eyes ACR is a sterile, isotonic buffered solution containing the active ingredients naphazoline hydrochloride (0.012%), zinc sulfate (0.25%) and glycerin (0.2%). It also contains boric acid, purified water, sodium chloride and sodium citrate. Edetate disodium and benzalkonium chloride are added as preservatives. Clear Eyes ACR is a triple-action formula that: (1) has an extra ingredient to clear away mucus buildup and relieve itching associated with allergies and colds, (2) immediately removes redness and (3) moisturizes irritated eyes. Clear Eyes ACR contains laboratory-tested and scientifically blended ingredients, including an effective vasoconstrictor which narrows swollen blood vessels and rapidly whitens reddened eyes in a formulation which also contains a lubricant and produces a refreshing, soothing effect. Clear Eyes ACR also contains an ocular astringent (zinc sulfate) that precipitates the sticky mucus buildup on the eye often associated with hay fever, allergies and colds, and this helps clear the mucus from the outer surface of the eye. Clear Eyes ACR is a sterile, isotonic solution compatible with the natural fluids of the eye.

Indications: For the temporary relief of redness due to minor eye irritation AND for protection against further irritation or dryness of the eye.

Warnings: To avoid contamination, do not touch tip of container to any surface. Replace cap after using. If you experience eye pain, changes in vision, continued redness or irritation of the eye, or if the condition worsens or persists for more than 72 hours, discontinue use and consult a doctor. If you have glaucoma, do not use this product except under the advice and supervision of a doctor. Overuse of this product may produce increased redness of the eye. If solution changes color or becomes cloudy, do not use. Keep this and all drugs out of the reach of children.

Directions: Instill 1 or 2 drops in the affected eye(s), up to four times daily.

How Supplied: In 0.5-fl-oz and 1.0-fl-oz plastic dropper bottles.
(FAN 2348)

Shown in Product Identification Guide, page 419

EAR DROPS BY MURINE®
[myūr 'ēn]
See Murine Ear Wax Removal System/Murine Ear Drops.

MURINE® EAR WAX REMOVAL SYSTEM/MURINE® EAR DROPS
[myūr 'ēn]
Carbamide Peroxide
Ear Wax Removal Aid

Description: MURINE EAR DROPS contains the active ingredient carbamide peroxide, 6.5%. It also contains alcohol (6.3%), anhydrous glycerin, polysorbate 20 and other ingredients in a buffered vehicle. The MURINE EAR WAX REMOVAL SYSTEM includes a 1.0-fl-oz soft bulb ear syringe. This system is a complete, medically approved system to safely remove ear wax. Application of carbamide peroxide drops followed by warm-water irrigation is an effective, medically recommended way to help loosen excessive and/or hardened ear wax.

Actions: The carbamide peroxide formula in MURINE EAR DROPS is an aid in the removal of wax from the ear canal. Anhydrous glycerin penetrates and softens wax while the release of oxygen from carbamide peroxide provides a mechanical action resulting in the loosening of the softened wax accumulation. It is usually necessary to remove the loosened wax by gently flushing the ear with warm water, using the soft bulb ear syringe provided.

Indications: The MURINE EAR WAX REMOVAL SYSTEM is indicated for occasional use as an aid to soften, loosen and remove excessive ear wax.

Warnings: DO NOT USE if you have ear drainage or discharge, ear pain, irritation or rash in the ear or are dizzy: Con-sult a doctor. DO NOT USE if you have an injury or perforation (hole) of the eardrum or after ear surgery, unless directed by a doctor.
DO NOT USE for more than 4 days; if excessive ear wax remains after use of this product, consult a doctor. Avoid contact with the eyes. If accidental contact with eyes occurs, flush eyes with water and consult a doctor. KEEP THIS AND ALL MEDICINES OUT OF THE REACH OF CHILDREN.

Directions: FOR USE IN THE EAR ONLY. Adults and children over 12 years of age: Tilt head sideways and place 5 to 10 drops in ear. Tip of applicator should not enter ear canal. Keep drops in ear for several minutes by keeping head tilted or placing cotton in the ear. Use twice daily for up to 4 days if needed, or as directed by a doctor. Any wax remaining after treatment may be removed by gently flushing the ear with warm water, using a soft bulb ear syringe. Children under 12 years: Consult a doctor.

Note: When the ear canal is irrigated, the tip of the ear syringe should not obstruct the flow of water leaving the ear canal.

How Supplied: The MURINE EAR WAX REMOVAL SYSTEM contains 0.5-fl-oz drops and a 1.0-fl-oz soft bulb ear syringe.
Also available in 0.5-fl-oz drops only, MURINE EAR DROPS.
(FAN 2369)

Shown in Product Identification Guide, page 420

MURINE®
[myūr 'ēn]
Lubricating Eye Drops

Description: Murine eye lubricant is a sterile, buffered solution containing the active ingredients 0.5% polyvinyl alcohol and 0.6% povidone. Also contains benzalkonium chloride, dextrose, disodium edetate, potassium chloride, purified water, sodium bicarbonate, sodium chloride, sodium citrate and sodium phosphate (mono- and dibasic). Murine is a sterile, hypotonic solution formulated to more closely match the natural tear fluid of the eye for gentle, soothing relief from minor eye irritation while moisturizing and relieving dryness. Use as desired to temporarily relieve minor eye irritation, dryness and burning.

Indications: For the temporary relief or prevention of further discomfort due to minor eye irritations and symptoms related to dry eyes.

Warnings: To avoid contamination, do not touch tip of container to any surface. Replace cap after using. If you experience eye pain, changes in vision, continued redness or irritation of the eye, or if the condition worsens or persists for more than 72 hours, discontinue use and consult a doctor. If solution changes color or becomes cloudy, do not use. Keep this and all drugs out of the reach of children.

Directions: Instill 1 or 2 drops in the affected eye(s) as needed.

How Supplied: In 0.5-fl-oz and 1.0-fl-oz plastic dropper bottles. (FAN 2345)

Shown in Product Identification Guide, page 419

MURINE® PLUS
[*myūr 'ēn*]
Lubricating Redness Reliever Eye Drops

Description: Murine Plus is a sterile, non-staining, buffered solution containing the active ingredients 0.5% polyvinyl alcohol, 0.6% povidone and 0.05% tetrahydrozoline hydrochloride. Also contains benzalkonium chloride, dextrose, disodium edetate, potassium chloride, purified water, sodium bicarbonate, sodium chloride, sodium citrate and sodium phosphate (mono- and dibasic). Murine Plus is a sterile, hypotonic, ophthalmic solution formulated to more closely match the natural fluid of the eye. It contains demulcents for gentle, soothing relief from minor eye irritation as well as the sympathomimetic agent, tetrahydrozoline hydrochloride, which produces local vasoconstriction in the eye. Thus, the drug effectively narrows swollen blood vessels locally and provides symptomatic relief of edema and hyperemia of conjunctival tissues due to eye allergies, minor local irritations and conjunctivitis. Use up to four times daily, to remove redness due to minor eye irritation. The effect of Murine Plus is prompt (apparent within minutes) and sustained.

Indications: For the temporary relief or prevention of further discomfort due to minor eye irritations and symptoms related to dry eyes PLUS removal of redness.

Warnings: To avoid contamination, do not touch tip of container to any surface. Replace cap after using. If you experience eye pain, changes in vision, continued redness or irritation of the eye, or if the condition worsens or persists for more than 72 hours, discontinue use and consult a doctor. If you have glaucoma, do not use this product except under the advice and supervision of a doctor. Overuse of this product may produce increased redness of the eye. If solution changes color or becomes cloudy, do not use. Keep this and all drugs out of the reach of children.

Directions: Instill 1 or 2 drops in the affected eye(s), **up to four times daily.**

How Supplied: In 0.5-fl-oz and 1.0-fl-oz plastic dropper bottles. (FAN 2345)

Shown in Product Identification Guide, page 420

PEDIALYTE®
[*pē 'dē-ah-līt* ″]
Oral Electrolyte Maintenance Solution

Usage: To quickly restore fluids and minerals lost in diarrhea and vomiting; for maintenance of water and electrolytes following corrective parenteral therapy for severe diarrhea.

Features:
- Ready To Use—no mixing or dilution necessary.
- Balanced electrolytes to replace stool losses and provide maintenance requirements.
- Provides glucose to promote sodium and water absorption.
- Unflavored form available for younger infants; Bubble Gum and Fruit-flavored forms available to enhance compliance in older infants and children.
- Plastic liter bottles are resealable and easy to pour.
- No coloring added.
- Widely available in grocery, drug and convenience stores.

Availability:

1 liter (33.8-fl-oz) plastic bottles; 8 per case; Unflavored, No. 336; Fruit-flavored, No. 365; Bubble Gum-flavored, No. 51752.

8-fl-oz bottles; 4 six-packs per case; Unflavored, No. 160. For hospital use, Pedialyte is available in the Ross Hospital Formula System.

Dosage: See Administration Guide to restore fluids and minerals lost in diarrhea and vomiting (Pedialyte Unflavored, Bubble Gum-flavored or Fruit-flavored) and management of mild to moderate dehydration secondary to moderate to severe diarrhea (Rehydralyte® Oral Electrolyte Rehydration Solution). Pedialyte (Unflavored, Bubble Gum-flavored or Fruit-flavored) or Rehydralyte should be offered frequently in amounts tolerated. Total daily intake should be adjusted to meet individual needs, based on thirst and response to therapy. The suggested intakes for maintenance are based on water requirements for ordinary energy expenditure.[1] The suggested intakes for replacement are based on fluid losses of 5% or 10% of body weight, including maintenance requirement. [See table on next page.]

Composition: Unflavored Pedialyte (Bubble Gum-flavored and Fruit-flavored Pedialyte have similar composition and nutrient value. For specific information, see product label.)

Ingredients: (Pareve, Ⓤ) Water, dextrose, potassium citrate, sodium chloride and sodium citrate.

Provides:	Per 8 Fl Oz	Per Liter	Per 32 Fl Oz
Sodium (mEq)	10.6	45	42.4
Potassium (mEq)	4.7	20	18.8
Chloride (mEq)	8.3	35	33.2
Citrate (mEq)	7.1	30	28.4
Dextrose (g)	5.9	25	23.6
Calories	24	100	96

(FAN 3004-01)

REHYDRALYTE®
[*rē-hī 'drə-līt* ″]
Oral Electrolyte Rehydration Solution

Usage: To restore fluids and minerals lost during moderate to severe diarrhea.

Features:
- Ready To Use—no mixing or dilution necessary.
- Safe, economical alternative to IV therapy.
- 75 mEq of sodium per liter for effective replacement of fluid deficits.
- 2½% glucose solution to promote sodium and water absorption and provide energy.
- Available in pharmacies.

Availability: 8-fl-oz bottles; 4 six-packs per case; No. 162.

Dosage: (See Administration Guide under Pedialyte®.)

Ingredients: (Pareve, Ⓤ) Water, dextrose, sodium chloride, potassium citrate and sodium citrate.

Provides:	Per 8 Fl Oz	Per Liter
Sodium (mEq)	17.7	75
Potassium (mEq)	4.7	20
Chloride (mEq)	15.4	65
Citrate (mEq)	7.1	30
Dextrose (g)	5.9	25
Calories	24	100

(FAN 3037-01)

SELSUN BLUE®
[*sel 'sun blü*]
**Dandruff Shampoo
(selenium sulfide lotion, 1%)**

Description: Selsun Blue is a non-prescription anti-dandruff shampoo containing the active ingredient selenium sulfide, 1%, in a freshly scented, pH-balanced formula to leave hair clean and manageable. Available in Regular, Extra Conditioning and Medicated Treatment formulas.

Inactive Ingredients:
Regular hair formula—Ammonium laureth sulfate, ammonium lauryl sulfate, citric acid, cocamide DEA, cocamidopropyl betaine, DMDM hydantoin, FD&C blue No. 1, fragrance, hydroxypropyl methylcellulose, magnesium aluminum silicate, purified water, sodium chloride and titanium dioxide.
Extra Conditioning formula—Aloe, ammonium laureth sulfate, ammonium lauryl sulfate, citric acid, cocamide DEA, di (hydrogenated) tallow phthalic acid amide, dimethicone, DMDM hydantoin, FD&C blue No. 1, fragrance, hydroxypropyl methylcellulose, purified

Continued on next page

If desired, additional information on any Ross product will be provided upon request to Ross Products Division, Abbott Laboratories, Columbus, Ohio 43215-1724.

Ross—Cont.

water, sodium citrate, sodium isostearoyl lactylate and titanium dioxide.

Medicated Treatment formula — Ammonium laureth sulfate, ammonium lauryl sulfate, citric acid, cocamide DEA, cocamidopropyl betaine, DMDM hydantoin, D&C red No. 33, FD&C blue No. 1, fragrance, hydroxypropyl methylcellulose, magnesium aluminum silicate, menthol, purified water, sodium chloride and TEA-lauryl sulfate.

Clinical testing has shown Selsun Blue to be as safe and effective as other leading shampoos in helping control dandruff symptoms with regular use. May be used on color-treated or permed hair, if used as directed.

Directions: Shake well. Shampoo and rinse thoroughly. For best results, use regularly, at least twice a week or as directed by a doctor.

Warnings: For external use only. Avoid contact with the eyes. If contact occurs, rinse eyes thoroughly with water. If condition worsens or does not improve after regular use of this product as directed, consult a doctor. Keep this and all drugs out of the reach of children.

How Supplied: 4-, 7- and 11-fl-oz plastic bottles.
(FAN 2342-02)

Shown in Product Identification Guide, page 420

SELSUN GOLD FOR WOMEN®
[*sel 'sun gōld*]
Dandruff Shampoo
(selenium sulfide lotion, 1%)

Description: Selsun Gold for Women is a non-prescription anti-dandruff shampoo containing the active ingredient selenium sulfide, 1%. This formula allows you to shampoo, condition and control dandruff flaking and itching with one shampoo. This formula contains patented ingredients to leave hair soft, shiny and manageable. You won't need a separate conditioner to have beautiful hair. May be used on color-treated or permed hair, if used as directed.

Inactive Ingredients: Ammonium lauryl sulfate, ammonium laureth sulfate, citric acid, cocamide DEA, di (hydrogenated) tallow phthalic acid amide, dimethicone, DMDM hydantoin, hydroxypropyl methylcellulose, purified water, sodium citrate and fragrance.

Directions: Shake well. Shampoo and rinse thoroughly. For best results, use regularly, at least twice a week or as directed by a doctor.

Warnings: For external use only. Avoid contact with the eyes. If contact occurs, rinse eyes thoroughly with water. If condition worsens or does not improve after regular use of this product as directed, consult a doctor. Keep this and all drugs out of the reach of children.

How Supplied: 4-, 7- and 11-fl-oz plastic bottles.
(FAN 2336-01)

Shown in Product Identification Guide, page 420

TRONOLANE®
[*tron 'ə-lān*]
Anesthetic Cream for Hemorrhoids

Description: The active ingredient in Tronolane cream is the topical anesthetic agent, pramoxine hydrochloride, 1% (chemically unrelated to the benzoate esters of the "caine" type), which is chemically designated as a 4-n-butoxyphenyl gammamor-pholinopropyl-ether hydrochloride. Also contains the following inactive ingredients: A nongreasy cream base containing beeswax, cetyl alcohol, cetyl esters wax, glycerin, methylparaben, propylparaben, sodium lauryl sulfate and zinc oxide.

Tronolane cream contains a rapidly acting topical anesthetic producing analgesia that lasts up to 5 hours. Because the drug is chemically unrelated to other anesthetics, cross-sensitization is unlikely. Patients who are already sensitized to the "caine" anesthetics can generally use Tronolane cream.

The emollient/emulsion base of Tronolane cream provides soothing lubrication. Tronolane cream is in a nondrying base that is nongreasy and nonstaining to undergarments.

Indications: Tronolane cream is indicated for the temporary relief of the pain, burning, itching and discomfort that accompany hemorrhoids.

Warnings: If condition worsens or does not improve within 7 days, consult a doctor. Do not exceed the recommended daily dosage, unless directed by a doctor. In case of bleeding, consult a doctor promptly. Do not put this product into the rectum by using fingers or any mechanical device or applicator. Certain persons can develop allergic reactions to ingredients in this product. If the symptom being treated does not subside, or if redness, irritation, swelling, pain or other symptoms develop or increase, discontinue use and consult a doctor. As with any drug, if you are pregnant or nursing a baby, seek the advice of a health care professional before using this

Pedialyte, Rehydralyte Administration Guide

For Infants and Young Children

Age	2 Weeks	3 Months	6 Months	9	1	1½	2	2½ Years	3	3½	4
Approximate Weight[2]											
(lb)	7	13	17	20	23	25	28	30	32	35	38
(kg)	3.2	6.0	7.8	9.2	10.2	11.4	12.6	13.6	14.6	16.0	17.0
PEDIALYTE UNFLAVORED, BUBBLE GUM— FLAVORED or FRUIT— FLAVORED fl oz/day for maintenance*	13 to 16	28 to 32	34 to 40	38 to 44	41 to 46	45 to 50	48 to 53	51 to 56	54 to 58	56 to 60	57 to 62
REHYDRALYTE fl oz/day for Replacement for 5% Dehydration (including maintenance)*	18 to 21	38 to 42	47 to 53	53 to 59	58 to 63	64 to 69	69 to 74	74 to 79	78 to 82	83 to 87	85 to 90
REHYDRALYTE fl oz/day for Replacement for 10% Dehydration (including maintenance)*	23 to 26	48 to 52	60 to 66	68 to 74	75 to 80	83 to 88	90 to 95	97 to 102	102 to 106	110 to 114	113 to 118

Administration Guide does not apply to infants less than 1 week of age. For children over 4 years, maintenance intakes may exceed 2 liters daily.

1. Extrapolated from Barness L: Nutrition and nutritional disorders, in Behrman RE, Vaughan VC III: *Nelson Textbook of Pediatrics*, ed 12. Philadelphia: WB Saunders Co, 1983, pp 136-138.
2. Weight based on the 50th percentile of weight for age of the National Center for Health Statistics (NCHS) reference data. Hamill PVV, Drizd TA, Johnson CL, et al: Physical growth: National Center for Health Statistics percentiles. *Am J Clin Nutr* 1979; 32:607-629.
* Fluid intakes do not take into account ongoing stool losses. Fluid loss in the stool should be replaced by consumption of an extra amount of Pedialyte or Rehydralyte equal to stool losses, in addition to the amounts given in this Administration Guide.

product. Keep this and all drugs out of the reach of children.

Dosage and Administration (Directions): Adults—When practical, cleanse the affected area with mild soap and warm water and rinse thoroughly or cleanse by patting or blotting with an appropriate cleansing pad. Gently dry by patting or blotting with toilet tissue or a soft cloth before application of this product. Apply externally to the affected area up to five times daily. Children under 12 years of age—Consult a doctor.

How Supplied: Tronolane cream is available in 1-oz and 2-oz tubes. (FAN 2365-02)
Shown in Product Identification Guide, page 420

TRONOLANE®
[tron ′ə-lān]
Hemorrhoidal Suppositories

Description: The active ingredients in Tronolane suppositories are zinc oxide, 5%, and hard fat, 95%. Zinc oxide (an astringent) and hard fat (a skin protectant) afford temporary relief of hemorrhoidal itching and burning and protect irritated hemorrhoidal areas.

Indications: Tronolane suppositories are indicated for the temporary relief of the itching and burning associated with hemorrhoids and the protection of irritated hemorrhoidal areas.

Warnings: If condition worsens or does not improve within 7 days, consult a doctor. Do not exceed the recommended daily dosage, unless directed by a doctor. In case of bleeding, consult a doctor promptly. As with any drug, if you are pregnant or nursing a baby, seek the advice of a health care professional before using this product. **Do not store above 86°F.** Keep this and all drugs out of the reach of children.

Dosage and Administration (Directions): Adults—When practical, cleanse the affected area with mild soap and warm water and rinse thoroughly or cleanse by patting or blotting with an appropriate cleansing pad. Gently dry by patting or blotting with toilet tissue or a soft cloth before application of this product. Remove foil wrapper before inserting into the rectum. Use up to six times daily or after each bowel movement. Children under 12 years of age—Consult a doctor.

How Supplied: Tronolane suppositories are available in 10- and 20-count boxes. (FAN 2365)
Shown in Product Identification Guide, page 420

If desired, additional information on any Ross product will be provided upon request to Ross Products Division, Abbott Laboratories, Columbus, Ohio 43215-1724.

Rydelle Laboratories
Division of S. C. Johnson
& Son, Inc.
1525 HOWE STREET
RACINE, WI 53403

AVEENO® ANTI-ITCH
[ah-ve ′no]
CREAM AND LOTION
(External analgesic/Skin protectant)

AVEENO® Anti-Itch Cream provides fast temporary relief of the itching and pain associated with many minor skin irritations such as chicken pox rash, poison ivy/oak/sumac, and insect bites. Unlike hydrocortisone products, AVEENO® Anti-Itch Cream contains calamine to dry up weepy rashes and help control further spreading and promote healing. Aveeno's soothing oatmeal-enriched formula is non-greasy and invisible when rubbed into the skin.

Directions: Adults and children 2 years and older: Apply no more than 4 times daily. Children under 2: Consult a physician.

Warnings: For external use only. Avoid contact with eyes. If condition does not improve or recurs within 7 days, discontinue use and consult a physician. Keep out of children's reach. If ingested, contact a physician or poison control center. Store at 59°–86°F.

Active Ingredients: CALAMINE 3.0%, PRAMOXINE HCl 1.0%, CAMPHOR 0.3% IN A BASE OF WATER, GLYCERIN, DISTEARYLDIMONIUM CHLORIDE, PETROLATUM, OATMEAL FLOUR, ISOPROPYL PALMITATE, CETYL ALCOHOL, DIMETHICONE, SODIUM CHLORIDE.

How Supplied: 1 oz. tube of cream and 4 oz. bottle of lotion.
Shown in Product Identification Guide, page 420

AVEENO® BATH TREATMENTS
[ah-ve ′no]
REGULAR FORMULA AND MOISTURIZING FORMULA FOR DRY, ITCHY SKIN

AVEENO® BATH TREATMENTS contain colloidal oatmeal, a natural oat derivative developed especially for soothing and cleaning itchy, sore, sensitive skin.
AVEENO® BATH TREATMENTS contain no soaps that may be harmful to the skin. They cleanse naturally because of their unique adsorptive properties.
AVEENO® BATH TREATMENTS can be used for prompt temporary relief of itch due to dry skin, rashes, psoriasis, hemorrhoidal and genital irritations, poison ivy/oak, and sunburn. They are safe for use on children and can be used for prompt temporary relief of itch due to chicken pox, diaper rash, prickly heat and hives.

Ingredients: AVEENO® Bath Regular: 100% colloidal oatmeal; AVEENO®

Bath Moisturizing Formula: 43% colloidal oatmeal, mineral oil.
Shown in Product Identification Guide, page 420

AVEENO® CLEANSING BAR
[ah-ve ′no]
FOR COMBINATION SKIN

AVEENO® Cleansing Bar For Combination Skin is made especially for itchy, sensitive skin that is irritated by ordinary soaps.
More than 50% of this mild skin cleanser is colloidal oatmeal, noted for its soothing and protective qualities.
AVEENO® Cleansing Bar is completely soap-free. It leaves no harsh alkaline film to irritate delicate skin, and it leaves skin feeling soft and comfortable.

Ingredients: AVEENO® Colloidal Oatmeal, 51%; in a sudsing soap-free base containing a mild surfactant.
Shown in Product Identification Guide, page 420

AVEENO® CLEANSING BAR
[ah-ve ′no]
FOR ACNE-PRONE SKIN

AVEENO® Cleansing Bar For Acne-Prone Skin is a unique soap-free cleanser made with natural oatmeal. It absorbs and removes excess oil, but it won't overdry skin.

Ingredients: AVEENO® Colloidal Oatmeal, 51% in a sudsing soap-free base containing a mild surfactant.
Shown in Product Identification Guide, page 420

AVEENO® CLEANSING BAR
[ah-ve ′no]
FOR DRY SKIN

AVEENO® Cleansing Bar For Dry Skin is a unique, soap-free cleanser for itchy, dry, sensitive skin that is irritated by ordinary soaps. It contains over 15% skin-softening emollients to help replace natural skin oils and 51% colloidal oatmeal, recommended for its soothing and protective qualities.

Ingredients: AVEENO® Colloidal Oatmeal, 51%, in a sudsing soap-free base containing vegetable oils, glycerine, and a mild surfactant.
Shown in Product Identification Guide, page 420

AVEENO® MOISTURIZING CREAM
[ah-véno]
Soothing Therapy for Dry, Itchy Skin

Aveeno® Moisturizing Cream has been clinically proven to relieve dry skin. The natural colloidal oatmeal in Aveeno Cream allows it to go beyond soothing and moisturizing dry skin to provide prompt temporary relief from persistent itch. Aveeno Cream is noncomedogenic

Continued on next page

Rydelle—Cont.

and contains no fragrance, parabens, or lanolin which can cause allergic reactions. Cream formula is especially effective for extra-dry hands, feet and elbows.

Active Ingredient: Colloidal oatmeal 1% in a base of water, glycerin, distearyldimonium chloride, petrolatum, isopropyl palmitate, 1-hexadecanol, dimethicone, sodium chloride, phenylcarbinol. For External Use Only.

How Supplied: 4 oz. jar.
Shown in Product Identification Guide, page 420

AVEENO® MOISTURIZING LOTION
[ah-ve'no]
FOR RELIEF OF DRY, ITCHY SKIN

AVEENO® Moisturizing Lotion has been clinically proven to relieve dry skin. It contains natural colloidal oatmeal to relieve the itch often associated with dry skin. It is noncomedogenic and contains no fragrance, parabens, or lanolin which can cause allergic reactions.

Active Ingredient: Colloidal oatmeal 1%.
Also Contains: Water, glycerin, distearyldimonium chloride, petrolatum, isopropyl palmitate, cetyl alcohol, dimethicone, sodium chloride, phenylcarbinol.
Shown in Product Identification Guide, page 420

AVEENO® SHOWER AND BATH OIL
[ah-ve'no]
FOR RELIEF OF DRY, ITCHY SKIN

AVEENO® Shower and Bath Oil combines the lubricating properties of mineral oil with the natural anti-itch benefits of colloidal oatmeal for the relief of dry, itchy skin. It contains no fragrance, parabens or lanolin which can cause allergic reactions.

Active Ingredient: Colloidal oatmeal 4%.
Also contains: Mineral oil, laureth-4, quaternium-18 hectorite, phenylcarbinol, silica, benzaldehyde.
Shown in Product Identification Guide, page 420

RHULICREAM®
(External analgesic/Skin protectant)

Rhulicream® works on contact to provide fast, soothing, temporary relief of the itching and pain associated with many minor skin irritations. Apply this non-greasy calamine formula after exposure to poison ivy/oak/sumac to dry and help control further spreading and promote healing.

Directions: Adults and children 2 years and older: Apply to affected area

no more than 4 times daily. Children under 2: Consult a physician.

Warnings: For external use only. Avoid contact with eyes. If condition does not improve or recurs within 7 days, discontinue use and consult a physician. Keep out of children's reach. If ingested contact a physician or poison control center. Store at 59°–86°F.

Active Ingredients: CALAMINE 3.0%, PRAMOXINE HCl 1.0%, CAMPHOR 0.3% IN A BASE OF WATER, GLYCERIN, DISTEARYLDIMONIUM CHLORIDE, PETROLATUM, ISOPROPYL PALMITATE, CETYL ALCOHOL, DIMETHICONE, SODIUM CHLORIDE.

How Supplied: 2 oz. tube.
Shown in Product Identification Guide, page 420

RHULIGEL®
(External analgesic)

Rhuligel® provides fast, cooling, temporary relief of the itching and pain associated with many minor skin irritations, including poison ivy/oak/sumac, insect bites, and sunburn. Clear Rhuligel® is non-greasy and invisible on the skin. Won't stain clothing.

Directions: Adults and children 2 years and older: Apply to affected area no more than 4 times daily. Children under 2: Consult a physician.

Warnings: For external use only. Avoid contact with eyes. If condition does not improve or recurs within 7 days, discontinue use and consult a physician. Keep out of children's reach. If ingested contact a physician or poison control center. Store at 59°–86°F.

Active Ingredients: Benzyl Alcohol 2%, Menthol 0.3%, Camphor 0.3% in a base of SD Alcohol 23A 31% w/w, Purified Water, Propylene Glycol, Carbomer 940, Triethanolamine, Benzophenone-4, EDTA.

How Supplied: 2 oz. tube.
Shown in Product Identification Guide, page 420

RHULISPRAY®
(External analgesic/Skin protectant)

Rhulispray® works on contact to provide fast, cooling, temporary relief of the itching and pain associated with many minor skin irritations. Calamine-based formula dries the oozing and weeping of poison ivy/oak/sumac. Convenient spray action eliminates the need to touch delicate inflamed skin.

Directions: Shake well before use. Adults and children 2 years and older: Apply to affected area no more than 4 times daily. Children under 2: Consult a physician.

Warnings: For external use only. Avoid contact with eyes. If condition does not improve or recurs within 7 days, discontinue use and consult a physician.

Keep out of children's reach. If ingested contact a physician or poison control center. Store at 59°–86°F.

Caution: Flammable. Contents under pressure. Do not puncture or incinerate. Intentional misuse by deliberately concentrating and inhaling the contents can be harmful or fatal. Do not use near an open flame. May burst at temperatures above 120°F.

Active Ingredients (in concentrate): Calamine 13.8%, Benzocaine 5.0%, Camphor 0.7% in a base of Benzyl Alcohol, Hydrated Silica, Isobutane, Isopropyl Alcohol 70% w/w (concentrate), Oleyl Alcohol, Sorbitan Trioleate.

How Supplied: 4 oz. aerosol.
Shown in Product Identification Guide, page 420

Sandoz Pharmaceuticals/ Consumer Division
59 ROUTE 10
EAST HANOVER, NJ 07936

ACID MANTLE® CREME
[ă'sĭd-mănt'l]
Acid pH

Description: Restores and maintains protective acidity of the skin. Provides relief of mildly irritated skin due to exposure to soaps, detergents, chemicals and alkalis. Aids in the treatment of diaper rash; bath dermatitis; winter eczema and dry, rough, scaly skin of varied causes.

Ingredients: Water, cetostearyl alcohol, white petrolatum, glycerin, synthetic beeswax, light mineral oil, sodium lauryl sulfate, aluminum sulfate, calcium acetate, methylparaben, white potato dextrin.

Caution: For external use only. Avoid contact with the eyes.

Directions: Apply several times daily, especially after wet work.

How Supplied: 1 oz. tubes; 4 oz. and 1 lb. jars.

BiCOZENE® Creme External Analgesic
[bī-cō-zēn]

Active Ingredients: Benzocaine 6%, resorcinol 1.67% in a specially prepared cream base.

Inactive Ingredients: Castor Oil, Chlorothymol, Ethanolamine Stearates, Glycerin, Glyceryl Borate, Glyceryl Stearates, Parachlorometaxylenol, Polysorbate 80, Sodium Stearate, Triglycerol Diisostearate, Perfume.

Indications: For the temporary relief of pain and itching associated with minor burns, sunburn, minor cuts, scrapes, insect bites or minor skin irritations.

Actions: Benzocaine is a topical anesthetic and resorcinol is a topical antipruritic, at the concentrations used in BiCozene Creme. Both exert their actions by depressing cutaneous sensory receptors.

Warnings: Do not apply over large areas of the body. Caution: Use only as directed. Keep away from the eyes. Not for prolonged use. If the symptoms persist for more than seven days or clear up and reoccur within a few days, or if a rash or irritation develops, discontinue use and consult a physician. For external use only. **KEEP THIS AND ALL DRUGS OUT OF THE REACH OF CHILDREN.** In case of accidental ingestion, seek professional assistance or contact a Poison Control Center immediately.

Drug Interaction Precautions: No known drug interaction.

Dosage and Administration: Adults and children 2 years of age and older: apply to affected area not more than 3 to 4 times daily. Children under 2 years of age: consult a physician. Apply liberally to affected area as needed, several times a day.

How Supplied: BiCozene Creme is available in 1-ounce tubes.

Shown in Product Identification Guide, page 420

CAMA® ARTHRITIS PAIN RELIEVER
[kă 'măh]

Description: Each CAMA Inlay-Tab contains: aspirin USP, 500 mg (7.7 grains); magnesium oxide, USP, 150 mg; dried aluminum hydroxide gel, USP, equivalent to 125 mg aluminum hydroxide. Other ingredients: colloidal silicon dioxide, croscarmellose sodium, hydrogenated vegetable oil, methylcellulose, methylparaben, microcrystalline cellulose, polyethylene glycol, povidone, pregelatinized starch, starch, Yellow 6, Yellow 10.

Indications: For the temporary relief of minor arthritic pain.

Warnings: Children and teenagers should not use this medicine for chicken pox or flu symptoms before a doctor is consulted about Reye syndrome, a rare but serious illness reported to be associated with aspirin. If redness or swelling is present, consult a doctor because these could be signs of a serious condition. Do not take this drug if you have asthma unless directed by a doctor. Do not take this product if you have stomach problems (such as heartburn, upset stomach, or stomach pain) that persists or recurs, or if you have ulcers or bleeding problems, unless directed by a doctor. If pain persists for more than 10 days, consult a physician immediately. As with any drug, if you are pregnant or nursing a baby, seek the advice of a health professional before using this product. **IT IS ESPECIALLY IMPORTANT NOT TO**

USE ASPIRIN DURING THE LAST 3 MONTHS OF PREGNANCY UNLESS SPECIFICALLY DIRECTED TO DO SO BY A DOCTOR BECAUSE IT MAY CAUSE PROBLEMS IN THE UNBORN CHILD OR COMPLICATIONS DURING DELIVERY. Stop taking this product if ringing in the ears, loss of hearing, or dizziness occur. Do not take this product if you are presently taking a prescription drug for anticoagulation (thinning the blood), diabetes, arthritis, gout or if you have an aspirin allergy unless directed by a doctor. **Keep this and all medicines out of the reach of children. In case of accidental overdose, contact a physician immediately.**

Directions For Use: Adults: 2 tablets with a full glass of water every 6 hours. Not to exceed 8 tablets in 24 hours unless directed by a physician. Do not use in children under 12 years of age except under the advice and supervision of a physician.

How Supplied: CAMA Arthritis Pain Reliever Tablets (white with salmon inlay), imprinted "Cama 500" on one side, "Dorsey" on the other, in bottles of 100.

DORCOL® CHILDREN'S COUGH SYRUP
[door 'call]

Description: Each teaspoonful (5 ml) of DORCOL Children's Cough Syrup contains pseudoephedrine hydrochloride 15 mg, guaifenesin 50 mg, dextromethorphan hydrobromide 5 mg. Other ingredients: benzoic acid, Blue 1, edetate disodium, flavors, glycerin, propylene glycol, purified water, Red 40, sodium hydroxide, sucrose, tartaric acid.

Indications: Temporarily relieves your child's cough due to minor throat and bronchial irritation as may occur with the common cold. Helps loosen phlegm (mucus) and thin bronchial secretions to rid the bronchial passageways of bothersome mucus. Helps drain bronchial tubes and makes coughs more productive. Temporarily relieves nasal stuffiness due to the common cold, hay fever or upper respiratory allergies, and promotes nasal and/or sinus drainage.

Warnings: Keep this and all drugs out of the reach of children. In case of accidental overdose, seek professional assistance or contact a Poison Control Center immediately.
Except under the advice and supervision of a physician: Do not give your child more than the recommended dosage because at higher doses nervousness, dizziness or sleeplessness may occur. Do not give this preparation if your child has high blood pressure, heart disease, diabetes or thyroid disease. Do not give this product for persistent or chronic cough such as occurs with asthma or where cough is accompanied by excessive secretions. A persistent cough may be a sign of a serious condition. If cough or other

symptoms persist for more than one week, tend to recur or are accompanied by high fever, rash or persistent headache, consult a physician before continuing use.
Drug Interaction Precaution: Do not give this product to a child who is taking a prescription drug for high blood pressure or depression, without consulting a physician.

Directions For Use: Children under 2 years—consult physician.
By age:
Children 2 to under 6 years: 1 teaspoonful every 4 hours.
Children 6 to under 12 years: 2 teaspoonfuls every 4 hours.
By weight:
Children 25 to 45 pounds: 1 teaspoonful every 4 hours.
Children 46 to 85 pounds: 2 teaspoonfuls every 4 hours.
Unless directed by a physician, do not exceed 4 doses in 24 hours.

Professional Labeling: The suggested dosage for pediatric patients is:
3–12 months 3 drops/Kg of body weight every 4 hours
12–24 months 7 drops (0.2 ml)/Kg of body weight every 4 hours
Maximum 4 doses in 24 hours.

How Supplied: DORCOL Children's Cough Syrup (grape colored), in 4 fl oz and 8 fl oz plastic bottles with tamper-evident band around child-resistant cap.
Shown in Product Identification Guide, page 420

DORCOL® CHILDREN'S DECONGESTANT LIQUID
[door 'call]

Description: Each teaspoonful (5 ml) of DORCOL Children's Decongestant Liquid contains pseudoephedrine hydrochloride 15 mg. Other ingredients: benzoic acid, edetate disodium, flavors, purified water, sodium hydroxide, sorbitol, sucrose, Yellow 6, Yellow 10.

Indications: For temporary relief of nasal congestion due to the common cold, hay fever or other upper respiratory allergies, or associated with sinusitis. Reduces swelling of nasal passages; shrinks swollen membranes.

Warnings: Keep this and all drugs out of the reach of children. In case of accidental overdose, seek professional assistance or contact a Poison Control Center immediately. Do not give your child more than the recommended dosage because at higher doses nervousness, dizziness, or sleeplessness may occur. If symptoms do not improve within seven days or are accompanied by high fever, consult a physician before continuing use. Do not give this preparation if your child has high blood pressure, heart disease, diabetes, or thyroid disease unless directed by a doctor.

Continued on next page

Sandoz—Cont.

Drug Interaction Precaution: Do not give this product to a child who is taking a prescription drug for high blood pressure or depression without first consulting the child's doctor.

Directions For Use: Children under 2 years—consult physician.
By age:
Children 2 to under 6 years: 1 teaspoonful every 4 to 6 hours.
Children 6 years and older: 2 teaspoonfuls every 4 to 6 hours.
By weight:
Children 25 to 45 pounds: 1 teaspoonful every 4 hours.
Children 46 to 85 pounds: 2 teaspoonfuls every 4 hours.
Unless directed by a physician, do not exceed 4 doses in 24 hours.

Professional Labeling: The suggested dosage for pediatric patients is:
3–12 months 3 drops/Kg of body weight every 4–6 hours
12–24 months 7 drops (0.2 ml)/Kg of body weight every 4–6 hours
Maximum of 4 doses in 24 hours.

How Supplied: DORCOL Children's Decongestant Liquid (pale orange), in 4 fl oz bottles with tamper-evident band around child-resistant cap.

DORCOL® CHILDREN'S LIQUID COLD FORMULA
[*door 'call*]

Description: Each teaspoonful (5 ml) of DORCOL Children's Liquid Cold Formula contains: pseudoephedrine hydrochloride 15 mg and chlorpheniramine maleate 1 mg. Other ingredients: benzoic acid, Blue 1, flavors, purified water, Red 40, sorbitol, sucrose, Yellow 10. May also contain sodium hydroxide.

Indications: For temporary relief of nasal congestion, runny nose and sneezing due to the common cold, hay fever or other upper respiratory allergies. Temporarily relieves itchy, watery eyes or itching of the nose or throat due to hay fever or other upper respiratory allergies.

Warnings: Keep this and all drugs out of the reach of children. In case of accidental overdose, seek professional assistance or contact a Poison Control Center immediately.
Do not give your child more than the recommended dosage because at higher doses nervousness, dizziness, or sleeplessness may occur. Do not give this preparation if your child has high blood pressure, a breathing problem such as chronic bronchitis, heart disease, diabetes, thyroid disease, or glaucoma unless directed by a doctor. If symptoms do not improve within 7 days or are accompanied by high fever, consult a physician before continuing use. May cause drowsiness. Sedatives and tranquilizers may increase the drow-

siness effect. Do not give this product to children who are taking sedatives or tranquilizers without first consulting the child's doctor. May cause excitability, especially in children.
Drug Interaction Precaution: Do not give this product to a child who is taking a prescription drug for high blood pressure or depression, without first consulting the child's doctor.

Directions For Use: Children under 6 years—consult physician.
By age:
Children 6 to under 12 years: 2 teaspoonfuls every 4 to 6 hours.
By weight:
Children 45 to 85 pounds: 2 teaspoonfuls every 4 to 6 hours.
Unless directed by a physician, do not exceed 4 doses in 24 hours.

Professional Labeling: The suggested dosage for pediatric patients is:
3–12 months 2 drops/Kg of body weight every 4–6 hours
12–24 months 5 drops (0.2 ml)/Kg of body weight every 4–6 hours
2–6 years 1 teaspoonful every 4–6 hours
Maximum of 4 doses in 24 hours.

How Supplied: DORCOL Children's Liquid Cold Formula (light brown), in 4 fl oz bottles with tamper-evident band around child-resistant cap.

EX–LAX® Chocolated Laxative Tablets

Active Ingredient: Yellow phenolphthalein, 90 mg. phenolphthalein per tablet.

Inactive Ingredients: Cocoa, Confectioners' Sugar, Hydrogenated Palm Kernel Oil, Lecithin, Nonfat Dry Milk, Vanillin.

Indication: For relief of occasional constipation (irregularity).

Caution: Do not take any laxative when abdominal pain, nausea, or vomiting are present. Frequent or prolonged use of this or any other laxative may result in dependence on laxatives. If skin rash appears, do not use this or any other preparation containing phenolphthalein.

Warnings: Keep this and all drugs out of the reach of children. In case of accidental overdose, seek professional assistance or contact a poison control center immediately. As with any drug, if you are pregnant or nursing a baby, seek the advice of a health care professional before using this product.

Dosage and Administration: Adults and children 12 years old and over: Chew 1 to 2 tablets, preferably at bedtime. Children over 6 years: Chew ½ tablet.

How Supplied: Available in boxes of 6, 18, 48, and 72 chewable chocolate-flavored tablets.

Shown in Product Identification Guide, page 420

EX–LAX® Laxative Pills
Regular Strength Ex-Lax® **Laxative Pills**
Extra Gentle Ex-Lax® Laxative Pills
Maximum Relief Formula Ex-Lax® Laxative Pills
Ex-Lax® Gentle Nature® Laxative Pills

Active Ingredients: Regular Strength Ex-Lax Laxative Pills—Yellow phenolphthalein, 90 mg. phenolphthalein per pill. **Extra Gentle Ex-Lax Laxative Pills**—Docusate sodium, 75 mg. and yellow phenolphthalein, 65 mg. per pill. **Maximum Relief Formula Ex-Lax Laxative Pills**—Yellow phenolphthalein, 135 mg. phenolphthalein per pill. **Ex-Lax Gentle Nature Laxative Pills**—Sennosides, 20 mg. per pill.

Inactive Ingredients: Regular Strength Ex-Lax Laxative Pills—Acacia, Alginic Acid, Carnauba Wax, Colloidal Silicon Dioxide, Dibasic Calcium Phosphate, Iron Oxides, Magnesium Stearate, Microcrystalline Cellulose, Sodium Benzoate, Sodium Lauryl Sulfate, Starch, Stearic Acid, Sucrose, Talc, Titanium Dioxide. **Extra Gentle Ex-Lax Laxative Pills**—Acacia, Croscarmellose Sodium, Dibasic Calcium Phosphate, Colloidal Silicon Dioxide, Magnesium Stearate, Microcrystalline Cellulose, Red 7, Stearic Acid, Sucrose, Talc, Titanium Dioxide. **Maximum Relief Formula Ex-Lax Laxative Pills**—Acacia, Alginic Acid, Blue No. 1, Carnauba Wax, Colloidal Silicon Dioxide, Dibasic Calcium Phosphate, Magnesium Stearate, Microcrystalline Cellulose, Povidone, Sodium Benzoate, Sodium Lauryl Sulfate, Starch, Stearic Acid, Sucrose, Talc, Titanium Dioxide. **Ex-Lax Gentle Nature Laxative Pills**—Alginic Acid, Colloidal Silicon Dioxide, Dibasic Calcium Phosphate, Magnesium Stearate, Microcrystalline Cellulose, Pregelatinized Starch, Sodium Lauryl Sulfate, Stearic Acid.

Indication: For relief of occasional constipation (irregularity).

Caution: Do not take any laxative when abdominal pain, nausea, or vomiting are present. Frequent or prolonged use of this or any other laxative may result in dependence on laxatives. If skin rash appears, do not use this or any other preparation containing phenolphthalein.

Warnings: Keep this and all drugs out of the reach of children. In case of accidental overdose, seek professional assistance or contact a Poison Control Center immediately. As with any drug, if you are pregnant or nursing a baby, seek the advice of a health care professional before using this product.

Dosage and Administration: Regular Strength Ex-Lax Laxative Pills, Extra Gentle Ex-Lax Laxative Pills, and Ex-Lax Gentle Nature Laxative Pills—Adults and children 12 years old and over: Take 1 to 2 pills with a glass of water, preferably at bedtime. Consult with a physician for children under 12 years of age. **Maximum Relief Formula Ex-Lax Laxative Pills**—Adults and children over 12 years of age, take 1 to 2 pills with a glass of water, preferably at bedtime. Consult with a physician for children under 12 years of age.

How Supplied: Extra Strength Ex-Lax Laxative Pills—Available in boxes of 8, 30, and 60 pills. **Extra Gentle Ex-Lax Laxative Pills and Maximum Relief Formula Ex-Lax Laxative Pills**—Available in boxes of 24 pills. **Ex-Lax Gentle Nature Laxative Pills**—Available in boxes of 16 pills.
Shown in Product Identification Guide, page 420

GAS-X® AND EXTRA STRENGTH GAS-X®
Antiflatulent, Anti-Gas Tablets

Active Ingredients: GAS-X®—Each tablet contains 80 mg. simethicone. EXTRA STRENGTH GAS-X®—Each tablet contains 125 mg. simethicone.

Inactive Ingredients: calcium phosphates dibasic and tribasic, calcium silicate, colloidal silicon dioxide, compressible sugar, microcrystalline cellulose and talc. GAS-X cherry creme flavored tablets also contain Red 30. Extra Strength GAS-X peppermint creme and Extra Strength GAS-X cherry creme flavored tablets also contain Red 30 and Yellow 10.

Indications: For relief of the pain and pressure symptoms of excess gas in the digestive tract, which is often accompanied by complaints of bloating, distention, fullness, pressure, pain, cramps or excess anal flatus.

Actions: GAS-X acts in the stomach and intestines to disperse and reduce the formation of mucus-trapped gas bubbles. The GAS-X defoaming action reduces the surface tension of gas bubbles so that they are more easily eliminated.

Warning: Keep this and all medicines out of the reach of children.

Drug Interaction Precautions: No known drug interaction.

Dosage and Administration: Adults: Chew thoroughly and swallow one or two tablets as needed after meals and at bedtime. Do not exceed six GAS-X tablets or four EXTRA STRENGTH GAS-X tablets in 24 hours, except under the advice and supervision of a physician.

Professional Labeling: GAS-X may be useful in the alleviation of postoperative gas pain, and for use in endoscopic examination.

How Supplied: GAS-X is available in peppermint creme and cherry creme flavored, chewable, scored tablets in boxes of 36 tablets and 12 tablets. EXTRA STRENGTH GAS-X is available in peppermint creme and cherry creme flavored, chewable, scored tablets in boxes of 18 tablets and 48 tablets.
Shown in Product Identification Guide, pages 420 and 421

TAVIST-1® TABLETS

Description: Each tablet contains: clemastine fumarate, USP, 1.34 mg (equivalent to 1 mg clemastine). Other ingredients: lactose, povidone, starch, stearic acid, and talc.

Indications: Temporarily reduces runny nose and relieves sneezing, itching of the nose or throat, and itchy, watery eyes due to hay fever or other upper respiratory allergies.

Warnings: May cause drowsiness; alcohol, sedatives, and tranquilizers may increase the drowsiness effect. Do not take this product if you are taking sedatives or tranquilizers without first consulting your doctor. Use caution when driving a motor vehicle or operating machinery. May cause excitability especially in children. Do not take this product if you have asthma, glaucoma, emphysema, chronic pulmonary disease, shortness of breath, difficulty in breathing, or difficulty in urination due to enlargement of the prostate gland unless directed by a doctor. As with any drug, if you are pregnant or nursing a baby, seek the advice of a health professional before using this product. Keep this and all drugs out of reach of children. In case of accidental overdose, seek professional assistance or contact a Poison Control Center immediately.

Directions: Adults and children 12 years of age and over: Take one tablet every 12 hours, not to exceed 2 tablets in 24 hours, or as directed by a doctor. Children under 12 years: Consult a doctor.

How Supplied: Tavist-1 tablets (white) imprinted "Tavist-1" on both sides in blister packs of 8 and 16.
Shown in Product Identification Guide, page 421

TAVIST-D® TABLETS

Description: Each tablet contains: clemastine fumarate, USP, 1.34 mg (equivalent to 1 mg clemastine) immediate release and 75 mg phenylpropanolamine hydrochloride, USP, extended release. Other ingredients: Colloidal silicon dioxide, dibasic calcium phosphate, lactose, magnesium stearate, methylcellulose, polyethylene glycol, povidone, starch, synthetic polymers, titanium dioxide and Yellow 10.

Indications: For the temporary relief of nasal congestion associated with upper respiratory allergies or sinusitis when accompanied by other symptoms of hay fever or allergies, including runny nose, sneezing, itchy nose or throat or itchy, watery eyes.

Warnings: May cause drowsiness; alcohol, sedatives, and tranquilizers may increase the drowsiness effect. Avoid alcoholic beverages while taking this product. Do not take this product if you are taking sedatives or tranquilizers without first consulting your doctor. Use caution when driving a motor vehicle or operating machinery. May cause excitability especially in children. **Do not exceed recommended dosage because at higher doses nervousness, dizziness, or sleeplessness may occur.** Do not take this product for more than 7 days. If symptoms do not improve or are accompanied by fever, consult a doctor. Do not take this product if you have asthma, diabetes, glaucoma, heart disease, emphysema, chronic pulmonary disease, shortness of breath, difficulty in breathing, or difficulty in urination due to enlargement of the prostate gland unless directed by a doctor. As with any drug, if you are pregnant or nursing a baby, seek the advice of a health professional before using this product. Keep this and all drugs out of reach of children. In case of accidental overdose, seek professional assistance or contact a Poison Control Center immediately.

Drug Interaction Precaution: Do not take this product if you are presently taking a decongestant or prescription drug for high blood pressure or depression, without first consulting your doctor.

Directions: Adults and children 12 years of age and over: Take one tablet swallowed whole every 12 hours, not to exceed 2 tablets in 24 hours, or as directed by a doctor. Children under 12 years: Consult a doctor.

How Supplied: Tavist-D tablets (white) imprinted "Tavist-D" on both sides, in blister packs of 8 and 16.
Shown in Product Identification Guide, page 421

THERAFLU®
Flu and Cold Medicine
Flu, Cold & Cough Medicine

Description: Each packet of TheraFlu Flu and Cold Medicine contains: acetaminophen 650 mg, pseudoephedrine hydrochloride 60 mg, and chlorpheniramine maleate 4 mg. Each packet of TheraFlu Flu, Cold & Cough Medicine also contains dextromethorphan hydrobromide 20 mg. Other ingredients: ascorbic acid (vitamin C), citric acid, natural lemon flavors, sodium citrate, sucrose, titanium dioxide, tribasic calcium phosphate, pregelatinized starch, Yellow 6, and Yellow 10.

Indications: Provides temporary relief of the symptoms associated with flu, common cold and other upper respiratory infections including: headache, body-aches, fever, minor sore throat pain, nasal and sinus congestion, runny nose and

Continued on next page

Sandoz—Cont.

sneezing. TheraFlu Flu, Cold & Cough Medicine also suppresses coughs due to minor throat and bronchial irritation.

Warnings: Keep this and all drugs out of the reach of children. In case of accidental overdose, contact a doctor or a Poison Control Center immediately. Prompt medical attention is critical for adults as well as children even if you do not notice any signs or symptoms.

Do not take this product for more than 7 days. Do not exceed recommended dosage because at higher doses nervousness, dizziness, or sleeplessness may occur. May cause excitability, especially in children. Unless directed by a doctor, do not take this product if you have heart disease, high blood pressure, thyroid disease, diabetes, glaucoma, a breathing problem such as emphysema or chronic bronchitis, or difficulty in urination due to enlargement of the prostate gland.

Unless directed by a doctor, do not take this product for fever for more than 3 days. If pain or fever persists or gets worse, if new symptoms occur, or if redness or swelling is present, consult a doctor because these could be signs of a serious condition. If sore throat is severe, persists for more than 2 days, is accompanied or followed by fever, headache, rash, nausea, or vomiting, consult a doctor promptly.

May cause marked drowsiness. Alcohol, sedatives, and tranquilizers may increase the drowsiness effect. Avoid alcoholic beverages while taking this product. Do not take this product if you are taking sedatives or tranquilizers without first consulting your doctor. Use caution when driving a motor vehicle or operating machinery.

Do not take the Flu, Cold & Cough formula for persistent or chronic cough such as occurs with smoking, asthma, or emphysema, or if cough is accompanied by excessive phlegm (mucus) unless directed by a doctor. A persistent cough may be a sign of a serious condition. If cough persists for more than 1 week, tends to recur, or is accompanied by a fever, rash, or persistent headache, consult a doctor.

As with any drug, if you are pregnant or nursing a baby, seek the advice of a health professional before using this product.

Drug Interaction Precaution: Do not take this product if you are presently taking a prescription drug for high blood pressure or depression without first consulting your doctor.

Dosage and Administration: Adults and children 12 years and over—dissolve one packet in 6 oz. cup of hot water. Sip while hot. Microwave Heating Instructions: Add contents of packet and 6 oz. of cool water to a microwave safe cup and stir briskly. Microwave on high 1½ minutes or until hot. Do not boil water or overheat and remember to stir liquid between reheatings. Sweeten to taste if de-

sired. May repeat every 4 hours, but not to exceed 4 doses in 24 hours.

How Supplied: TheraFlu Flu and Cold Medicine powder in foil packets, 6 or 12 packets per carton. TheraFlu Flu, Cold & Cough Medicine powder in foil packets, 6 or 12 packets per carton.

Shown in Product Identification Guide, page 421

THERAFLU®
MAXIMUM STRENGTH NIGHTTIME
Flu, Cold & Cough Medicine

Description: Each packet of TheraFlu Maximum Strength Nighttime Flu, Cold & Cough Medicine contains: acetaminophen 1000 mg, dextromethorphan HBr 30 mg, pseudoephedrine HCl 60 mg, and chlorpheniramine maleate 4 mg. Other ingredients: ascorbic acid (Vitamin C), citric acid, natural lemon flavors, maltol, pregelatinized starch, silicon dioxide, sodium citrate, sucrose, titanium dioxide, tribasic calcium phosphate, Yellow 6 and Yellow 10.

Indications: Provides temporary relief of the symptoms associated with flu, common cold and other upper respiratory infections including: headache, body aches, fever, minor sore throat pain, nasal and sinus congestion, runny nose, sneezing, watery and itchy eyes. TheraFlu Maximum Strength Flu, Cold, & Cough Medicine also suppresses coughs due to minor throat and bronchial irritation.

Warnings: Keep this and all drugs out of the reach of children. In case of accidental overdose, contact a doctor or a Poison Control Center immediately. Prompt medical attention is critical for adults as well as children even if you do not notice any signs or symptoms.

Do not take this product for more than 7 days. Do not exceed recommended dosage because at higher doses nervousness, dizziness, or sleeplessness may occur. May cause excitability, especially in children. Unless directed by a doctor, do not take this product if you have heart disease, high blood pressure, thyroid disease, diabetes, glaucoma, a breathing problem such as emphysema or chronic bronchitis, or difficulty in urination due to enlargement of the prostate gland.

A persistent cough may be a sign of a serious condition. If cough persists for more than one week, tends to recur, or is accompanied by a fever, rash, or persistent headache, consult a doctor. Do not take this product for persistent or chronic cough such as occurs with smoking, asthma, or emphysema, or if cough is accompanied by excessive phlegm (mucus) unless directed by a doctor.

Unless directed by a doctor, do not take this product for fever for more than 3 days. If pain or fever persists or gets worse, if new symptoms occur, or if redness or swelling is present, consult a doctor because these could be signs of a serious condition. If sore throat is severe,

persists for more than 2 days, is accompanied or followed by fever, headache, rash, nausea, or vomiting, consult a doctor promptly.

May cause marked drowsiness. Alcohol, sedatives, and tranquilizers may increase the drowsiness effect. Avoid alcoholic beverages while taking this product. Do not take this product if you are taking sedatives or tranquilizers without first consulting your doctor. Use caution when driving a motor vehicle or operating machinery.

As with any drug, if you are pregnant or nursing a baby, seek the advice of a health professional before using this product.

Drug Interaction Precaution: Do not take this product if you are presently taking a prescription drug for high blood pressure or depression without first consulting your doctor.

Directions: Adults and children 12 years and over: Dissolve one packet in 6 oz. cup of hot water. Sip while hot. Microwave Heating Instructions: Add contents of packet and 6 oz. of cool water to a microwave safe cup and stir briskly. Microwave on high 1½ minutes or until water is hot. Do not boil water or overheat and remember to stir liquid between reheatings. Sweeten to taste if desired. May repeat every 6 hours, but not to exceed 4 doses in 24 hours.

How Supplied: TheraFlu Maximum Strength Nighttime Flu, Cold, & Cough Medicine powder in foil packets, 6 or 12 packets per carton.

Shown in Product Identification Guide, page 421

THERAFLU®
MAXIMUM STRENGTH
NON-DROWSY FORMULA
Flu, Cold & Cough Medicine

Description: Each packet of TheraFlu Maximum Strength Non-Drowsy Formula contains: acetaminophen 1000 mg, dextromethorphan 30 mg, pseudoephedrine HCl 60 mg. Other Ingredients: ascorbic acid (Vitamin C), citric acid, natural lemon flavors, maltol, pregelatinized starch, silicon dioxide, sodium citrate, sucrose, titanium dioxide, tribasic calcium phosphate, Yellow 6 and Yellow 10.

Indications: Provides temporary relief of the symptoms associated with flu, common cold, and other upper respiratory infections including: headache, body aches, fever, minor sore throat pain, nasal and sinus congestion, runny nose, sneezing, watery and itchy eyes. TheraFlu Maximum Strength Non-Drowsy Formula also suppresses coughs due to minor throat and bronchial irritation.

Warnings: Keep this and all drugs out of the reach of children. In case of accidental overdose, seek professional assistance or contact a Poison Control Center immediately. Prompt medical attention is critical for adults as well as children even if you do not notice any signs or symptoms.

Do not take this product for more than 7 days. Do not exceed recommended dosage because at higher doses nervousness, dizziness, or sleeplessness may occur. Unless directed by a doctor, do not take this product if you have heart disease, high blood pressure, thyroid disease, diabetes, or difficulty in urination due to enlargement of the prostate gland.

A persistent cough may be the sign of a serious condition. If cough persists for more than 1 week, tends to recur, or is accompanied by a fever, rash, or persistent headache, consult a doctor. Do not take this product for persistent or chronic cough such as occurs with smoking, asthma, or emphysema, or if cough is accompanied by excessive phlegm (mucus) unless directed by a doctor.

Unless directed by a doctor, do not take this product for fever for more than 3 days. If pain or fever persists or gets worse, if new symptoms occur, or if redness or swelling is present, consult a doctor, because these could be signs of a serious condition. If sore throat is severe, persists for more than 2 days, is accompanied or followed by fever, headache, rash, nausea, or vomiting, consult a doctor promptly.

As with any drug, if you are pregnant or nursing a baby, seek the advice of a health professional before using this product.

Drug Interaction Precaution: Do not take this product if you are presently taking a prescription drug for high blood pressure or depression without first consulting your doctor.

Directions: Adults and children 12 years and over: Dissolve one packet in 6 oz. cup of hot water; sip while hot. Microwave Heating Instructions: Add contents of packet and 6 oz. of cool water to a microwave safe cup and stir briskly. Microwave on high 1 1/2 minutes or until hot. Do not boil or overheat, and remember to stir liquid between reheatings. Sweeten to taste if desired. May repeat every 6 hours, but not to exceed 4 doses in 24 hours.

Shown in Product Identification Guide, page 421

TRIAMINIC® ALLERGY TABLETS
[trī"ah-mĭn'ĭc]

Description: Each tablet contains: phenylpropanolamine hydrochloride 25 mg and chlorpheniramine maleate 4 mg. Other ingredients: calcium stearate, calcium sulfate, colloidal silicon dioxide, methylcellulose, methylparaben, microcrystalline cellulose, polyethylene glycol, povidone, pregelatinized starch, titanium dioxide, Yellow 10.

Indications: For the temporary relief of runny nose, nasal congestion, sneezing, itching of the eyes, nose or throat and watery eyes as may occur in hay fever or other upper respiratory allergies (allergic rhinitis).

Warnings: Do not take this product if you have high blood pressure, heart disease, diabetes, thyroid disease, asthma, glaucoma, a breathing problem such as emphysema or chronic bronchitis, or difficulty in urination due to enlargement of the prostate gland or are taking a prescription drug for high blood pressure or depression unless directed by a doctor. Do not exceed the recommended dosage because at higher doses nervousness, dizziness or sleeplessness may occur, or take for more than 7 days. This preparation may cause drowsiness; alcohol, sedatives and tranquilizers may increase the drowsiness effect; avoid alcoholic beverages; do not operate machinery or drive a motor vehicle while taking this product; this preparation may cause excitability, especially in children. If symptoms do not improve within seven days or are accompanied by high fever, consult a doctor. As with any drug, if you are pregnant or nursing a baby, seek the advice of a health professional before using this product. Keep this and all drugs out of the reach of children. In case of accidental overdose, seek professional assistance or contact a Poison Control Center immediately.

Directions: Adults and children over 12 years of age—1 tablet every 4 hours. Children 6 to under 12 years, ½ tablet every 4 hours. Unless directed by physician, do not exceed 6 doses in 24 hours or give to children under 6 years.

How Supplied: Triaminic Allergy Tablets (yellow), scored, in blister packs of 24.

TRIAMINIC® CHEWABLES
[trī"ah-mĭn'ĭc]

Description: Each TRIAMINIC Chewable contains: phenylpropanolamine hydrochloride 6.25 mg, chlorpheniramine maleate 0.5 mg. Other ingredients: calcium stearate, citric acid, flavors, magnesium trisilicate, mannitol, microcrystalline cellulose, saccharin sodium, sucrose, Yellow 6, Yellow 10.

Indications: For the temporary relief of children's nasal congestion, runny nose, and sneezing due to the common cold or hay fever.

Warnings: Do not exceed recommended dosage because at higher doses nervousness, dizziness, or sleeplessness may occur. Do not give this product to children for more than 7 days. If symptoms do not improve or are accompanied by fever, consult a doctor. Do not give this product to children who have heart disease, high blood pressure, thyroid disease, diabetes, asthma, a breathing problem such as chronic bronchitis, or who have glaucoma, unless directed by a doctor. May cause drowsiness. Sedatives and tranquilizers may increase the drowsiness effect. May cause excitability.

Drug Interaction Precaution: Do not give this product to a child who is taking a

prescription drug for high blood pressure or depression, without first consulting the child's doctor. Keep this and all drugs out of the reach of children. In case of accidental overdose, seek professional assistance or contact a Poison Control Center immediately.

Dosage: Children 6 to 12 years—2 tablets every 4 hours. Children under 6, consult your physician.

Professional Labeling: The suggested dosage for children 2 to 6 years is 1 tablet every 4 hours.

How Supplied: TRIAMINIC Chewables (hexagonal, yellow), in blister packs of 24. Orange flavor.

TRIAMINIC® COLD TABLETS
[trī"ah-mĭn'ĭc]

Description: Each tablet contains: phenylpropanolamine hydrochloride 12.5 mg and chlorpheniramine maleate 2 mg. Other ingredients: calcium stearate, colloidal silicon dioxide, flavor, lactose, methylcellulose, methylparaben, microcrystalline cellulose, polyethylene glycol, povidone, pregelatinized starch, Red 40, saccharin sodium, titanium dioxide, Yellow 6.

Indications: For the temporary relief of nasal congestion due to the common cold, hay fever or other upper respiratory allergies and symptoms associated with sinusitis. Helps decongest sinus openings, sinus passages, promotes nasal and/or sinus drainage, temporarily restores freer breathing through the nose. For temporary relief of runny nose, sneezing, itching of the nose or throat and itchy and watery eyes as may occur in allergic rhinitis (such as hay fever).

Warnings: Do not take this product if you have high blood pressure, heart disease, diabetes, thyroid disease, glaucoma, a breathing problem such as emphysema or chronic bronchitis, or difficulty in urination due to enlargement of the prostate gland or are taking a prescription drug for high blood pressure or depression unless directed by a doctor. Do not exceed the recommended dosage because at higher doses nervousness, dizziness or sleeplessness may occur or take for more than 7 days. This preparation may cause drowsiness; alcohol, sedatives and tranquilizers may increase the drowsiness effect; avoid alcoholic beverages; do not operate machinery or drive a motor vehicle while taking this product; this preparation may cause excitability, especially in children. If symptoms do not improve within seven days or are accompanied by high fever, consult a doctor. As with any drug, if you are pregnant or nursing a baby, seek the advice of a health professional before using this product. Keep this and all drugs out of the reach of children. In case of accidental overdose, seek professional assistance

Continued on next page

Sandoz—Cont.

or contact a Poison Control Center immediately.

Directions: Adults and children 12 years of age and older: 2 tablets every 4 hours. Children 6 to under 12 years, 1 tablet every 4 hours. Unless directed by physician, do not exceed 6 doses in 24 hours or give to children under 6 years.

How Supplied: Triaminic Cold Tablets (orange) imprinted "DORSEY" on one side, "TRIAMINIC" on the other, in blister packs of 24.

Shown in Product Identification Guide, page 421

TRIAMINIC® EXPECTORANT
[*trī"ah-mĭn'ĭc*]

Description: Each teaspoonful (5 ml) of TRIAMINIC Expectorant contains: phenylpropanolamine hydrochloride 6.25 mg and guaifenesin 50 mg in a palatable, citrus-flavored alcohol-free liquid. Other ingredients: benzoic acid, edetate disodium, flavors, purified water, saccharin, saccharin sodium, sodium hydroxide, sorbitol, sucrose, Yellow 6, Yellow 10.

Indications: Relieves chest congestion by loosening phlegm to help clear bronchial passageways. Temporarily relieves stuffy nose.

Warnings: Keep this and all drugs out of the reach of children. In case of accidental overdose, seek professional assistance or contact a Poison Control Center immediately.
Do not exceed recommended dosage because at higher doses nervousness, dizziness, or sleeplessness may occur. Do not take for more than 7 days. If syptoms persist, are accompanied by fever, rash or persistent headache, or if cough recurs, consult a doctor. A persistent cough may be a sign of a serious condition. Do not take this product: 1) if cough is accompanied by excessive phlegm (sputum), 2) for persistent or chronic cough such as occurs with smoking, asthma, chronic bronchitis or emphysema, or 3) if you have heart disease, high blood pressure, thyroid disease, diabetes, difficulty in urination due to enlargement of the prostate gland, or are taking a prescription drug for high blood pressure or depression.
As with any drug, if you are pregnant or nursing a baby, seek the advice of a health professional before using this product.

Dosage and Administration: Adults and children 12 and over (96+ lbs)—4 teaspoons every 4 hours. Children 6 to under 12 years (48–95 lbs)—2 teaspoons every 4 hours. Children 2 to under 6 years (24–47 lbs)—1 teaspoon every 4 hours. Unless directed by physician, do not exceed 6 doses in 24 hours or give to children under 2 years of age. For convenience, a True-Dose® dosage cup is provided with each 4 fl. oz. and 8 fl. oz. bottle.

Professional Labeling: The suggested dosage for pediatric patients is:
3–12 months 1.25 ml (¼ tsp)
(12–17 lbs)   every 4 hours
12–24 months 2.5 ml (½ tsp)
(18–23 lbs)   every 4 hours

How Supplied: TRIAMINIC Expectorant (yellow), in 4 fl oz and 8 fl oz plastic bottles with tamper-evident band around child-resistant cap. Citrus flavored, Alcohol free.

Shown in Product Identification Guide, page 421

TRIAMINIC® NITE LIGHT®
Nighttime Cough and Cold Medicine for Children
[*tri"ah-min'ic*]

Description: Each teaspoonful (5 ml) of Triaminic® Nite Light® contains: Pseudoephedrine hydrochloride 15 mg, chlorpheniramine maleate 1 mg, dextromethorphan hydrobromide 7.5 mg in a palatable, grape-flavored, alcohol-free liquid. Other ingredients: benzoic acid, Blue 1, citric acid, flavors, propylene glycol, purified water, Red 33, dibasic sodium phosphate, sorbitol, sucrose.

Indications: Temporarily relieves cold symptoms, including coughs due to minor throat and bronchial irritation, runny nose, stuffy nose, sneezing, itching nose or throat and itchy, watery eyes.

Warnings: Keep this and all drugs out of the reach of children. In case of accidental overdose, seek professional assistance or contact a Poison Control Center immediately.
Do not exceed recommended dosage because at higher doses nervousness, dizziness, or sleeplessness may occur. Do not take for more than 7 days. If symptoms persist, are accompanied by fever, rash or persistent headache, or if cough recurs, consult a doctor. A persistent cough may be a sign of a serious condition. Do not take this product: 1) if cough is accompanied by excessive phlegm (sputum), 2) for persistent or chronic cough such as occurs with smoking, asthma or emphysema, or 3) if you have heart disease, high blood pressure, thyroid disease, diabetes, glaucoma, a breathing problem such as emphysema or chronic bronchitis, or difficulty in urination due to enlargement of the prostate gland, 4) if you are taking a prescription drug for high blood pressure or depression, or 5) if you are taking sedatives or tranquilizers, unless directed by a doctor. May cause excitability, especially in children. May cause drowsiness. Alcohol, sedatives or tranquilizers may increase drowsiness. Avoid driving or operating machinery while taking this product.
As with any drug, if you are pregnant or nursing a baby, seek the advice of a health professional before using this product.

Dosage and Administration: Adults and children 12 and over (96+ lbs.)—4

teaspoons every 6 hours. Children 6 to under 12 years (48–95 lbs.)—2 teaspoons every 6 hours. Unless directed by physician, do not exceed 4 doses in 24 hours or give to children under 6 years of age. For convenience, a True-Dose® dosage cup is provided with each 4 fl. oz. and 8 fl. oz. bottle.

Professional Labeling: The suggested dosage for pediatric patients is:
3 to under   ¼ teaspoon or 1.25 ml
12 months
(12–17 lbs.)
12 months to   ½ teaspoon or 2.5 ml
under 2 years
(18–23 lbs.)
2 to under   1 teaspoon or 5 ml
6 years

How Supplied: Triaminic® Nite Light® Nighttime Cough and Cold Medicine for Children (purple), in 4 fl. oz. and 8 fl. oz. plastic bottles packaged in cartons with tamper-evident band around child-resistant cap. Grape flavored. Alcohol free.

Shown in Product Identification Guide, page 421

TRIAMINIC®
Sore Throat Formula
[*trī"ah-mĭn'ĭc*]

Description: Each teaspoonful (5 ml) of Triaminic Sore Throat Formula contains: acetaminophen, USP 160 mg, dextromethorphan hydrobromide, USP 7.5 mg, and pseudoephedrine hydrochloride, USP 15 mg. in a palatable, grape-flavored, alcohol-free liquid. Other ingredients: benzoic acid, Blue 1, dibasic sodium phosphate, edetate disodium, flavors, glycerin, polyethylene glycol, propylene glycol, purified water, Red 33, Red 40, sucrose, tartaric acid.

Indications: Temporarily relieves sore throat pain and other minor aches and pains, quiets coughs due to minor throat and bronchial irritations, relieves stuffy noses, and reduces fever.

Warnings: Keep this and all drugs out of the reach of children. In case of accidental overdose, seek professional assistance or contact a Poison Control Center immediately. Prompt medical attention is critical for adults as well as for children even if you do not notice any signs or symptoms.
Do not exceed recommended dosage because at higher doses nervousness, dizziness, or sleeplessness may occur. Do not take this product for more than 4 days. If symptoms persist or new ones occur, if sore throat is severe or persists for more than 2 days, if fever persists for more than 3 days, if symptoms are accompanied by rash, fever, nausea, vomiting, persistent headache or if cough recurs, consult a doctor. A persistent cough may be the sign of a serious condition. Do not take this product: 1) if cough is accompanied by excessive phlegm (mucus), 2) for persistent or chronic cough such as occurs with smoking, asthma or emphy-

sema, or 3) if you have heart disease, high blood pressure, thyroid disease, diabetes, difficulty in urination due to enlargement of the prostate gland, or are taking a prescription drug for high blood pressure or depression, unless directed by a doctor.

As with any drug, if you are pregnant or nursing a baby, seek advice from a health professional before using this product.

Dosage and Administration: Adults and children 12 and over (96+lbs)—4 teaspoons every 6 hours. Children 6 to under 12 years (48–95 lbs)—2 teaspoons every 6 hours. Children 2 to under 6 years (24–47 lbs)—1 teaspoon every 6 hours. Unless directed by a physician, do not exceed 4 doses in 24 hours or give to children under 2 years of age. For convenience, a True-Dose® dosage cup is provided with each 4 fl. oz and 8 fl. oz. bottle.

Professional Labeling: The suggested dosage for pediatric patients is:

3–12 months	1.25 ml (¼ tsp)
(12–17 lbs)	every 6 hours
12–24 months	2.5 ml (½ tsp)
(18–23 lbs)	every 6 hours
2–6 years	5 ml (1 tsp)
(24–47 lbs)	every 6 hours

How Supplied: Triaminic Sore Throat Formula (purple), in 4 fl. oz. and 8 fl. oz. plastic bottles with tamper-evident band around child resistant cap. Grape flavored, alcohol-free.

Shown in Product Identification Guide, page 421

TRIAMINIC® SYRUP
[*trī"ah-mĭn'ĭc*]

Description: Each teaspoonful (5 ml) of TRIAMINIC Syrup contains: phenylpropanolamine hydrochloride 6.25 mg and chlorpheniramine maleate 1 mg in a palatable, orange-flavored, alcohol-free liquid. Other ingredients: benzoic acid, edetate disodium, flavors, purified water, sodium hydroxide, sorbitol, sucrose. Contains FD&C Yellow No. 6 as a color additive.

Indications: Temporarily relieves cold and allergy symptoms, including runny nose, stuffy nose, sneezing, itching nose or throat, and itchy, watery eyes.

Warnings: Keep this and all drugs out of the reach of children. In case of accidental overdose, seek professional assistance or contact a Poison Control Center immediately.

Do not exceed recommended dosage because at higher doses nervousness, dizziness or sleeplessness may occur. Do not take for more than 7 days. If symptoms persist or are accompanied by fever, consult a doctor. Do not take this product: 1) if you have heart disease, high blood pressure, thyroid disease, diabetes, glaucoma, a breathing problem such as emphysema or chronic bronchitis, or difficulty in urination due to enlargement of the prostate gland, 2) if you are taking a prescription drug for high blood pressure

---

or depression, or 3) if you are taking sedatives or tranquilizers, unless directed by a doctor. May cause excitability, especially in children. May cause drowsiness. Alcohol, sedatives or tranquilizers may increase drowsiness. Avoid driving or operating machinery while taking this product.

As with any drug, if you are pregnant or nursing a baby, seek the advice of a health professional before using this product.

Dosage and Administration: Adults and children 12 and over (96+ lbs)—4 teaspoons every 4 hours. Children 6 to under 12 years (48–95 lbs)—2 teaspoons every 4 hours. Unless directed by physician, do not exceed 6 doses in 24 hours. Consult physician for dosage under 6 years of age. For convenience, a True-Dose® dosage cup is provided with each 4 fl. oz. and 8 fl. oz. bottle.

Professional Labeling: The suggested dosage for pediatric patients is:

3–12 months	1.25 ml (¼ tsp)
(12–17 lbs)	every 4 hours
12–24 months	2.5 ml (½ tsp)
(18–23 lbs)	every 4 hours
2–6 years	5 ml (1 tsp)
(24–47 lbs)	every 4 hours

How Supplied: TRIAMINIC Syrup (orange), in 4 fl oz and 8 fl oz plastic bottles with tamper-evident band around child-resistant cap. Orange flavored. Alcohol-free.

Shown in Product Identification Guide, page 421

TRIAMINIC-DM® SYRUP
[*trī"ah-mĭn'ĭc*]

Description: Each teaspoonful (5 ml) of TRIAMINIC-DM Syrup contains: phenylpropanolamine hydrochloride 6.25 mg and dextromethorphan hydrobromide 5 mg in a palatable, berry-flavored alcohol-free liquid. Other ingredients: benzoic acid, Blue 1, flavors, propylene glycol, purified water, Red 40, sodium chloride, sorbitol, sucrose.

Indications: Temporarily quiets coughs due to minor throat and bronchial irritation, and relieves stuffy nose. The decongestant and antitussive are provided in an alcohol-free and antihistamine-free formula.

Warnings: Keep this and all drugs out of the reach of children. In case of accidental overdose, seek professional assistance or contact a Poison Control Center immediately.

Do not exceed recommended dosage because at higher doses nervousness, dizziness, or sleeplessness may occur. Do not take for more than 7 days. If symptoms persist, are accompanied by fever, rash or persistent headache or if cough recurs, consult a doctor. A persistent cough may be a sign of a serious condition. Do not take this product: 1) if cough is accompanied by excessive phlegm (sputum), 2) for persistent or chronic cough such as oc-

---

curs with smoking, asthma or emphysema, or 3) if you have heart disease, high blood pressure, thyroid disease, diabetes, difficulty in urination due to enlargement of the prostate gland, or are taking a prescription drug for high blood pressure or depression, unless directed by a doctor.

As with any drug, if you are pregnant or nursing a baby, seek the advice of a health professional before using this product.

Dosage and Administration: Adults and children 12 and over (96+ lbs)—4 teaspoons every 4 hours. Children 6 to under 12 years (48–95 lbs)—2 teaspoons every 4 hours. Children 2 to under 6 years (24–47 lbs) 1 teaspoon every 4 hours. Unless directed by physician, do not exceed 6 doses in 24 hours or give to children under 2 years of age. For convenience, a True-Dose® dosage cup is provided with each 4 fl. oz. and 8 fl. oz. bottle.

Professional Labeling: The suggested dosage for pediatric patients is:

3–12 months	1.25 ml (¼ tsp)
(12–17 lbs)	every 4 hours
12–24 months	2.5 ml (½ tsp)
(18–23 lbs)	every 4 hours

How Supplied: TRIAMINIC-DM Syrup (dark red), in 4 fl oz and 8 fl oz plastic bottles with tamper-evident band around child-resistant cap. Berry flavored. Alcohol-free.

Shown in Product Identification Guide, page 421

TRIAMINIC–12® TABLETS
[*trī"ah-mĭn'ĭc*]

Description: Each tablet contains: phenylpropanolamine hydrochloride 75 mg and chlorpheniramine maleate 12 mg. Other ingredients: carnauba wax, colloidal silicon dioxide, lactose, methylcellulose, polyethylene glycol, povidone, Red 30, stearic acid, titanium dioxide, Yellow 6. Triaminic-12 Tablets contain the nasal decongestant phenylpropanolamine, and the antihistamine chlorpheniramine, in a formulation providing 12 hours of symptomatic relief.

Indications: For the temporary relief of nasal congestion due to the common cold, hay fever or other upper respiratory allergies and symptoms associated with sinusitis. Helps decongest sinus openings, sinus passages; promotes nasal and/or sinus drainage; temporarily restores freer breathing through the nose. For temporary relief of running nose, sneezing, itching of the nose or throat and itchy and watery eyes as may occur in allergic rhinitis (such as hay fever).

Warnings: Do not give this product to children under 12 years except under the advice and supervision of a physician. Do not take this product if you are taking another medication containing phenylpropanolamine. Do not take this preparation if you have high blood pressure,

Continued on next page

Sandoz—Cont.

heart disease, diabetes, thyroid disease, asthma, glaucoma, emphysema, chronic pulmonary disease, shortness of breath, difficulty in breathing or difficulty in urination due to enlargement of the prostate gland except under the advice and supervision of a physician. Do not exceed the recommended dosage because at higher doses nervousness, dizziness or sleeplessness may occur. This preparation may cause drowsiness; alcohol may increase the drowsiness effect; this preparation may cause excitability, especially in children. If symptoms do not improve within seven days or are accompanied by high fever, consult a physician before continuing use. As with any drug, if you are pregnant or nursing a baby, seek the advice of a health professional before using this product. Keep this and all drugs out of the reach of children. In case of accidental overdose, seek professional assistance or contact a Poison Control Center immediately.

Caution: Avoid driving a motor vehicle or operating heavy machinery. Avoid alcoholic beverages while taking this product.

Drug Interaction Precaution: Do not take this product if you are presently taking a prescription antihypertensive or antidepressant drug containing a monoamine oxidase inhibitor except under the advice and supervision of a physician.

Directions: Adults and children over 12 years of age—1 tablet swallowed whole every 12 hours. Unless directed by physician, do not exceed 2 tablets in 24 hours.

Note: The nonactive portion of the tablet that supplies the active ingredients may occasionally appear in your stool as a soft mass.

How Supplied: Triaminic-12 Tablets (orange) imprinted "DORSEY" on one side, "TRIAMINIC-12" on the other, in blister packs of 10 and 20.
Shown in Product Identification Guide, page 421

TRIAMINICIN® TABLETS
[$tr\bar{\imath}''ah$-$m\breve{\imath}n$ '$\breve{\imath}$-$s\breve{\imath}n$]

Description: Each tablet contains: phenylpropanolamine hydrochloride 25 mg and chlorpheniramine maleate 4 mg and acetaminophen 650 mg. Other ingredients: colloidal silicon dioxide, croscarmellose sodium, hydroxypropyl cellulose, lactose, magnesium stearate, methylcellulose, methylparaben, polyethylene glycol, povidone, pregelatinized starch, Red 40, titanium dioxide, Yellow 10.

Indications: Temporarily relieves runny nose, sneezing, itching of the nose or throat, and itchy, watery eyes due to hay fever or other upper respiratory allergies (allergic rhinitis). Temporarily

relieves nasal congestion due to hay fever or other upper respiratory allergies or symptoms associated with sinusitis. Temporarily relieves nasal congestion, runny nose and sneezing associated with the common cold. For the temporary relief of occasional minor aches, pains, headache and for the reduction of fever associated with the common cold.

Warnings: Do not take this product if you have high blood pressure, heart disease, diabetes, thyroid disease, glaucoma, a breathing problem such as emphysema or chronic bronchitis, or difficulty in urination due to enlargement of the prostate gland or are taking a prescription drug for high blood pressure or depression unless directed by a doctor. Do not exceed recommended dosage because at higher doses nervousness, dizziness, or sleeplessness may occur. This preparation may cause drowsiness; alcohol, sedatives and tranquilizers may increase the drowsiness effect; avoid alcoholic beverages; do not operate machinery or drive a motor vehicle while taking this product; this preparation may cause excitability, especially in children. Do not take this product for more than 7 days. If symptoms do not improve, new ones occur, or if fever persists for more than 3 days (72 hours) or recurs, consult a doctor. As with any drug, if you are pregnant or nursing a baby, seek the advice of a health professional before using this product. Keep this and all drugs out of the reach of children. In case of accidental overdose, seek professional assistance or contact a Poison Control Center immediately. Prompt medical attention is critical for adults as well as for children even if you do not notice any signs or symptoms.

Directions: Adults and children 12 years and older: Take 1 tablet every 4 hours. Unless directed by a doctor, do not exceed 6 doses in 24 hours or give to children under 12 years.

How Supplied: TRIAMINICIN Tablets (yellow) imprinted "DORSEY" on one side, "TRIAMINICIN" on the other, in blister packs of 12, 24 and 48, and bottles of 100 tablets.
Shown in Product Identification Guide, page 421

TRIAMINICOL® MULTI-SYMPTOM COLD TABLETS
[$tr\bar{\imath}''ah$-$m\breve{\imath}n$ '$\breve{\imath}$-$call$]

Description: Each tablet contains: phenylpropanolamine hydrochloride 12.5 mg, chlorpheniramine maleate 2 mg and dextromethorphan hydrobromide 10 mg. Other ingredients: calcium stearate, colloidal silicon dioxide, lactose, methylcellulose, methylparaben, microcrystalline cellulose, polyethylene glycol, povidone, pregelatinized starch, Red 40, titanium dioxide.

Indications: For the temporary relief of nasal congestion due to the common cold, hay fever or other upper respiratory

allergies and symptoms associated with sinusitis. Helps decongest sinus openings, sinus passages, promotes nasal and/or sinus drainage, temporarily restores freer breathing through the nose. For temporary relief of runny nose, sneezing, itching of the nose or throat and itchy and watery eyes as may occur in allergic rhinitis (such as hay fever). For temporary relief of cough due to minor throat and bronchial irritation as may occur with the common cold or with inhaled irritants.

Warnings: Do not take this product: 1) if cough is accompanied by excessive secretions, 2) for persistent cough such as occurs with smoking, asthma or emphysema, or 3) if you have high blood pressure, heart disease, diabetes, thyroid disease, glaucoma, a breathing problem such as emphysema or chronic bronchitis, or difficulty in urination due to enlargement of the prostate gland or are taking a prescription drug for high blood pressure or depression unless directed by a doctor. Do not exceed recommended dosage because at higher doses nervousness, dizziness, or sleeplessness may occur or take for more than 7 days. This preparation may cause drowsiness; alcohol, sedatives, and tranquilizers may increase the drowsiness effect; avoid alcoholic beverages; do not operate machinery or drive a motor vehicle while taking this product; this preparation may cause excitability, especially in children. If symptoms do not improve within seven days or are accompanied by fever, rash or persistant headache or if cough recurs, consult a doctor. As with any drug, if you are pregnant or nursing a baby, seek the advice of a health professional before using this product. Keep this and all drugs out of the reach of children. In case of accidental overdose, seek professional assistance or contact a Poison Control Center immediately.

Directions: Adults and children 12 years of age and older: 2 tablets every 4 hours. Children 6 to under 12 years, 1 tablet every 4 hours. Unless directed by physician, do not exceed 6 doses in 24 hours or give to children under 6 years.

How Supplied: Triaminicol Tablets (cherry red) imprinted "DORSEY" on one side, "TRIAMINICOL" on the other, in blister packs of 24.
Shown in Product Identification Guide, page 421

TRIAMINICOL® MULTI-SYMPTOM RELIEF
[$tr\bar{\imath}''ah$-$m\breve{\imath}n$ '$\breve{\imath}$-$call$]

Description: Each teaspoonful (5 ml) of TRIAMINICOL Multi-Symptom Relief contains: phenylpropanolamine hydrochloride 6.25 mg, chlorpheniramine maleate 1 mg, dextromethorphan hydrobromide 5 mg in a palatable, cherry flavored alcohol-free liquid. Other ingredients: benzoic acid, flavors, propylene glycol, purified water, Red 40, saccharin sodium, sodium chloride, sorbitol, sucrose.

Indications: Temporarily relieves cold symptoms, including coughs due to minor throat and bronchial irritation, runny nose, stuffy nose, sneezing, itching nose or throat and itchy, watery eyes.

Warnings: Keep this and all drugs out of the reach of children. In case of accidental overdose, seek professional assistance or contact a Poison Control Center immediately.

Do not exceed recommended dosage because at higher doses nervousness, dizziness, or sleeplessness may occur. Do not take for more than 7 days. If symptoms persist, are accompanied by fever, rash or persistent headache, or if cough recurs, consult a doctor. A persistent cough may be a sign of a serious condition. Do not take this product: 1) if cough is accompanied by excessive phlegm (sputum), 2) for persistent or chronic cough such as occurs with smoking, asthma or emphysema, or 3) if you have heart disease, high blood pressure, thyroid disease, diabetes, glaucoma, a breathing problem such as emphysema or chronic bronchitis, or difficulty in urination due to enlargement of the prostate gland, 4) if you are taking a prescription drug for high blood pressure or depression, or 5) if you are taking sedatives or tranquilizers, unless directed by a doctor. May cause excitability, especially in children. May cause drowsiness. Alcohol, sedatives or tranquilizers may increase drowsiness. Avoid driving or operating machinery while taking this product.

As with any drug, if you are pregnant or nursing a baby, seek the advice of a health professional before using this product.

Dosage and Administration: Adults and children 12 and over (96+ lbs)— 4 teaspoons every 4 hours. Children 6 to under 12 years (48–95 lbs)—2 teaspoons every 4 hours. Unless directed by physician, do not exceed 6 doses in 24 hours or give to children under 6 years of age. For convenience, a True-Dose® Dosage cup is provided with each 4 fl. oz. and 8 fl. oz. bottle.

Professional Labeling: The suggested dosage for pediatric patients is:

3–12 months	1.25 ml (¼ tsp)	
(12–17 lbs)	every 4 hours	
12–24 months	2.5 ml (½ tsp)	
(18–23 lbs)	every 4 hours	
2–6 years	5 ml (1 tsp)	
(24–47 lbs)	every 4 hours	

How Supplied: TRIAMINICOL Multi-Symptom Relief (red), in 4 fl oz and 8 fl oz plastic bottles with tamper-evident band around child-resistant cap. Cherry flavored. Alcohol-free.

Shown in Product Identification Guide, page 421

URSINUS® INLAY–TABS®
[yur "sīgn 'us]

Description: Each URSINUS Inlay-Tab contains: pseudoephedrine hydrochloride 30 mg and aspirin (USP) 325 mg. Other ingredients: calcium stearate, lactose, microcrystalline cellulose, pregelatinized starch, sodium starch, Yellow 6, Yellow 10.

Indications: For the temporary relief of nasal congestion due to the common cold, hay fever or symptoms associated with sinusitis. For the temporary relief of occasional minor aches, pains and headache and for the reduction of fever associated with the common cold.

Warnings: Children and teenagers should not use this medicine for chicken pox or flu symptoms before a doctor is consulted about Reye syndrome, a rare but serious illness reported to be associated with aspirin. Unless directed by a doctor: 1) Do not take this product if you are allergic to aspirin or if you have asthma, or if you have stomach distress, ulcers or bleeding problems; 2) Do not take this product if you have heart disease, thyroid disease, or difficulty in urination due to enlargement of the prostate gland, and 3) Do not exceed recommended dosage because at higher doses nervousness, dizziness, or sleeplessness may occur. Do not take this product for more than 7 days. If symptoms do not improve, are accompanied by fever, or new symptoms occur, consult a doctor. Stop taking this product if ringing in the ears or other symptoms occur. As with any drug, if you are pregnant or nursing a baby, seek the advice of a health professional before using this product. **IT IS ESPECIALLY IMPORTANT NOT TO USE ASPIRIN DURING THE LAST 3 MONTHS OF PREGNANCY UNLESS SPECIFICALLY DIRECTED TO DO SO BY A DOCTOR BECAUSE IT MAY CAUSE PROBLEMS IN THE UNBORN CHILD OR COMPLICATIONS DURING DELIVERY.**

Drug Interaction Precaution: Do not take this product if you are presently taking a prescription drug for high blood pressure or depression without first consulting your doctor. Do not take this product if you are presently taking a prescription drug for anticoagulation (thinning the blood), diabetes, arthritis or gout unless directed by a doctor. **Keep this and all medicines out of the reach of children. In case of accidental overdose, contact a physician immediately.**

Directions for Use: Adults and children 12 years and older: 2 tablets with a full glass of water every 4 hours while symptoms persist or as directed by a physician. Do not take more than 4 doses in 24 hours. For chicken pox or flu see Warnings.

How Supplied: URSINUS INLAY-TABS (white with yellow inlay), in bottles of 24.

Sanofi Winthrop Pharmaceuticals
**90 PARK AVENUE
NEW YORK, NY 10016**

DRISDOL®
**brand of ergocalciferol oral solution, USP (in propylene glycol)
Vitamin D Supplement**

Description: 200 International Units (5 µg) per drop. (Contains 8000 IU ergocalciferol per gram. The dropper supplied delivers 40 drops per mL.)

Indication: For the prevention of vitamin D deficiency in infants, children, and adults.

Warnings: As with any drug, if you are pregnant or nursing a baby, seek the advice of a health professional before using this product. Keep this and all drugs out of the reach of children. In case of accidental overdose, seek professional assistance or contact a poison control center immediately.

Dosage: 2 drops daily. This dose provides the US Recommended Daily Allowance for vitamin D for infants, children, and adults.

How Supplied: Bottles of 2 fl oz (NDC 0024-0391-02)

ZEPHIRAN® CHLORIDE
**brand of benzalkonium chloride
ANTISEPTIC
AQUEOUS SOLUTION 1:750
TINTED TINCTURE 1:750
SPRAY—TINTED TINCTURE 1:750**

Description: ZEPHIRAN Chloride, brand of benzalkonium chloride, NF, a mixture of alkylbenzyldimethylammonium chlorides, is a cationic quaternary ammonium surface-acting agent. It is very soluble in water, alcohol, and acetone. Aqueous solutions of ZEPHIRAN Chloride are neutral to slightly alkaline, generally colorless, and nonstaining. They have a bitter taste, aromatic odor, and foam when shaken. ZEPHIRAN Chloride Tinted Tincture 1:750 contains alcohol 50 percent and acetone 10 percent by volume. ZEPHIRAN Chloride Spray—Tinted Tincture 1:750 contains alcohol 92 percent. The Tinted Tincture and Spray also contain an orange-red coloring agent.

Clinical Pharmacology: ZEPHIRAN Chloride solutions are rapidly acting anti-infective agents with a moderately long duration of action. They are active

Continued on next page

This product information was effective as of October 31, 1993. Current detailed information may be obtained directly from Sanofi Winthrop Pharmaceuticals by writing to 90 Park Avenue, New York, NY 10016.

Sanofi Winthrop—Cont.

against bacteria and some viruses, fungi, and protozoa. Bacterial spores are considered to be resistant. Solutions are bacteriostatic or bactericidal according to their concentration. The exact mechanism of bactericidal action is unknown but is thought to be due to enzyme inactivation. Activity generally increases with increasing temperature and pH. Gram-positive bacteria are more susceptible than gram-negative bacteria (TABLE 1).

TABLE 1
Highest Dilution of ZEPHIRAN Chloride Aqueous Solution Destroying the Organism in 10 but not in 5 Minutes

Organisms	20°C
Streptococcus pyogenes	1:75,000
Staphylococcus aureus	1:52,500
Salmonella typhosa	1:37,500
Escherichia coli	1:10,500

Pseudomonas is the most resistant gram-negative genus. Using the AOAC Use-Dilution Confirmation Method, no growth was obtained when *Staphylococcus aureus*, *Salmonella choleraesuis*, and *Pseudomonas aeruginosa* (strain PRD-10) were exposed for ten minutes at 20°C to ZEPHIRAN Chloride Aqueous Solution 1:750 and Tinted Tincture 1:750.

ZEPHIRAN Chloride Aqueous Solution 1:750 has been shown to retain its bactericidal activity following autoclaving for 30 minutes at 15 lb pressure, freezing, and then thawing.

The tubercle bacillus may be resistant to aqueous ZEPHIRAN Chloride solutions but is susceptible to the 1:750 tincture (AOAC Method, 10 minutes at 20°C).

ZEPHIRAN Chloride solutions also demonstrate deodorant, wetting, detergent, keratolytic, and emulsifying activity.

Indications and Usage: ZEPHIRAN Chloride aqueous solutions in appropriate dilutions (see Recommended Dilutions) are indicated for the antisepsis of skin, mucous membranes, and wounds. They are used for preoperative preparation of the skin, surgeons' hand and arm soaks, treatment of wounds, preservation of ophthalmic solutions, irrigations of the eye, body cavities, bladder, urethra, and vaginal douching.
ZEPHIRAN Chloride Tinted Tincture 1:750 and Spray are indicated for preoperative preparation of the skin and for treatment of minor skin wounds and abrasions.

Contraindication: The use of ZEPHIRAN Chloride solutions in occlusive dressings, casts, and anal or vaginal packs is inadvisable, as they may produce irritation or chemical burns.

Warnings: Sterile Water for Injection, USP, should be used as diluent in preparing diluted aqueous solutions intended for use on deep wounds or for irrigation of body cavities. Otherwise, freshly distilled water should be used. Tap water, containing metallic ions and organic matter, may reduce antibacterial potency. Resin deionized water should not be used since it may contain pathogenic bacteria.

Organic, inorganic, and synthetic materials and surfaces may adsorb sufficient quantities of ZEPHIRAN Chloride to significantly reduce its antibacterial potency in solutions. This has resulted in serious contamination of solutions of ZEPHIRAN Chloride with viable pathogenic bacteria. Solutions should not be stored in bottles stoppered with cork closures, but rather in those equipped with appropriate screw-caps. Cotton, wool, rayon, and other materials should not be stored in ZEPHIRAN Chloride solutions. Gauze sponges and fiber pledgets used to apply solutions of ZEPHIRAN Chloride to the skin should be sterilized and stored in separate containers. Only immediately prior to application should they be immersed in ZEPHIRAN Chloride solutions.

Since ZEPHIRAN Chloride solutions are inactivated by soaps and anionic detergents, thorough rinsing is necessary if these agents are employed prior to their use.

Antiseptics such as ZEPHIRAN Chloride solutions must not be relied upon to achieve complete sterilization, because they do not destroy bacterial spores and certain viruses, including the etiologic agent of infectious hepatitis, and may not destroy *Mycobacterium tuberculosis* and other rare bacterial strains.

ZEPHIRAN Chloride Tinted Tincture 1:750 and Spray contain flammable organic solvents and should not be used near an open flame or cautery.

If solutions stronger than 1:3000 enter the eyes, irrigate immediately and repeatedly with water. Prompt medical attention should then be obtained. Concentrations greater than 1:5000 should not be used on mucous membranes, with the exception of the vaginal mucosa (see Recommended Dilutions).

Precautions: In preoperative antisepsis of the skin, ZEPHIRAN Chloride solutions should not be permitted to remain in prolonged contact with the patient's skin. Avoid pooling of the solution on the operating table.

ZEPHIRAN Chloride solutions that are used on inflamed or irritated tissues must be more dilute than those used on normal tissues (see Recommended Dilutions). ZEPHIRAN Chloride Tinted Tincture 1:750 and Spray, which contain irritating organic solvents, should be kept away from the eyes or other mucous membranes.

Preoperative periorbital skin or head prep should be performed only before the patient, or eye, is anesthetized.

Adverse Reactions: ZEPHIRAN Chloride solutions in normally used concentrations have low systemic and local toxicity and are generally well tolerated, although a rare individual may exhibit hypersensitivity.

Directions for Use:
General: For most surgical applications, the recommended concentration of ZEPHIRAN Chloride Aqueous Solution or ZEPHIRAN Chloride Tinted Tincture is 1:750 (0.13 percent). Liberal use of the solution is recommended to compensate for any adsorption of ZEPHIRAN Chloride by cotton or other materials.

To use ZEPHIRAN Chloride Spray—Tinted Tincture 1:750, remove protective cap, hold in an UPRIGHT position several inches away from the surgical field or injured area, and apply by spraying freely.

Preoperative preparation of skin: ZEPHIRAN Chloride solutions 1:750 are recommended as an antiseptic for use on unbroken skin in the preoperative preparation of the surgical field. Detergents and soaps should be thoroughly rinsed from the skin before applying ZEPHIRAN Chloride solutions. The detergent action of ZEPHIRAN Chloride solutions, particularly when used alternately with alcohol, leaves the skin smooth and clean. When ZEPHIRAN Chloride solutions are applied by friction (using several changes of sponges), dirt, skin fats, desquamating epithelium, and superficial bacteria are effectively removed, thus exposing the underlying skin to the antiseptic activity of the solutions.

The following procedure has been found satisfactory for preparation of the surgical field. On the day prior to surgery, the operative site is shaved and then scrubbed thoroughly with ZEPHIRAN Chloride Aqueous Solution 1:750. Immediately before surgery, ZEPHIRAN Chloride Tinted Tincture 1:750 or Spray is applied to the site in the usual manner (see Precautions). If the red tinted solution turns yellow during the preparation of patient's skin for surgery, it usually indicates the presence of soap (alkali) residue which is incompatible with ZEPHIRAN solutions. Therefore, rinse thoroughly and reapply the antiseptic. Because ZEPHIRAN Chloride Tinted Tincture 1:750 contains alcohol and acetone, its cleansing action on the skin is particularly effective and it dries more rapidly than the aqueous solution. The Tinted Tincture is recommended when it is desirable to outline the operative site.

Recommended Dilutions: For specific directions, see TABLES 2 and 3.
Surgery
Preoperative preparation of skin: Aqueous solution 1:750 and Tinted Tincture 1:750 or Spray
Surgeons' hand and arm soaks: Aqueous solution 1:750
Treatment of minor wounds and lacerations: Tinted Tincture 1:750 or Spray
Irrigation of deep infected wounds: Aqueous solution 1:3000 to 1:20,000
Denuded skin and mucous membranes: Aqueous solution 1:5000 to 1:10,000

TABLE 2
Correct Use of ZEPHIRAN Chloride

ZEPHIRAN Chloride solutions must be prepared, stored, and used correctly to achieve and maintain their antiseptic action. Serious inactivation and contamination of ZEPHIRAN Chloride solutions may occur with misuse.

CORRECT DILUENTS	INCOMPATIBILITIES	PREFERRED FORM
Sterile Water for Injection is recommended for irrigation of body cavities. *Sterile distilled water* is recommended for irrigating traumatized tissue and in the eye. *Freshly distilled water* is recommended for skin antisepsis. *Resin deionized water* should not be used because the deionizing resins can carry pathogens (especially gram-negative bacteria); they also inactivate quaternary ammonium compounds. *Stored water* is not recommended since it may contain many organisms. *Saline* should not be used since it may decrease the antibacterial potency of ZEPHIRAN Chloride solutions.	Anionic detergents and soaps should be thoroughly rinsed from the skin or other areas prior to use of ZEPHIRAN Chloride solutions because they reduce the antibacterial activity of the solutions. Serum and protein material also decrease the activity of ZEPHIRAN Chloride solutions. Corks should not be used to stopper bottles containing ZEPHIRAN Chloride solutions. Fibers or fabrics when stored in ZEPHIRAN Chloride solutions adsorb ZEPHIRAN from the surrounding liquid. Examples are: Cotton　　　Gauze sponges Wool　　　Rayon 　　Rubber materials Applicators or sponges, intended for a skin prep, should be stored separately and dipped in ZEPHIRAN Chloride solutions immediately before use. Under certain circumstances the following commonly encountered substances are incompatible with ZEPHIRAN Chloride solutions: Iodine　　　Aluminum Silver nitrate　Caramel Fluorescein　Kaolin Nitrates　　Pine oil Peroxide　　Zinc sulfate Lanolin　　Zinc oxide Potassium　Yellow oxide 　permanganate　of mercury	ZEPHIRAN Chloride Tinted Tincture 1:750 is recommended for preoperative skin preparation because it contains alcohol and acetone which enhance its cleansing action and promote rapid drying. ZEPHIRAN Chloride Tinted Tincture 1:750, containing acetone, is recommended when it is desirable to outline the operative site. (Aqueous solutions of ZEPHIRAN Chloride used in skin preparation have a tendency to "run off" the skin.) Caution: Because of the flammable organic solvents in ZEPHIRAN Chloride Tinted Tincture 1:750 and Spray, these products should be kept away from open flame or cautery.

Obstetrics and Gynecology

Preoperative preparation of skin: Aqueous solution 1:750 and Tinted Tincture 1:750 or Spray

Vaginal douche and irrigation: Aqueous solution 1:2000 to 1:5000

Postepisiotomy care: Aqueous solution 1:5000 to 1:10,000

Breast and nipple hygiene: Aqueous solution 1:1000 to 1:2000

Urology

Bladder and urethral irrigation: Aqueous solution 1:5000 to 1:20,000

Bladder retention lavage: Aqueous solution 1:20,000 to 1:40,000

Dermatology

Oozing and open infections: Aqueous solution 1:2000 to 1:5000

Wet dressings by irrigation or open dressing (Use in occlusive dressings is inadvisable.): Aqueous solution 1:5000 or less

Ophthalmology

Eye irrigation: Aqueous solution 1:5000 to 1:10,000

Preservation of ophthalmic solutions: Aqueous solution 1:5000 to 1:7500

[See table above.]

TABLE 3
Dilutions of ZEPHIRAN Chloride
Aqueous Solution 1:750

Final Dilution	ZEPHIRAN Chloride Aqueous Solution 1:750 (parts)	Distilled Water (parts)
1:1000	3	1
1:2000	3	5
1:2500	3	7
1:3000	3	9
1:4000	3	13
1:5000	3	17
1:10,000	3	37
1:20,000	3	77
1:40,000	3	157

Accidental Ingestion: If ZEPHIRAN Chloride solution, particularly a concentrated solution, is ingested, marked local irritation of the gastrointestinal tract, manifested by nausea and vomiting, may occur. Signs of systemic toxicity include restlessness, apprehension, weakness, confusion, dyspnea, cyanosis, collapse, convulsions, and coma. Death occurs as a result of paralysis of the respiratory muscles.

Treatment: Immediate administration of several glasses of a mild soap solution, milk, or egg whites beaten in water is recommended. This may be followed by gastric lavage with a mild soap solution. Alcohol should be avoided as it promotes absorption.

To support respiration, the airway should be clear and oxygen should be administered, employing artificial respiration if necessary. If convulsions occur, a

Continued on next page

This product information was effective as of October 31, 1993. Current detailed information may be obtained directly from Sanofi Winthrop Pharmaceuticals by writing to 90 Park Avenue, New York, NY 10016.

Sanofi Winthrop—Cont.

short-acting barbiturate may be given parenterally with caution.

How Supplied:
ZEPHIRAN Chloride Aqueous Solution 1:750
  Bottles of 8 fl oz (NDC 0024-2521-04) and 1 gallon (NDC 0024-2521-08)
ZEPHIRAN Chloride Tinted Tincture 1:750 (*flammable*)
  Bottles of 1 gallon (NDC 0024-2523-08)
ZEPHIRAN Chloride Spray—Tinted Tincture 1:750 (*flammable*)
  Bottles of 1 fl oz (NDC 0024-2527-01) and 6 fl oz (NDC 0024-2527-03)

ZW-83-H

Schering-Plough HealthCare Products
LIBERTY CORNER, NJ 07938

A AND D® MEDICATED DIAPER RASH OINTMENT

Description: An ointment containing White Petrolatum and Zinc Oxide. Also contains: Benzoic Acid, Benzyl Alcohol, Cholecalciferol, Cod Liver Oil, Cyclomethicone, Glyceryl Monostearate, Light Mineral Oil, Magnesium Aluminum Silicate, Ozokerite, Propylparaben.

Indications: Helps treat and prevent diaper rash. Protects chafed skin due to diaper rash and helps seal out wetness.

Dosage and Administration: Change wet and soiled diapers promptly, cleanse the diaper area and allow to dry. Apply ointment liberally as often as necessary, with each diaper change, especially at bedtime or anytime when exposure to wet diapers is prolonged.

Warning: Keep this and all drugs out of the reach of children. In case of accidental ingestion, seek professional assistance or contact a Poison Control Center immediately.

How Supplied: A and D® Medicated Ointment is available in 1 ½-ounce (42.5g) and 4-ounce (113g) tubes.
Store between 15° and 30°C (59° and 86°F).

Shown in Product Identification Guide, page 422

A and D® Ointment

Description: An ointment containing the emollients, lanolin and petrolatum. Also contains: Cholecalciferol, Fish Liver Oil, Fragrance, Mineral Oil, Paraffin.

Indications: *Diaper rash*—**A and D Ointment** provides prompt, soothing relief for diaper rash and helps heal baby's tender skin; forms a moistureproof shield that helps protect against urine and detergent irritants; comforts baby's skin and helps prevent chafing. *Chafed Skin*—**A and D Ointment** helps skin retain its vital natural moisture; quickly soothes chafed skin in adults and children and helps prevent abnormal dryness.

Abrasions and Minor Burns—**A and D Ointment** soothes and helps relieve the smarting and pain of abrasions and minor burns, encourages healing and prevents dressings from sticking to the injured area.

Warning: Keep this and all drugs out of the reach of children. In case of accidental ingestion, seek professional assistance or contact a poison control center immediately.

Dosage and Administration: Apply as needed or consult your physician.

How Supplied: A and D Ointment is available in 1½-ounce (42.5 g) and 4-ounce (113 g) tubes and 1-pound (454 g) jars and 2.5 oz. pumps.

Shown in Product Identification Guide, page 422

AFRIN®
[*a 'frin*]
Nasal Spray 0.05%
Nasal Spray Pump 0.05%
Cherry Scented Nasal Spray 0.05%
Menthol Nasal Spray 0.05%
Extra Moisturizing Nasal Spray .05%
Nose Drops 0.05%
Children's Strength Nose Drops 0.025%

Description: AFRIN products contain oxymetazoline hydrochloride, the longest acting topical nasal decongestant available. Each ml of AFRIN Nasal Spray, Nasal Spray Pump, and Nose Drops contains Oxymetazoline Hydrochloride, USP 0.5 mg (0.05%); Benzalkonium Chloride, Glycine, Phenylmercuric Acetate (0.002%), Sorbitol, and Water. Each ml of AFRIN Extra Moisturizing Nasal Spray contains Oxymetazoline Hydrochloride, USP 0.5 mg (0.05%), Benzalkonium Chloride, Benzyl Alcohol, Edetate Disodium, Polyethylene Glycol 1450, Propylene Glycol, Sodium Phosphate Dibasic, Sodium Phosphate Monobasic, Water.
Each ml of AFRIN Children's Strength Nose Drops contains Oxymetazoline Hydrochloride, USP 0.25 mg (0.025%); Benzalkonium Chloride, Glycine, Phenylmercuric Acetate (0.002%), Sorbitol, and Water.
AFRIN Menthol Nasal Spray contains cooling aromatic vapors of menthol, eucalyptol, camphor and polysorbate, in addition to the ingredients of AFRIN Nasal Spray.
AFRIN Cherry Scented Nasal Spray contains artificial cherry flavor in addition to the ingredients in regular AFRIN.
AFRIN Extra Moisturizing Nasal Spray's Unique Formula won't burn or sting nasal passages. It also soothes and moisturizes dry nasal passages.

Indications: For temporary relief of nasal congestion associated with colds, hay fever and sinusitis.

Actions: The sympathomimetic action of AFRIN products constricts the smaller arterioles of the nasal passages, producing a prolonged, gentle and predictable decongesting effect. In just a few minutes a single dose, as directed, provides prompt, temporary relief of nasal congestion that lasts up to 12 hours. AFRIN products last up to 3 or 4 times longer than most ordinary nasal sprays.
AFRIN products used at bedtime help restore freer nasal breathing through the night.

Warnings: Do not exceed recommended dosage because burning, stinging, sneezing or increase of nasal discharge may occur. Do not use these products for more than 3 days. If nasal congestion persists, consult a physician. As with any drug, if you are pregnant or nursing a baby, seek the advice of a health professional before using this product. The use of the dispensers by more than one person may spread infection. Keep these and all medicines out of the reach of children. In case of accidental ingestion, seek professional assistance or contact a Poison Control Center immediately.

Dosage and Administration: Because AFRIN has a long duration of action, twice-a-day administration—in the morning and at bedtime—is usually adequate.
AFRIN Nasal Spray, Extra Moisturizing Nasal Spray, Cherry Scented Nasal Spray and Menthol Nasal Spray, 0.05%—For adults and children 6 years of age and over: With head upright, spray 2 or 3 times into each nostril twice daily—morning and evening. To spray, squeeze bottle quickly and firmly. Do not tilt head backward while spraying. Wipe nozzle clean after use. Not recommended for children under six.
Afrin Nasal Spray Pump, 0.05%—For adults and children 6 years of age and over: Two or three sprays in each nostril twice daily—morning and bedtime. Remove protective cap. Hold bottle with thumb at base and nozzle between first and second fingers. With head upright, insert metered pump spray nozzle in nostril. Depress pump 2 or 3 times, all the way down, with a firm even stroke and sniff deeply. Repeat in other nostril. Do not tilt head backward while spraying. Wipe tip clean after each use. Before using the first time, remove the protective cap from the tip and prime the metered pump by depressing pump firmly several times.
AFRIN Nose Drops—For adults and children 6 years of age and over: Tilt head back, apply 2 or 3 drops into each nostril twice daily—morning and evening. Immediately bend head forward toward knees. Hold a few seconds, then return to upright position. Wipe dropper clean after each use. Not recommended for children under six.
AFRIN Children's Strength Nose Drops—Children 2 through 5 years of age: Tilt head back, apply 2 or 3 drops into each nostril twice daily—morning and evening. Promptly move head forward toward knees. Hold a few seconds, then return child to upright position.

Wipe dropper clean after each use. For children under 2 years, use only as directed by a physician.

How Supplied: AFRIN Nasal Spray 0.05% (1:2000), 15 ml and 30 ml plastic squeeze bottles.
AFRIN Nasal Spray Pump 0.05% (1:2000), 15 ml spray pump bottles.
AFRIN Extra Moisturizing Nasal Spray 0.05%, 15 ml plastic squeeze bottle.
AFRIN Cherry Scented Nasal Spray 0.05% (1:2000), 15 ml plastic squeeze bottle.
AFRIN Menthol Nasal Spray 0.05% (1:2000), 15 ml plastic squeeze bottle.
AFRIN Nose Drops, 0.05% (1:2000), 20 ml dropper bottle.
AFRIN Children's Strength Nose Drops, 0.025% (1:4000), 20 ml dropper bottle.
Store all nasal sprays and nose drops between 2° and 30°C (36° and 86°F).
Shown in Product Identification Guide, page 422

AFRIN®
[a'frin]
Saline Mist

Ingredients: Water, Sodium Chloride, Disodium Phosphate, Sodium Phosphate, Benzalkonium Chloride, Phenyl Mercuric Acetate (0.002%) (preservative).

Indications: Provides soothing moisture to dry, inflamed nasal membranes due to colds, allergies, low humidity, and other minor nasal irritations. Afrin Saline Mist loosens and thins mucus secretions to aid removal of mucus from nose and sinuses. Afrin Saline Mist can be used as often as needed, and is safe to use with cold, allergy, and sinus medications.

Directions: For infants, children, and adults, 2 to 6 sprays/drops in each nostril as often as needed or as directed by a physician. For a fine mist, keep bottle upright; for nose drops, keep bottle upside down; for a stream, keep bottle horizontal. Wipe nozzle clean after use.
Keep out of the reach of children. If you are pregnant or nursing a baby, seek the advice of a health professional before using this product.
The use of this dispenser by more than one person may spread infection.
CONTAINS NO ALCOHOL
Shown in Product Identification Guide, page 422

AFTATE® Antifungal
Aerosol Liquid
Aerosol Powder
Gel
Powder

Active Ingredient: Tolnaftate 1% (Also contains: Aerosol Spray Liquid-36% alcohol; Aerosol Spray Powder-14% alcohol.)

How Supplied:
AFTATE for Athlete's Foot
Sprinkle Powder—2.25 oz. bottle
Aerosol Spray Powder—3.5 oz can
Gel—.5 oz. tube
Aerosol Spray Liquid—4 oz. can
AFTATE for Jock Itch
Aerosol Spray Powder—3.5 oz. can
Sprinkle Powder—1.5 oz. bottle
Gel—.5 oz. tube
Shown in Product Identification Guide, page 422

CHLOR-TRIMETON®
[klor-tri'mĕ-ton]
4 Hour Allergy Tablets
8 Hour Allergy Tablets
12 Hour Allergy Tablets

Active Ingredients: Each 4 Hour Allergy Tablet contains: 4 mg chlorpheniramine maleate, USP; also contains: Corn Starch, D&C Yellow No. 10 Aluminum Lake, Lactose, Magnesium Stearate. Each 8 Hour Allergy Tablet contains: 8 mg chlorpheniramine maleate; also contains: Acacia, Butylparaben, Calcium Phosphate, Calcium Sulfate, Carnauba Wax, Corn Starch, D&C Yellow No. 10 Aluminum Lake, FD&C Yellow No. 6 Aluminum Lake, FD&C Yellow No. 6, Lactose, Magnesium Stearate, Neutral Soap, Oleic Acid, Potato Starch, Rosin, Sugar, Talc, White Wax, Zein.
Each 12 Hour Allergy Tablet contains: 12 mg chlorpheniramine maleate; also contains: Acacia, Butylparaben, Calcium Phosphate, Calcium Sulfate, Carnauba Wax, Corn Starch, D&C Yellow No. 10 Aluminum Lake, FD&C Blue No. 2 Aluminum Lake, FD&C Yellow No. 6, FD&C Yellow No. 6 Aluminum Lake, Lactose, Magnesium Stearate, Neutral Soap, Oleic Acid, Potato Starch, Rosin, Sugar, Talc, White Wax, Zein.

Indications: For effective relief of sneezing, itchy, watery eyes, itchy throat, and runny nose due to hay fever and other upper respiratory allergies.

Warnings: May cause excitability especially in children. Do not give the 8 Hour or 12 Hour Allergy Tablets to children under 12 years, or 4 Hour Allergy Tablets to children under 6 years except under the advice and supervision of a doctor. Do not take this product, unless directed by a doctor, if you have a breathing problem such as emphysema or chronic bronchitis, or if you have glaucoma, difficulty in urination due to enlargement of the prostate gland. May cause drowsiness; alcohol may increase the drowsiness effect. Avoid alcoholic beverages while taking this product. Do not take this product if you are taking sedatives or tranquilizers, without first consulting your doctor. Use caution when driving a motor vehicle or operating machinery. As with any drug, if you are pregnant or nursing a baby, seek the advice of a health professional before using this product. Keep this and all drugs out of the reach of children. In case of

accidental overdose, seek professional assistance or contact a Poison Control Center immediately.

Dosage and Administration: 4 Hour Allergy Tablets—Adults and Children 12 years of age and over: Oral dosage is one tablet (4 mg) every 4 to 6 hours, not to exceed 6 tablets in 24 hours. Children 6 to under 12 years of age: Oral dosage is one half the adult dose (2 mg) (break tablet in half) every 4 to 6 hours, not to exceed 3 whole tablets (12 mg) in 24 hours, or as directed by a doctor. Children under 6 years of age: consult a doctor.
8 Hour Allergy Tablets—Adults and Children 12 years and over—One tablet every 8 to 12 hours. Do not take more than one tablet every 8 hours or 3 tablets in 24 hours.
12 Hour Allergy Tablets—Adults and children 12 years and over—One tablet every 12 hours. Do not exceed 2 tablets in 24 hours.

How Supplied: CHLOR-TRIMETON 4 Hour Allergy Tablets, box of 24, bottles of 100.
CHLOR-TRIMETON 8 Hour Allergy Tablets, boxes of 15, bottles of 100.
CHLOR-TRIMETON 12 Hour Allergy Tablets, boxes of 10 and 24, bottles of 100.
Store between 2° and 30°C (36° and 86°F). Protect from excessive moisture.
Shown in Product Identification Guide, page 422

CHLOR-TRIMETON®
[klor-tri 'mĕ-ton]
Allergy-Sinus Headache Caplets

Active Ingredients (per Caplet): 500 mg acetaminophen, 2 mg chlorpheniramine maleate, 12.5 mg phenylpropanolamine hydrochloride. **Also contains:** Carnauba Wax, Cellulose, Hydroxypropyl Methylcellulose, Magnesium Stearate, PEG, Povidone.

Indications: CHLOR-TRIMETON caplets provide effective, temporary relief of sinus pain and nasal congestion, sneezing, itchy, watery eyes, itchy throat, and runny nose due to hay fever and other upper respiratory allergies.

Directions: ADULTS AND CHILDREN 12 YEARS OF AGE AND OVER—Oral dosage is two caplets every 6 hours, not to exceed 8 caplets in 24 hours, or as directed by a doctor. Swallow one caplet at a time.
CHILDREN UNDER 12 YEARS OF AGE: Consult a doctor.

Warnings: Do not take this product for pain or congestion for more than 7 days, and do not take for fever for more than 3 days unless directed by a doctor. If pain or fever persists or gets worse, if new

Continued on next page

Information on Schering-Plough HealthCare Products appearing on these pages is effective as of November 1993.

Schering-Plough—Cont.

symptoms occur, or if redness or swelling is present, consult your physician because these could be signs of a serious condition. May cause excitability, especially in children. Do not exceed recommended dosage because at higher doses nervousness, dizziness, or sleeplessness may occur. Do not take this product, unless directed by a doctor, if you have a breathing problem such as emphysema or chronic bronchitis, or if you have glaucoma, heart disease, high blood pressure, thyroid disease, diabetes, or difficulty in urination due to enlargement of the prostate gland. May cause drowsiness; alcohol, sedatives, and tranquilizers may increase the drowsiness effect. Avoid alcoholic beverages while taking this product. Do not take this product if you are taking sedatives or tranquilizers without first consulting your doctor. Use caution when driving a motor vehicle or operating machinery. As with any drug, if you are pregnant or nursing a baby, seek the advice of a health professional before using this product. Keep this and all drugs out of the reach of children. In case of accidental overdose, seek professional assistance or contact a Poison Control Center immediately. Prompt medical attention is critical for adults as well as for children even if you do not notice any signs or symptoms.

Drug Interaction Precaution: Do not take this product if you are presently taking a prescription drug containing a monoamine oxidase inhibitor (MAOI) (certain drugs for depression or psychiatric or emotional conditions), without first consulting your doctor. If you are uncertain whether your prescription drug contains an MAOI, consult a health professional before taking this product. Do not take this product if you are taking an appetite-controlling medication containing phenylpropanolamine without first consulting your doctor.
Store between 2° and 30°C (36° and 86°F). Protect from excessive moisture.

Shown in Product Identification Guide, page 422

CHLOR-TRIMETON®
[*klortri 'mĕ-ton*]
4 Hour Allergy/Decongestant Tablets
12 Hour Allergy/Decongestant Tablets

Active Ingredients: Each 4 Hour Allergy/Decongestant Tablet contains: 4 mg chlorpheniramine maleate, USP and 60 mg pseudoephedrine sulfate; also contains: Corn Starch, FD&C Blue No. 1, Lactose, Magnesium Stearate, Povidone. Each 12 Hour Allergy/Decongestant Tablet contains: 8 mg chlorpheniramine maleate and 120 mg pseudoephedrine sulfate; also contains: Acacia, Butylparaben, Calcium Sulfate, Carnauba Wax, Corn Starch, D&C Yellow No. 10 Aluminum Lake, FD&C Blue No. 1 Aluminum Lake, FD&C Yellow No. 6 Aluminum Lake, Gelatin, Lactose, Magnesium Stearate, Neutral Soap, Oleic Acid, Povidone, Rosin, Sugar, Talc, White Wax, Zein.

Indications: For effective temporary relief of sneezing, itchy, watery eyes, itchy throat, and runny nose due to hay fever and other upper respiratory allergies. Helps decongest sinus openings and sinus passages; relieves sinus pressure. Temporarily restores freer breathing through the nose.

Warnings: May cause excitability, especially in children. Do not exceed recommended dosage because at higher doses nervousness, dizziness, or sleeplessness may occur. Do not take this product for more than 7 days. If symptoms do not improve or are accompanied by fever, consult a doctor. Do not take this product, unless directed by a doctor, if you have a breathing problem such as emphysema or chronic bronchitis, or if you have glaucoma, heart disease, high blood pressure, thyroid disease, diabetes, or difficulty in urination due to enlargement of the prostate gland. May cause drowsiness; alcohol, sedatives, and tranquilizers may increase the drowsiness effect. Avoid alcoholic beverages while taking this product. Do not take this product if you are taking sedatives or tranquilizers without first consulting your doctor. Use caution when driving a motor vehicle or operating machinery. As with any drug, if you are pregnant or nursing a baby, seek the advice of a health professional before using this product. Keep this and all drugs out of the reach of children. In case of accidental overdose, seek professional assistance or contact a Poison Control Center immediately.

Drug Interaction Precaution: Do not use this product if you are taking a prescription drug containing a monoamine oxidase inhibitor (MAOI) (certain drugs for depression or psychiatric or emotional conditions), without first consulting your doctor. If you are uncertain whether your prescription drug contains an MAOI, consult a health professional before taking this product.

Dosage and Administration: 4 Hour Allergy/Decongestant Tablets —ADULTS AND CHILDREN 12 YEARS OF AGE AND OVER: Oral dosage is one tablet every 4 to 6 hours, not to exceed 4 tablets in 24 hours, or as directed by a doctor. CHILDREN 6 TO UNDER 12 YEARS OF AGE: Oral dosage is one half the adult dose (break tablet in half) every 4 to 6 hours, not to exceed 2 whole tablets in 24 hours, or as directed by a doctor. CHILDREN UNDER 6 YEARS OF AGE: Consult a doctor. 12 Hour Allergy/Decongestant Tablets—ADULTS AND CHILDREN 12 YEARS AND OVER: one tablet every 12 hours. Do not exceed 2 tablets in 24 hours.

How Supplied: CHLOR-TRIMETON 4 Hour Allergy/Decongestant Tablets— boxes of 24. CHLOR-TRIMETON 12 Hour Allergy/Decongestant Tablets boxes of 10.
Store these CHLOR-TRIMETON Products between 2° and 30°C (36°and 86°F); and protect from excessive moisture.

Shown in Product Identification Guide, page 422

CHOOZ® ANTACID GUM

Active Ingredients: 500 mg. of calcium carbonate per tablet.

Inactive Ingredients: Sucrose, gum base, glucose, corn starch, peppermint oil, hydrated silica, gelatin, glycerin, acacia, carnauba wax, beeswax, sodium benzoate.

Indications: For relief from acid indigestion, sour stomach, heartburn, and upset stomach associated with these symptoms. Five tablets provide 100% of the adult U.S. Recommended Daily Allowance for calcium. Chooz Antacid Gum is dietically sodium-free, an important benefit for those watching their sodium and salt consumption.

Warnings: Adults—Do not take more than 14 tablets in a 24-hour period. Do not use the maximum dosage of this product for more than 2 weeks except under the advice and supervision of a physician. Children 6 to 12 years—Do not take more than 8 tablets in a 24-hour period. Keep this and all drugs out of reach of children.

Dosage and Administration: Adults chew 1 to 2 tablets every 2 to 4 hours. Children 6 to 12 years of age chew 1 tablet every 2 to 4 hours. Or take as directed by physician.

How Supplied: Tablets—individually foil-backed safety sealed blister packaging in boxes of 16 tablets.
Shown in Product Identification Guide, page 422

COMPLEX 15®
Therapeutic Moisturizing Lotion
Contains Phospholipids
Formulated For Mild To Severe Dry Skin

Ingredients: Water, Caprylic/Capric Triglyceride, Glycerin, Glyceryl Stearate, Dimethicone, PEG-50 Stearate, Squalane, Cetyl Alcohol, Glycol Stearate, Myristyl Myristate, Stearic Acid, Lecithin, C10–30 Cholesterol/Lanosterol Esters, Diazolidinyl Urea, Carbomer, Magnesium Aluminum Silicate, Sodium Hydroxide, BHT, Tetrasodium EDTA
COMPLEX 15® Therapeutic Moisturizing Lotion is formulated for mild to severe dry skin with a system modeled from nature. It contains lecithin, a phospholipid water-binding agent found naturally in the skin. Each phospholipid molecule holds 15 molecules of water, restoring the natural moisture balance. COMPLEX 15 Therapeutic Moisturizing Lotion is nongreasy and absorbs quickly into the skin. COMPLEX 15 Therapeutic Moisturizing Lotion is unscented, contains no parabens, lanolin, or mineral oil.

COMPLEX 15 Therapeutic Moisturizing Lotion is proven to be hypoallergenic and noncomedogenic.

Directions: Apply to the hands and body as needed, or as directed by a physician. Avoid contact with eyes.

FOR EXTERNAL USE ONLY

How Supplied: COMPLEX 15® Therapeutic Moisturizing Lotion is available in 8 fluid ounce bottles (0085-4115-08).

Shown in Product Identification Guide, page 422

COMPLEX 15®
Therapeutic Moisturizing
Face Cream Contains Phospholipids

Ingredients: Water, Caprylic/Capric Triglyceride, Glycerin, Squalane, Glyceryl Stearate, Propylene Glycol, PEG-50 Stearate, Cetyl Alcohol, Dimethicone, Glycol Stearate, Myristyl Myristate, Stearic Acid, Carbomer, Magnesium Aluminum Silicate, Diazolidinyl Urea, Lecithin, Sodium Hydroxide, C10–30 Cholesterol/Lanosterol Esters, BHT, Tetrasodium EDTA

COMPLEX 15® Therapeutic Moisturizing Face Cream is formulated for mild to severe dry skin with a system modeled from nature. It contains lecithin, a phospholipid water-binding agent found naturally in the skin. Each phospholipid molecule holds 15 molecules of water, restoring the natural moisture balance. COMPLEX 15 Therapeutic Moisturizing Face Cream is nongreasy and absorbs quickly into the skin. COMPLEX 15 Therapeutic Moisturizing Face Cream is unscented, contains no parabens, lanolin or mineral oil. COMPLEX 15 Therapeutic Moisturizing Face Cream is proven to be hypoallergenic and noncomedogenic.

Directions: Apply to the face as needed or as directed by a physician. Avoid contact with eyes.

FOR EXTERNAL USE ONLY

How Supplied: COMPLEX 15® Moisturizing Face Cream is available in 2.5 oz. tubes (0085-4100-25).

Shown in Product Identification Guide, page 422

CORICIDIN® Tablets
[*kor-a-see 'din*]
CORICIDIN 'D'® Decongestant Tablets

Active Ingredients: CORICIDIN Tablets—2 mg chlorpheniramine maleate, 325 mg (5 gr) acetaminophen.
CORICIDIN 'D' Decongestant Tablets—2 mg chlorpheniramine maleate, 12.5 mg phenylpropanolamine hydrochloride, 325 mg (5 gr) acetaminophen.

Inactive Ingredients: CORICIDIN Tablets—Acacia, Butylparaben, Calcium Sulfate, Carnauba Wax, Cellulose, Corn Starch, FD&C Red No. 40 Aluminum Lake, FD&C Yellow No. 6 Aluminum Lake, Lactose, Magnesium Stearate, Povidone, Sugar, Talc, Titanium Dioxide, White Wax.
CORICIDIN 'D' Decongestant Tablets—Acacia, Butylparaben, Calcium Sulfate, Carnauba Wax, Cellulose, Corn Starch, Magnesium Stearate, Povidone, Sugar, Talc, Titanium Dioxide, White Wax.

Indications: CORICIDIN Tablets temporarily relieve minor aches, pains and headache, and reduce the fever associated with colds or flu; temporarily relieve sneezing, runny nose and itchy water eyes due to hay fever, other upper respiratory allergies or the common cold. CORICIDIN 'D' Tablets temporarily relieve minor aches and pains, and reduce the fever associated with a cold or flu, temporarily relieve sneezing and stuffy/runny nose associated with the common cold; provide temporary relief of sinus headache and pressure and reduce swelling of nasal passages.

Warnings: CORICIDIN Tablets: Do not take this product for pain for more than 10 days (adults) or 5 days (children 6 to under 12 years of age) and do not take for fever for more than 3 days unless directed by a doctor. If pain or fever persists or gets worse, if new symptoms occur, or if redness or swelling is present, consult a doctor because these could be signs of a serious condition. May cause excitability especially in children. Do not take this product, unless directed by a doctor, if you have a breathing problem such as emphysema or chronic bronchitis, or if you have glaucoma or difficulty in urination due to enlargement of the prostate gland. May cause drowsiness; alcohol, sedatives, and tranquilizers may increase the drowsiness effect. Avoid alcoholic beverages while taking this product. Do not take this product if you are taking sedatives or tranquilizers, without first consulting your doctor. Use caution when driving a motor vehicle or operating machinery. As with any drug, if you are pregnant or nursing a baby, seek the advice of a health professional before using this product. Keep this and all drugs out of the reach of children. In case of accidental overdose, seek professional assistance or contact a Poison Control Center immediately. Prompt medical attention is critical for adults as well as for children even if you do not notice any signs or symptoms.
CORICIDIN 'D' Decongestant Tablets: Do not take this product for pain or congestion for more than 7 days (adults) or 5 days (children 6 through 12 years of age), and do not take for fever for more than 3 days unless directed by a doctor. If pain or fever persists or gets worse, if new symptoms occur, or if redness or swelling is present, consult your physician because these could be signs of a serious condition.
May cause excitability, especially in children. Do not exceed recommended dosage because at higher doses nervousness, dizziness, or sleeplessness may occur. Do not take this product, unless directed by a doctor, if you have a breathing problem such as emphysema or chronic bronchitis, or if you have glaucoma, heart disease, high blood pressure, thyroid disease, diabetes, or difficulty in urination due to enlargement of the prostate gland. May cause drowsiness; alcohol, sedatives, and tranquilizers may increase the drowsiness effect. Avoid alcoholic beverages while taking this product. Do not take this product if you are taking sedatives or tranquilizers without first consulting your doctor. Use caution when driving a motor vehicle or operating machinery. As with any drug, if you are pregnant or nursing a baby, seek the advice of a health care professional before using this product. Keep this and all drugs out of the reach of children. In case of accidental overdose, seek professional assistance or contact a Poison Control Center immediately. Prompt medical attention is critical for adults as well as for children even if you do not notice any signs or symptoms.

Drug Interaction Precaution: Do not take this product if you are taking a prescription drug containing a monoamine oxidase inhibitor (MAOI) (certain drugs for depression or psychiatric or emotional conditions), without first consulting your doctor. If you are uncertain whether your prescription drug contains an MAOI, consult a health professional before taking this product. Do not take this product if you are taking an appetite-controlling medication containing phenylpropanolamine without first consulting your doctor.

Dosage and Administration: Coricidin Tablets—ADULTS AND CHILDREN 12 YEARS OF AGE AND OVER: oral dosage is 2 tablets every 4 to 6 hours, not to exceed 12 tablets in 24 hours, or as directed by a doctor. CHILDREN 6 TO UNDER 12 YEARS OF AGE: oral dosage is 1 tablet every 4 to 6 hours, not to exceed 5 tablets in 24 hours, or as directed by a doctor. CHILDREN UNDER 6 YEARS OF AGE: consult a doctor.
Coricidin 'D' Decongestant Tablets—ADULTS AND CHILDREN 12 YEARS OF AGE AND OVER: oral dosage is 2 tablets ever 4 hours not to exceed 12 tablets in 24 hours, or as directed by a doctor.
CHILDREN 6 TO UNDER 12 YEARS OF AGE: oral dosage is 1 tablet every 4 hours not to exceed 5 tablets in 24 hours, or as directed by a doctor. CHILDREN UNDER 6 YEARS OF AGE: consult a doctor.

How Supplied: CORICIDIN Tablets—12, 48, and 100, blisters of 24.
CORICIDIN 'D' Decongestant Tablets—12, 48, and 100, blisters of 24.
Store the tablets between 2° and 30°C (36° and 86°F).

Shown in Product Identification Guide, page 423
Continued on next page

Information on Schering-Plough HealthCare Products appearing on these pages is effective as of November 1993.

Schering-Plough—Cont.

CORRECTOL®
Laxative
Tablets & Caplets

Active Ingredients: Tablets and Caplets—Yellow phenolphthalein, 65 mg. and docusate sodium, 100 mg. per tablet/caplet.

Inactive Ingredients: Butylparaben, calcium gluconate, calcium sulfate, carnauba wax, D&C Red No. 7 calcium lake, gelatin, magnesium stearate, sugar, talc, titanium dioxide, wheat flour, white wax, and other ingredients.

Indications: For relief of occasional constipation or irregularity. CORRECTOL generally produces bowel movement in 6 to 8 hours.

Actions: Yellow phenolphthalein—stimulant laxative; docusate sodium—fecal softener.

Warnings: Not to be taken in case of nausea, vomiting, abdominal pain, or signs of appendicitis. Take only as needed —as frequent or continued use of laxatives may result in dependence on them. If skin rash appears, do not use this or any other preparation containing phenolphthalein. Keep out of children's reach.

Dosage and Administration
Dosage: Adults—1 or 2 tablets or caplets daily as needed, at bedtime or on arising. Children over 6 years—1 tablet or caplet daily as needed.

How Supplied: Tablets—Individual foil-backed safety sealed blister packaging in boxes of 15, 30 , 60 and 90 tablets. Caplets—Individual foil-backed safety sealed blister packaging in boxes of 30 and 60 caplets.
Shown in Product Identification Guide, page 423

CORRECTOL® EXTRA GENTLE
Stool Softener

Active Ingredient: Docusate sodium 100 mg. per soft gel.
Also Contains—D&C Red No. 33, FD&C Red No. 40, FD&C Yellow No. 6, gelatin, glycerin, polyethylene glycol 400, propylene glycol, sorbitol.

Indications: For relief of constipation without cramps for sensitive systems. Correctol Extra Gentle will work gradually to return you to regularity in 1 to 3 days.

Warning: Keep out of reach of children.

Directions: Adults: For gradual relief of constipation, take 2 soft gels daily, as needed. Children 6–12: Take 1 daily, as needed.

How Supplied: Tablets—individual foil-backed safety sealed blister packaging in boxes of 30 tablets.
Store below 86°F. Protect from freezing.
Shown in Product Identification Guide, page 423

DI–GEL®
Antacid · Anti-Gas
Tablets/Liquid

DI-GEL Tablets: Active Ingredients: (Per Tablet)—Simethicone 20 mg., Calcium Carbonate 280 mg., Magnesium Hydroxide 128 mg. **Inactive Ingredients:** D & C yellow No. 10 aluminum lake, dextrin, FD&C yellow No. 6 aluminum lake, flavor, magnesium stearate, mannitol, povidone, stearic acid, sucrose, talc.
Dietetically sodium free, calcium rich.

DI-GEL Liquid: Active Ingredients—per teaspoonful (5 ml): Simethicone 20 mg., aluminum hydroxide (equivalent to aluminum hydroxide dried gel USP) 200 mg., magnesium hydroxide 200 mg. **Also contains:** Flavor, hydroxypropyl methylcellulose, methylcellulose, methylparaben, propylparaben, sodium saccharin, sorbitol, water.
Dietetically sodium free.

Indications: For fast, temporary relief of acid indigestion, heartburn, sour stomach and accompanying painful gas symptoms.

Actions: The antacid system in DI-GEL relieves and soothes acid indigestion, heartburn and sour stomach. At the same time, the simethicone "defoamers" eliminate gas.
When air becomes entrapped in the stomach, heartburn and acid indigestion can result, along with sensations of fullness, pressure and bloating.

Warnings: Do not take more than 20 teaspoonfuls or 24 tablets in a 24 hour period, or use the maximum dosage of this product for more than 2 weeks, except under the advice and supervision of a physician. If you have kidney disease do not use this product except under the advice and supervision of a physician. May cause constipation or have a laxative effect. Keep this and all drugs out of the reach of children.

Drug Interaction: (Liquid Only) This product should not be taken if patient is presently taking a prescription antibiotic drug containing any form of tetracycline.

Dosage and Administration: Two teaspoonfuls or tablets every 2 hours, or after or between meals and at bedtime, not to exceed 20 teaspoonfuls or 24 tablets per day, or as directed by a physician.

How Supplied:
DI-GEL Liquid in Mint Flavor - 6 and 12 fl. oz. bottles, safety sealed and Lemon/Orange Flavors - 12 fl. oz. bottles, safety sealed.

DI-GEL Tablets in Mint and Lemon/Orange Flavors - In boxes of 30 and 90 in handy portable safety sealed blister packaging. Also available in Mint 60-tablet bottles.
Shown in Product Identification Guide, page 423

DRIXORAL® Cough Liquid Caps
Cough Suppressant
Liquid Caps

Description: Each Drixoral Cough Liquid Cap contains 30 mg Dextromethorphan Hydrobromide. Also contains: FD&C Blue No. 1, FD&C Red No. 40, Gelatin, Glycerin, Polyethylene Glycol 400, Povidone, Propylene Glycol, Sorbitol, Water.

Indications: Temporarily relieves coughs due to minor throat and bronchial irritations as may occur with a cold. Each DRIXORAL Cough Liquid Cap contains a maximum strength dose of cough suppressant—control daytime and nighttime coughs without narcotic side effects.

Warnings: A persistent cough may be a sign of a serious condition. If cough persists for more than 1 week, tends to recur, or is accompanied by fever, rash or persistent headache, consult a doctor. Do not take this product for persistent or chronic cough such as occurs with smoking, asthma, emphysema, or if cough is accompanied by excessive phlegm (mucus) unless directed by a doctor. As with any drug, if you are pregnant or nursing a baby, seek the advice of a health professional before using this product. Keep this and all drugs out of the reach of children. In case of accidental overdose, seek professional assistance or contact a Poison Control Center immediately.

Drug Interaction Precaution: Do not take this product if you are taking a prescription drug containing a monoamine oxidase inhibitor (MAOI) (certain drugs for depression or psychiatric or emotional conditions), without first consulting your doctor. If you are uncertain whether your prescription drug contains an MAOI, consult a health professional before taking this product.

Dosage and Administration: Adults: Swallow one liquid cap (30 mg.) with water every 6 to 8 hours, not to exceed 4 liquid caps (120 mg.) in 24 hours, or as directed by a doctor. This product is not for children under 12 years of age.
Store before 86°. Protect from freezing. Protect from excessive moisture.

How Supplied: DRIXORAL COUGH Liquid Caps are available in boxed of 10's and 20's.
Shown in Product Identification Guide, page 423

DRIXORAL® COLD & ALLERGY
[dricks-or 'al]
Sustained-Action Tablets

Description: EACH DRIXORAL COLD & ALLERGY SUSTAINED-ACTION TABLET CONTAINS: 120 mg of pseudoephedrine sulfate and 6 mg of dex-brompheniramine maleate. Half of the medication is released after the tablet is swallowed and the remaining amount of medication is released hours later providing continuous long-lasting relief for 12 hours. Also contains: Acacia, Butylparaben, Calcium Sulfate, Carnauba Wax, Corn Starch, D&C Yellow No. 10 Aluminum Lake, FD&C Blue No. 1 Aluminum Lake, FD&C Yellow No. 6 Aluminum Lake, Gelatin, Lactose, Magnesium Stearate, Neutral Soap, Oleic Acid, Povidone, Rosin, Sugar, Talc, White Wax, Zein.

Indications: The decongestant (pseudoephedrine sulfate) temporarily relieves nasal congestion due to the common cold, hay fever or other upper respiratory allergies, and associated with sinusitis. Helps decongest sinus openings and sinus passages. Reduces swelling of nasal passages; shrinks swollen membranes; and temporarily restores freer breathing through the nose. The antihistamine (dexbrompheniramine maleate) alleviates runny nose, sneezing, itching of the nose or throat, and itchy and watery eyes as may occur in allergic rhinitis (such as hay fever).

Warnings: If symptoms do not improve within 7 days or are accompanied by fever, consult a physician before continuing use. May cause excitability especially in children. Do not exceed recommended dosage because at higher doses nervousness, dizziness, or sleeplessness may occur. Do not take this product if you have asthma, glaucoma, emphysema, chronic pulmonary disease, high blood pressure, thyroid disease, diabetes, or difficulty in urination due to enlargement of the prostate gland or give this product to children under 12 years, unless directed by a physician. May cause drowsiness; alcohol may increase the drowsiness effect. Avoid alcoholic beverages while taking this product. Use caution when driving a motor vehicle or operating machinery. Keep this and all drugs out of the reach of children. In case of accidental overdose, seek professional assistance or contact a Poison Control Center immediately. As with any drug, if you are pregnant or nursing a baby, seek the advice of a health professional before using this product.

Drug Interaction Precaution: Do not take this product if you are presently taking a prescription drug for high blood pressure or depression, without first consulting your physician.

Dosage and Administration: ADULTS AND CHILDREN 12 YEARS AND OVER—one tablet every 12 hours. Do not exceed two tablets in 24 hours.

How Supplied: DRIXORAL Cold & Allergy Sustained-Action Tablets, green, sugar-coated tablets branded in black with the product name, boxes of 10, 20, and 40, bottle of 100.

Store between 2° and 25°C (36° and 77°F).
Shown in Product Identification Guide, page 423

DRIXORAL® NON-DROWSY FORMULA
[*dricks-or 'al*]
Long-Acting Nasal Decongestant

DRIXORAL NON-DROWSY FORMULA Long-Acting Nasal Decongestant Tablets contain 120 mg pseudoephedrine sulfate, a nasal decongestant, in a special timed-release tablet providing up to 12 hours of continuous relief . . . without drowsiness. Also contains: Acacia, Butylparaben, Calcium Sulfate, Carnauba Wax, Corn Starch, FD&C Blue No. 1 Aluminum Lake, Gelatin, Lactose, Magnesium Stearate, Neutral Soap, Oleic Acid, Povidone, Rosin, Sugar, Talc, White Wax, Zein.

Indications: For temporary relief of nasal congestion due to the common cold, hay fever or other upper respiratory allergies, and nasal congestion associated with sinusitis. Helps decongest sinus openings and sinus passages.

Directions: Adults and Children 12 Years and Over—One tablet every 12 hours. Do not exceed two tablets in 24 hours. DRIXORAL NON-DROWSY FORMULA is not recommended for children under 12 years of age.

Each Extended-Release Tablet Contains: 120 mg pseudoephedrine sulfate. Half the dose is released after the tablet is swallowed and the other half is released hours later, providing continuous relief for up to 12 hours.

Warnings: Do not exceed recommended dosage because at higher doses, nervousness, dizziness, or sleeplessness may occur. Do not take this product if you have heart disease, high blood pressure, thyroid disease, diabetes, difficulty in urination due to enlargement of the prostate gland, or give this product to children under 12 years unless directed by a physician. If symptoms do not improve within 7 days or are accompanied by fever, consult your physician before continuing use. Keep this and all drugs out of the reach of children. In case of accidental overdose, seek professional assistance or contact a Poison Control Center immediately. As with any drug, if you are pregnant or nursing a baby, seek the advice of a health professional before using this product.

Drug Interaction Precautions: Do not take this product if you are presently taking a prescription drug for high blood pressure or depression, without first consulting your physician.

How Supplied: DRIXORAL NON-DROWSY FORMULA Long-Acting Nasal Decongestant Tablets are available in boxes of 10's and 20's.
Store between 2°C and 25°C (36° and 77°F).

Protect from excessive moisture.
Shown in Product Identification Guide, page 423

DRIXORAL® COLD & FLU
[*dricks-or 'al*]
Extended-Release Tablets

Active Ingredients: 500 mg Acetaminophen, 3 mg Dexbrompheniramine Maleate, 60 mg Pseudoephedrine Sulfate.

Also Contains: Calcium Phosphate, Carnauba Wax, D&C Yellow No. 10 Aluminum Lake, FD&C Blue No. 1 Aluminum Lake, FD&C Yellow No. 6 Aluminum Lake, Hydroxypropyl Methylcellulose, Magnesium Stearate, Methylparaben, PEG, Propylparaben, Stearic Acid.
DRIXORAL® COLD & FLU Extended-Release Tablets combine a nasal decongestant and an antihistamine with a nonaspirin analgesic in a special 12-hour continuous-acting timed-release tablet.

Indications: The *decongestant* temporarily relieves nasal congestion due to the common cold, hay fever or other upper respiratory allergies, and associated with sinusitis. Reduces swelling of nasal passages; shrinks swollen membranes; and temporarily restores freer breathing through the nose. Also helps decongest sinus openings, sinus passages. The *nonaspirin analgesic* temporarily relieves occasional minor aches, pains, and headache and reduces fever due to the common cold. The *antihistamine* alleviates running nose, sneezing, itching of the nose or throat, and itchy and watery eyes as may occur in allergic rhinitis (such as hay fever).

Directions: ADULTS AND CHILDREN 12 YEARS AND OVER—two tablets every 12 hours. Do not exceed four tablets in 24 hours. Children under 12 years of age: consult a doctor.

Warnings: Do not take this product for more than 7 days. If symptoms do not improve, or are accompanied by fever that lasts for more than three days (72 hours) or recurs, or if new symptoms occur, consult a physician before continuing use. If pain or fever persists or gets worse, or if redness or swelling is present, consult a physician because these could be signs of a serious condition. May cause excitability especially in children. Do not exceed recommended dosage because at higher doses nervousness, dizziness, or sleeplessness may occur. Do not take this product if you have asthma, glaucoma, emphysema, chronic pulmonary disease, shortness of breath, difficulty in breathing, heart disease, high blood pressure, thyroid disease, diabetes difficulty in urina-

Continued on next page

Information on Schering-Plough HealthCare Products appearing on these pages is effective as of November 1993.

Schering-Plough—Cont.

tion due to enlargement of the prostate gland, or give this product to children under 12 years unless directed by a physician. May cause drowsiness; alcohol, sedatives, and tranquilizers may increase the drowsiness effect. Avoid alcoholic beverages while taking this product. Use caution when driving a motor vehicle or operating machinery. Keep this and all drugs out of the reach of children. In case of accidental overdose, seek professional assistance or contact a Poison Control Center immediately. Prompt medical attention is critical for adults as well as for children even if you do not notice any signs or symptoms. As with any drug, if you are pregnant or nursing a baby, seek the advice of a health professional before using this product.

Drug Interaction Precaution: Do not take this product if you are presently taking a prescription drug for high blood pressure or depression, sedatives or tranquilizers, without first consulting your physician.

How Supplied: DRIXORAL COLD & FLU Extended-Release Tablets are available in boxes of 12's and 24's and bottles of 48.
Store between 2° and 25°C (36° and 77°F).
Protect from excessive moisture.
Shown in Product Identification Guide, page 423

DRIXORAL® SINUS
[*dricks-or 'al*]
Nasal decongestant/Pain reliever/Antihistamine

DRIXORAL® SINUS Extended-Release Tablets combine a nasal decongestant, and a non-aspirin analgesic, with an antihistamine in a special 12-hour continuous-acting timed-release tablet.

Indications: The *decongestant* temporarily relieves nasal congestion due to sinusitis, the common cold, and hay fever or other upper respiratory allergies. Helps decongest sinus openings, sinus passages; relieves sinus pressure. Reduces swelling of nasal passages; shrinks swollen membranes; and temporarily restores freer breathing through the nose. The *non-aspirin analgesic* temporarily relieves occasional headaches, minor aches and pains, and reduces fever due to the common cold. The *antihistamine* alleviates runny nose, sneezing, itching of the nose or throat, and itchy and watery eyes as may occur in allergic rhinitis (such as hay fever).

Each Drixoral Sinus Extended-Release Tablet Contains: 60 mg of pseudoephedrine sulfate, 3 mg of dexbrompheniramine maleate, and 500 mg of acetaminophen. These ingredients are released continuously, providing long-lasting relief for 12 hours. Also contains: Calcium Phosphate, Carnauba Wax, D&C Yellow No. 10 Aluminum Lake, FD&C Yellow No. 6 Aluminum Lake, Hydroxypropyl Methylcellulose, Magnesium Stearate, Methylparaben, PEG, Propyparaben, Stearic Acid.

Directions: ADULTS AND CHILDREN 12 YEARS AND OVER—two tablets every 12 hours. Do not exceed four tablets in 24 hours. Children under 12 years of age: consult a physician.
Store between 2° and 25°C (36° and 77°F).

Warnings: Do not take this product for more than 7 days. If symptoms do not improve, or are accompanied by fever that lasts for more than three days (72 hours) or recurs, or if new symptoms occur, consult a physician before continuing use. If pain or fever persists or gets worse, or if redness or swelling is present, consult a physician because these could be signs of a serious condition. May cause excitability especially in children. Do not exceed recommended dosage because at higher doses nervousness, dizziness, or sleeplessness may occur. Do not take this product if you have asthma, glaucoma, emphysema, chronic pulmonary disease, shortness of breath, difficulty in breathing, heart disease, high blood pressure, thyroid disease, diabetes, difficulty in urination due to enlargement of the prostate gland, or give this product to children under 12 years unless directed by a physician. May cause drowsiness; alcohol, sedatives, and tranquilizers may increase the drowsiness effect. Avoid alcoholic beverages while taking this product. Use caution when driving a motor vehicle or operating machinery. Keep this and all drugs out of the reach of children. In case of accidental overdose, seek professional assistance or contact a Poison Control Center immediately. Prompt medical attention is critical for adults as well as for children even if you do not notice any signs or symptoms. As with any drug, if you are pregnant or nursing a baby, seek the advice of a health care professional before using this product.

Drug Interaction Precaution: Do not take this product if you are presently taking a prescription drug for high blood pressure or depression, sedatives, or tranquilizers, without first consulting your physician.

How Supplied: DRIXORAL SINUS Extended-Release Tablets are available in boxes of 12's and 24's.
Shown in Product Identification, Guide, page 423

DUOFILM® LIQUID

Active Ingredient: Salicylic Acid 17% (w/w).

Inactive Ingredients: Alcohol 15.8% w/w, castor oil, ether 42.6% w/w, ethyl lactate, and polybutene in flexible collodion.

Indications: For the removal of common and plantar warts. Common warts can be easily recognized by the rough, cauliflower-like appearance of the surface. Plantar warts are found on the bottom of the foot.

Warnings: For external use only. Do not use this product on irritated skin, on any area that is infected or reddened, if you are a diabetic, or if you have poor blood circulation. If discomfort persists, see your doctor. Do not use on moles, birthmarks, warts with hair growing from them, genital warts, or warts on the face or mucous membranes. Keep out of reach of children. If DuoFilm Liquid gets in eyes, flush with water for 15 minutes. Avoid inhaling vapors. DuoFilm Liquid is extremely flammable. Keep away from fire or flame. Cap bottle tightly when not in use. Store at room temperature away from heat.

Directions: Wash affected area. May soak wart in warm water for 5 minutes. Dry area thoroughly.
Apply one thin layer (with brush applicator) at a time to sufficiently cover each wart. Let dry. Repeat this procedure once or twice daily as needed (until wart is removed) for up to 12 weeks.
Note: Adhesive bandage may be used to cover treated area.

How Supplied: DuoFilm Liquid is available in ½ fluid oz. spill-resistant bottles with brush applicator for pinpoint application.
Shown in Product Identification Guide, page 423

DUOFILM®PATCH

Active Ingredient: Salicylic Acid 40% in a rubber-based vehicle.

Indications: For the concealment and removal of common warts. Common warts can be easily recognized by the rough, cauliflower-like appearance of the surface.

Warnings: For external use only. Do not use this product on irritated skin, on any area that is infected or reddened, if you are a diabetic, or if you have poor blood circulation. If discomfort persists, see your doctor. Do not use on moles, birthmarks, warts with hair growing from them, genital warts, or warts on the face or mucous membranes. Keep out of reach from children.

Directions: Wash affected area. Soak in warm water for five minutes. Dry area thoroughly. Apply Medicated Patch (packet A). If necessary, cut patch to fit wart. Repeat procedure every 48 hours as needed (until wart is removed) for up to 12 weeks.
Note: Self-adhesive cover-up patches (packet B) may be used to conceal Medicated Patch and wart.

How Supplied: DuoFilm Patch includes 54 Medicated Patches of varying sizes, with 20 self-adhesive Cover-Up patches for concealment while treatment is ongoing.

Shown in Product Identification Guide, page 423

DUOPLANT® GEL

Active Ingredient: Salicylic Acid 17% (w/w).

Inactive Ingredients: Alcohol 57.6% w/w, ether 16.42% w/w, ethyl lactate, hydroxypropyl cellulose, and polybutene in flexible collodion, USP.

Indications: For the removal of plantar and common warts. Plantar warts are found on the bottom of the foot. Common warts can be easily recognized by the rough, cauliflower-like appearance of the surface.

Warnings: For external use only. Do not use this product on irritated skin, on any area that is infected or reddened, if you are a diabetic, or if you have poor blood circulation. If discomfort persists, see your doctor. Do not use on moles, birthmarks, warts with hair growing from them, genital warts, or warts on the face or mucous membranes. Keep out of reach of children. If DuoPlant Gel gets in eyes, flush with water for 15 minutes. Avoid inhaling vapors. DuoPlant Gel is extremely flammable. Keep away from fire or flame. Keep tube tightly capped when not in use. Store at room temperature away from heat.

Directions: Wash affected area. May soak wart in warm water for five minutes. Dry area thoroughly. Apply a thin layer to sufficiently cover each wart. Let dry. Repeat this procedure once or twice daily as needed (until wart is removed) for up to 12 weeks.
Note: Adhesive bandage may be used to cover treated area.

How Supplied: DuoPlant Gel is available in ½ oz. tubes with applicator tip for pinpoint application.

Shown in Product Identification Guide, page 423

DURATION
12 Hour Nasal Spray 0.05%
12 Hour Nasal Spray Pump 0.05%

Description: DURATION products contain oxymetazoline hydrochloride, the longest acting topical nasal decongestant available. Each ml of DURATION Nasal Spray and Nasal Spray Pump contains Oxymetazoline Hydrochloride, USP 0.5 mg (0.05%), Benzalkonium Chloride, Glycine, Phenylmercuric Acetate (0.002%), Sorbitol and Water.

Indications: Fast relief for up to 12 hours of nasal congestion due to colds, hay fever and sinusitis.

Actions: The sympathomimetic action of DURATION products constricts the smaller arterioles of the nasal passages, producing a prolonged, gentle and predictable decongesting effect. In just a few minutes a single dose, as directed, provides prompt, temporary relief of nasal congestion that lasts up to 12 hours. DURATION products last up to 3 times longer than most ordinary nasal sprays.

Warnings: Do not exceed recommended dosage because symptoms may occur such as burning, stinging, sneezing or increase of nasal discharge. Do not use this product for more than three days. If symptoms persist, consult a physician. As with any drug, if you are pregnant or nursing a baby, seek the advice of a health professional before using this product. The use of the dispenser by more than one person may spread infection. Keep this and all medications out of the reach of children. In case of accidental ingestion, seek professional assistance or contact a Poison Control Center immediately.

Dosage and Administration: DURATION 12 Hour Nasal Spray, 0.05%—For adults and children 6 years of age and over: With head upright, spray 2 or 3 times into each nostril twice daily—morning and evening. To spray, squeeze bottle quickly and firmly. Do not tilt head backward while spraying. Wipe nozzle clean after use. Not recommended for children under six.
DURATION Nasal Spray Pump, 0.05%—For adults six years of age and over: Before using first time, remove protective cap. Prime the metered pump by depressing several times. Hold bottle with thumb at base and nozzle between first and second fingers. With head upright (do not tilt backward), insert metered pump-spray nozzle into nostril. Depress pump completely 2 or 3 times. Sniff deeply. Repeat in other nostril. Wipe tip clean after use. Not recommended for children under six.
Store between 2° and 30°C (36° and 86°F).

How Supplied: DURATION 12 Hour Nasal Spray 0.05%—½ oz and 1 oz plastic squeeze bottles
DURATION 12 Hour Nasal Spray Pump—½ oz metered dose pump spray bottle

Shown in Product Identification Guide, page 423

FEEN-A-MINT®
Laxative Gum/Pills

Active Ingredients: Gum—yellow phenolphthalein 97.2 mg. per tablet. Pills—yellow phenolphthalein 65 mg., and docusate sodium 100 mg. per pill.

Indications: For relief of occasional constipation or irregularity. FEEN-A-MINT generally produces bowel movement in 6 to 8 hours.

Inactive Ingredients: Gum—Acacia, butylated hydroxyanisole, carnauba wax, corn starch, gelatin, glucose, glycerin, gum base, peppermint oil, sodium benzoate, sugar, water, white wax.
Pills—Butylparaben, calcium gluconate, calcium sulfate, carnauba wax, gelatin, magnesium stearate, sugar, talc, tita-nium dioxide, wheat flour, white wax and other ingredients.

Warning: Do not take any laxative in case of nausea, vomiting, or abdominal pain. Take only as needed as frequent or continued use of laxatives may result in dependence on them. If skin rash appears, do not take this or any other preparation containing phenolphthalein. Keep out of the reach of children. In case of accidental overdose, seek professional assistance or contact a Poison Control Center immediately.

How Supplied: Gum—Individual foil-backed safety sealed blister packaging in boxes of 5 and 16 tablets.
Pills—Safety sealed boxes of 15, 30, and 60 tablets.

Shown in Product Identification Guide, page 423

FEMCARE™
Clotrimazole
Vaginal Cream
Antifungal

Active Ingredient: Clotrimazole 1%

Inactive Ingredients: Benzyl alcohol, cetearyl, alcohol, cetyl esters wax, octyldodecanol, polysorbate 60, purified water, sorbitan monostearate.

Indications: FemCare™ will cure most recurrent vaginal yeast (Candida) infections. FemCare™ usually starts to relieve the itching and other symptoms of vaginal yeast infection within 3 days. If the patient does not improve in 3 days or if the patient does not get well in 7 days, a condition other than yeast infection may exist. The patient should discontinue use of the product and consult a doctor. Also, if symptoms recur within a 2-month period, patient should consult a doctor.

Important: In order to kill the yeast completely, FEMCARE must be used the full seven days, even if symptoms are relieved sooner.

Warnings:
• Do not use if you have abdominal pain, fever, or a foul-smelling vaginal discharge. You may have a condition which is more serious than a yeast infection. Contact your doctor immediately.
• Do not use if this is your first experience with vaginal itch and discomfort. See your doctor.
• If there is no improvement within 3 days, you may have a condition other than a yeast infection. Stop using this product and see your doctor.
• If you may have been exposed to the human immunodeficiency virus (HIV,

Continued on next page

Information on Schering-Plough HealthCare Products appearing on these pages is effective as of November 1993.

Schering-Plough—Cont.

the virus that causes AIDS) and are now having recurrent vaginal infections, especially infections that don't clear up easily with proper treatment, see your doctor promptly to determine the cause of your symptoms and to receive proper medical care.

- If your symptoms return within two months or if you have infections that do not clear up easily with proper treatment, consult your doctor. You could be pregnant or there could be a serious underlying medical cause for your infections, including diabetes or a damaged immune system (including damage from infection with HIV - the virus that causes AIDS). (PLEASE READ EDUCATIONAL PAMPHLET FOUND INSIDE THIS PACKAGE).
- Do not use during pregnancy except under the advice and supervision of a doctor.
- This medication is for vaginal use only. It is not for use in the mouth or the eyes. In case accidentally swallowed, seek professional assistance or contact a Poison Control Center immediately.
- Keep this and all drugs out of reach of chilren. This product is not be used on children less than 12 years of age.

Dosage: Fill the applicator with the cream and then insert one applicatorful of cream into the vagina every day, preferably at bedtime. Repeat this procedure for seven consecutive days.

Shown in Product Identification Guide, page 423

FEMCARE™
Clotrimazole
Vaginal Inserts
Antifungal

Active Ingredient: Each insert contains Clotrimazole 100 mg.

Inactive Ingredients: Corn starch, lactose magnesium stearate, povidone.

Indications: FemCare™ will cure most recurrent vaginal yeast (Candida) infections. FemCare™ usually starts to relieve the itching and other symptoms of vaginal yeast infection within 3 days. If the patient does not improve in 3 days or if the patient does not get well in 7 days, a condition other than yeast infection may exist. The patient should discontinue use of the product and consult a doctor. Also, if symptoms recur within a 2 month period, patient should consult a doctor.

Important: In order to kill the yeast completely, FEMCARE must be used the full seven days, even if symptoms are relieved sooner.

Warnings:
- Do not use if you have abdominal pain, fever, or a foul-smelling vaginal discharge. You may have a condition which is more serious than a yeast infection. Contact your doctor immediately.

- Do not use if this is your first experience with vaginal itch and discomfort. See your doctor.
- If there is no improvement within 3 days, you may have a condition other than a yeast infection. Stop using this product and see your doctor.
- If you may have been exposed to the human immunodeficiency virus (HIV, the virus that causes AIDS) and are now having recurrent vaginal infections, especially infections that don't clear up easily with proper treatment, see your doctor promptly to determine the cause of your symptoms and to receive proper medical care.
- If your symptoms return within two months or if you have infections that do not clear up easily with proper treatment, consult your doctor. You could be pregnant or there could be a serious underlying medical cause for your infections, including diabetes or a damaged immune system (including damage from infection with HIV - the virus that causes AIDS). (PLEASE READ EDUCATIONAL PAMPHLET FOUND INSIDE PACKAGE).
- Do not use during pregnancy except under the advice and supervision of a doctor.
- This medication is for vaginal use only. It is not for use in the mouth or the eyes. In case accidentally swallowed, seek professional assistance or contact a Poison Control Center immediately.
- Keep this and all drugs out of reach of children. This product is not be used on children less than 12 years of age.

Dosage: Using the applicator, place one insert into the vagina, preferably at bedtime. Repeat this procedure for seven consecutive days.

Shown in Product Identification Guide, page 423

GYNE-LOTRIMIN®
Clotrimazole
Vaginal Cream
Antifungal

Active Ingredient: Clotrimazole 1%

Inactive Ingredients: Benzyl alcohol, cetearyl alcohol, cetyl esters wax, octyldodecanol, polysorbate 60, purified water, sorbitan monostearate.

Indications: Gyne-Lotrimin® will cure most recurrent vaginal yeast (Candida) infections. Gyne-Lotrimin® usually starts to relieve the itching and other symptoms of vaginal yeast infection within 3 days. If the patient does not improve in 3 days or if the patient does not get well in 7 days, a condition other than yeast infection may exist. The patient should discontinue use of the product and consult a doctor. Also, if symptoms recur within a 2-month period, patient should consult a doctor.

Important: In order to kill the yeast completely, GYNE-LOTRIMIN must be used the full seven days, even if symptoms are relieved sooner.

Warnings:
- Do not use if you have abdominal pain, fever, or a foul-smelling vaginal discharge. You may have a condition which is more serious than a yeast infection. Contact your doctor immediately.
- Do not use if this is your first experience with vaginal itch and discomfort. See your doctor.
- If there is no improvement within 3 days, you may have a condition other than a yeast infection. Stop using this product and see your doctor.
- If you may have been exposed to the human immunodeficiency virus (HIV, the virus that causes AIDS) and are now having recurrent vaginal infections, especially infections that don't clear up easily with proper treatment, see your doctor promptly to determine the cause of your symptoms and to receive proper medical care.
- If your symptoms return within two months or if you have infections that do not clear up easily with proper treatment, consult your doctor. You could be pregnant or there could be a serious underlying medical cause for your infections, including diabetes or a damaged immune system (including damage from infection with HIV—the virus that causes AIDS). (PLEASE READ EDUCATIONAL PAMPHLET FOUND INSIDE PACKAGE.)
- Do not use during pregnancy except under the advice and supervision of a doctor.
- This medication is for vaginal use only. It is not for use in the mouth or the eyes. In case accidentally swallowed, seek professional assistance or contact a Poison Control Center immediately.
- Keep this and all drugs out of reach of children. This product is not be used on children less than 12 years of age.

Dosage: Fill the applicator with the cream and then insert one applicatorful of cream into the vagina every day, preferably at bedtime. Repeat this procedure for seven consecutive days. For relief of external vulvar itching, squeeze a small amount of cream onto your finger and gently spread the cream onto the irritated area of the vulva. Use once or twice a day for up to 7 days as needed to relieve external vulvar itching. THE CREAM SHOULD NOT BE USED FOR VULVAR ITCHING DUE TO CAUSES OTHER THAN A YEAST INFECTION. *Cream also available with 7 disposable applicators and 7 pre-filled applicators.

Shown in Product Identification Guide, page 423

GYNE-LOTRIMIN®
Clotrimazole
Vaginal Inserts
Antifungal

Active Ingredient: Each insert contains Clotrimazole 100 mg.

Inactive Ingredients: Corn starch, lactose, magnesium stearate, povidone.

Indications: Gyne-Lotrimin® will cure most vaginal yeast (Candida) infections. Gyne-Lotrimin® usually starts to relieve the itching and other symptoms of vaginal yeast infection within 3 days. If the patient does not improve in 3 days or if the patient does not get well in 7 days, a condition other than yeast infection may exist. The patient should discontinue use of the product and consult a doctor. Also, if symptoms recur within a 2-month period, patient should consult a doctor.

Important: In order to kill the yeast completely, GYNE-LOTRIMIN must be used the full seven days, even if symptoms are relieved sooner.

Warnings:
- Do not use if you have abdominal pain, fever, or a foul-smelling vaginal discharge. You may have a condition which is more serious than a yeast infection. Contact your doctor immediately.
- Do not use if this is your first experience with vaginal itch and discomfort. See your doctor.
- If there is no improvement within 3 days, you may have a condition other than a yeast infection. Stop using this product and see your doctor.
- If you may have been exposed to the human immunodeficiency virus (HIV, the virus that causes AIDS) and are now having recurrent vaginal infections, especially infections that don't clear up easily with proper treatment, see your doctor promptly to determine the cause of your symptoms and to receive proper medical care.
- If your symptoms return within two months or if you have infections that do not clear up easily with proper treatment, consult your doctor. You could be pregnant or there could be a serious underlying medical cause for your infections, including diabetes or a damaged immune system (including damage from infection with HIV—the virus that causes AIDS). (PLEASE READ EDUCATIONAL PAMPHLET FOUND INSIDE PACKAGE.)
- Do not use during pregnancy except under the advice and supervision of a doctor.
- This medication is for vaginal use only. It is not for use in the mouth or the eyes. In case accidentally swallowed, seek professional assistance or contact a Poison Control Center immediately.
- Keep this and all drugs out of reach of children. This product is not to be used on children less than 12 years of age.

Dosage: Using the applicator, place one insert into the vagina, preferably at bedtime. Repeat this procedure for seven consecutive days.

*Inserts also available in a combination pack, which includes external vulvar cream for the relief of associated external vulvar itching and irritation.

Shown in Product Identification Guide, page 423

GYNE–MOISTRIN®
Vaginal Moisturizing Gel

Description: Gyne-Moistrin Vaginal Moisturizing Gel was specially developed to soothe and relieve vaginal dryness. Gyne-Moistrin provides natural feeling moisture and lubrication. It is clear, colorless, odorless and proven to be non-irritating. Gyne-Moistrin is water-based, greaseless and non-staining; and it contains no hormones or medication, so it can be used as often as needed.

Actions: When used as directed, Gyne-Moistrin will relieve vaginal dryness. Gyne-Moistrin forms a non-occlusive layer of moisture over the vaginal epithelium, gradually hydrating a dry irritated area. Gyne-Moistrin can be used as often as needed.
Externally, in the vulvar area, Gyne-Moistrin will also moisturize tissues.

Ingredients: Polyglycerylmethacrylate, water, propylene glycol, methylparaben, propylparaben.

Warnings: Gyne-Moistrin is not a contraceptive. Does not harm condoms.

Directions: Gyne-Moistrin may be applied externally and internally according to personal preference using fingertip application or the reusable applicator.
FOR FINGERTIP APPLICATION: Squeeze out small amount of gel to cover fingertip and apply to the vaginal opening and external area as needed. Actual amount applied may be increased or decreased according to personal preference.
FOR INTERNAL USE: Remove reusable applicator from sealed wrapper. Fill with gel to line on applicator. Gently insert front end well into vagina; push end of applicator to fully release gel; remove applicator. Actual amount used may be increased or decreased according to personal preference. Wash applicator in warm soapy water then thoroughly rinse and dry before and after each use.
Store at room temperature.

How Supplied: Gyne-Moistrin is available in 1.5 oz. and 2.5 oz. tubes.
Shown in Product Identification Guide, page 424

LOTRIMIN® AF ANTIFUNGAL
[lo-tre-min]
Clotrimazole
Cream 1%
Solution 1%
Lotion 1%

Description: Lotrimin® AF Cream 1% is a white fully vanishing homogeneous cream containing 1% clotrimazole. The cream contains no sensitizing parabens and is totally grease free and non-staining.

Lotrimin® AF Solution 1% is a non-aqueous liquid, containing polyethylene glycol.
Lotrimin® AF Lotion 1% is a light penetrating buffered emulsion also containing no common sensitizing agents and is greaseless and nonstaining.

Indications: Lotrimin® AF Cream, Solution and Lotion contain 1% clotrimazole, a synthetic broad-spectrum antifungal agent. Clotrimazole is used for the treatment of dermal infections caused by a variety of pathogenic dermatophytes, yeasts and *Malassezia furfur*. The primary action of clotrimazole is against dividing and growing organisms. Lotrimin® AF was first made available as an over-the-counter drug in 1990 and is indicated for superficial dermatophyte infections: athlete's foot (tinea pedis), jock itch (tinea cruris) and ringworm (tinea corporis). Lotrimin® remains on prescription for topical candidiasis due to *Candida albicans* and tinea versicolor due to *Malassezia furfur*.

Directions: Cleanse skin with soap and water and dry thoroughly. Apply a thin layer over affected area morning and evening or as directed by a physician. For athlete's foot, pay special attention to the spaces between the toes. It is also helpful to wear well-fitting, ventilated shoes and to change shoes and socks at least once daily. Best results in athlete's foot and ringworm are usually obtained with 4 weeks use of this product, and in jock itch, with 2 weeks use. If satisfactory results have not occurred within these times, consult a physician or pharmacist. Children under 12 years of age should be supervised in the use of this product. This product is not effective on the scalp or nails.

How Supplied: Lotrimin® AF Antifungal Cream is available in a 0.42 oz. tube (12 grams) and a 0.84 oz. tube (24 grams).
Inactive ingredients include: benzyl alcohol, cetearyl alcohol, cetyl esters wax, octyldodecanol, polysorbate, sorbitan monostearate and water.
Lotrimin® AF Antifungal Solution is available in a 0.33 fl. oz. (10 milliliters) bottle. Inactive ingredients include PEG.
Lotrimin® AF Antifungal Lotion is available in a 0.66 fl. oz. (20 milliliters) bottle. Inactive ingredients include benzyl alcohol, cetearyl alcohol, cetyl esters wax, octyldodecanol, polysorbate, sodium biphosphate, sodium phosphate dibasic, sorbitan monostearate and water.

Storage: Keep Lotrimin® AF products between 2° and 30°C (36° and 86°F).
Shown in Product Identification Guide, page 424

Continued on next page

Information on Schering-Plough HealthCare Products appearing on these pages is effective as of November 1993.

Schering-Plough—Cont.

LOTRIMIN® AF ANTIFUNGAL
Miconazole Nitrate 2%
Athlete's Foot Spray Liquid
Athlete's Foot Spray Powder
Athlete's Foot Powder
Jock Itch Spray Powder

Active Ingredients:
SPRAY LIQUID contains Miconazole Nitrate 2%. Also contains: Alcohol SD-40 (17% w/w), Cocamide DEA, Isobutane, Propylene Glycol, Tocopherol (vitamin E).
SPRAY POWDER (Athlete's Foot/Jock Itch) contains Miconazole Nitrate 2%. Also contains: Alcohol SD-40 (10% w/w), Isobutane, Stearalkonium Hectorite, Talc.
POWDER contains Miconazole Nitrate 2%. Also contains: Talc.

Indications: LOTRIMIN AF Athlete's Foot Spray Liquid, Spray Powder and Powder are proven clinically effective in the treatment of athlete's foot (tinea pedis), jock itch (tinea cruris) and ringworm (tinea corporis). For effective relief of the itching, cracking, burning, scaling and discomfort that can accompany these conditions.
LOTRIMIN AF Powder also aids in the drying of naturally moist areas.
LOTRIMIN AF Jock Itch Spray Powder cures jock itch (tinea cruris). For effective relief of the itching, burning, scaling and discomfort associated with jock itch.

Warnings: For Athlete's Foot Spray Powder, Spray Liquid and Jock Itch Spray Powder: Do not use on children under 2 years of age except under the advice and supervision of a doctor. For external use only. If irritation occurs or if there is no improvement within 4 weeks (for athlete's foot or ringworm) or within 2 weeks (for jock itch), discontinue use and consult a doctor or a pharmacist. Avoid spraying in eyes. Contents under pressure. Do not puncture or incinerate. Flammable mixture: do not use or store near heat or open flames. Do not use while smoking. Exposure to temperatures above 120°F may cause bursting. Never throw container into fire or incinerator. Use only as directed. Intentional misuse by deliberately concentrating and inhaling contents may be harmful or fatal. Keep this and all drugs out of the reach of children. In case of accidental ingestion, seek professional assistance or contact a Poison Control Center immediately.
Lotrimin AF Powder: Do not use on children under 2 years of age except under the advice and supervision of a doctor. For external use only. If irritation occurs, or if there is no improvement within 4 weeks (for athlete's foot or ringworm) or within 2 weeks (for jock itch) discontinue use and consult a doctor or pharmacist. Keep this and all drugs out of the reach of children. In case of accidental ingestion, seek professional assis-

tance or contact a Poison Control Center immediately.

Directions: For Athlete's Foot Spray Liquid, Spray Powder and Jock Itch Spray Powder: Cleanse skin with soap and water and dry thoroughly. Shake can well before using. Hold can about six inches from the area to be treated. Apply a thin layer over affected area morning and night or as directed by a doctor. For athlete's foot, pay special attention to spaces between the toes. It is helpful to wear well fitting, ventilated shoes and to change socks and shoes at least once daily. Best results in athlete's foot and ringworm are usually obtained with 4 weeks use of this product and in jock itch with 2 weeks use. If satisfactory results have not occurred within these times, consult a doctor or pharmacist. Children under 12 years of age should be supervised in the use of this product. This product is not effective on the scalp or nails.
Powder: Cleanse skin with soap and water and dry thoroughly. Sprinkle powder liberally over affected area morning and night or as directed by a physician. For athlete's foot, pay special attention to the spaces between the toes. It is also helpful to wear well-fitting, ventilated shoes and to change socks and shoes at least once daily. Best results in athlete's foot and ringworm are usually obtained with 4 weeks use of this product and in jock itch with 2 weeks use. If satisfactory results have not occurred within these times, consult a doctor or pharmacist. Children under 12 years of age should be supervised in the use of this product. This product is not effective on the scalp or nails.
Store between 2° and 30° C (36° and 86°F).

How Supplied: LOTRIMIN AF Athlete's Foot Spray Powder and Jock Itch Spray Powder—3.5 oz. cans. LOTRIMIN AF Spray Liquid—4 oz. can. LOTRIMIN AF POWDER—3 oz. plastic bottle.

SHADE SUNBLOCK GEL SPF 30

Active Ingredients: Ethylhexyl p-methoxycinnamate, homosalate, oxybenzone.

Other Ingredients: SD alcohol 40 (73% V/V), water, PVP/VA copolymer, tetrahydroxypropyl ethylenediamine, acrylates/C10-30 alkyl acrylate crosspolymer, acrylates/octylacrylamide copolymer.

Indications: PABA-FREE Shade SPF 30 Oil-Free Clear Gel is clinically tested to protect your skin from the sun's burning UVA and UVB rays. This clean, clear gel vanishes quickly without any greasy residue. It leaves your skin feeling fresh and clean while providing 30 times your natural protection against sunburn. This unique formula blocks UVB rays that are primarily responsible for sunburn and long-term skin damage caused by overexposure to the sun. It also protects your skin against the deeper penetrating

UVA rays that have been associated with skin damage resulting premature aging and wrinkling. Regular use of Shade 30 Oil-Free Clear Gel may help prevent skin cancer caused by long-term overexposure to the sun.

Non-greasy/Non-oily: Fresh, clear, lightweight greaseless formula that absorbs quickly—feels cool. Specially formulated for people with normal to oily skin.

Waterproof Maintains its degree of protection (SPF 30) for 80 minutes or more in the water.

Non-acnegenic/Non-comedogenic: Won't clog pores or cause blemishes.

Fragrance-free: Free of fragrances that may irritate those with sensitive skin.

Hypoallergenic: Won't irritate or sting sensitive skin like some protective sunscreens. Gentle enough for children's delicate skin.

Warnings: Flammable, do not use near heat or flame. Avoid contact with eyes, if skin irritation or rash develops discontinue use.

Directions for Use: Smooth evenly and liberally on all exposed areas. To ensure maximum protection, reapply often especially after swimming or excessive perspiration.

How Supplied: 4 oz. plastic bottles.
Shown in Product Identification Guide, page 424

SHADE® SUNBLOCK LOTION SPF 45

Active Ingredients: Ethylhexyl p-methoxycinnamate, octocrylene, oxybenzone, 2-ethylhexyl salicylate.

Other Ingredients: Water, sorbitan isostearate, sorbitol, octadecene/MA copolymer, triethanolamine, stearic acid, benzyl alcohol, barium sulfate, dimethicone, methylparaben, imidazolidinyl urea, phenethyl alcohol, propylparaben, carbomer, disodium EDTA.

Indications: PABA-FREE Shade 45 is clinically tested to protect your skin from the sun's burning UVA and UVB rays. This ultra moisturizing formula keeps your skin feeling soft yet provides 45 times your natural protection against sunburn. It blocks UVB rays that are primarily responsible for sunburn and long-term skin damage caused by overexposure to the sun. It also protects your skin against the deeper penetrating UVA rays that have been associated with skin damage resulting in premature aging and wrinkling. Regular use of Shade 45 may help prevent skin cancer caused by long-term overexposure to the sun.

Moisturizing: Rich moisturizing formula helps keep your skin feeling smooth, soft and supple.

Waterproof: Maintains its degree of protection (SPF 45) for 80 minutes or more in the water.

Non-comedogenic: Won't clog pores.

Hypoallergenic: Won't irritate or sting sensitive skin like some protective sunscreens. Gentle enough for children's delicate skin.

Fragrance Free: Free of fragrances that may irritate those with sensitive skin.

Warnings: Avoid contact with eyes. If skin irritation or rash develops, discontinue use.

Directions for Use: Smooth evenly and liberally on all exposed areas. To ensure maximum protection, reapply often especially after swimming or excessive perspiration.

How Supplied: 4 oz. plastic bottles
Shown in Product Identification Guide, page 424

SHADE® UVAGUARD™

Active Ingredients: Octyl methoxycinnamate, 7.5%; avobenzone (Parsol® 1789), 3%; oxybenzone, USP, 3%.

Other Ingredients: Benzyl alcohol, carbomer-941, dimethicone, edetate disodium, glyceryl stearate SE, isopropyl myristate, methylparaben, octadecene/MA copolymer, propylparaben, purified water, sorbitan monooleate, sorbitol, stearic acid and trolamine.

Indications: While all sunscreens protect your skin from the sun's burning rays, Shade® UVAGUARD™ sunscreen, with the patented ingredient Parsol®1789, offers extra protection from the UVA rays that may contribute to skin damage and premature aging of the skin. Shade UVAGUARD is clinically tested to provide 15 times your natural sunburn protection (UVB). And the moisturizing formula of Shade UVAGUARD keeps your skin feeling soft and is PABA-free. Regular use of Shade UVAGUARD may help reduce the chance of acute and long-term skin damage associated with exposure to UVA and UVB rays. Overexposure to the sun may lead to premature aging of the skin and skin cancer.

Water-resistant: Maintains its degree of protection (SPF 15) for 40 minutes or more in water.

Fragrance-free: Free of fragrance that may irritate those with sensitive skin.

Moisturizing: Moisturizing formula helps keep your skin feeling smooth and soft.

Non-comedogenic: Won't clog pores.

Warnings: Do not use if sensitive to cinnamates, benzophenones or any other ingredient in this product. Avoid contact with the eyes, if contact occurs, rinse eyes thoroughly with water. For external use only, not to be swallowed. Discontinue use if signs of irritation or rash ap-

pear. Keep this and all drugs out of the reach of children. In case of accidental ingestion, seek professional assistance or contact a Poison Control Center immediately.

Directions for Use: Shake well before using. Before sun exposure, apply evenly and liberally on all exposed areas and reapply after 40 minutes in the water or after excessive sweating. There is no recommended dosage for children under six (6) months of age except under the advice and supervision of a physician.

How Supplied: 4 oz. plastic bottles.

ST. JOSEPH®
ADULT CHEWABLE ASPIRIN
Low Strength Tablets (81 mg. each)

Active Ingredient: Each St. Joseph Adult Chewable Aspirin Tablet contains 81 mg. aspirin in a chewable, orange flavored form.

Inactive Ingredients: Corn Starch, FD&C Yellow No. 6 Aluminum Lake, Flavor, Hydrogenated Vegetable Oil, Maltodextrin, Mannitol, Saccharin.

Indications: St. Joseph® Adult Chewable Aspirin Tablets provide safe, effective, temporary relief from: Headaches, muscular aches, minor aches and pain associated with overexertion; sprains; menstrual cramps; neuralgia; bursitis; and discomforts of fever due to colds.

Warnings: Children and teenagers should not use this medicine for chicken pox or flu symptoms before a doctor is consulted about Reye Syndrome, a rare but serious illness reported to be associated with aspirin. If symptoms persist, or new ones occur, consult your doctor. NOTE: SEVERE OR PERSISTENT SORE THROAT, HIGH FEVER, HEADACHE, NAUSEA OR VOMITING, MAY BE SERIOUS, DISCONTINUE USE AND CONSULT YOUR DOCTOR IF NOT RELIEVED IN 24 HOURS. Do not take this product for more than five days unless directed by your doctor. Do not exceed recommended dosage. When using St. Joseph Adult Chewable Aspirin, do not give any other medications containing aspirin unless directed by your doctor. As with any drug, if you are pregnant or nursing a baby, seek the advice of a health professional before using this product. **IT IS ESPECIALLY IMPORTANT NOT TO USE ASPIRIN THE LAST 3 MONTHS OF PREGNANCY UNLESS SPECIFICALLY DIRECTED TO DO SO BY A DOCTOR BECAUSE IT MAY CAUSE PROBLEMS IN THE UNBORN CHILD OR COMPLICATIONS DURING DELIVERY.** Keep this and all drugs out of reach of children. In case of accidental overdose, seek professional assistance or contact a Poison Control Center immediately.

Dosage and Administration: Take from 4 to 8 tablets (325 mg. to 650 mg.) every 4 hours as needed. Do not exceed 48

tablets in 24 hours. For professional dosage see below.

Professional Labeling: Aspirin for Myocardial Infarction.

Indication: Aspirin is indicated to reduce the risk of death and/or nonfatal myocardial infarction in patients with a previous infarction or unstable angina pectoris.

Clinical Trials: The indication is supported by the results of six large randomized, multicenter, placebo-controlled studies[1-7] involving 10,816 predominantly male post–myocardial infarction (MI) patients and one randomized placebo-controlled study of 1,266 men with unstable angina. Therapy with aspirin was begun at intervals after the onset of acute MI varying from less than three days to more than five years and continued for periods of from less than one year to four years. In the unstable angina study, treatment was started within one month after the onset of unstable angina and continued for 12 weeks, and complicating conditions, such as congestive heart failure, were not included in the study. Aspirin therapy in MI patients was associated with about a 20% reduction in the risk of subsequent death and/or nonfatal reinfarction, a median absolute decrease of 3% from the 12% to 22% event rates in the placebo groups. In the aspirin-treated unstable angina patients, the reduction in risk was about 50%, a reduction in the event rate of 5% from the 10% rate in the placebo group over the 12 weeks of study.

Daily dosage of aspirin in the post–myocardial infarction studies was 300 mg in one study and 900–1,500 mg in five studies. A dose of 325 mg was used in the study of unstable angina.

Adverse Reactions: Gastrointestinal Reactions: Doses of 1,000 mg per day of aspirin caused gastrointestinal symptoms and bleeding that, in some cases, were clinically significant. In the largest postinfarction study (the Aspirin Myocardial Infarction Study [AMIS] with 4,500 people), the percentage of incidences of gastrointestinal symptoms for the aspirin (1,000 mg of a standard, solid-tablet formulation) and placebo-treated subjects, respectively, were stomach pain (14.5%, 4.4%), heartburn, (11.9%, 4.8%), nausea and/or vomiting (7.6%, 2.1%), hospitalization for GI disorder (4.9%, 3.5%). In the AMIS and other trials, aspirin-treated patients had increased rates of gross gastrointestinal bleeding. Symptoms and signs of gastrointestinal irritation were not significantly increased in subjects treated for unstable angina with buffered aspirin in solution.

Continued on next page

Information on Schering-Plough HealthCare Products appearing on these pages is effective as of November 1993.

Schering-Plough—Cont.

Cardiovascular and Biochemical: In the AMIS trial, the dosage of 1,000 mg per day of aspirin was associated with small increases in systolic blood pressure (BP) (average 1.5 to 2.1 mm) and diastolic BP (0.5 to 0.6 mm), depending upon whether maximal or last available readings were used. Blood urea nitrogen and uric acid levels were also increased, but by less than 1.0 mg percent. Subjects with marked hypertension or renal insufficiency had been excluded from the trial so that the clinical importance of these observations for such subjects or for any subjects treated over more prolonged periods is not known. It is recommended that patients placed on long-term aspirin treatment, even at doses of 300 mg per day, be seen at regular intervals to assess changes in these measurements.

Dosage and Administration: Although most of the studies used dosage exceeding 300 mg, two trials used only 300 mg daily and pharmacologic data indicate that this dose inhibits platelet function fully. Therefore, 300 mg or 325 mg (4 tablets) aspirin dose daily is a reasonable routine dose that would minimize gastrointestinal adverse reactions.

References:
1. Elwood PC, et al: A randomized controlled trial of acetylsalicylic acid in the secondary prevention of mortality from myocardial infarction, *BR Med J.* 1974;1;436–440.
2. The Coronary Drug Project Research Group: Aspirin in coronary heart disease. *J Chronic Dis.* 1976;29:625–642.
3. Breddin K, et al: Secondary prevention of myocardial infarction: a comparison of acetylsalicylic acid, phenprocoumon or placebo. *Homeostasis.* 1979;470:263–268.
4. Aspirin Myocardial Infarction Study Research Group: A randomized, controlled trial of aspirin in persons recovered from myocardial infarction, *JAMA.* 1980;245:661–669.
5. Elwood PC, and Sweetnam, PM: Aspirin and secondary mortality after myocardial infarction. *Lancet.* December 22–29, 1979, pp 1313–1315.
6. The Persantine-Aspirin Reinfarction Study Research Group: Persantine and aspirin in coronary heart disease. *Circulation.* 1980;62:449–460.
7. Lewis HD. et al: Protective effects of aspirin against acute myocardial infarction and death in men with unstable angina: Results of a Veterans Administration Cooperative Study, *N Engl J Med* 1983;309:396–403.

How Supplied: Chewable, orange flavored tablets in plastic bottles of 36 tablets each.

Shown in Product Identification Guide, page 424

TINACTIN® Antifungal
[*tin-ak 'tin*]
Cream 1%
Solution 1%
Powder 1%
Powder (1%) Aerosol
Liquid (1%) Aerosol
Deodorant Powder Aerosol 1%
Jock Itch Cream 1%
Jock Itch Spray Powder 1%

Description: TINACTIN Cream 1% is a white homogeneous, nonaqueous preparation containing the highly active synthetic fungicidal agent, tolnaftate. Each gram contains 10 mg tolnaftate solubilized in BHT, Carbomer, Monoamylamine, PEG-8, Propylene Glycol, and Titanium Dioxide.

TINACTIN Jock Itch Cream 1% is a smooth white homogeneous cream containing the highly active synthetic fungicidal agent, tolnaftate. Each gram contains 10 mg tolnaftate finely dispersed in a water-washable emulsion containing: Cetearyl Alcohol, Ceteareth-30, Chlorocresol, Mineral Oil, Petrolatum, Propylene Glycol, Sodium Phosphate and Water. Phosphoric acid and sodium hydroxide used to adjust pH.

TINACTIN Solution 1% contains in each ml tolnaftate 10 mg, BHT, and PEG. The solution solidifies at low temperatures but liquefies readily when warmed, retaining its potency.

TINACTIN Liquid Aerosol contains 91 mg tolnaftate in a vehicle of Alcohol SD-40-2 (36% w/w), BHT and PPG-12 Buteth-16. The spray deposits solution containing a concentration of 1% tolnaftate.

Each gram of **TINACTIN Powder 1%** contains tolnaftate 10 mg in a vehicle of corn starch and talc.

TINACTIN Powder Aerosol contains 91 mg tolnaftate in a vehicle of Alcohol SD-40-2 (14% w/w), BHT, Hydrocarbon Propellant, PPG-12 Buteth-16 and Talc. The spray deposits a white clinging powder containing a concentration of 1% tolnaftate.

TINACTIN Deodorant Powder Aerosol contains tolnaftate in a vehicle of SD Alcohol 40 (14% w/w), talc, PPG-12-Buteth-16, starch/acrylates/acrylamide copolymer, fragrance, BHT. The spray deposits a white clinging powder containing a concentration of 1% tolnaftate.

TINACTIN Jock Itch Spray Powder contains 91 mg tolnaftate in a vehicle of Alcohol SD-40-2 (14% w/w), BHT, Hydrocarbon Propellant, PPG-12 Buteth-16, Talc. The spray deposits a white clinging powder containing a concentration of 1% tolnaftate.

Indications: TINACTIN Cream, Solution, Liquid Aerosol and **TINACTIN Jock Itch Cream** are highly active antifungal agents that are effective in killing superficial fungi of the skin which cause tinea pedis (athlete's foot), tinea cruris (jock itch) and tinea corporis (body ringworm).

TINACTIN Powder, Powder Aerosol, Deodorant Powder Aerosol and

TINACTIN Jock Itch Spray Powder are effective in killing superficial fungi of the skin which cause tinea cruris (jock itch) and/or tinea pedis (athlete's foot). All forms begin to relieve burning, itching and soreness quickly. The powder and powder aerosol forms aid the drying of naturally moist areas. The deodorant powder aerosol provides additional protection against odor and wetness.

Actions: The active ingredient in TINACTIN, tolnaftate, is a highly active synthetic fungicidal agent that is effective in the treatment of superficial fungous infections of the skin. It is inactive systemically, virtually nonsensitizing, and does not ordinarily sting or irritate intact or broken skin, even in the presence of acute inflammatory reactions. TINACTIN products are odorless, greaseless, and do not stain or discolor the skin, hair, or nails.

Warnings: Keep these and all drugs out of the reach of children. Do not use in children under 2 years of age except under the advice and supervision of a physician.

TINACTIN Powder Aerosol, Deodorant Powder Aerosol and **Liquid Aerosol:** Avoid spraying in eyes. Contents under pressure. Do not puncture or incinerate. Flammable mixture, do not use or store near heat or open flame. Exposure to temperatures above 120°F may cause bursting. Never throw container into fire or incinerator. Use only as directed. Intentional misuse by deliberately concentrating and inhaling the contents can be harmful or fatal.

Warnings: If irritation occurs or symptoms do not improve within 10 days, discontinue use and consult your physician or podiatrist.

TINACTIN products are for external use only. Keep out of eyes.

TINACTIN is not effective on nail or scalp infections.

In case of accidental ingestion, seek professional assistance or contact a Poison Control Center immediately.

Dosage and Administration: Children under 12 years of age should be supervised in the use of TINACTIN.

TINACTIN Cream and **TINACTIN Jock Itch Cream**—Wash and dry infected area. Then apply a thin layer of cream and massage gently.

Best results in athlete's foot and body ringworm are usually obtained with 4 weeks use of this product and in jock itch, with 2 weeks use. Continue treatment for two weeks after symptoms disappear. To help prevent recurrence of athlete's foot, bathe daily, dry carefully and apply TINACTIN Powder or Powder Aerosol.

TINACTIN Solution—Wash and dry infected area morning and evening. Then apply two or three drops, and massage gently to cover the infected area. Best results in athlete's foot and body ringworm are usually obtained with 4 weeks use of this product and in jock itch, with 2 weeks use. Continue treatment for two weeks after symptoms disappear. To prevent recurrence of athlete's foot, bathe daily, dry carefully and apply TINACTIN Powder or Powder Aerosol.

TINACTIN Liquid Aerosol—Wash and dry infected area. Spray from a distance of 6 to 10 inches morning and evening or as directed by a doctor. For athlete's foot, spray between toes and on feet. For jock itch, spray infected area. Best results in athlete's foot are usually obtained with 4 weeks use of this product and in jock itch, with 2 weeks use. Continue treatment for two weeks after symptoms disappear. To help prevent reinfection of athlete's foot, bathe daily, dry carefully and apply **TINACTIN Powder** daily.

TINACTIN Powder—Wash and dry infected area. Sprinkle powder liberally on all areas of infection and in shoes or socks morning and evening or as directed by a doctor. Best results in athlete's foot are usually obtained with 4 weeks use of this product and in jock itch, with 2 weeks use. Continue treatment for two weeks after symptoms disappear. To prevent recurrence of athlete's foot, bathe daily, dry carefully and apply **TINACTIN Powder.**

TINACTIN Powder Aerosol, Deodorant Powder Aerosol and **TINACTIN Jock Itch Spray Powder**—Wash and dry infected area. Shake container well before using. Spray liberally from a distance of 6 to 10 inches onto affected area morning and night or as directed by a doctor. Best results in athlete's foot are usually obtained with 4 weeks use of this product and in jock itch, with 2 weeks use. To help prevent recurrence of athlete's foot, bathe daily, dry carefully and apply **TINACTIN Powder Aerosol** or **TINACTIN Deodorant Powder Aerosol.**

How Supplied: TINACTIN Antifungal Cream 1%, 15 g (½ oz) and 30 g (1 oz) collapsible tube with dispensing tip. **TINACTIN Antifungal Solution 1%,** 10 ml (⅓ oz) plastic squeeze bottle. **TINACTIN Antifungal Liquid (1%) Aerosol,** 113 g (4 oz) spray can. **TINACTIN Antifungal Powder 1%,** 45 g (1.5 oz) and 90 g (3.0 oz) plastic containers. **TINACTIN Antifungal Powder (1%) Aerosol,** 100 g (3.5 oz) and 150 g (5.0 oz) spray containers. TINACTIN Antifungal Deodorant Powder Aerosol 100 g (3.5 oz.) spray container. **TINACTIN Antifungal Jock Itch Cream 1%,** 15 g (½ oz) collapsible tube with dispensing tip. **TINACTIN Antifungal Jock Itch Spray Powder (1%),** 100 g (3.5 oz) spray can.

Store TINACTIN products between 36° and 86°F (2° and 30°C).

Shown in Product Identification Guide, page 424

Scot-Tussin Pharmacal Co., Inc.
P.O. BOX 8217
CRANSTON, RI 02920-0217

The following SCOT-TUSSIN® may be taken by individuals with diabetes, heart condition and/or high blood pressure and/or on Sugar restricted diet.

SCOT-TUSSIN SUGAR-FREE DM
Antitussive-Antihistaminic
Dextromethorphan
Chlorpheniramine Maleate

(Dextromethorphan 15 mg/5 ml, chlorpheniramine maleate 2 mg/5 ml). No alcohol, sorbitol, saccharin, or decongestant.
#036

SCOT-TUSSIN® SUGAR-FREE ALLERGY RELIEF FORMULA
Antihistaminic
Diphenhydramine HCl

(Diphenhydramine HCl 12.5 mg/5 ml). No alcohol, sorbitol, saccharin, dye.
#047-04

SCOT-TUSSIN® SUGAR-FREE COUGH CHASERS Lozenges
Antitussive
Dextromethorphan

No sodium, dye. DM 2.5 mg/lozenge.
#044-20

SCOT-TUSSIN® SUGAR-FREE; ALCOHOL-FREE EXPECTORANT
Guaifenesin

(Guaifenesin 100 mg/5 ml). No alcohol, sorbitol, sodium, dye, saccharin.
#006-04

SmithKline Beecham Consumer Healthcare, L.P.
Unit of SmithKline Beecham, Inc.
POST OFFICE BOX 1467
PITTSBURGH, PA 15230

A-200®₁
Pediculicide Shampoo Concentrate

Description:

Active Ingredients:
  Pyrethrins 0.30%
* Piperonyl Butoxide Technical 3.00%

**Inert Ingredients: 96.70%
  TOTAL 100.00%
* Equivalent to min. 2.4% (butylcarbityl) (6 propylpiperonyl) ether and 0.6% Related compounds.

**Contains petroleum distrillate
† Tested under Laboratory conditions.

Indications: A-200 is indicated for the treatment of head lice, body lice, and pubic (crab) lice.

Actions: A-200 is an effective pediculicide to kill head lice (pediculus humanus capitis), body lice (pediculus humanus corporis), and pubic (crab) lice (phthirus pubis).

Warning: A-200 should be used with caution by ragweed sensitized-persons.

Precautions: This product is for external use on humans only. It is harmful if swallowed. If accidently swallowed, call a physician or Poison Control Center immediately. It should not be inhaled. It should be kept out of the eyes and contact with mucous membranes should be avoided. If accidental contact with eyes occurs, flush eyes immediately with plenty of water. Call a physician if eye irritation persists. In case of infection or skin irritation, discontinue use immediately and consult a physician. Consult a physician before using this product if infestation of eyebrows or eyelashes occurs. Avoid contamination of feed or foodstuffs. Keep out of reach of children.

Storage and Disposal: Do not contaminate water, food or feed by storage or disposal. Do not transport or store below 32°F. Do not reuse empty container. Wrap in several layers of newspaper and discard in trash.

Directions for Use: It is a violation of Federal law to use the product in a manner inconsistent with its labeling. 1. Shake well. Apply undiluted A-200 to dry hair and scalp or any other infested areas and wet entirely. Do not use on eyelashes or eyebrows. 2. Allow A-200 shampoo to remain on area for 10 minutes before washing thoroughly with warm water and soap or regular shampoo. 3. Dead lice and eggs should be removed with special A-200 precision comb provided. 4. Repeat treatment in 7–10 days to kill any newly hatched lice. Do not exceed two consecutive applications within 24 hours.
Since lice infestations are spread by contact, it is important that each family member be examined carefully. If infested, they should be treated promptly to avoid spread or reinfestation of previously treated individuals. To eliminate infestation, all personal head gear, scarfs, coats, and bed linen should be laundered in hot water or dry cleaned. Carpets, upholstery, and mattresses should be vacuumed thoroughly. Combs and brushes should be soaked in hot water (above 130°) for 5 to 10 minutes.

How Supplied: In 2 and 4 fl. oz. unbreakable plastic bottles. An A-200 precision comb that removes nits and patient instruction booklet in English and Spanish are included in each carton. Also available in combination with A-200 Lice Treatment Kit.

Shown in Product Identification Guide, page 424

Continued on next page

SmithKline Beecham—Cont.

CĒPACOL®/CĒPACOL MINT
[sē 'pə-cŏl]
Mouthwash/Gargle

Description: Cēpacol Mouthwash contains: Ceepryn® (cetylpyridinium chloride) 0.05%. Also contains: Alcohol 14%, Edetate Disodium, FD&C Yellow No. 5 (tartrazine) as a color additive, Flavors, Glycerin, Polysorbate 80, Saccharin, Sodium Biphosphate, Sodium Phosphate, and Water.
Cēpacol Mint Mouthwash contains: Ceepryn® (cetylpyridinium chloride) 0.05%. Also contains: Alcohol 14.5%, D&C Yellow No. 10, FD&C Green No. 3, Flavor, Glucono Delta-Lactone, Glycerin, Poloxamer 407, Saccharin Sodium, Sodium Gluconate, and Water.

Actions: Cēpacol/Cēpacol Mint is a soothing, pleasant-tasting mouthwash/gargle. It kills germs that cause bad breath for a fresher, cleaner mouth. Cēpacol/Cēpacol Mint has a low surface tension, approximately ½ that of water. This property is the basis of the spreading action in the oral cavity as well as its foaming action. Cēpacol/Cēpacol Mint leaves the mouth feeling fresh and clean and helps provide soothing, temporary relief of dryness and minor mouth irritations.

Uses: Recommended as a mouthwash and gargle for daily oral care; as an aromatic mouth freshener to provide a clean feeling in the mouth; as a soothing, foaming rinse to freshen the mouth.
Used routinely before dental procedures, helps give patient confidence of not offending with mouth odor. Often employed as a foaming and refreshing rinse before, during, and after instrumentation and dental prophylaxis. Convenient as a mouth-freshening agent after taking dental impressions. Helpful in reducing the unpleasant taste and odor in the mouth following gingivectomy.
Used in hospitals as a mouthwash and gargle for daily oral care. Also used to refresh and soothe the mouth following emesis, inhalation therapy, and intubations, and for swabbing the mouths of patients incapable of personal care.

Warning: Keep out of the reach of children.

Directions for Use: Rinse vigorously before or after brushing or any time to freshen the mouth. Particularly useful after meals or before social engagements. Cēpacol/Cēpacol Mint leaves the mouth feeling refreshingly clean.
Use full strength every two or three hours as a soothing, foaming gargle, or as directed by a physician or dentist. May also be mixed with warm water.
Product label directions are as follows: Use full strength. Rinse mouth thoroughly before or after brushing or whenever desired or use as directed by a physician or dentist.

How Supplied:
Cēpacol Mouthwash: 12 oz, 18 oz, 24 oz, and 32 oz. 4 oz trial size.
Shown in Product Identification Guide, page 424

CĒPACOL®
[sē 'pə-cŏl]
Dry Throat Lozenges
Cherry Flavor

Description: Each lozenge contains Menthol 3.6 mg. Also contains: Benzyl Alcohol, Cetylpyridinium Chloride, D&C Red No. 33, FD&C Red No. 40, Flavor, Liquid Glucose, and Sucrose.

Actions: Menthol provides a cooling sensation to aid in symptomatic relief of minor throat irritations.

Indications: Cēpacol Cherry Flavor Lozenges provide temporary relief of occasional dry, scratchy throat.

Warnings: If sore throat is severe, persists for more than 2 days, is accompanied or followed by fever, headache, rash, nausea, or vomiting, consult a physician promptly. If sore mouth symptoms do not improve in 7 days, see your dentist or physician promptly. Do not administer to children under 6 years of age unless directed by physician or dentist. Keep this and all drugs out of the reach of children. In case of accidental overdose, seek professional assistance or contact a Poison Control Center immediately. As with any drug, if you are pregnant or nursing a baby, seek the advice of a health professional before using this product.

Dosage and Administration: Adults and children 6 years of age and older: Allow product to dissolve slowly in the mouth. May be repeated every 2 hours as needed or as directed by a dentist or physician. Do not exceed 10 lozenges per day.

How Supplied:
18 lozenges in 2 pocket packs of 9 each. Store at room temperature, below 86°F (30°C). Protect contents from humidity.
Shown in Product Identification Guide, page 424

CĒPACOL®
[sē-pə-cŏl]
Dry Throat Lozenges
Honey-Lemon Flavor

Description: Each lozenge contains Menthol 3.6 mg. Also contains: Benzyl Alcohol, Caramel, Cetylpyridinium Chloride, FD&C Yellow No. 6, D&C Yellow No. 10, Flavors, Liquid Glucose, and Sucrose.

Actions: Menthol provides a cooling sensation to aid in symptomatic relief of minor throat irritations.

Indications: Cēpacol Honey-Lemon Flavor Lozenges provide temporary relief of occasional dry, scratchy throat.

Warnings: If sore throat is severe, persists for more than 2 days, is accompanied or followed by fever, headache, rash, nausea, or vomiting, consult a physician promptly. If sore mouth symptoms do not improve in 7 days, see your dentist or physician promptly. Do not administer to children under 6 years of age unless directed by physician or dentist. Keep this and all drugs out of the reach of children. In case of accidental overdose, seek professional assistance or contact a Poison Control Center immediately. As with any drug, if you are pregnant or nursing a baby, seek the advice of a health professional before using this product.

Dosage and Administration: Adults and children 6 years of age and older: Allow product to dissolve slowly in the mouth. May be repeated every 2 hours as needed or as directed by a dentist or physician.

How Supplied:
18 lozenges in 2 pocket packs of 9 each. Store at room temperature, below 86°F (30°C). Protect contents from humidity.
Shown in Product Identification Guide, page 424

CĒPACOL®
[sē-pə-cŏl]
Dry Throat Lozenges
Menthol-Eucalyptus Flavor

Description: Each lozenge contains Menthol 5.0 mg. Also contains: Benzyl Alcohol, Cetylpyridinium Chloride, Eucalyptol, Liquid Glucose, and Sucrose.

Actions: Menthol provides a cooling sensation to aid in symptomatic relief of minor throat irritations.

Indications: Cēpacol Menthol-Eucalyptus Flavor Lozenges provide temporary relief of occasional dry, scratchy throat.

Warnings: If sore throat is severe, persists for more than 2 days, is accompanied or followed by fever, headache, rash, nausea, or vomiting, consult a physician promptly. If sore mouth symptoms do not improve in 7 days, see your dentist or physician promptly. Do not administer to children under 6 years of age unless directed by physician or dentist. Keep this and all drugs out of the reach of children. In case of accidental overdose, seek professional assistance or contact a Poison Control Center immediately. As with any drug, if you are pregnant or nursing a baby, seek the advice of a health professional before using this product.

Dosage and Administration: Adults and children 6 years of age and older: Allow product to dissolve slowly in the mouth. May be repeated every 2 hours as needed or as directed by a dentist or physician.

How Supplied:
18 lozenges in 2 pocket packs of 9 each. Store at room temperature, below 86°F (30°C). Protect contents from humidity.
Shown in Product Identification Guide, page 424

CĒPACOL®
[sē′pǝ-cŏl]
Dry Throat Lozenges
Original Flavor

Description: Each lozenge contains Ceepryn® (cetylpyridinium chloride) 0.07%, Benzyl Alcohol 0.3%. Also contains: FD&C Yellow No. 5 (tartrazine) as a color additive, Flavor, Glucose, and Sucrose.

Actions: Cetylpyridinium chloride (Ceepryn) is a cationic quaternary ammonium compound, which is a surface-active agent. Aqueous solutions of cetylpyridinium chloride have a surface tension lower than that of water.
Cetylpyridinium chloride in the concentration used in Cēpacol is nonirritating to tissues.

Indications: For soothing, temporary relief of dryness of the mouth and throat.

Warnings: Severe sore throat or sore throat accompanied by high fever, headache, nausea, or vomiting, or any sore throat or mouth irritations persisting more than 2 days may be serious. Consult a physician promptly. Persons with a high fever or persistent cough should not use this preparation unless directed by a physician. Do not administer to children under 6 years of age unless directed by a physician or dentist. If sensitive to any of the ingredients, do not use. Keep this and all drugs out of the reach of children. In case of accidental overdose, seek professional assistance or contact a Poison Control Center immediately. As with any drug, if you are pregnant or nursing a baby, seek the advice of a health professional before using this product.

Dosage and Administration: Adults and children 6 years and older, dissolve 1 lozenge in the mouth every 2 hours, if needed. For children under 6 years, consult a physician or dentist.

How Supplied:
Trade Package: 18 lozenges in 2 pocket packs of 9 each.
Professional Package: 648 lozenges in 72 blisters of 9 each.
Store at room temperature, below 86°F (30°C). Protect contents from humidity.
Shown in Product Identification Guide, page 424

CĒPACOL®
[sē′pǝ-cŏl]
Anesthetic Lozenges (Troches)

Description: Each lozenge contains Benzocaine 10 mg, Ceepryn® (cetylpyridinium chloride) 0.07%. Also contains: FD&C Blue No. 1, FD&C Yellow No. 5 (tartrazine) as a color additive, Flavors, Glucose, and Sucrose.

Actions: Cetylpyridinium chloride (Ceepryn) is a cationic quaternary ammonium compound, which is a surface-active agent. Aqueous solutions of cetylpyridinium chloride have a surface tension lower than that of water.
Cetylpyridinium chloride in the concentration used in Cēpacol is nonirritating to tissues.
Cēpacol Anesthetic Lozenges stimulate salivation to relieve dryness of the mouth and provide a mild anesthetic effect for pain relief.

Indications: For fast, temporary relief of minor sore throat pain. For temporary relief of minor pain and discomfort associated with tonsillitis and pharyngitis.

Warnings: If sore throat is severe, persists for more than 2 days, is accompanied or followed by fever, headache, rash, nausea, or vomiting, consult a physician promptly. Keep this and all drugs out of the reach of children. In case of accidental overdose, seek professional assistance or contact a Poison Control Center immediately. As with any drug, if you are pregnant or nursing a baby, seek the advice of a health professional before using this product.

Dosage and Administration: Adults and children 6 years and older, dissolve 1 lozenge in the mouth every 2 hours, if needed. For children under 6 years, consult a physician or dentist.

How Supplied:
Trade Package: 18 lozenges in 2 pocket packs of 9 each.
Professional Package: 324 lozenges in 36 blisters of 9 each.
Store at room temperature, below 86°F (30°C). Protect contents from humidity.
Shown in Product Identification Guide, page 424

CĒPASTAT®
[sē′pǝ-stăt]
Sore Throat Lozenges
Cherry Flavor and Extra Strength

Description: Each Cherry Flavor lozenge contains: Phenol 14.5 mg. Also contains: Antifoam Emulsion, D&C Red No. 33, FD&C Yellow No. 6, Flavor, Gum Crystal, Mannitol, Menthol, Saccharin Sodium, and Sorbitol.
Each Extra Strength lozenge contains: Phenol 29 mg. Also contains: Antifoam Emulsion, Caramel, Eucalyptus Oil, Gum Crystal, Mannitol, Menthol, Saccharin Sodium, and Sorbitol.

Actions: Phenol is a recognized topical anesthetic. The sugar-free formula should not promote tooth decay as sugar-based lozenges can.

Indications: For fast, temporary relief of minor sore throat pain.

Warnings: If sore throat is severe, persists for more than 2 days, is accompanied or followed by fever, headache, rash, nausea, or vomiting, consult a physician promptly. If sore mouth symptoms do not improve in 7 days, see your dentist or physician promptly. Keep this and all drugs out of the reach of children. In case of accidental overdose, seek professional assistance or contact a Poison Control Center immediately. As with any drug, if you are pregnant or nursing a baby, seek the advice of a health professional before using this product.

Note to Diabetics: Each lozenge contributes approximately 8 calories from 2 grams of sorbitol.

Dosage and Administration:
Lozenges–Cherry Flavor
Adults and children 12 years of age and older: Allow the lozenge to dissolve slowly in the mouth. May be repeated every 2 hours, or as directed by a dentist or physician. Children 6 to under 12 years of age: Allow lozenge to dissolve slowly in the mouth. May be repeated every 2 hours, not to exceed 10 lozenges per day, or as directed by a dentist or physician. Children under 6 years of age: Consult a dentist or physician.
Lozenges–Extra Strength
Adults and children 12 years of age and older: Allow the lozenge to dissolve slowly in the mouth. May be repeated every 2 hours, or as directed by a dentist or physician. Children 6 to under 12 years of age: Allow lozenge to dissolve slowly in the mouth. May be repeated every 2 hours, not to exceed 10 lozenges per day, or as directed by a dentist or physician. Children under 6 years of age: Consult a dentist or physician.

How Supplied:
Lozenges–Cherry Flavor
Trade package: Boxes of 18 lozenges as 2 pocket packs of 9 lozenges each.
Professional package: 648 lozenges in 72 blisters of 9 lozenges each.
Lozenges–Extra Strength
Trade package: Boxes of 18 lozenges as 2 pocket packs of 9 lozenges each.
Professional package: 648 lozenges in 72 blisters of 9 lozenges each.
Store at room temperature, below 86°F (30°C). Protect contents from humidity.
Shown in Product Identification Guide, page 424

Orange Flavor
CITRUCEL®
[sĭt′rǝ-sĕl]
(Methylcellulose)
Bulk-forming Fiber Laxative

Description: Each 19 g adult dose (approximately one heaping measuring tablespoonful) contains Methylcellulose 2 g. Each 9.5 g child's dose (one-half the adult dose) contains Methylcellulose 1 g. Methylcellulose is a nonallergenic fiber. Also contains: Citric Acid, FD&C Yellow No. 6, Orange Flavors (natural and artificial), Potassium Citrate, Riboflavin, Sucrose, and other ingredients. Each adult dose contains approximately 3 mg of so-

Continued on next page

SmithKline Beecham—Cont.

dium, 105 mg of potassium, and contributes 60 calories from Sucrose.

Actions: Promotes elimination by providing additional fiber (bulk) to the diet. This product generally produces bowel movement in 12 to 72 hours.

Indications: For relief of constipation (irregularity). May also be used for relief of constipation associated with other bowel disorders such as irritable bowel syndrome, diverticular disease, and hemorrhoids as well as for bowel management during postpartum, postsurgical, and convalescent periods when recommended by a physician.

Contraindications: Intestinal obstruction, fecal impaction, known hypersensitivity to formula ingredients.

Precautions: Patients should be instructed to consult their physician before using any laxative if they have noticed a sudden change in bowel habits which persists for two weeks. Unless directed by a physician, patients should be advised not to use laxative products when abdominal pain, nausea, or vomiting is present. Patients should also be advised to discontinue use and consult a physician if rectal bleeding or failure to have a bowel movement occurs after use of any laxative product.

Dosage and Administration: Adults and children older than 12 years of age: *one heaping measuring* tablespoonful stirred briskly into 8 ounces of cold water one to three times a day at the first sign of constipation. Children 6 to under 12 years: *one-half the adult dose stirred briskly into 4 ounces of cold water, one to three times a day. The mixture should be administered promptly and drinking additional water is helpful. Children under 6 years: use only as directed by a physician.* Continued use for two or three days may be necessary for full benefit.

How Supplied:
16 oz, 24 oz, and 30 oz containers.
Boxes of 20 single-dose packets.
Store below 86°F (30°C). Protect contents from humidity; keep tightly closed.

Shown in Product Identification Guide, page 424

Sugar Free Orange Flavor
CITRUCEL®
[sĭt′rə-sĕl]
(Methylcellulose)
Bulk-forming Fiber Laxative

Description: Each 10.2 g adult dose (approximately one rounded measuring tablespoonful) contains Methylcellulose 2 g. Each 5.1 g child's dose (one-half the adult dose) contains Methylcellulose 1 g. Methylcellulose is a nonallergenic fiber. Also contains: Aspartame*, Dibasic Cal-

*NutraSweet and the NutraSweet symbol are trademarks of the NutraSweet Company.

cium Phosphate, FD&C Yellow No. 6, Malic Acid, Maltodextrin, Orange Flavors (natural and artificial), Potassium Citrate and Riboflavin. Each 10.2 g dose contributes 24 calories from Maltodextrin.

Actions: Promotes elimination by providing additional fiber (bulk) to the diet. This product generally produces bowel movement in 12 to 72 hours.

Indications: For relief of constipation (irregularity). May also be used for relief of constipation associated with other bowel disorders such as irritable bowel syndrome, diverticular disease, and hemorrhoids as well as for bowel management during postpartum, postsurgical, and convalescent periods when recommended by a physician.

Contraindications: Intestinal obstruction, fecal impaction, known hypersensitivity to formula ingredients.

Warning: Individuals with phenylketonuria and other individuals who must restrict their intake of phenylalanine should be warned that each 10.2 g adult dose contains aspartame which provides 52 mg of phenylalanine.

Precautions: Patients should be instructed to consult their physician before using any laxative if they have noticed a sudden change in bowel habits which persists for two weeks. Unless directed by a physician, patients should be advised not to use laxative products when abdominal pain, nausea, or vomiting is present. Patients should also be advised to discontinue use and consult a physician if rectal bleeding or failure to have a bowel movement occurs after use of any laxative product.

Dosage and Administration: Adults and children older than 12 years of age: one rounded measuring tablespoonful stirred briskly into 8 ounces of cold water, one to three times a day at the first sign of constipation. Children 6 to 12 years of age: one-half the adult dose stirred briskly into 4 ounces of cold water one to three times a day. The mixture should be administered promptly and drinking additional water is helpful. Continued use for two or more days may be necessary for full benefit.

How Supplied:
8.6 oz and 16.9 oz containers.
Store below 86°F (30°C). Protect contents from humidity; keep tightly closed.

Shown in Product Identification Guide, page 424

CLEAR BY DESIGN®
Medicated Acne Gel for Sensitive Skin

Product Information: CLEAR BY DESIGN contains benzoyl peroxide, an effective anti-acne agent available without a prescription in a lower 2.5% strength. CLEAR BY DESIGN is as effec-

tive as 10% benzoyl peroxide but with less of the irritation and redness that you may get with the higher strengths. Greaseless, colorless CLEAR BY DESIGN is invisible while it works fast. Helps prevent new acne pimples and blackheads from forming.

Directions: Wash problem areas thoroughly but gently and dry well. Using fingertips, apply CLEAR BY DESIGN to all affected and surrounding areas of face, neck, and body. Apply one or two times a day or as directed by a physician.

Warnings: Persons with a known allergy to benzoyl peroxide should not use this medication. To test for an allergy, apply CLEAR BY DESIGN on a small affected area once a day for two days. If discomforting irritation or undue dryness occurs during treatment, reduce frequency of use or amount. If excessive itching, redness, burning, swelling, irritation or dryness occurs, discontinue use and consult a physician. Avoid contact with eyes, lips and mouth. May bleach hair or dyed fabrics. Keep tightly closed. Keep this and all drugs out of reach of children. Store at controlled room temperature (59°–86°F). Avoid excessive heat. FOR EXTERNAL USE ONLY

Formula: Active Ingredient: Benzoyl Peroxide, 2.5% in a gel base. Inactive Ingredients: Purified water, carbomer 940, dioctyl sodium sulfosuccinate, sodium hydroxide, and edetate disodium.

How Supplied: Available in 1.5 oz. tubes.

Shown in Product Identification Guide, page 425

CONTAC
Day & Night Allergy/Sinus

Product Information: Contac Day & Night Allergy/Sinus includes 15 day caplets and 5 night caplets in each package to provide:
• 5 days of relief from stuffy nose, sinus pressure and headache pain without drowsiness.
• 5 nights of relief from stuffy, runny nose, sinus pressure, sneezing and headache pain to let your rest.

Day Caplets
Product Benefits: Contac Day Caplets provide an ANALGESIC and a DECONGESTANT.

Indications: For temporary relief of sinus pressure, nasal congestion, and headache pain.

Directions: Adults and children 12 and older: Take one white Day caplet every 6 hours. Children under 12, use only as directed by a doctor. DO NOT EXCEED A TOTAL OF 4 CAPLETS (whether all Day or all Night or a combination of each) IN 24 HOURS. ALL CAPLETS SHOULD BE TAKEN AT LEAST 6 HOURS APART.

Warnings: Do not exceed recommended dosage because at higher doses, dizziness, sleeplessness, or nervousness may occur. Do not use this product if: symptoms do not improve within 7 days, worsen, recur, or are accompanied by fever, redness, or swelling; fever lasts for more than 3 days; you have high blood pressure, heart disease, diabetes, thyroid disease, or difficulty in urination due to an enlarged prostrate gland; unless directed by a doctor. As with any drug, if you are pregnant or nursing a baby, seek the advice of a health professional before using this product. Keep this and all drugs out of reach of children. In case of accidental overdose, seek professional assistance or contact a poison control center immediately. Prompt medical attention is critical for adults as well as for children even if you do not notice any signs or symptoms.

Drug Interaction Precaution: Do not take if you are presently taking a prescription drug for high blood pressure or depression, without first consulting a doctor.

Active Ingredients: Each caplet contains:
Acetaminophen 650 mg
Pseudoephedrine Hydrochloride 60 mg

Inactive Ingredients: Hydroxypropyl Methylcellulose, Magnesium Stearate, Microcrystalline Cellulose, Polyethylene Glycol, Polysorbate 80, Silicon Dioxide, Starch, Stearic Acid, Titanium Dioxide.

How Supplied: Consumer package of 15 Day Caplets and 5 Night Caplets (see following Night Caplet listing).

Night Caplets
Product Benefits: Contac Night Caplets provide an ANALGESIC, an ANTIHISTAMINE, and a DECONGESTANT

Indication: For temporary relief of sinus pressure, nasal congestion, runny nose, sneezing, itchy watery eyes; and headache pain.

Directions: Adults and children 12 and older: Take one green Night caplet every 6 hours. Children under 12, use only as directed by a doctor. DO NOT EXCEED A TOTAL OF 4 CAPLETS (whether all Day or all Night or combination of each) IN 24 HOURS. ALL CAPLETS SHOULD BE TAKEN AT LEAST 6 HOURS APART.

Warnings: Do not exceed recommended dosage, because at higher doses, dizziness, sleeplessness or nervousness may occur. Do not use this product if: symptoms do not improve within 7 days, worsen, recur, or are accompanied by fever, redness, or swelling; fever lasts more than 3 days; you have chronic pulmonary disease, high blood pressure, asthma, heart disease, diabetes, thyroid disease, glaucoma, shortness of breath, difficulty in breathing, emphysema, or difficulty in urination due to an enlarge prostrate gland. May cause marked drowsiness; use caution when driving a motor vehicle or operation machinery. Alcohol, sedatives or tranquilizers will increase drowsiness; avoid alcholic beverages. May cause excitability especially

in children. As with any drug, if you are pregnant or nursing a baby, seek the advice of a health professional before using this product. Keep this and all drugs out of reach of children. In case of accidental overdose, seek professional assistance or contact a poison control center immediately. Prompt medical attention is critical for adults as well as for children even if you do not notice any signs or symptoms.

Drug Interaction Precaution: Do not take if you are presently taking a prescription drug for high blood pressure or depression, without first consulting a doctor.

Active Ingredients: Each caplet contains:
Acetaminophen 650 mg
Pseudoephedrine Hydrochloride 60 mg
Diphenhydramine Hydrochloride 50 mg

Inactive Ingredients: D&C Yellow 10, FD&C Blue 1, Hydroxypropyl Methylcellulose, Magnesium Stearate, Microcrystalline Cellulose, Polyethylene Glycol, Polysorbate 80, Silicon Dioxide, Starch, Stearic Acid, Titanium Dioxide.

How Supplied: Consumer package of 5 Night Caplets and 15 Day Caplets (see previous Day Caplet listing).
Note: There are other CONTAC products. Make sure this is the one you are interested in.
Shown in Product Identification Guide, page 425

CONTAC
Day & Night Cold/Flu

Composition:

Product Information: Contac Day & Night Cold/Flu includes 15 day caplets and 5 night caplets in each package to provide:
● 5 days of relief from stuffy nose, coughing and aches and pains without drowsiness
● 5 nights of relief from stuffy runny, nose, sneezing and aches and pains to let you rest.

Day Caplets

Product Benefits: Contac Day Caplets provide an ANALGESIC, a DECONGESTANT, and a COUGH SUPPRESSANT.

Indications: For temporary relief of nasal congestion, fever, coughs, minor aches and pains due to the common cold and flu.

Directions: Adults and children 12 and older: Take one yellow Day caplet every 6 hours. Children under 12, use only as directed by a doctor.
DO NOT EXCEED A TOTAL OF 4 CAPLETS (whether all Day or all Night or combination of each) IN 24 HOURS. ALL CAPLETS SHOULD BE TAKEN AT LEAST 6 HOURS APART.

Warnings: Do not exceed recommended dosage because at higher doses, dizziness, sleeplessness, or nervousness

may occur. A persistent cough may be a sign of a serious condition. Do not use this product if: cough or other symptoms do not improve within 7 days, worsen, recur, or are accompanied by fever, rash, redness, swelling or persistent headache; fever lasts for more than 3 days; you have high blood pressure, heart disease, diabetes, thyroid disease, or difficulty in urination due to an enlarged prostate gland; you have persistent or chronic cough such as occurs with smoking, asthma, emphysema or if cough is accompanied by excessive phlegm (mucus), unless directed by a doctor. As with any drug, if you are pregnant or nursing a baby, seek the advice of a health professional before using this product. Keep this and all drugs out of reach of children. In case of accidental overdose, seek professional assistance or contact a poison control center immediately. Prompt medical attention is critical for adults as well as for children even if you do not notice any signs or symptoms.

Drug Interaction Precaution: Do not take if you are presently taking a prescription drug for high blood pressure or depression, without first consulting a doctor. Do not use this product if you are taking a prescription drug containing a monoamine oxidose inhibitor (MAOI) (certain drugs for depression or psychiatric or emotional conditions), without first consulting your doctor. If you are uncertain whether your prescription drug contains an MAOI, consult a health professional before taking this product.

Active Ingredients: Each caplet contains:
Acetaminophen 650 mg.,
Pseudoephedrine Hydrochloride 60 mg.,
Dextromethorphan Hydrobromide 30 mg.

Inactive Ingredients: D&C Yellow 10 FD&C Yellow 6, Hydroxypropyl Methylcellulose, Magnesium Stearate, Microcrystalline Cellulose, Polyethylene Glycol, Polysorbate 80, Silicon Dioxide, Starch, Stearic Acid, Titanium Dioxide.

How Supplied: Consumer package of 15 Day Caplets and 5 Night Caplets (see following Night Caplet listing).

Night Caplets

Product Benefits: Contac Night Caplets provide an ANALGESIC, an ANTIHISTAMINE, and a DECONGESTANT.

Indications: For temporary relief of nasal congestion, fever, minor aches and pains, runny nose, and sneezing, due to the common cold and flu.

Directions: Adults and children 12 and older: Take one blue Night caplet every 6 hours. Children under 12, use only as directed by a doctor. DO NOT EXCEED A TOTAL OF 4 CAPLETS (whether all Day or all Night or combination of each) IN 24 HOURS. ALL CAPLETS SHOULD BE TAKEN AT LEAST 6 HOURS APART.

Continued on next page

SmithKline Beecham—Cont.

Warnings: Do not exceed recommended dosage, because at higher doses, dizziness, sleeplessness, or nervousness may occur. Do not use this product if: cough or other symptoms do not improve within 7 days, worsen, recur, or are accompanied by fever, redness, swelling; fever lasts more than three days; you have chronic pulmonary disease, high blood pressure, asthma, heart disease, diabetes, thyroid disease, glaucoma, shortness of breath, difficulty in breathing, emphysema, or difficulty in urination due to an enlarged prostate gland. May cause marked drowsiness; use caution when driving a motor vehicle or operating machinery. Alcohol, sedatives or tranquilizers will increase drowsiness; avoid alcoholic beverages. May cause excitability especially in children. As with any drug, if you are pregnant or nursing a baby, seek the advice of a health professional before using this product. Keep this and all drugs out of reach of children. In case of accidental overdose, seek professional assistance or contact a poison control center immediately. Prompt medical attention is critical for adults as well as for children even if you do not notice any signs or symptoms.

Drug Interaction Precaution: Do not take if you are presently taking a prescription drug for high blood pressure or depression, without first consulting a doctor.

Active Ingredients: Each caplet contains:
Acetaminophen 650 mg.,
Pseudoephedrine Hydrochloride 60 mg.,
Diphenhydramine Hydrochloride 50 mg.

Inactive Ingredients: FD&C Blue 1, Hydroxypropyl Methylcellulose, Magnesium Stearate, Microcrystalline Cellulose, Polyethylene Glycol, Polysorbate 80, Silicon Dioxide, Starch, Stearic Acid, Titanium Dioxide.

How Supplied: Consumer package of 5 Night Caplets and 15 Day Caplets (see previous Day Caplet listing).
Note: There are other CONTAC products. Make sure this is the one you are interested in.
Shown in Product Identification Guide, page 425

CONTAC®
MAXIMUM STRENGTH
Continuous Action Nasal Decongestant/Antihistamine 12 Hour Caplets

Composition: [See table on page 705.]

Product Information: Each CONTAC Maximum Strength continuous action caplet provides up to 12 hours of relief. Part of the caplet goes to work right away for fast relief; the rest is released gradually to provide up to 12 hours of prolonged relief. With just *one* caplet in the morning and *one* at bedtime, you feel better all day, sleep better at night, breathing freely without congestion. CONTAC Maximum Strength provides:

● A NASAL DECONGESTANT which helps clear nasal passages, shrinks swollen membranes and helps decongest sinus openings.
● AN ANTIHISTAMINE at the maximum level to help relieve itchy, watery eyes, sneezing, and runny nose.

Indications: For temporary relief of nasal congestion due to the common cold, hay fever or other upper respiratory allergies, and nasal congestion associated with sinusitis.

Directions: One caplet every 12 hours. Do not exceed 2 caplets in 24 hours.
NOTE: The nonactive portion of the caplet that supplies the active ingredients may occasionally appear in your stool as a soft mass.
This carton is protected by a clear overwrap printed with "safety-sealed"; do not use if overwrap is missing or broken.

TAMPER-RESISTANT PACKAGING FEATURES FOR YOUR PROTECTION:
● Each caplet is encased in a plastic cell with a foil back; do not use if cell or foil is broken.
● The name CONTAC appears on each caplet; do not use this product if the CONTAC name is missing.

Warnings: Do not give this product to children under 12 years except under the advice and supervision of a physician. Do not exceed recommended dosage because at higher doses nervousness, dizziness, or sleeplessness may occur. Do not take this product if you have high blood pressure, heart disease, diabetes or thyroid disease except under the advice and supervision of a physician. If symptoms do not improve within 7 days or are accompanied by high fever, consult a physician before continuing use. Do not take this product if you have asthma, glaucoma or difficulty in urination due to enlargement of the prostate gland except under the advice and supervision of a physician. Do not take this product if you are taking another medication containing phenylpropanolamine. Avoid alcoholic beverages while taking this product. Do not drive or operate heavy machinery. May cause drowsiness. May cause excitability, especially in children. Keep this and all drugs out of reach of children. In case of accidental overdose, seek professional assistance or contact a poison control center immediately. As with any drug, if you are pregnant or nursing a baby, seek the advice of a health professional before using this product. Store at controlled room temperature (59°–86°F).

Drug Interaction Precaution: Do not take this product if you are presently taking a prescription antihypertensive or antidepressant drug containing monoamine oxidase inhibitor except under the advice and supervision of a physician.

Formula: Active Ingredients: Each Maximum Strength caplet contains Phenylpropanolamine Hydrochloride 75 mg.; Chlorpheniramine Maleate 12 mg. (which is a higher dose of antihistamine than CONTAC capsules). **Inactive Ingredients (listed for individuals with specific allergies):** Acetylated Monoglycerides, Colloidal Silicon Dioxide, Ethylcellulose, Hydroxypropyl Methylcellulose, Lactose, Stearic Acid, Titanium Dioxide.

How Supplied: Consumer packages of 10, 20 and 40 caplets.
Note: There are other CONTAC products. Make sure this is the one you are interested in.
Shown in Product Identification Guide, page 425

CONTAC®
Continuous Action Nasal Decongestant/Antihistamine 12 Hour Capsules

Composition: [See table on next page.]

Product Information: Each CONTAC continuous action capsule contains over 600 "tiny time pills." Some go to work right away. The rest are scientifically timed to dissolve slowly to give up to 12 hours of relief. With just *one* capsule in the morning and *one* at bedtime, you feel better all day, sleep better at night, breathing freely without congestion. CONTAC provides:

● A NASAL DECONGESTANT which helps clear nasal passages, shrinks swollen membranes and helps decongest sinus openings.
● AN ANTIHISTAMINE to help relieve itchy, watery eyes, sneezing, and runny nose.

Indications: For temporary relief of nasal congestion due to the common cold, hay fever or other upper respiratory allergies, and nasal congestion associated with sinusitis.

Directions: One capsule every 12 hours. Do not exceed 2 capsules in 24 hours.
This carton is protected by a clear overwrap printed with "safety-sealed"; do not use if overwrap is missing or broken.

TAMPER-RESISTANT PACKAGING FEATURES FOR YOUR PROTECTION:
● Each capsule is encased in a plastic cell with a foil back; do not use if cell or foil is broken.
● Each CONTAC capsule is protected by a red Perma-Seal™ band which bonds the two capsule halves together; do not use if capsule or band is broken.

Warnings: Do not give this product to children under 12 years except under the advice and supervision of a physician. Do not exceed recommended dosage because at higher doses nervousness, dizziness, or sleeplessness may occur. Do not take this product if you have high blood pressure, heart disease, diabetes or thyroid disease except under the advice and supervision of a physician. If symptoms do not im-

CONTAC	CONTAC Maximum Strength Continuous Action Decongestant Caplets	CONTAC Continuous Action Decongestant Capsules	CONTAC Severe Cold and Flu Formula Caplets (each 2 caplet dose)	CONTAC Severe Cold and Flu Hot Medicine Drink (each Packet dose)	CONTAC Severe Cold and Flu Non-Drowsy Formula caplets (each 2 caplet dose)	CONTAC Day & Night Cold & Flu Day Caplets	CONTAC Day & Night Cold & Flu Night Caplets
Phenylpropanolamine HCl	75.0 mg	75.0 mg	25.0 mg	—	—	—	—
Chlorpheniramine Maleate	12.0 mg	8.0 mg	4.0 mg	4.0 mg	—	—	—
Pseudoephedrine HCl	—	—	—	60.0 mg	60.0 mg	60.0 mg	60.0 mg
Acetaminophen	—	—	1000.0 mg	650.0 mg	650.0 mg	650.0 mg	650.0 mg
Dextropmethorphan Hydrobromide	—	—	30.0 mg	20.0 mg	30.0 mg	30.0 mg	—
Diphenhydramine HCl	—	—	—	—	—	—	50.0 mg

prove within 7 days or are accompanied by a high fever, consult a physician before continuing use. Do not take this product if you have asthma, glaucoma or difficulty in urination due to enlargement of the prostate gland except under the advice and supervision of a physician. Do not take this product if you are taking another medication containing phenylpropanolamine. Avoid alcoholic beverages while taking this product. Do not drive or operate heavy machinery. May cause drowsiness. May cause excitability, especially in children. Keep this and all drugs out of reach of children. In case of accidental overdose, seek professional assistance or contact a poison control center immediately. As with any drug, if you are pregnant or nursing a baby, seek the advice of a health professional before using this product. Store at controlled room temperature (59°–86°F). Protect against excess moisture.

Drug Interaction Precaution: Do not take this product if you are presently taking a prescription antihypertensive or antidepressant drug containing monoamine oxidase inhibitor except under the advice and supervision of a physician.

Each Capsule Contains: Phenylpropanolamine Hydrochloride 75 mg. and Chlorpheniramine Maleate 8 mg. Also Contains: Benzyl Alcohol, Butylparaben, Carboxymethylcellulose Sodium, D&C Red No. 33, D&C Red 27, D&C Red 30, D&C Yellow No. 10, Edetate Calcium Disodium, FD&C Red No. 3, FD&C Red 40, FD&C Yellow No. 6, Gelatin, Methylparaben, Pharmaceutical Glaze, Polysorbate 80, Propylparaben, Sodium Lauryl Sulfate, Sodium Propionate, Starch, Sucrose and other ingredients.

How Supplied: Consumer packages of 10, 20 and 40 capsules.
Note: There are other CONTAC products. Make sure this is the one you are interested in.

Shown in Product Identification Guide, page 425

CONTAC®
Severe Cold and Flu Formula Caplets
Analgesic • Decongestant
Antihistamine • Cough Suppressant

Composition: [See table above.]

Product Information: Two caplets every 6 hours to help relieve the discomforts of severe colds with flu-like symptoms.

Product Benefits: CONTAC Severe Cold and Flu Formula contains a Non-Aspirin Analgesic, a Decongestant, an Antihistamine and a Cough Suppressant. These safe and effective ingredients provide temporary relief from these major cold symptoms: fever, body aches and pains, minor sore throat pain, headache, runny nose, postnasal drip, sneezing, itchy, watery eyes, nasal and sinus congestion, and temporarily relieves cough due to the common cold.

Directions: Adults (12 years and over): Two caplets every 6 hours, not to exceed 8 caplets in any 24 hour period.
This carton is protected by a clear overwrap printed with "safety-sealed". Do not use if overwrap is missing or broken.
TAMPER-RESISTANT PACKAGING FEATURES FOR YOUR PROTECTION:
• Caplets are encased in a plastic cell with a foil back; do not use if cell or foil is broken.
• The letters SCF appear on each caplet; do not use this product if these letters are missing.

Warnings: Do not administer to children under 12. Do not take this product for more than 7 days or for fever for more than 3 days unless directed by a doctor. If symptoms do not improve or are accompanied by fever, consult a doctor. A persistent cough may be a sign of a serious condition. If cough persists for more than one week, tends to recur or is accompanied by fever, rash, or persistent headache, consult a doctor. Do not take this product for persistent or chronic coughs such as occurs with smoking, asthma,

emphysema, or if cough is accompanied by excessive phlegm (mucus), unless directed by a doctor. Do not exceed recommended dosage because at higher doses nervousness, dizziness, or sleeplessness may occur. May cause excitability, especially in children. Do not take this product if you have asthma, glaucoma, heart disease, high blood pressure, emphysema, chronic pulmonary disease, shortness of breath, difficulty in breathing, diabetes, thyroid disease, or difficulty in urination due to enlargement of the prostate gland unless directed by a doctor. Do not take this product if you are taking another medication containing phenylpropanolamine. May cause marked drowsiness. Alcohol may increase the drowsiness effect. Avoid alcoholic beverages while taking this product. Use caution when driving a motor vehicle or operating machinery. Keep this and all medication out of the reach of children. As with any drug, if you are pregnant or nursing a baby, seek the advice of a health professional before using this product. In case of accidental overdose, contact a physician or poison control center immediately. Prompt medical attention is critical for adults as well as for children even if you do not notice any signs or symptoms.

Drug Interaction Precaution: Do not take this product if you are presently taking a prescription drug for high blood pressure or depression without first consulting your doctor.

Formula: Active Ingredients: Each caplet contains Acetaminophen, 500 mg., Dextromethorphan Hydrobromide, 15 mg.; Phenylpropanolamine Hydrochloride, 12.5 mg.; Chlorpheniramine Maleate, 2 mg. **Inactive Ingredients (listed for individuals with specific allergies):** Cellulose, FD&C Blue 1, Hydroxypropyl Methylcellulose, Polyethylene Glycol, Polysorbate 80, Povidone, Sodium Starch Glycolate, Starch, Stearic Acid, Titanium Dioxide.

Continued on next page

SmithKline Beecham—Cont.

How Supplied: Consumer packages of 16 and 30 caplets.

Note: There are other CONTAC products. Make sure this is the one you are interested in.

Shown in Product Identification Guide, page 425

CONTAC
Severe Cold and Flu
Non-Drowsy Formula
Caplets
**Decongestant * Analgesic
Cough Suppressant**

Product Information: Two caplets every 6 hours to help relieve, without drowsiness, the discomfort of severe colds with flu-like symptoms.

Product Benefits: Contac Severe Cold and Flu Non-Drowsy Formula contains a NON-ASPIRIN ANALGESIC, a DECONGESTANT, and a COUGH SUPPRESSANT. These safe and effective ingredients provide temporary relief from nasal and sinus congestion, coughing, fever, headache and minor aches associated with the common cold, sore throat and flu, without drowsiness.

Directions: Adults (12 years and older.) Two caplets every 6 hours, not to exceed 8 caplets in any 24-hour period. TAMPER-RESISTANT PACKAGING FEATURES FOR YOUR PROTECTION:
* Caplets are encased in a plastic cell with a foil back; do not use if cell or foil is broken.
* The letters ND SCF appear on each caplet, do not use this product if these letters are missing.

Warnings: Do not administer to children under 12. Do not take this product for more than 7 days or for fever for more than 3 days unless directed by a doctor. If sore throat is severe, persists for more than 2 days, is accompanied or followed by fever, headache, rash, nausea or vomiting, consult a doctor promptly. A persistent cough may be a sign of a serious condition. If cough persists for more than one week, tends to recur or is accompanied by high fever, rash, or persistent headache, consult a doctor. Do not take this product for persistent or chronic cough such as occurs with smoking, asthma, emphysema, or if cough is accompanied by excessive phlegm (mucus) unless directed by a doctor. Do not take this product if you have asthma, glaucoma, heart disease, high blood pressure, emphysema, chronic pulmonary disease, shortness of breath, difficulty in breathing, diabetes, thyroid disease, or difficulty in urination due to enlargement of the prostrate gland unless directed by a doctor. Keep this and all medication out of the reach of children. As with any drug, if you are pregnant or nursing a baby, seek the advice of a health professional before using this product. In case of accidental overdose, contact a doctor or poison control center immediately. Prompt medical attention is critical for adults as well as for children even if you do not notice any signs or symptoms.

Drug Interaction Precaution: Do not take this product if you are presently taking a prescription drug for high blood pressure or monoamine oxidase inhibitor (MAOI) for depression or for two weeks after stopping use of a MAOI without first consulting your doctor.

Formula: Active Ingredients: Each tablet contains Acetaminophen 325 mg, Dextromethorphan Hydrobromide 15 mg, Pseudoephedrine Hydrochloride. Inactive Ingredients (listed for those with specific allergies): Colloidal Silicon Dioxide, Croscarmellose Sodium, Hydroxypropyl Methylcellulose, Microcrystalline Cellulose, Polyethylene Glycol, Polysorbate 80, Pregelatinized Starch, Stearic Acid, Titanium Dioxide.

How Supplied: Consumer package of 16 and 30 caplets.
Note: There are other Contac products. Make sure this is the one you are interested in.

Shown in Product Identification Guide, page 425

DEBROX® Drops

Description: Carbamide peroxide 6.5%. Also contains citric acid, glycerin, propylene glycol, sodium stannate, water, and other ingredients.

Actions: DEBROX®, used as directed, cleanses the ear with sustained microfoam. DEBROX Drops foam on contact with earwax due to the release of oxygen.

Indications: DEBROX Drops provide a safe, nonirritating method of softening and removing earwax.

Directions: FOR USE IN THE EAR ONLY. Adults and children over 12 years of age: tilt head sideways and place 5 to 10 drops into ear. Tip of applicator should not enter ear canal. Keep drops in ear for several minutes by keeping head tilted or placing cotton in the ear. Use twice daily for up to four days if needed, or as directed by a doctor. Any wax remaining after treatment may be removed by gently flushing the ear with warm water, using a soft rubber bulb ear syringe. Children under 12 years of age: consult a doctor.

Warnings: Do not use if you have ear drainage or discharge, ear pain, irritation or rash in the ear, or are dizzy, unless directed by a physician. Do not use if you have an injury or perforation (hole) of the eardrum or after ear surgery unless directed by a physician. Do not use for more than four consecutive days. If excessive earwax remains after use of this product, consult a physician. Consult a physician prior to use in children under 12.

Cautions: Avoid exposing bottle to excessive heat and direct sunlight. Keep tip on bottle when not in use. Avoid contact with eyes. Keep this and all drugs out of the reach of children. In case of accidental ingestion, seek professional assistance or contact a poison control center immediately.

How Supplied: DEBROX Drops are available in ½- or 1-fl-oz plastic squeeze bottles with applicator spouts.

Shown in Product Identification Guide, page 425

ECOTRIN®
Enteric-Coated Aspirin
Antiarthritic, Antiplatelet

Description: 'Ecotrin' is enteric-coated aspirin (acetylsalicylic acid, ASA) available in tablet and caplet forms in 81 mg, 325 mg and 500 mg dosage units. The enteric coating covers a core of aspirin and is designed to resist disintegration in the stomach, dissolving in the more neutral-to-alkaline environment of the duodenum. Such action helps to protect the stomach from injury that may result from ingestion of plain, buffered or highly buffered aspirin (see SAFETY).

Indications: 'Ecotrin' is indicated for:
* conditions requiring chronic or long-term aspirin therapy for pain and/or inflammation, e.g., rheumatoid arthritis, juvenile rheumatoid arthritis, systemic lupus erythematosus, osteoarthritis (degenerative joint disease), ankylosing spondylitis, psoriatic arthritis, Reiter's syndrome and fibrositis,
* antiplatelet indications of aspirin (see the ANTIPLATELET-EFFECT section) and
* situations in which compliance with aspirin therapy may be affected because of the gastrointestinal side effects of plain, i.e., non-enteric-coated, or buffered aspirin.

Dosage: For analgesic or anti-inflammatory indications, the OTC maximum dosage for aspirin is 4000 mg per day in divided doses, i.e., up to 650 mg every 4 hours or 1000 mg every 6 hours.
For antiplatelet effect dosage: see the ANTIPLATELET EFFECT section.
Under a physician's direction, the dosage can be increased or otherwise modified as appropriate to the clinical situation. When 'Ecotrin' is used for anti-inflammatory effect, the physician should be attentive to plasma salicylate levels, and may also caution the patient to be alert to the development of tinnitus as an indicator of elevated salicylate levels. It should be noted that patients with a high frequency hearing loss (such as may occur in older individuals) may have difficulty perceiving the tinnitus. Tinnitus would then not be a reliable indicator in such individuals.

Inactive Ingredients: Cellulose, Cellulose Acetate Phthalate, D&C Yellow 10, Diethyl Phthalate, FD&C Yellow 6,

Silicon Dioxide, Sodium Starch Glycolate, Starch, Stearic Acid, Titanium Dioxide, and trace amounts of other inactive ingredients.

Bioavailability: The bioavailability of aspirin from 'Ecotrin' has been demonstrated in a number of salicylate excretion studies. The studies show levels of salicylate (and metabolites) in urine excreted over 48 hours for 'Ecotrin' do not differ statistically from plain, i.e., non-enteric-coated, aspirin.

Plasma studies, in which 'Ecotrin' has been compared with plain aspirin in steady-state studies over eight days, also demonstrate that 'Ecotrin' provides plasma salicylate levels not statistically different from plain aspirin.

Information regarding salicylate levels over a range of doses was generated in a study in which 24 healthy volunteers (12 male and 12 female) took daily (divided) doses of either 2600 mg, 3900 mg, or 5200 mg of 'Ecotrin'. Plasma salicylate levels generally acknowledged to be anti-inflammatory (15 mg/dL.) were attained at daily doses of 5200 mg, on Day 2 by females and Day 3 by males. At 3900 mg, anti-inflammatory levels were attained at Day 3 by females and Day 4 by males. Dissolution of the enteric coating occurs at a neutral-to-basic pH and is therefore dependent on gastric emptying into the duodenum. With continued dosing, appropriate plasma levels are maintained.

Safety: The safety of 'Ecotrin' has been demonstrated in a number of endoscopic studies comparing 'Ecotrin', plain aspirin, buffered aspirin and highly buffered aspirin preparations. In these studies, all forms of aspirin were dosed to the OTC maximum (3900–4000 mg per day) for up to 14 days. The normal healthy volunteers participating in these studies were gastroscoped before and after the courses of treatment and 14-day drug-free periods followed active drug. Compared to all the other preparations, there was less gastric damage at a statistically significant level during the 'Ecotrin' courses. There was also statistically less duodenal damage when compared with the plain, i.e., non-enteric-coated, aspirin.

Details of studies demonstrating the safety and bioavailability of 'Ecotrin' are available to health care professionals. Write: Professional Services Department, SmithKline Beecham Consumer Healthcare, L.P., P.O. Box 1467, Pittsburgh, Pa. 15230.

Warning:
Consumer Warning: Children and teenagers should not use this medicine for chicken pox or flu symptoms before a doctor is consulted about Reye Syndrome, a rare but serious illness reported to be associated with aspirin. If under medical care, or with a history of ulcers, consult a physician before taking this product. If pain persists for more than 10 days, or if redness is present, or in arthritic or rheumatic conditions affecting children under 12, consult a physician immediately. Discontinue use if dizzi-

ness, ringing in ears, or impaired hearing occurs. If you experience persistent or unexplained stomach upset, consult a physician. Keep this and all drugs out of children's reach. In case of accidental overdose, seek professional assistance or contact a poison control center immediately. As with any medicine, if you are pregnant or nursing a baby, seek the advice of a health professional before using this product. **IT IS ESPECIALLY IMPORTANT NOT TO USE ASPIRIN DURING THE LAST 3 MONTHS OF PREGNANCY UNLESS SPECIFICALLY DIRECTED TO DO SO BY A DOCTOR BECAUSE IT MAY CAUSE PROBLEMS IN THE UNBORN CHILD OR COMPLICATIONS DURING DELIVERY.** Store at controlled room temperature (59°-86°F.).

Drug Interaction Precaution: Do not take this product if you are taking a prescription drug for anticoagulation (thinning of the blood), diabetes, gout, or arthritis unless directed by a physician.

Professional Warning: There have been occasional reports in the literature concerning individuals with impaired gastric emptying in whom there may be retention of one or more 'Ecotrin' tablets over time. This unusual phenomenon may occur as a result of outlet obstruction from ulcer disease alone or combined with hypotonic gastric peristalsis. Because of the integrity of the enteric coating in an acidic environment, these tablets may accumulate and form a bezoar in the stomach. Individuals with this condition may present with complaints of early satiety or of vague upper abdominal distress. Diagnosis may be made by endoscopy or by abdominal films which show opacities suggestive of a mass of small tablets *(Ref.: Bogacz, K. and Caldron, P.: Enteric-coated Aspirin Bezoar: Elevation of Serum Salicylate Level by Barium Study. Amer. J. Med. 1987:83, 783–6.).* Management may vary according to the condition of the patient. Options include: gastrotomy and alternating slightly basic and neutral lavage *(Ref.: Baum, J.: Enteric-Coated Aspirin and the Problem of Gastric Retention. J. Rheum., 1984:11, 250–1.).* While there have been no clinical reports, it has been suggested that such individuals may also be treated with parenteral cimetidine (to reduce acid secretion) and then given sips of slightly basic liquids to effect gradual dissolution of the enteric coating. Progress may be followed with plasma salicylate levels or via recognition of tinnitus by the patient.

It should be kept in mind that individuals with a history of partial or complete gastrectomy may produce reduced amounts of acid and therefore have less acidic gastric pH. Under these circumstances, the benefits offered by the acid-resistant enteric coating may not exist.

Antiplatelet Effect Aspirin may be recommended to reduce the risk of death and/or nonfatal myocardial infarction (MI) in patients with a previous infarction or unstable angina pectoris and its

use in reducing the risk of transient ischemic attacks in men.
Labeling for both indications follows:
ASPIRIN FOR MYOCARDIAL INFARCTION
Indication: Aspirin is indicated to reduce the risk of death and/or nonfatal myocardial infarction in patients with a previous infarction or unstable angina pectoris.

Clinical Trials: The indication is supported by the results of six, large, randomized multicenter, placebo-controlled studies involving 10,816 predominantly male, post-myocardial infarction (MI) patients and one randomized placebo-controlled study of 1,266 men with unstable angina.[1–7] Therapy with aspirin was begun at intervals after the onset of acute MI varying from less than three days to more than five years and continued for periods of from less than one year to four years. In the unstable angina study, treatment was started within one month after the onset of unstable angina and continued for 12 weeks, and patients with complicating conditions such as congestive heart failure were not included in the study.

Aspirin therapy in MI patients was associated with about a 20 percent reduction in the risk of subsequent death and/or nonfatal reinfarction, a median absolute decrease of 3 percent from the 12 to 22 percent event rates in the placebo groups. In aspirin-treated unstable angina patients, the reduction in risk was about 50 percent, a reduction in event rate to 5% from the 10% in the placebo group over the 12 weeks of the study.

Daily dosage of aspirin in the post-myocardial infarction studies was 300 mg in one study and 900 to 1500 mg in five studies. A dose of 325 mg was used in the study of unstable angina.

Adverse Reactions
Gastrointestinal Reactions: Doses of 1000 mg per day of plain aspirin caused gastrointestinal symptoms and bleeding that in some cases were clinically significant. In the largest postinfarction study (the Aspirin Myocardial Infarction Study [AMIS] with 4,500 people), the percentage incidences of gastrointestinal symptoms of a standard, solid-tablet formulation and placebo-treated subjects, respectively, were: stomach pain (14.5%; 4.4%); heartburn (11.9%; 4.8%); nausea and/or vomiting (7.6%; 2.1%); hospitalization for gastrointestinal disorder (4.9%; 3.5%). In the AMIS and other trials, plain aspirin-treated patients had increased rates of gross gastrointestinal bleeding. Symptoms and signs of gastrointestinal irritation were not significantly increased in subjects treated for unstable angina with buffered aspirin in solution.

Cardiovascular and Biochemical: In the AMIS trial, the dosage of 1000 mg per day of plain aspirin was associated with small increases in systolic blood pressure (BP) (average 1.5 to 2.1 mmHg) and dia-

Continued on next page

SmithKline Beecham—Cont.

stolic BP (0.5 to 0.6 mmHg), depending upon whether maximal or last available readings were used. Blood urea nitrogen and uric acid levels were also increased, but by less than 1.0 mg%. Subjects with marked hypertension or renal insufficiency had been excluded from the trial so that the clinical importance of these observations for such subjects or for any subjects treated over more prolonged periods is not known. It is recommended that patients placed on long-term aspirin treatment, even at doses of 300 mg per day, be seen at regular intervals to assess changes in these measurements.

Sodium in Buffered Aspirin for Solution Formulations: One tablet daily of buffered aspirin in solution adds 553 mg of sodium to that in the diet and may not be tolerated by patients with active sodium-retaining states such as congestive heart or renal failure. This amount of sodium adds about 30 percent to the 70 to 90 meq intake suggested as appropriate for dietary hypertension in the 1984 Report of the Joint National Committee on Detection, Evaluation, and Treatment of High Blood Pressure.[8]

Dosage and Administration: Although most of the studies used dosages exceeding 300 mg daily, two trials used only 300 mg and pharmacologic data indicate that this dose inhibits platelet function fully. Therefore, 300 mg or a conventional 325 mg aspirin dose daily is a reasonable, routine dose that would minimize gastrointestinal adverse reactions for both solid oral dosage forms (buffered and plain aspirin) and buffered aspirin in solution.

References:
1. Elwood, P.C., et al.: A Randomized Controlled Trial of Acetylsalicylic Acid in the Secondary Prevention of Mortality from Myocardial Infarction, *Br. Med. J.* 1:436–440, 1974.
2. The Coronary Drug Project Research Group: Aspirin in Coronary Heart Disease, *J. Chronic Dis.* 29:625–642, 1976.
3. Breddin, K., et al.: Secondary Prevention of Myocardial Infarction: A Comparison of Acetylsalicylic Acid, Phenprocoumon or Placebo, *Homeostasis* 470:263–268, 1979.
4. Aspirin Myocardial Infarction Study Research Group: A Randomized Controlled Trial of Aspirin in Persons Recovered from Myocardial Infarction, *J.A.M.A.* 243:661–669, 1980.
5. Elwood, P.C., and Sweetnam, P.M.: Aspirin and Secondary Mortality After Myocardial Infarction, *Lancet* pp. 1313–1315, Dec. 22–29, 1979.
6. The Persantine-Aspirin Reinfarction Study Research Group, Persantine and Aspirin in Coronary Heart Disease, *Circulation* 62: 449–469, 1980.
7. Lewis, H.D., et al.: Protective Effects of Aspirin Against Acute Myocardial Infarction and Death in Men with Unstable Angina, Results of a Veterans Ad-

ministration Cooperative Study, *N. Engl. J. Med.* 309:396–403, 1983.
8. 1984 Report of the Joint National Committee on Detection, Evaluation, and Treatment of High Blood Pressure, U.S. Department of Health and Human Services and U.S. Public Health Service, National Institutes of Health. NIH Pub. No. 84–1088.

Aspirin for Transient Ischemic Attacks

Indication For reducing the risk of recurrent transient ischemic attacks (TIAs) or stroke in men who have had transient ischemia of the brain due to fibrin platelet emboli. There is inadequate evidence that aspirin or buffered aspirin is effective in reducing TIAs in women at the recommended dosage. There is no evidence that aspirin or buffered aspirin is of benefit in the treatment of completed strokes in men or women.

Clinical Trials The indication is supported by the results of a Canadian study[1] in which 585 patients with threatened stroke were followed in a randomized clinical trial for an average of 26 months to determine whether aspirin or sulfinpyrazone, singly or in combination, was superior to placebo in preventing transient ischemic attacks, stroke or death. The study showed that, although sulfinpyrazone had no statistically significant effect, aspirin reduced the risk of continuing transient ischemic attacks, stroke or death by 19 percent and reduced the risk of stroke or death by 31 percent. Another aspirin study carried out in the United States with 178 patients showed a statistically significant number of "favorable outcomes," including reduced transient ischemic attacks, stroke and death.[2]

Precautions Patients presenting with signs and/or symptoms of TIAs should have a complete medical and neurologic evaluation. Consideration should be given to other disorders that resemble TIAs. Attention should be given to risk factors: it is important to evaluate and treat, if appropriate, other diseases associated with TIAs and stroke, such as hypertension and diabetes.

Concurrent administration of absorbable antacids at therapeutic doses may increase the clearance of salicylates in some individuals. The concurrent administration of nonabsorbable antacids may alter the rate of absorption of aspirin, thereby resulting in a decreased acetylsalicylic acid/salicylate ratio in plasma. The clinical significance of these decreases in available aspirin is unknown. Aspirin at dosages of 1,000 mg per day has been associated with small increases in blood pressure, blood urea nitrogen, and serum uric acid levels. It is recommended that patients placed on long-term aspirin treatment be seen at regular intervals to assess changes in these measurements.

Adverse Reactions: At dosages of 1,000 mg or higher of aspirin per day, gastrointestinal side effects include stomach pain, heartburn, nausea and/or vomit-

ing, as well as increased rates of gross gastrointestinal bleeding.

Dosage and Administration Adult dosage for men is 1,300 mg a day, in divided doses of 650 mg twice a day or 325 mg four times a day.

References:
1. The Canadian Cooperative Study Group: Randomized Trial of Aspirin and Sulfinpyrazone in Threatened Stroke, *N. Engl. J. Med.* 299:53, 1978.
2. Fields, W. S., et al.: Controlled Trial of Aspirin in Cerebral Ischemia, *Stroke* 8:301–316, 1980.

How Supplied:
'Ecotrin' Tablets
 81 mg in bottle of 36
 325 mg in bottles of 100*, 250 and 1000.
 500 mg in bottles of 60*, 150 and 300.
'Ecotrin' Caplets
 325 mg in bottles of 100.
 500 mg in bottles of 60.
* Without child-resistant caps.

TAMPER-RESISTANT PACKAGE FEATURES FOR YOUR PROTECTION:
- Bottle has imprinted seal under cap.
- The words ECOTRIN LOW or ECOTRIN REG or ECOTRIN MAX appear on each tablet or caplet (see product illustration printed on carton).
- **DO NOT USE THIS PRODUCT IF ANY OF THESE TAMPER-RESISTANT FEATURES ARE MISSING OR BROKEN.**

Comments or Questions? Call Toll-Free 800-245-1040 weekdays.
Shown in Product Identification Guide, page 425

FEOSOL® CAPSULES
Hemantinic

Description: 'Feosol' Capsules provide the body with ferrous sulfate—iron in its most efficient form—for simple iron deficiency and iron-deficiency anemia when the need for such therapy has been determined by a physician. The special targeted-release capsule formulation—ferrous sulfate in pellets—reduces stomach upset, a common problem with iron.

Formula: Active ingredients: Each capsule contains 159 mg. of dried ferrous sulfate USP (50 mg. of elemental iron), equivalent to 250 mg. of ferrous sulfate USP. **Inactive Ingredients** (listed for individuals with specific allergies): Benzyl Alcohol, Cetylpyridinium Chloride, D&C Red 33, Yellow 10, FD&C Blue 1, D&C Red 7, Red 40, Gelatin, Glyceryl Stearates, Iron Oxide, Polyethylene Glycol, Povidone, Sodium Lauryl Sulfate, Starch, Sucrose, White Wax and trace amounts of other inactive ingredients.

Dosage: Adults: 1 or 2 capsules daily or as directed by a physician.
Children: As directed by a physician.
TAMPER-RESISTANT PACKAGING FEATURES:
- The carton is protected by a clear overwrap printed with "safety sealed", do

not use if overwrap is missing or broken.

- Each capsule is encased in a plastic cell with a foil back; do not use if cell or foil is broken.
- Each FEOSOL capsule is protected by a red Perma-Seal™ band which bonds the two capsule halves together; do not use if capsule is broken or band is missing or broken.

WARNINGS: Do not exceed recommended dosage. The treatment of any anemic condition should be under the advice and supervision of a physician. Iron-containing medication may occasionally cause constipation or diarrhea. Since oral iron products interfere with absorption of oral tetracycline antibiotics, these products should not be taken within two hours of each other. **Keep this and all drugs out of the reach of children. In case of accidental overdose, seek professional assistance or contact a poison control center immediately.** As with any drug, if you are pregnant or nursing a baby, seek the advice of a health professional before using this product.

> Manufactured with methylchloroform, a substance which harms public health and environment by destroying ozone in the upper atmosphere.

Store at controlled room temperature (59°–86°F.).

How Supplied: Packages of 30 and 60 capsules; in Single Unit Packages of 100 capsules (intended for institutional use only).

Also available in Tablets and Elixir.

Shown in Product Idenficiation Guide, page 425

FEOSOL® ELIXIR
Hemantinic

Description: 'Feosol' Elixir, an unusually palatable iron elixir, provides the body with ferrous sulfate—iron in its most efficient form. The standard elixir for simple iron deficiency and iron-deficiency anemia when the need for such therapy has been determined by a physician.

Formula: Active Ingredients: Each 5 ml. (1 teaspoonful) contains ferrous sulfate USP, 220 mg. (44 mg. of elemental iron); alcohol, 5%.
Inactive Ingredients (listed for individuals with specific allergies): Citric Acid, FD&C Yellow 6 (Sunset Yellow) as a color additive, Flavors, Glucose, Saccharin Sodium, Sucrose, Purified Water.

Dosage: Adults—1 to 2 teaspoonsful three times daily preferably between meals. Children—½ to 1 teaspoonful three times daily preferably between meals. Infants—as directed by physician. Mix with water or fruit juice to avoid

temporary staining of teeth; do not mix with milk or wine-based vehicles.

TAMPER-RESISTANT PACKAGE FEATURE:
IMPRINTED SEAL AROUND BOTTLE CAP: DO NOT USE IF BROKEN.

Warnings: The treatment of any anemic condition should be under the advice and supervision of a physician. Since oral iron products interfere with absorption of oral tetracycline antibiotics, these products should not be taken within two hours of each other. Occasional gastrointestinal discomfort (such as nausea) may be minimized by taking with meals and by beginning with one teaspoonful the first day, two the second, etc. until the recommended dosage is reached. Iron-containing medication may occasionally cause constipation or diarrhea, and liquids may cause temporary staining of the teeth (this is less likely when diluted). **Keep this and all drugs out of reach of children. In case of accidental overdose, seek professional assistance or contact a poison control center immediately.** As with any drug, if you are pregnant or nursing a baby, seek the advice of a health professional before using this product.
Avoid storing at high temperature (greater than 100°F.).
Protect from freezing.

How Supplied: A clear orange liquid in 16 fl. oz. bottles.

Also available: 'Feosol' Tablets, 'Feosol' Capsules
NOTE: There are other Feosol products. Make sure this is the one you are interested in.

Shown in Product Identification Guide, page 425

FEOSOL® TABLETS
Hemantinic

Description: 'Feosol' Tablets provide the body with ferrous sulfate, iron in its most efficient form, for iron deficiency and iron-deficiency anemia when the need for such therapy has been determined by a physician. The distinctive triangular-shaped tablet has a coating to prevent oxidation and improve palatability.

Formula: Active Ingredients: Each tablet contains 200 mg. of dried ferrous sulfate USP (65 mg. of elemental iron), equivalent to 325 mg. (5 grains) of ferrous sulfate USP. **Inactive Ingredients** (listed for individuals with specific allergies): Calcium Sulfate, D&C Yellow 10, FD&C Blue 2, Glucose, Hydroxypropyl Methylcellulose, Mineral Oil, Polyethylene Glycol, Sodium Lauryl Sulfate, Starch, Stearic Acid, Talc, Titanium Dioxide, and trace amounts of other inactive ingredients.

Dosage: Adults—one tablet 3 to 4 times daily, after meals and upon retiring or as directed by a physician. Children 6 to 12 years—one tablet three times a day after meals or as directed by

a physician. Children under 6 years and infants—use 'Feosol' Elixir.

TAMPER-RESISTANT PACKAGE FEATURES:
- Bottle has imprinted seal under cap. Do not use if missing or broken.
- FEOSOL Tablets are triangular shaped (see product illustration printed on carton).

CAUTION: DO NOT USE THIS PRODUCT IF ANY OF THESE TAMPER-RESISTANT FEATURES ARE MISSING OR BROKEN.
Comments or Questions?
Call toll-free 800-245-1040 weekdays.

Warnings: Do not exceed recommended dosage. The treatment of any anemic condition should be under the advice and supervision of a physician. Since oral iron products interfere with absorption of oral tetracycline antibiotics, these products should not be taken within two hours of each other. Occasional gastrointestinal discomfort (such as nausea) may be minimized by taking with meals and by beginning with one tablet the first day, two the second, etc. until the recommended dosage is reached. Iron-containing medication may occasionally cause constipation or diarrhea. **Keep this and all drugs out of reach of children. In case of accidental overdose, seek professional assistance or contact a poison control center immediately.** As with any drug, if you are pregnant or nursing a baby, seek the advice of a health professional before using this product.
Avoid storing at high temperature (greater than 100°F.).

How Supplied: Bottles of 100 tablets; in Single Unit Packages of 100 tablets (intended for institutional use only).
Also available in Capsules and Elixir.

Shown in Product Identification Guide, page 425

GAVISCON® Antacid Tablets
[găv 'ĭs-kŏn]

Composition: Each chewable tablet contains the following active ingredients: Aluminum hydroxide dried gel... 80 mg Magnesium trisilicate .... 20 mg and the following inactive ingredients: alginic acid, calcium stearate, flavor, sodium bicarbonate, starch (may contain cornstarch), and sucrose.

Actions: Unique formulation produces soothing foam which floats on stomach contents. Foam containing antacid precedes stomach contents into the esophagus when reflux occurs to help protect the sensitive mucosa from further irritation. GAVISCON® acts locally without neutralizing entire stomach contents to help maintain integrity of the digestive process. Endoscopic studies indicate that GAVISCON Antacid Tablets are equally as effective in the erect or supine patient.

Indications: GAVISCON is specifically formulated for the temporary relief

Continued on next page

SmithKline Beecham—Cont.

of heartburn (acid indigestion) due to acid reflux. GAVISCON is not indicated for the treatment of peptic ulcers.

Directions: Chew two to four tablets four times a day or as directed by a physician. Tablets should be taken after meals and at bedtime or as needed. For best results follow by a half glass of water or other liquid. DO NOT SWALLOW WHOLE.

Warnings: Do not take more than 16 tablets in a 24-hour period or 16 tablets daily for more than 2 weeks, except under the advice and supervision of a physician. Do not use this product except under the advice and supervision of a physician if you are on a sodium-restricted diet. Each GAVISCON Tablet contains approximately 0.8 mEq sodium.

Drug Interaction Precautions: Do not take this product if you are presently taking a prescription antibiotic drug containing any form of tetracycline.
Store at a controlled room temperature in a dry place.
Keep this and all drugs out of the reach of children. In case of accidental overdose, seek professional assistance or contact a poison control center immediately.

How Supplied: Available in bottles of 100 tablets and in foil-wrapped 2s in boxes of 30 tablets.

Issued 2/87

Shown in Product Identification Guide, page 425

GAVISCON® EXTRA STRENGTH RELIEF FORMULA Antacid Tablets
[găv 'ĭs-kŏn]

Composition: Each chewable tablet contains the following active ingredients:
Aluminum hydroxide .... 160 mg
Magnesium carbonate .... 105 mg
and the following inactive ingredients: alginic acid, calcium stearate, flavor, mannitol, sodium bicarbonate, stearic acid, and sucrose.

Directions: Chew 2 to 4 tablets four times a day or as directed by a physician. Tablets should be taken after meals and at bedtime or as needed. For best results follow by a half glass of water or other liquid. DO NOT SWALLOW WHOLE.

> **FDA Approved Uses:** For the relief of heartburn, sour stomach, and/or acid indigestion, and upset stomach associated with heartburn, sour stomach, and/or acid indigestion.

Warnings: Do not take more than 16 tablets in a 24-hour period or 16 tablets daily for more than 2 weeks, except under the advice and supervision of a physician. Do not use this product except under the advice and supervision of a physician if you are on a sodium-restricted

diet. Each tablet contains approximately 1.3 mEq sodium.

Drug Interaction Precautions: Do not take this product if you are presently taking a prescription antibiotic drug containing any form of tetracycline.
Store at a controlled room temperature in a dry place.
Keep this and all drugs out of the reach of children.
In case of accidental overdose, seek professional assistance or contact a poison control center immediately.

How Supplied: Available in bottles of 100 tablets and in foil-wrapped 2s in boxes of 30.

Shown in Product Identification Guide, page 425

GAVISCON® EXTRA STRENGTH RELIEF FORMULA
Liquid Antacid
[găv 'ĭs-kŏn]

Composition: Each 2 teaspoonfuls (10 mL) contains the following active ingredients:
Aluminum hydroxide.................. 508 mg
Magnesium carbonate................. 475 mg
And the following inactive ingredients: butylparaben, edetate disodium, flavor, glycerin, propylparaben, saccharin sodium, simethicone emulsion, sodium alginate, sorbitol solution, water, and xanthan gum.

> **FDA Approved Uses:** For the relief of heartburn, sour stomach and/or acid indigestion, and upset stomach associated with heartburn, sour stomach and/or acid indigestion.

Directions: SHAKE WELL BEFORE USING. Take 2 to 4 teaspoonfuls four times a day or as directed by a physician. GAVISCON Extra Strength Relief Formula Liquid should be taken after meals and at bedtime, followed by half a glass of water. Dispense product only by spoon or other measuring device.

Warnings: Except under the advice and supervision of a physician, do not take more than 16 teaspoonfuls in a 24-hour period or 16 teaspoonfuls daily for more than 2 weeks. May have laxative effect. Do not use this product if you have a kidney disease; do not use this product if you are on a sodium-restricted diet. Each teaspoonful contains approximately 0.9 mEq sodium.

Drug Interaction Precautions: Do not take this product if you are presently taking a prescription antibiotic drug containing any form of tetracycline.
Keep tightly closed. Avoid freezing. Store at a controlled room temperature.
Keep this and all drugs out of the reach of children.
In case of accidental overdose, seek professional assistance or contact a poison control center immediately.

How Supplied: Available in 12 fl oz (355 mL) bottles.

Shown in Product Identification Guide, page 425

GAVISCON® Liquid Antacid
[găv 'ĭs-kŏn]

Composition: Each tablespoonful (15 ml) contains the following active ingredients:
Aluminum hydroxide .... 95 mg
Magnesium carbonate .... 358 mg
And the following inactive ingredients: D&C Yellow #10, edetate disodium, FD&C Blue #1, flavor, glycerin, paraben preservatives, saccharin sodium, sodium alginate, sorbitol solution, water, and xanthan gum.

> **FDA Approved Uses:** For the relief of heartburn, sour stomach and/or acid indigestion, and upset stomach associated with heartburn, sour stomach and/or acid indigestion.

Directions: SHAKE WELL BEFORE USING. Take 1 or 2 tablespoonfuls four times a day or as directed by a physician. GAVISCON Liquid should be taken after meals and at bedtime, followed by half a glass of water. Dispense product only by spoon or other measuring device.

Warnings: Except under the advice and supervision of a physician, do not take more than 8 tablespoonfuls in a 24-hour period or 8 tablespoonfuls daily for more than 2 weeks. May have laxative effect. Do not use this product if you have a kidney disease; do not use this product if you are on a sodium-restricted diet. Each tablespoonful of GAVISCON Liquid contains approximately 1.7 mEq sodium.

Drug Interaction Precautions: Do not take this product if you are presently taking a prescription antibiotic drug containing any form of tetracycline.
Keep tightly closed. Avoid freezing. Store at a controlled room temperature.
Keep this and all drugs out of the reach of children.
In case of accidental overdose, seek professional assistance or contact a poison control center immediately.

How Supplied: Bottles of 12 fluid ounce (355 ml) and 6 fluid ounce (177 ml).

Shown in Product Identification Guide, page 425

GAVISCON®-2 Antacid Tablets
[găv 'ĭs-kŏn]

Composition: Each chewable tablet contains the following active ingredients:
Aluminum hydroxide dried gel...160 mg
Magnesium trisilicate .... 40 mg
and the following inactive ingredients: alginic acid, calcium stearate, flavor, sodium bicarbonate, starch (may contain cornstarch), and sucrose.

Indications: GAVISCON® is specifically formulated for the temporary relief of heartburn (acid indigestion) due to acid reflux. GAVISCON is not indicated for the treatment of peptic ulcers.

Directions: Chew one to two tablets four times a day or as directed by a physician. Tablets should be taken after meals and at bedtime or as needed. For best results follow by a half glass of water or other liquid. DO NOT SWALLOW WHOLE.

Warnings: Do not take more than eight tablets in a 24-hour period or eight tablets daily for more than 2 weeks, except under the advice and supervision of a physician. Do not use this product except under the advice and supervision of a physician if you are on a sodium-restricted diet. Each GAVISCON-2 Tablet contains approximately 1.6 mEq sodium.

Drug Interaction Precautions: Do not take this product if you are presently taking a prescription antibiotic drug containing any form of tetracycline.
Store at a controlled room temperature in a dry place.
Keep this and all drugs out of the reach of children. In case of accidental overdose, seek professional assistance or contact a poison control center immediately.

How Supplied: Boxes of 48 foil-wrapped tablets.

Issued 2/87

Shown in Product Identification Guide, page 425

GERITOL COMPLETE™ Tablets
[jer 'e-tol]
High Potency Multi-Vitamin/Mineral

Active Ingredients (Per Tablet): Vitamin A (6000 IU as Beta Carotene); Vitamin E (30 IU); Vitamin C (60 mg.); Folic Acid (400 mcg.); Vitamin B_1 (1.5 mg.); Vitamin B_2 (1.7 mg.); Niacin (20 mg.); Vitamin B_6 (2 mg.); Vitamin B_{12} (6 mcg.); Vitamin D (400 IU); Biotin (45 mcg.); Pantothenic Acid (10 mg.); Vitamin K (25 mcg.); Calcium (162 mg.); Phosphorus (125 mg.); Iodine (150 mcg.); Iron (18 mg.); Magnesium (100 mg.); Copper (2 mg.); Manganese (2.5 mg.); Potassium (37.5 mg.); Chloride (34 mg.); Chromium (15 mcg.); Molybdenum (15 mcg.); Selenium (15 mcg.); Zinc (15 mcg.); Nickel (5 mcg.); Silicon (80 mcg.); Tin (10 mcg.); Vanadium (10 mcg.).

Inactive Ingredients: Crospovidone, Gelatin, Glycerides of Stearic and Palmitic acids, Hydroxypropyl cellulose, Hydroxypropyl methylcellulose, Magnesium stearate, Microcrystalline cellulose, Polyethylene glycol, Silicon dioxide, Stearic acid, FD&C Red #40, FD&C Blue #2, FD&C Yellow #6, Titanium dioxide.

Indications: For use as a dietary supplement.

Actions: Help treat and prevent iron deficiency.

Warnings: Keep out of reach of children.

Precaution: Alcoholics and individuals with chronic liver or pancreatic disease may have enhanced iron absorption with the potential for iron overload.
NOTE: Unabsorbed iron may cause some darkening of the stool.

Symptoms and Treatment of Oral Overdose: Toxicity and symptoms are primarily due to iron overdose. Abdominal pain, nausea, vomiting and diarrhea may occur, with possible subsequent acidosis and cardiovascular collapse with severe poisoning. If an overdose is suspected, immediately seek professional assistance by contacting your physician, the local poison control center, or the Rocky Mt. Poison Control Center at 303-592-1710 (Collect), 24 hours a day.

Dosage and Administration (Adults): One (1) tablet daily after mealtime.

How Supplied: Bottles of 14, 40, 100, and 180 tablets.

GERITOL EXTEND™ Tablets or Caplets
Nutritional Supplement

Active Ingredients (per tablet); Vitamin A (3333 IU, including 1250 IU from Beta Carotene); Vitamin D (200 IU); Vitamin E (15 IU); Vitamin C (60 mg); Folic Acid (0.2 mg); Vitamin B_1 (1.2 mg); Vitamin B_2 (1.4 mg); Niacin (15 mg); Vitamin B_6 (2.0 mg); Vitamin B_{12} (2 mcg); Vitamin K (80 mcg); Calcium (130 mg); Phosphorus (100 mg); Magnesium (35 mg); Zinc (15 mg); Iodine (150 mcg); Iron (10 mg); Selenium (70 mcg)

Inactive Ingredients: Croscarmelose Sodium, Gelatin, Glycerides of Stearic and Palmitic Acids, Hydroxypropyl Methylcellulose, Magnesium Stearate, Microcrystalline Cellulose, Polyethylene Glycol, Silicon Dioxide, Stearic Acid, FD&C Red #40, FD&C Blue #2, Titanium Dioxide.

Indications: For use as a dietary supplement. Recommended for active adults over 50.

Actions: Help treat and prevent iron deficiency.

Warnings: Keep out of reach of children.

Precaution: Alcoholics and individuals with chronic liver or pancreatic disease may have enhanced iron absorption with the potential for iron overload.
NOTE: Unabsorbed iron may cause some darkening of the stool.

Symptoms and Treatment of Oral Overdose: Toxicity and symptoms are primarily due to iron overdose. Abdominal pain, nausea, vomiting, and diarrhea may occur with possible subsequent acidosis and cardiovascular collapse with severe poisoning. If an overdose is suspected, immediately seek professional assistance by contacting your physician, the local poison control center, or the Rocky Mountain Poison Control Center at 303-592-1710 (collect), 24 hours a day.

Dosage and Administration (Adults 50+): One (1) tablet/caplet daily after mealtime.

How Supplied: Bottles of 40 and 100 tablets or caplets in blister-pack cartons.

GERITOL® Liquid
[jer 'e-tol]
High Potency Vitamin & Iron Tonic

Active Ingredients Per Dose (½ fluid ounce): Iron (as ferric ammonium citrate) 18 mg; Thiamine (B_1) 2.5 mg; Riboflavin (B_2) 2.5 mg; Niacinamide 50 mg; Panthenol 2 mg; Pyridoxine (B_6) 0.5 mg; Methionine 25 mg; Choline Bitartrate 50 mg.

Inactive Ingredients: Alcohol, Benzoic acid, Caramel color, Citric acid, Invert sugar, Sucrose, Water, Flavors.

Indications: For use as a dietary supplement.

Actions: Help treat and prevent iron deficiency.

Warnings: Keep out of reach of children.

Precaution: Alcohol accelerates absorption of ferric iron. Alcoholics and individuals with chronic liver or pancreatic disease may have enhanced iron absorption with the potential for iron overload.
NOTE: Unabsorbed iron may cause some darkening of the stool.

Symptoms and Treatment of Oral Overdose: Toxicity and symptoms are primarily due to iron overdose. Abdominal pain, nausea, vomiting and diarrhea may occur, with possible subsequent acidosis and cardiovascular collapse with severe poisoning. If an overdose is suspected, immediately seek professional assistance by contacting your physician, the local poison control center, or the Rocky Mt. Poison Control Center at 303-592-1710 (Collect), 24 hours a day.

Dosage and Administration (Adults): As an iron supplement and for normal menstrual needs: One (1) tablespoonful (0.5 fl. oz.) daily at mealtime. For iron deficiency: One (1) tablespoonful (0.5 fl. oz.) three times daily at mealtime or as directed by a physician.

How Supplied: Bottles of 4 oz., and 12 oz.

7001M
11/14/83

GLY-OXIDE® Liquid

Description: GLY-OXIDE® Liquid contains carbamide peroxide 10%. Also contains citric acid, flavor, glycerin, propylene glycol, sodium stannate, water, and other ingredients.

Continued on next page

SmithKline Beecham—Cont.

Actions: GLY-OXIDE® Liquid has an oxygen-rich formula that works to relieve the pain of canker sores by cleaning and debriding damaged tissue so natural healing can occur.

Administration: Do not dilute. Apply directly from bottle. Replace tip on bottle when not in use.

Indications: For local treatment and hygienic prevention of minor oral inflammation such as canker sores, denture irritation, and postdental procedure irritation. Place several drops on affected area four times daily, after meals and at bedtime, or as directed by a dentist or physician; expectorate after two or three minutes. Or place 10 drops onto tongue, mix with saliva, swish for several minutes, and expectorate.

As an adjunct to oral hygiene (orthodontics, dental appliances) after regular brushing, swish 10 or more drops vigorously. Continue for two to three minutes; expectorate.

When normal oral hygiene is inadequate or impossible (total care geriatrics, etc), swish 10 or more drops vigorously after meals and expectorate.

Precautions: Severe or persistent oral inflammation, denture irritation, or gingivitis may be serious. If these conditions or unexpected side effects occur, consult a dentist or physician immediately.

Avoid contact with eyes. Protect from heat and direct light. Keep this and all drugs out of the reach of children. In case of accidental overdose, seek professional assistance or contact a poison control center immediately.

How Supplied: GLY-OXIDE® Liquid is available in ½-fl-oz and 2-fl-oz non-spill, plastic squeeze bottles with applicator spouts.

Shown in Product Identification Guide, page 425

MASSENGILL® Douches
[mas 'sen-gil]

PRODUCT OVERVIEW

Key Facts
Massengill is the brand name for a line of douches which are recommended for routine cleansing and for temporary relief of vaginal itching and irritation. Massengill Disposable douches are available in two Vinegar & Water formulas (Extra Mild and Extra Cleansing), a Baking Soda formula, four Cosmetic solutions (Country Flowers, Fresh Baby Powder Scent (formerly Belle Mai), Mountain Breeze and Spring Rain Freshness) and a Medicated formula (with povidone-iodine). Massengill also is available in a Medicated liquid concentrate (povidone-iodine) and a Non-Medicated liquid concentrate and powder form.

Major Uses: Massengill's Vinegar & Water, Baking Soda & Water, and Cos-metic douches are recommended for routine douching, or for cleansing following menstruation, prescribed use of vaginal medication or use of contraceptives. Massengill Medicated is recommended in a seven day regimen for the symptomatic relief of minor itching and irritation associated with vaginitis due to Candida albicans, Trichomonas vaginalis, and Gardnerella vaginalis.

Safety Information: Do not douche during pregnancy unless directed by a physician. Douching does not prevent pregnancy. Do not use this product and consult your physician if you are experiencing any of the following symptoms: unusual vaginal discharge, painful and/or frequent urination, lower abdominal pain, or you or your sex partner has genital sores or ulcers.

Massengill Vinegar & Water, Baking Soda & Water, and Cosmetic Douches—If irritation occurs, discontinue use.

Massengill Medicated — Women with iodine-sensitivity should not use this product. If symptoms persist after seven days, or if redness, swelling or pain develop, consult a physician. Do not use while nursing unless directed by a physician.

PRODUCT INFORMATION

MASSENGILL®
[mas 'sen-gil]
Disposable Douches
MASSENGILL®
Liquid Concentrate
MASSENGILL® Powder

Ingredients:
DISPOSABLES: Extra Mild Vinegar and Water—Water and Vinegar.

Extra Cleansing Vinegar and Water—Water, Vinegar, Puraclean™ (Cetylpyridinium Chloride), Diazolidinyl Urea, Disodium EDTA.

Baking Soda and Water—Sanitized Water, Sodium Bicarbonate (Baking Soda).

Fresh Baby Powder Scent (formerly Belle-Mai Powder) Water, SD Alcohol 40, Lactic Acid, Sodium Lactate, Octoxynol-9, Cetylpyridinium Chloride, Propylene Glycol (and) Diazolidinyl Urea (and) Methylparaben (and) Propylparaben, Disodium EDTA, Fragrance, FD&C Blue #1.

Country Flowers—Water, SD Alcohol 40, Lactic Acid, Sodium Lactate, Octoxynol-9, Cetylpyridinium Chloride, Propylene Glycol (and) Diazolidinyl Urea (and), Methylparaben (and) Propylparaben, Disodium EDTA, Fragrance, D&C Red #28, FD&C Blue #1.

Mountain Breeze—Water, SD Alcohol 40, Lactic Acid, Sodium Lactate, Octoxynol-9, Cetylpyridinium Chloride, Propylene Glycol (and) Diazolidinyl Urea (and) Methylparaben (and) Propylparaben, Disodium EDTA, Fragrance, D&C Yellow #10, FD&C Blue #1.

Spring Rain freshness—Water, SD Alcohol 40, Lactic Acid, Sodium Lactate, Octoxynol-9, Cetylpyridinium Chloride, Propylene Glycol (and) Methylparaben (and) Propylparaben, Disodium EDTA, fragrance.

LIQUID CONCENTRATE: Water, SD Alcohol 40, Lactic Acid, Sodium Bicarbonate, Octoxynol-9, Methyl Salicylate, Liquid Menthol, Eucalyptol, Thymol, D&C Yellow #10, FD&C Yellow #6 (Sunset Yellow).

POWDER: Sodium Chloride, Ammonium alum, PEG-8, Phenol, Methyl Salicylate, Eucalyptus Oil, Menthol, Thymol, D&C Yellow #10, FD&C Yellow #6 (Sunset Yellow).

FLORAL POWDER: Sodium Chloride, Ammonium alum, Octoxynol-9, SD Alcohol 23-A, Fragrance, and FD&C Yellow #6 (Sunset Yellow).

Indications: Recommended for routine cleansing at the end of menstruation, after use of contraceptive creams or jellies (check the contraceptive package instructions first) or to rinse out the residue of prescribed vaginal medication (as directed by physician).

Actions: The buffered acid solutions of Massengill Douches are valuable adjuncts to specific vaginal therapy following the prescribed use of vaginal medication or contraceptives and in feminine hygiene.

Directions:
DISPOSABLES: Twist off flat, wing-shaped tab from bottle containing pre-mixed solution, attach nozzle supplied and use. The unit is completely disposable.

LIQUID CONCENTRATE: Fill cap ¾ full, to measuring line, and pour contents into douche bag containing 1 quart of warm water. Mix thoroughly.

POWDER: Dissolve two rounded teaspoonfuls in a douche bag containing 1 quart of warm water. Mix thoroughly.

Warning: Douching does not prevent pregnancy. If vaginal dryness or irritation occurs discontinue use. Do not use during pregnancy except under the advice and supervision of your physician. Use this product only as directed for routine cleansing. You should douche no more than twice a week except on the advice of your doctor.

An association has been reported between douching and pelvic inflammatory disease (PID), a serious infection of the reproductive system, which can lead to sterility and/or ectopic (tubal) pregnancy. PID requires immediate medical attention.

PID's most common symptoms are pain and/or tenderness in the lower part of the abdomen and pelvis. You may also experience a vaginal discharge, vaginal bleeding, nausea or fever. Other sexually transmitted diseases (STDs) have similar symptoms and/or frequent urination, genital sores or ulcers. Douches should not be used for self-treatment of any STDs or PID. If you suspect you have one of these infections or PID, stop using this product and see your doctor immediately.

Keep out of reach of children. In case of accidental ingestion, seek professional assistance by contacting your physician, the local poison control center, or the Rocky Mt. Poison Control Center at 303-592-1710 (collect), 24 hours a day.

How Supplied:
Disposable—6 oz. disposable plastic bottle.
Liquid Concentrate—4 oz., 8 oz., plastic bottles.
Powder—4 oz., 8 oz., 16 oz., Packettes —10's, 12's.

MASSENGILL® Medicated
[*mas 'sen-gil*]
Disposable Douche
MASSENGILL® Medicated
Liquid Concentrate

Active Ingredient:
DISPOSABLE: Cepticin™ (povidone-iodine)
LIQUID CONCENTRATE: Cepticin™ (povidone-iodine)

Indications: For symptomatic relief of minor vaginal irritation or itching associated with vaginitis due to Candida albicans, Trichomonas vaginalis, and Gardnerella vaginalis.

Action: Povidone-iodine is widely recognized as an effective broad spectrum microbicide against both gram negative and gram positive bacteria, fungi, yeasts and protozoa. While remaining active in the presence of blood, serum or bodily secretions, it possesses virtually none of the irritating properties of iodine.

Warnings: Douching does not prevent pregnancy. Do not use during pregnancy or while nursing except under the advice and supervision of your physician. If vaginal dryness or irritation occurs discontinue use.
Use this product only as directed. Do not use this product for routine cleansing.
An association has been reported between douching and pelvic inflammatory disease (PID), a serious infection of the reproductive system, which can lead to sterility and/or ectopic (tubal) pregnancy. PID requires immediate medical attention.
PID's most common symptoms are pain and/or tenderness in the lower part of the abdomen and pelvis. You may also experience and vaginal discharge, vaginal bleeding, nausea or fever. Other sexually transmitted diseases (STDs) have similar symptoms and/or frequent urination, genital sores, or ulcers. Douches should not be used for self-treatment of any STDs or PID. If you suspect you have one of these infections or PID, stop using this product and see your doctor immediately. Women with iodine sensitivity should not use this product. Keep out of the reach of children. In case of accidental ingestion, seek professional assistance by contacting your physician, the local poison control center, or the Rocky Mt. Poison

Control Center at 303-592-1710 (Collect), 24 hours a day.

Dosage and Administration:
DISPOSABLE: Dosage is provided as a single unit concentrate to be added to 6 oz. of sanitized water supplied in a disposable bottle. A specially designed nozzle is provided. After use, the unit is discarded. Use one bottle a day. Although symptoms may be relieved earlier, for maximum relief, use for seven days.
LIQUID CONCENTRATE: Pour one capful into douche bag containing one quart of water. Mix thoroughly. Use once daily. Although symptoms may be relieved earlier, for maximum relief, use for seven days.

How Supplied:
Disposable—6 oz. bottle of sanitized water with 0.17 oz. vial of povidone-iodine and nozzle.
Liquid Concentrate—4 oz., 8 oz. plastic bottles.
Shown in Product Identification Guide, page 426

MASSENGILL®
[*mas 'sen-gil*]
Unscented Soft Cloth Towelette

Inactive Ingredients: Water, Octoxynol-9, Lactic Acid, Sodium Lactate, Potassium Sorbate, Disodium EDTA, and Cetylpyridinium Chloride.

Indications: For cleansing and refreshing the external vaginal area.

Actions: Massengill Unscented Soft Cloth Towelettes safely cleanse the external vaginal area and do not contain fragrance. The towelette delivery system makes the application soft and gentle.

Warnings: For external use only. Avoid contact with eyes.

Directions: Remove towelette from foil packet, unfold, and gently wipe. Throw away towelette after it has been used once.

How Supplied: Sixteen individually wrapped, disposable towelettes per carton.

MASSENGILL® Medicated
[*mas 'sen-gil*]
Soft Cloth Towelette

Active Ingredient: Hydrocortisone (0.5%).
Inactive Ingredients: Diazolidinyl Urea, DMDM Hydantoin, Isopropyl Myristate, Methylparaben, Polysorbate 60, Propylene Glycol, Propylparaben, Sorbitan Stearate, Steareth-2, Steareth-21, Water.
Tamper Resistant: If foil packet is torn or broken, do not use.
Also available in non-medicated Baby Powder Scent and Unscented formulas to freshen and cleanse the external vaginal area.

Indications: Massengill Medicated Towelettes provide temporary soothing relief of minor external feminine itching associated with irritations. They can also be used for the temporary relief of itching associated with skin rashes. Other uses of this product should be only under the advice and supervision of a physician.

Action: Massengill Medicated Soft Cloth Towelettes contain hydrocortisone, a proven anti-inflammatory, anti-pruritic ingredient. The towelette delivery system makes the application soothing, soft, and gentle.

Warnings: For external use only. Avoid contact with eyes. if condition worsens, symptoms persist for more than 7 days, or symptoms recur within a few days, do not use this or any other hydrocortisone product unless you have consulted a physician. Do not use if you are experiencing a vaginal discharge—see a physician. Do not use this towelette for the treatment of diaper rash. See a physician.
Keep this and all drugs out of the reach of children. As with any drug, if you are pregnant or nursing a baby, seek the advice of a health professional before using this product. In case of accidental ingestion, seek professional assistance or contact a Poison Control Center immediately.
Avoid storing at extreme temperatures (below 40°F or greater than 100°F).

Directions: For adults and children two years of age and older. Remove towelette from foil packet and gently wipe. Throw away towelette after it has been used once. Apply to the affected area not more than 3 to 4 times daily. Children under 2 years of age: DO NOT USE, consult a physician.

How Supplied: Ten individually wrapped, disposable towelettes per carton.

NATURE'S REMEDY®
Natural Vegetable Laxative

Active Ingredients: Cascara Sagrada 150 mg, Aloe 100 mg.

Inactive Ingredients: Calcium Stearate, Cellulose, Lactose, Coating, Colors (contains FD&C Yellow No. 6).

Indications: For gentle, overnight relief of constipation.

Actions: Nature's Remedy has two natural active ingredients that give gentle, overnight relief of constipation. These ingredients, Cascara Sagrada and Aloe, gently stimulate the body's natural function.

Dosage and Administration: Adults, swallow two tablets daily along with a full glass of water; children (8–15 yrs.), one tablet daily; or as directed by a physician.

Continued on next page

SmithKline Beecham—Cont.

Warnings: Do not take any laxative when nausea, vomiting, abdominal pain, or other symptoms of appendicitis are present. Frequent or prolonged use of laxatives may result in dependence on them. As with any drug, if you are pregnant or nursing a baby, seek the advice of a health professional before using this product.
KEEP OUT OF THE REACH OF CHILDREN.

Symptoms and Treatment of Oral Overdosage: If an overdose is suspected, immediately seek professional assistance by contacting your physician, local poison control center, or the Rocky Mountain Poison Control Center at 303-592-1710 (Collect) 24 hours a day.

How Supplied: Beige, film-coated tablets with foil-backed blister packaging in boxes of 12s, 30s and 60s.
Shown in Product Identification Guide, page 426

N'ICE® Medicated Sugarless Sore Throat and Cough Lozenges
[nis]

Active Ingredient: Cherry—Each lozenge contains 5.0 mg. menthol in a sorbitol base. Citrus—Each lozenge contains 5.0 mg. menthol in a sorbitol base. Menthol Eucalyptus—Each lozenge contains 5.0 mg. menthol in a sorbitol base. Cool Peppermint—Each lozenge contains 5.0 mg. menthol in a sorbitol base. N'ICE 'N CLEAR Cherry Eucalyptus—Each lozenge contains 7.0 mg. menthol in a sorbitol base. N'ICE 'N CLEAR. Menthol Eucalyptus—Each lozenge contains 5.0 mg. menthol in a sorbitol base.

Inactive Ingredients: Cherry—Flavors, D&C Red 33, Sorbitol, Tartaric Acid, FD&C Yellow 6. Citrus—Citric Acid, Flavors, Saccharin Sodium, Sodium Citrate, Sorbitol, Yellow 10. Menthol Eucalyptus—Citric Acid, Flavors, Sorbitol. Cool Peppermint—Blue 1, Flavor, Maltitol Solution, Syrup, Sorbitol, Yellow 10. N'ICE 'N CLEAR Cherry Eucalyptus—Flavors, D&C Red 33, Sorbitol, Tartaric Acid, FD&C Yellow 6. N'ICE 'N CLEAR Menthol Eucalyptus—Citric Acid, Flavors, Sorbitol.

Indications: Temporarily suppresses cough due to minor throat and bronchial irritation associated with a cold or inhaled irritants. Temporarily relieves minor sore throat pain.

Warnings: Do not administer to children under six years of age unless directed by a doctor. A persistent cough may be a sign of a serious condition. If cough or sore throat is severe, persists for more than 2 days, or is accompanied or followed by difficulty in breathing, fever, headache, rash, swelling, nausea, or vomiting, do not use and consult a doctor promptly. Do not take this product for persistent or chronic cough such as occurs with smoking, asthma, emphysema, or if cough is accompanied by excessive phlegm (mucus) unless directed by a doctor. In case of accidental overdose, seek professional assistance. **Keep this and all medications out of the reach of children.** Do not exceed recommended dosage. Avoid storing at high temperature (greater than 100°F).

Drug Interaction: No know drug interaction.

Dosage and Administration: Cherry, Citrus, Menthol Eucalyptus, Cool Peppermint, N'ICE 'N CLEAR Cherry Eucalyptus, N'ICE 'N CLEAR Menthol Eucalyptus—Adults and children six and older: Let lozenge dissolve slowly in the mouth. Repeat every hour as needed, or as directed by a doctor, up to 10 lozenges per day.

Professional Labeling: For the temporary relief of pain associated with tonsillitis, pharyngitis, throat infections or stomatitis.

How Supplied: Available in packages of 2, 8, and 16 lozenges.

NOVAHISTINE® DMX
[nō "vă-hĭs 'tēn]
Cough/Cold Formula & Decongestant

Description: Each 5 mL teaspoonful of NOVAHISTINE DMX contains: Dextromethorphan Hydrobromide 10 mg, Guaifenesin 100 mg, Pseudoephedrine Hydrochloride 30 mg. Also contains: Alcohol 10%, FD&C Red No. 40, FD&C Yellow No. 6, Flavors, Glycerin, Hydrochloric Acid, Invert Sugar, Saccharin Sodium, Sodium Chloride, Sorbitol, and Water. Dextromethorphan hydrobromide, a synthetic nonnarcotic antitussive, is the dextrorotatory isomer of 3-methoxy-*N*-methylmorphinan. Guaifenesin is the glyceryl ether of guaiacol. Pseudoephedrine hydrochloride is the salt of a pharmacologically active stereoisomer of ephedrine (1-phenyl-2-methylamino-1-propanol).

Actions: Dextromethorphan hydrobromide suppresses the cough reflex by a direct effect on the cough center in the medulla of the brain. Although it is chemically related to morphine, it produces no analgesia or addiction. Its antitussive activity is about equal to that of codeine.
Pseudoephedrine hydrochloride is an orally effective nasal decongestant. It is a sympathomimetic amine with peripheral effects similar to epinephrine and central effects similar to, but less intense than, amphetamines. Therefore, it has the potential for excitatory side effects. Pseudoephedrine hydrochloride at the recommended oral dosage has little or no pressor effect in normotensive adults. Patients taking pseudoephedrine orally have not been reported to experience the rebound congestion sometimes experienced with frequent, repeated use of topical decongestants. Pseudoephedrine is not known to produce drowsiness. Guaifenesin acts as an expectorant by increasing respiratory tract fluid which reduces the viscosity of tenacious secretions, thus making expectoration easier.

Indications: NOVAHISTINE DMX is indicated for temporary relief of cough and nasal congestion; helps loosen phlegm and bronchial secretions. It is useful when exhausting, nonproductive cough accompanies respiratory tract congestion and in the symptomatic relief of upper respiratory congestion associated with the common cold, influenza, bronchitis, and sinusitis.

Contraindications: NOVAHISTINE DMX is contraindicated in patients with severe hypertension, severe coronary artery disease, and in patients on MAO inhibitor therapy. Patient idiosyncrasy to adrenergic agents may be manifested by insomnia, dizziness, weakness, tremor, or arrhythmias.
Nursing mothers: Pseudoephedrine is contraindicated in nursing mothers because of the higher than usual risk for infants from sympathomimetic amines.
Hypersensitivity: NOVAHISTINE DMX is contraindicated in patients with hypersensitivity or idiosyncrasy to sympathomimetic amines, dextromethorphan, or to other formula ingredients.

Warnings: At dosages higher than the recommended dose, nervousness, dizziness, sleeplessness, nausea, or headache may occur. Do not take for more than 7 days. A persistent cough may be a sign of a serious condition. If symptoms do not improve, recur, or are accompanied by fever, rash, or persistent headache, patients should be advised to consult their physician before continuing use. Do not use for persistent or chronic cough such as occurs with smoking, asthma, chronic bronchitis or emphysema, or where cough is accompanied by excessive phlegm (sputum) unless directed by a physician. Sympathomimetic amines should be used judiciously and sparingly in patients with hypertension, diabetes mellitus, cardiovascular disease (e.g. ischemic heart disease), increased intraocular pressure, hyperthyroidism, or prostatic hypertrophy. Sympathomimetics may produce central nervous system stimulation with convulsions or cardiovascular collapse with accompanying hypotension. See Contraindications.
Use in elderly: The elderly (60 years and older) are more likely to have adverse reactions to sympathomimetics. Overdosage of sympathomimetics in this age group may cause hallucinations, convulsions, CNS depression, and death.
Use in children: NOVAHISTINE DMX should not be used in children under 2 years except under the advice and supervision of a physician.
Use in pregnancy: Safety for use during pregnancy has not been established. As

with any drug, if you are pregnant or nursing a baby, seek the advice of a health professional before using this product.

If sensitive to any of the ingredients, do not use.

Keep this and all drugs out of the reach of children. In case of accidental overdose, seek professional assistance or contact a Poison Control Center immediately.

Adverse Reactions: Adverse reactions occur infrequently with usual oral doses of NOVAHISTINE DMX. When they occur, adverse reactions may include gastrointestinal upset and nausea. Because of the pseudoephedrine in NOVAHISTINE DMX, hyperreactive individuals may display ephedrine-like reactions such as tachycardia, palpitations, headache, dizziness or nausea. Sympathomimetic drugs have been associated with certain untoward reactions including fear, anxiety, tenseness, restlessness, tremor, weakness, pallor, respiratory difficulty, dysuria, insomnia, hallucinations, convulsions, CNS depression, arrhythmias, and cardiovascular collapse with hypotension.

Note: Guaifenesin interferes with the colorimetric determination of 5-hydroxyindoleacetic acid (5-HIAA) and vanillylmandelic acid (VMA).

Drug Interactions: NOVAHISTINE DMX should not be used in patients taking a prescription drug for hypertension or depression without the advice of a physician. MAO inhibitors and beta-adrenergic blockers increase the effects of pseudoephedrine (sympathomimetics). Sympathomimetics may reduce the antihypertensive effects of methyldopa, mecamylamine, reserpine, and veratrum alkaloids.

Dosage and Administration: Adults and children 12 years and over, 2 teaspoonfuls every 4 hours. Children 6 to under 12 years, 1 teaspoonful every 4 hours. Children 2 to under 6 years, $\frac{1}{2}$ teaspoonful every 4 hours. Not more than 4 doses every 24 hours. For children under 2 years of age, give only as directed by a physician.

How Supplied: As a red syrup in 4 fluid ounce bottles.

Keep tightly closed. Protect from excessive heat and light. Avoid freezing.

Shown in Product Identification Guide, page 426

NOVAHISTINE® Elixir
[nō "vă-hĭs 'tēn]
Cold & Hay Fever Formula

Description: Each 5 mL teaspoonful of NOVAHISTINE Elixir contains: Chlorpheniramine Maleate 2 mg, Phenylephrine Hydrochloride 5 mg. Also contains: Alcohol 5%, D&C Yellow No. 10, FD&C Blue No. 1, Flavors, Glycerin, Sodium Chloride, Sorbitol, and Water. Although considered sugar-free, each 5 mL contributes approximately 7 calories from sorbitol.

Actions: Phenylephrine is a nasal decongestant. Its effects are similar to epinephrine, but it is less potent on a weight basis, and has a longer duration of action. Phenylephrine produces peripheral effects similar to epinephrine, but has little or no central nervous system stimulation. After oral administration, nasal decongestion may occur within 15 or 20 minutes and persist for 2 to 4 hours. Chlorpheniramine maleate, an antihistaminic effective for the symptomatic relief of allergic rhinitis, possesses anticholinergic and sedative effects. Chlorpheniramine antagonizes many of the pharmacologic actions of histamine. It prevents released histamine from dilating capillaries and causing edema of the respiratory mucosa.

Indications: For the temporary relief of nasal congestion and eustachian tube congestion associated with the common cold, sinusitis, and hay fever (allergic rhinitis). Also provides temporary relief of runny nose, sneezing, itching of nose or throat, and itchy, watery eyes due to the common cold, hay fever (allergic rhinitis) or other upper respiratory allergies. May be given concomitantly, when indicated, with analgesics and antibiotics.

Contraindications: NOVAHISTINE Elixir is contraindicated in patients with severe hypertension, severe coronary artery disease, and in patients on MAO inhibitor therapy. Patient idiosyncrasy to adrenergic agents may be manifested by insomnia, dizziness, weakness, tremor, or arrhythmias.

NOVAHISTINE Elixir is also contraindicated in patients with narrow-angle glaucoma, urinary retention, peptic ulcer, asthma, emphysema, chronic pulmonary disease, shortness of breath, or difficulty in breathing.

Nursing mothers: Phenylephrine is contraindicated in nursing mothers.

Hypersensitivity: NOVAHISTINE Elixir is also contraindicated in patients with hypersensitivity or idiosyncrasy to sympathomimetic amines, antihistamines or to other formula ingredients.

Warnings: At dosages higher than the recommended dose, nervousness, dizziness, or sleeplessness may occur. If symptoms do not improve within 7 days or are accompanied by high fever, patients should be advised to consult their physician before continuing use. Sympathomimetic amines should be used judiciously and sparingly in patients with hypertension, diabetes mellitus, cardiovascular disease (e.g. ischemic heart disease), increased intraocular pressure, hyperthyroidism, or prostatic hypertrophy. Sympathomimetics may produce central nervous system stimulation with convulsions or cardiovascular collapse with accompanying hypotension. See Contraindications.

Use in elderly: The elderly (60 years and older) are more likely to have adverse reactions to sympathomimetics.

Overdosage of sympathomimetics in this age group may cause hallucinations, convulsions, CNS depression, and death.

Use in children: May cause excitability. NOVAHISTINE Elixir should not be used in children under 6 years except under the advice and supervision of a physician.

Use in pregnancy: Safety for use during pregnancy has not been established. As with any drug, if you are pregnant or nursing a baby, seek the advice of a health professional before using this product.

If sensitive to any of the ingredients, do not use.

Keep this and all drugs out of the reach of children. In case of accidental overdose, seek professional assistance or contact a Poison Control Center immediately.

Precautions: The antihistamine may cause drowsiness, and ambulatory patients who operate machinery or motor vehicles should be cautioned accordingly.

Adverse Reactions: Drugs containing sympathomimetic amines have been associated with certain untoward reactions, including fear, anxiety, tenseness, restlessness, tremor, weakness, pallor, respiratory difficulty, dysuria, insomnia, hallucinations, convulsions, CNS depression, arrhythmias, and cardiovascular collapse with hypotension. Individuals hyperreactive to phenylephrine may display ephedrine-like reactions such as tachycardia, palpitation, headache, dizziness, or nausea.

Phenylephrine is considered safe and relatively free of unpleasant side effects when taken at recommended dosage.

Patients sensitive to antihistamine drugs may experience mild sedation. Other side effects from antihistamines may include dry mouth, dizziness, weakness, anorexia, nausea, vomiting, headache, nervousness, polyuria, heartburn, diplopia, dysuria, and, very rarely, dermatitis.

Drug Interactions: NOVAHISTINE Elixir should not be used in patients taking a prescription drug for hypertension or depression without the advice of a physician. MAO inhibitors and beta-adrenergic blockers increase the effects of sympathomimetics. Sympathomimetics may reduce the antihypertensive effects of methyldopa, mecamylamine, reserpine, and veratrum alkaloids. Antihistamines have been shown to enhance one or more of the effects of tricyclic antidepressants, barbiturates, alcohol, and other central nervous system depressants.

Dosage and Administration: Adults and children 12 years and older, 2 teaspoonfuls every 4 hours; children 6 to under 12 years, 1 teaspoonful every 4 hours; children 2 to under 6 years, $\frac{1}{2}$ teaspoonful every 4 hours.

For children under 2 years, at the discretion of the physician.

Product label dosage is as follows: Adults and children 12 years and older, 2 tea-

Continued on next page

SmithKline Beecham—Cont.

spoonfuls every 4 hours. Children 6 to under 12 years, 1 teaspoonful every 4 hours. Not more than 6 doses every 24 hours. For children under 6 years, give only as directed by a physician.

How Supplied: NOVAHISTINE Elixir, as a green liquid in 4 fluid ounce bottles. Keep tightly closed. Protect from excessive heat and light. Avoid freezing.

Shown in Product Identification Guide, page 426

OS-CAL® 500 Chewable Tablets
[ăhs'kăl]
(calcium supplement)

Each Tablet Contains: 1,250 mg of calcium carbonate.
Elemental calcium........................ 500 mg
Ingredients: calcium carbonate, dextrose monohydrate, maltodextrin, microcrystalline cellulose, magnesium stearate, Bavarian cream flavor, sodium chloride, and coconut cream flavor.

Directions: One tablet two to three times a day with meals, or as recommended by your physician.

Two Tablets Provide: 1,000 mg calcium, 100% of U.S. RDA for adults and children 12 or more years of age.

Three Tablets Provide: 1,500 mg calcium, 115% of U.S. RDA for pregnant and lactating women.

Store at room temperature. Keep out of reach of children.

How Supplied: OS-CAL® 500 Chewable Tablets is available in bottles of 60 tablets.

Issued 5/91

Shown in Product Identification Guide, page 426

OS-CAL® 500 Tablets
[ăhs'kăl]
(calcium supplement)

Each Tablet Contains: 1,250 mg of calcium carbonate from oyster shell, an organic calcium source.
Elemental calcium .... 500 mg
Ingredients: oyster shell powder, corn syrup solids, talc, hydroxypropyl methylcellulose, cornstarch, sodium starch glycolate, calcium stearate, polysorbate 80, pharmaceutical glaze, titanium dioxide, methyl propyl paraben, polyethylene glycol, polyvinylpyrrolidone, carnauba wax, D&C Yellow #10, acetylated monoglyceride, edetate disodium, FD&C Blue #1, and simethicone emulsion.

Directions: One tablet two or three times a day with meals, or as recommended by your physician.

Two Tablets Provide: 1,000 mg calcium, 100% of U.S. RDA for adults and children 12 or more years of age.

Three Tablets Provide: 1,500 mg calcium, 115% of U.S. RDA for pregnant and lactating women.

Store at room temperature. Keep out of reach of children.

How Supplied: OS-CAL® 500 is available in bottles of 60 and 120 tablets.

Issued 10/87

Shown in Product Identification Guide, page 426

OS-CAL® 250+D Tablets
[ăhs'kăl]
(calcium supplement with vitamin D)

Each Tablet Contains: 625 mg of calcium carbonate from oyster shell, an organic calcium source.
Elemental calcium .... 250 mg
Vitamin D .... 125 USP Units

Ingredients: oyster shell powder, corn syrup solids, talc, cornstarch, hydroxypropyl methylcellulose, calcium stearate, polysorbate 80, titanium dioxide, methyl propyl paraben, polyethylene glycol, pharmaceutical glaze, vitamin D, polyvinylpyrrolidone, carnauba wax, D&C Yellow #10, acetylated monoglyceride, edetate disodium, FD&C Blue #1, simethicone emulsion, and edible gray ink.

Directions: One tablet three times a day with meals, or as recommended by your physician.

Three Tablets Provide:

		% U.S. RDA for Adults
Calcium	750 mg	75%
Vitamin D	375 Units	94%

Store at room temperature. Keep out of reach of children.

How Supplied: OS-CAL® 250+D is available in bottles of 100 and 240.

Issued 10/87

Shown in Product Identification Guide, page 426

OS-CAL® 500+D Tablets
[ăhs'kăl]
(calcium supplement with vitamin D)

Each Tablet Contains: 1,250 mg of calcium carbonate from oyster shell, an organic calcium source.
Elemental calcium .... 500 mg
Vitamin D .... 125 USP Units

Ingredients: oyster shell powder, corn syrup solids, talc, hydroxypropyl methylcellulose, cornstarch, sodium starch glycolate, calcium stearate, polysorbate 80, pharmaceutical glaze, titanium dioxide, methyl propyl paraben, polyethylene glycol, polyvinylpyrrolidone, vitamin D, carnauba wax, D&C Yellow #10, acetylated monoglyceride, edetate disodium, FD&C Blue #1, and simethicone emulsion.

Directions: One tablet two or three times a day with meals, or as recommended by your physician.

Two Tablets Provide: 1,000 mg calcium, 100% of U.S. RDA for adults and children 12 or more years of age.

Three Tablets Provide: 1,500 mg calcium, 115% of U.S. RDA for pregnant and lactating women and 94% of vitamin D.

Store at room temperature. Keep out of reach of children.

How Supplied: OS-CAL® 500+D is available in bottles of 60 and 120.

Issued 10/87

Shown in Product Identification Guide, page 426

OS-CAL® FORTIFIED Tablets
[ăhs'kăl]
(multivitamin and minerals supplement with added calcium)

Each Tablet Contains:
Vitamin A (palmitate) 1668 USP Units
Vitamin D .... 125 USP Units
Thiamine mononitrate
(vitamin B₁) .... 1.7 mg
Riboflavin (vitamin B₂)................ 1.7 mg
Pyridoxine hydrochloride
(vitamin B₆)................................ 2.0 mg
Ascorbic acid (vitamin C).......... 50.0 mg
dl-alpha-tocopherol acetate
(vitamin E) .... 0.8 IU
Niacinamide .... 15.0 mg
Calcium (from oyster shell) .... 250.0 mg
Iron (as ferrous fumarate)........... 5.0 mg
Magnesium (as oxide)................... 1.6 mg
Manganese (as sulfate)................ 0.3 mg
Zinc (as sulfate)............................ 0.5 mg

Ingredients: oyster shell powder, ascorbic acid, corn syrup solids, niacinamide, D&C Yellow #10 Aluminum Lake, ferrous fumarate, calcium stearate, FD&C Blue #1 Aluminum Lake, cornstarch, vitamin A palmitate, polysorbate 80, magnesium oxide, pyridoxine, thiamine, riboflavin, vitamin E, pharmaceutical glaze, methyl paraben, zinc sulfate, manganese sulfate, propylparaben, povidone, vitamin D, hydroxypropyl methylcellulose, carnauba wax, titanium dioxide, ethylcellulose, and acetylated monoglyceride.

Indication: Multivitamin and mineral supplement with added calcium.

Dosage: One tablet three times daily with meals or as directed by physician. In case of accidental overdose, seek professional assistance or contact a poison control center immediately.

Keep out of reach of children.
Store at room temperature.

How Supplied: Bottles of 100 tablets.

Issued 6/89

Shown in Product Identification Guide, page 426

SINE-OFF

Each tablet/ caplet contains:	SINE-OFF Tablets—Aspirin Formula	SINE-OFF Maximum Strength No Drowsiness Formula Caplets
Chlorpheniramine maleate	2.0 mg	—
Phenylpropanolamine HCl	12.5 mg	—
Aspirin	325.0 mg	—
Acetaminophen	—	500.0 mg
Pseudoephedrine HCl	—	30.0 mg

OXY ACNE MEDICATIONS
OXY–5® and OXY–10®
with SORBOXYL®
Benzoyl peroxide lotion 5% and 10% with silica oil absorber
Vanishing and Tinted Formulas

Description: Active Ingredient: Oxy-5: Benzoyl peroxide 5%. Oxy-10: Benzoyl peroxide 10%.

Inactive Ingredients: Oxy-5 Vanishing: Cetyl alcohol, citric acid, methylparaben, propylene glycol, propylparaben, silica (Sorboxyl®), sodium lauryl sulfate, sodium PCA, and water.
Oxy-5 Tinted: Cetyl alcohol, citric acid, iron oxides, methylparaben, propylene glycol, propylparaben, silica (Sorboxyl®), sodium lauryl sulfate, stearyl alcohol, sodium PCA, titanium dioxide and water.
Oxy-10 Vanishing: Cetyl alcohol, citric acid, methylparaben, propylene glycol, propylparaben, silica (Sorboxyl®), sodium citrate, sodium lauryl sulfate, and water.
Oxy-10 Tinted: Cetyl alcohol, citric acid, glyceryl stearate, iron oxides, methylparaben, propylene glycol, propylparaben, silica (Sorboxyl®), sodium citrate, sodium lauryl sulfate, stearic acid, titanium dioxide and water.

Indications: Topical medications for the treatment of acne vulgaris.

Action: Provides antibacterial activity against Propionibacterium acnes.

Additional Benefits: Absorbs excess skin oil up to 12 hours.
Vanishing formulas are colorless, odorless, greaseless lotions that vanish upon application. Tinted formulas are flesh tone, odorless, greaseless lotions.

Directions: Wash skin thoroughly and dry well. Shake well before using. Dab on Oxy 5 or Oxy 10, smoothing it into acne pimple areas of face, neck, and body (see Warnings). Apply once a day initially, then two or three times a day, or as directed by a physician.

Warnings: FOR EXTERNAL USE ONLY. Using other topical acne medications at the same time or immediately following use of this product may increase dryness or irritation of the skin. If this occurs only one medication should be used unless directed by a doctor. Do not use this medication if you have very sensitive skin or if you are sensitive to benzoyl peroxide. To test for sensitivity, apply to a small affected area once a day for two days. Follow label instructions and continue use if no discomfort or burning occurs. This product may cause irritation, characterized by redness, burning, itching, peeling, or possibly swelling. More frequent use or higher concentrations may aggrevate such irritation. Mild irritation may be reduced by using the product less frequently or in lower concentration. If irritation becomes severe, discontinue use. If irritation still continues, consult a doctor. Keep away from eyes, lips, and mouth. Keep this and all drugs out of reach of children. This product may bleach hair or dyed fabrics, including clothing and carpeting. Keep tightly closed. Store at room temperature, avoid excessive heat.

Symptoms and Treatment of Ingestion: These symptoms are based upon medical judgment, not on actual experience. Theoretically, ingestion of very large amounts may cause nausea, vomiting, abdominal discomfort, and diarrhea. If an oral overdose is suspected, contact a physician, the local poison control center, or the Rocky Mountain Poison Control Center at 303-592-1710 (Collect) 24 hours a day.
How Supplied: 1 fl. oz. plastic bottles.
Shown in Product Identification Guide, page 426

OXY 10® BENZOYL PEROXIDE WASH

Active Ingredient: Benzoyl peroxide 10%.

Inactive Ingredients: Citric acid, cocamidopropyl betaine, diazolidinyl urea, methylparaben, propylparaben, sodium citrate, sodium cocoyl isethionate, sodium lauroyl sarcosinate, water, and xanthan gum.

Indications: Antibacterial skin wash used as an aid in the treatment of acne vulgaris.

Actions: Promotes antibacterial activity against Propionibacterium acnes.

Additional Benefits: When used instead of regular soap, cleanses acne-prone skin and removes dirt, grime and excess skin oil.

Directions: Shake well. Wet area to be washed. Apply Oxy 10 Benzoyl Peroxide Wash and work into lather, massaging gently for 1 to 2 minutes. Rinse thoroughly. Use 2 to 3 times daily or as directed by a physician.

Warnings: FOR EXTERNAL USE ONLY. Using other topical acne medications at the same time or immediately following use of this product may increase dryness or irritation of the skin. If this occurs, only one medication should be used unless directed by a doctor. Do not use this medication if you have very sensitive skin or if you are sensitive to benzoyl peroxide. To test for sensitivity, apply to a small affected area once a day for two days. Follow label instructions and continue use if no discomfort or burning occurs. This product may cause irritation, characterized by redness, burning, itching, peeling, or possibly swelling. More frequent use or higher concentrations may aggravate such irritation. Mild irritation may be reduced by using the product less frequently or in a lower concentration. If irritation becomes severe, discontinue use; if irritation still continues, consult a doctor. Keep away from eyes, lips, and mouth. Keep this and all drugs out of reach of children. This product may bleach hair or dyed fabrics, including clothing and carpeting. Keep tightly closed. Store at room temperature; avoid excessive heat.

Symptoms and Treatment of Ingestion: These symptoms are based upon medical judgment, not on actual experience. Theoretically, ingestion of very large amounts may cause nausea, vomiting, abdominal discomfort, and diarrhea. If an oral overdose is suspected, contact a physician, the local poison control center, or the Rocky Mountain Poison Control Center at 303-592-1710 (Collect) 24 hours a day.

How supplied: 4 fl. oz. plastic bottles.
Shown in Product Identification Guide, page 426

SINE–OFF® Maximum Strength No Drowsiness Formula Caplets

Composition:
[See table above.]

Product Information: SINE-OFF Maximum Strength No Drowsiness Formula provides maximum strength relief from headache and sinus pain. Relieves pressure and congestion due to sinusitis, allergic sinusitis or the common cold. This formula contains acetaminophen, a non-aspirin pain reliever.
NO ANTIHISTAMINE DROWSINESS

Product Benefits: Eases headache, pain and pressure ● Promotes sinus drainage ● Shrinks swollen membranes to relieve congestion.

Directions: Adults and children over 12 years of age: 2 caplets every 6 hours,

Continued on next page

SmithKline Beecham—Cont.

not to exceed 8 caplets in any 24-hour period. Children under 12 should use only as directed by physician.

TAMPER-RESISTANT PACKAGE FEATURES FOR YOUR PROTECTION:

- Each caplet is encased in a clear plastic cell with a foil back.
- The name SINE-OFF appears on each caplet (see product illustration on front of carton).
- **DO NOT USE THIS PRODUCT IF ANY OF THESE TAMPER-RESISTANT FEATURES ARE MISSING OR BROKEN.**

Comments or Questions? Call Toll-Free 800-245-1040 Weekdays.

For maximum strength relief of headache and sinus pain, without antihistamine drowsiness. Relieves pressure and congestion due to sinusitis, or the common cold. This formula contains acetaminophen, a non-aspirin pain reliever.

Warnings: Do not exceed recommended dosage because dizziness, sleeplessness, or nervousness may occur. Do not take this product for more than 10 days. If symptoms do not improve or are accompanied by fever that lasts more than 3 days, or if new symptoms occur, consult a physician. Do not take this product if you have heart disease, high blood pressure, diabetes, thyroid disease, or difficulty in urination due to enlargement of the prostate gland unless directed by a physician. Keep this and all drugs out of reach of children. In case of accidental overdose, seek professional assistance or contact a poison control center immediately. Prompt medical attention is critical for adults as well as children even if you do not notice any signs or symptoms. As with any drug, if you are pregnant or nursing a baby, seek the advice of a health professional before using this product.

Drug Interaction Precaution: Do not take this product if you are presently taking a prescription drug for high blood pressure or depression, without first consulting your physician.

Avoid storing at high temperatures (greater than 100°F).

Active Ingredients: Each caplet contains: 30 mg. Pseudoephedrine Hydrochloride, 500 mg. Acetaminophen (500 mg. is a non-standard dosage of acetaminophen, as compared to the standard of 325 mg.).

Inactive Ingredients: Crospovidone, Hydroxypropyl Methylcellulose, Magnesium Stearate, Microcrystalline Cellulose, Polyethylene Glycol, Polysorbate 80, Povidone, FD&C Red 40, Starch, Titanium Dioxide.

How Supplied: Consumer packages of 24 caplets.

Note: There are other SINE-OFF products. Make sure this is the one you are interested in.

Also Available:
SINE-OFF® Tablets with Aspirin
SINE-OFF® Maximum Strength Allergy/Sinus Formula Caplets
Shown in Product Identification Guide, page 426

SINE–OFF® Sinus Medicine Tablets–Aspirin Formula
Relieves sinus headache and congestion.

Composition: [See table on page 717.]

Product Information: SINE-OFF relieves headache, pain, pressure and congestion due to sinusitis, allergic sinusitis, or the common cold.

Product Benefits: Eases headache, pain and pressure • Promotes sinus drainage • Shrinks swollen membranes to relieve congestion • Relieves postnasal drip.

Directions: Adults: 2 tablets every 4 hours, not to exceed 8 tablets in any 24-hour period. Children (6–12) one-half the adult dosage. Children under 6 years should use only as directed by a physician.

TAMPER-RESISTANT PACKAGE FEATURES FOR YOUR PROTECTION:

- Each tablet is encased in a clear plastic cell with a foil back.
- The name SINE-OFF appears on each tablet (see product illustration on front of carton).
- **DO NOT USE THIS PRODUCT IF ANY OF THESE TAMPER-RESISTANT FEATURES ARE MISSING OR BROKEN.**

Comments or Questions? Call Toll-Free 800-245-1040 Weekdays.

Warnings: Children and teenagers should not use this medicine for chicken pox or flu symptoms before a doctor is consulted about Reye Syndrome, a rare but serious illness. Do not take this product for more than 10 days. If symptoms do not improve or are accompanied by fever that lasts for more than 3 days, or if new symptoms occur, consult a doctor. Do not take this product if you have asthma, glaucoma, heart disease, high blood pressure, thyroid disease, diabetes, emphysema, chronic pulmonary disease, shortness of breath, difficulty in breathing or difficulty in urination due to enlargement of the prostate gland unless directed by a doctor. Do not take this product if you are allergic to aspirin, have stomach problems, ulcers or bleeding problems unless directed by a doctor. Do not exceed recommended dosage. At higher doses nervousness, dizziness or sleeplessness may occur. May cause excitability, especially in children. May cause drowsiness. Avoid alcoholic beverages while taking this product. Do not drive or operate heavy machinery. Keep

this and all drugs out of reach of children. In case of accidental overdose, seek professional assistance or contact a poison control center immediately. As with any drug, if you are pregnant or nursing a baby, seek the advice of a health professional before using this product. **IT IS ESPECIALLY IMPORTANT NOT TO USE ASPIRIN DURING THE LAST 3 MONTHS OF PREGNANCY UNLESS SPECIFICALLY DIRECTED TO DO SO BY A DOCTOR BECAUSE IT MAY CAUSE PROBLEMS IN THE UNBORN CHILD OR COMPLICATIONS DURING DELIVERY.**

Drug Interaction Precaution: Do not take this product if you are taking a prescription drug for anticoagulation (thinning the blood), high blood pressure, depression, diabetes, gout or arthritis unless directed by a doctor.

Store at controlled room temperature (59°–86°F.).

Each tablet contains: Active Ingredients: Aspirin, 325 mg.; Chlorpheniramine Maleate, 2 mg.; Phenylpropanolamine Hydrochloride, 12.5 mg.

Inactive Ingredients: Acacia, Calcium Sulfate, Carnauba Wax, D&C Yellow 10, Ethylcellulose, FD&C Yellow 6, Gelatin, Guar Gum, Polysorbate 80, Silicon Dioxide, Starch, Sucrose, Titanium Dioxide, and trace amounts of other inactive ingredients.

How Supplied: Consumer packages of 24, 48 and 100 tablets.

Note: There are other SINE-OFF products. Make sure this is the one you are interested in.

Also Available: SINE-OFF® Maximum Strength Allergy/Sinus Formula Caplets 24's. SINE-OFF® Maximum Strength No Drowsiness Formula Caplets 24's.
Shown in Product Identification Guide, page 426

SINGLET® For Adults
Decongestant/Antihistamine/Analgesic (pain reliever)/Antipyretic (fever reducer)

Description: Each pink Singlet tablet contains Pseudoephedrine Hydrochloride 60 mg, Chlorpheniramine Maleate 4 mg, and Acetaminophen 650 mg. Also contains: D&C Red No. 27, D&C Yellow No. 10, FD&C Blue No. 1, Hydroxypropyl Cellulose, Hydroxypropyl Methylcellulose 2910, Magnesium Stearate, Microcrystalline Cellulose, Polyethylene Glycol 8000, Pregelatinized Corn Starch, Sodium Starch Glycolate, Sucrose, and Titanium Dioxide.

Indications: For the temporary relief of nasal congestion, runny nose, occasional sinus headache, fever, sneezing, watery eyes or itching of the nose, throat, and eyes due to colds, hay fever, or other upper respiratory allergies.

Warnings: Do not take this product for more than 7 days. Unless directed by a physician, do not take this product if you have asthma, glaucoma, emphysema, chronic pulmonary disease, heart disease, high blood pressure, thyroid disease, diabetes, shortness of breath, difficulty in breathing, difficulty in urination due to enlargement of the prostate gland, or if you are presently taking a prescription drug for high blood pressure or depression. Do not exceed recommended dosage because severe liver damage, nervousness, dizziness, or sleeplessness may occur. May cause excitability. Consult your physician if symptoms persist, if new symptoms occur, or if redness or swelling is present, because these could be signs of a serious condition. Consult your physician if fever persists for more than 3 days (72 hours) or recurs. May cause drowsiness; alcohol, sedatives, and tranquilizers may increase the drowsiness effect. Avoid alcoholic beverages while taking this product. Do not take this product if you are taking sedatives or tranquilizers without first consulting your physician. Use caution when driving a motor vehicle or operating machinery. If sensitive to any of the ingredients, do not use.

As with any drug, if you are pregnant or nursing a baby, seek the advice of a health professional before using this product. KEEP THIS AND ALL DRUGS OUT OF THE REACH OF CHILDREN. In case of accidental overdose, seek professional assistance or contact a Poison Control Center immediately. Prompt medical attention is critical for adults as well as for children even if you do not notice any signs or symptoms.

Dosage and Administration: Adults and children 12 years and older: one tablet 3 to 4 times a day, taken with water, while symptoms persist. Do not take more than 1 tablet within a 4-hour period. Do not exceed 4 tablets in 24 hours. Children under 12 years of age: consult a physician.

Storage: Protect from excessive heat and moisture.

How Supplied: Bottles of 100.

SOMINEX®
[som 'in-ex]
Tablets and Caplets

Active Ingredients: Each tablet contains Diphenhydramine HCl, 25 mg. Each caplet contains Diphenhydramine HCl, 50 mg.

Inactive Ingredients Tablets: Dibasic Calcium Phosphate, Magnesium Stearate, Microcrystalline Cellulose, Silicon Dioxide, Starch, FD&C Blue #1.

Inactive Ingredients Caplets: Carnauba Wax, Crospovidone, Dibasic Calcium Phosphate, Hydroxypropyl Methylcellulose, Magnesium Stearate, Microcrystalline Cellulose, Polyethylene Glycol, Polysorbate 80, Silicon Dioxide, Starch, Titanium Dioxide, White Wax, FD&C Blue #1.

Indications: Helps to reduce difficulty falling asleep.

Action: An antihistamine with anticholinergic and sedative effects.

Directions: Take 50 mg. (2 tablets or 1 caplet) at bedtime if needed, or as directed by a doctor.

Warnings: Do not give to children under 12 years of age. If sleeplessness persists continuously for more than two weeks, consult your doctor. Insomnia may be a symptom of serious underlying medical illness. Avoid alcoholic beverages while taking this product. Do not take this product if you are taking sedatives or tranquilizers, without first consulting your doctor. Do not take this product if you have asthma, glaucoma, emphysema, chronic pulmonary disease, shortness of breath, difficulty in breathing, or difficulty in urination due to enlargement of the prostate gland unless directed by a doctor. As with any drug, if you are pregnant or nursing a baby, seek the advice of a health professional before using this product. Keep this and all drugs out of the reach of children. In case of accidental overdose, seek professional assistance or contact a poison control center immediately or the Rocky Mountain Poison Control Center at 303-592-1710 (Collect) 24 hours a day.

Drug Interaction: Monoamine oxidase (MAO) inhibitors prolong and intensify the anticholinergic effects of antihistamines. The CNS depressant effect is heightened by alcohol and other CNS depressant drugs.

Symptoms and Treatment of Oral Overdosage: Antihistamine overdosage reactions may vary from central nervous system depression to stimulation. Stimulation is particularly likely in children. Atropine-like signs and symptoms, such as dry mouth, fixed and dilated pupils, flushing, and gastrointestinal symptoms, may also occur.

How Supplied Tablets: Available in blister packs of 16, 32, and 72.

How Supplied Caplets: Available in blister packs of 8, 16, and 32.
Shown in Product Identification Guide, page 426

SOMINEX® Pain Relief Formula
[som 'in-ex]

Active Ingredients: Each tablet contains 500 mg. Acetaminophen and 25 mg. Diphenhydramine HCl.

Inactive Ingredients: Crospovidone, Povidone, Silicon Dioxide, Starch, Stearic Acid, FD&C Blue #1.

Indications: For sleeplessness with accompanying occasional minor aches, pains, or headache.

Action: An antihistamine with sedative effects combined with an internal analgesic.

Directions: Take two tablets thirty minutes before bedtime, or as directed by a physician.

Warnings: Do not give to children under 12 years of age. If symptoms persist continuously for more than 10 days, or if new ones occur, consult your physician. Do not exceed recommended dosage because severe liver damage may occur. Insomnia may be a symptom of serious underlying medical illness. Take this product with caution if alcohol is being consumed. Do not take this product for the treatment of arthritis, except under the advice and supervision of a physician. As with any drug, if you are pregnant or nursing a baby, seek the advice of a health professional before using this product. Keep this and all drugs out of the reach of children. In case of accidental overdose, seek professional assistance by contacting your physician, the local poison control center, or the Rocky Mountain Poison Control Center at 303-592-1710 (Collect), 24 hours a day. DO NOT TAKE THIS PRODUCT IF YOU HAVE ASTHMA, GLAUCOMA OR ENLARGEMENT OF THE PROSTATE GLAND, EXCEPT UNDER THE ADVICE AND SUPERVISION OF A PHYSICIAN.

Drug Interaction: Monoamine oxidase (MAO) inhibitors prolong and intensify the anticholinergic effects of antihistamines. The CNS depressant effect is heightened by alcohol and other CNS depressant drugs.

Symptoms and Treatment of Oral Overdosage: Antihistamine overdosage reactions may vary from central nervous system depression to stimulation. Stimulation is particularly likely in children. Atropine-like signs and symptoms, such as dry mouth, fixed and dilated pupils, flushing, and gastrointestinal symptoms, may also occur.

How Supplied: Available in blister packs of 16 tablets and bottles of 32 tablets.
Shown in Product Identification Guide, page 426

SUCRETS® Maximum Strength Wintergreen
SUCRETS® Wild Cherry Regular Strength
SUCRETS® Children's Cherry Flavored
Sore Throat Lozenges
[su 'krets]
SUCRETS® Regular Strength Original Mint
SUCRETS® Regular Strength Vapor Lemon
SUCRETS® Maximum Strength Vapor Black Cherry

Active Ingredient: Maximum Strength Wintergreen: Dyclonine Hydrochloride 3.0 mg. per lozenge. Wild Cherry, Regular Strength: Dyclonine Hydrochloride

Continued on next page

SmithKline Beecham—Cont.

2.0 mg. per lozenge. Children's Cherry: Dyclonine Hydrochloride 1.2 mg. per lozenge. Regular Strength–Original Mint: Hexylresorcinol 2.4 mg. per lozenge. Regular Strength–Vapor Lemon: Dyclonine Hydrochloride 2.0 mg. per lozenge. Maximum Strength–Vapor Black Cherry: Dyclonine Hydrochloride 3.0 mg. per lozenge.

Inactive Ingredients: Maximum StrengthWintergreen: Citric Acid, Corn Syrup, Silicon Dioxide, Sucrose, Yellow 10. Wild Cherry Regular Strength: Blue 1, Corn Syrup, Flavor, Red 40, Silicon Dioxide, Sucrose, Tartaric Acid. Children's Cherry: Blue 1, Citric Acid, Corn Syrup, Red 40, Silicon Dioxide, Sucrose. Regular Strength–Original Mint: Blue 1, Corn Syrup, Flavors, Silicon Dioxide, Sucrose, Yellow 10. Regular Strength–Vapor Lemon: Citric Acid, Corn Syrup, Flavors, Menthol, Silicon Dioxide, Sucrose, Yellow 10. Maximum Strength–Vapor Black Cherry: Blue 1, Corn Syrup, Flavor, Menthol, Red 40, Silicon Dioxide, Sucrose, Tartaric Acid.

Indications: For temporary relief of occasional minor sore throat pain and mouth irritations.

Actions: Dyclonine Hydrochloride's soothing anesthetic action relieves minor throat irritations.

Warnings: If sore throat is severe, persists more than 2 days, is accompanied or followed by fever, headache, rash, nausea, or vomiting, consult a doctor promptly. If sore mouth symptoms do not improve in 7 days, see your dentist or doctor promptly. KEEP THIS AND ALL MEDICINES OUT OF THE REACH OF CHILDREN.

Drug Interaction: No known drug interaction.

Symptoms and Treatment of Oral Overdosage: Reactions due to large overdosage are systemic and involve the central nervous system and cardiovascular system. Central nervous system reactions are characterized by excitation and/or depression. Nervousness, dizziness, blurred vision or tremors may occur. Reactions involving the cardiovascular system include depression of the myocardium, hypotension or bradycardia. Should a large overdose be suspected seek professional assistance. Call your physician, local poison control center or the Rocky Mountain Poison Control Center at 303-592-1710 (Collect), 24 hours a day.

Dosage and Administration: Adults and children 2 years of age or older: Allow to dissolve slowly in the mouth. Repeat every two hours as needed. Do not administer to children under 2 years of age unless directed by a doctor.

Professional Labeling: For the temporary relief of pain associated with ton-

sillitis, pharyngitis, throat infections or stomatitis.

How Supplied: Available in tins of 24 lozenges.

TELDRIN®
Chlorpheniramine Maleate
Timed-Release Allergy Capsules
Maximum Strength 12 mg.

Product Information: Hay fever and allergies are caused by grass and tree pollen, dust and pollution. TELDRIN provides up to 12 hours of relief from hay fever/upper respiratory allergy symptoms: sneezing, runny nose, itchy, watery eyes. TELDRIN is formulated to release some medication initially and the rest gradually over a prolonged period.

Directions: Adults and children over 12: Just one capsule in the morning, and one in the evening. Do not give to children under 12 without the advice and consent of a physician. Not to exceed 24 mg. (2 capsules) in 24 hours.
- The carton is protected by a clear overwrap printed with "safety sealed"; do not use if overwrap is missing or broken.

TAMPER-RESISTANT PACKAGING FEATURES FOR YOUR PROTECTION:
- Each capsule is encased in a plastic cell with a foil back; do not use if the cell or foil is broken.
- Each TELDRIN capsule is protected by a green PERMA-SEAL™ band which bonds the two capsule halves together; do not use if capsule or band is broken.

Warnings: Do not take this product if you have asthma, glaucoma, or difficulty in urination due to enlargement of the prostate gland, except under the advice and supervision of a physician. Do not drive or operate heavy machinery. May cause drowsiness. Avoid alcoholic beverages while taking this product. May cause excitability, especially in children. Keep this and all drugs out of the reach of children. In case of accidental overdose, seek professional assistance or contact a poison control center immediately. As with any drug, if you are pregnant or nursing a baby, seek the advice of a health professional before using this product.

Formula:
Active Ingredient: Each capsule contains Chlorpheniramine Maleate, 12 mg. Inactive Ingredients (listed for individuals with specific allergies): Benzyl Alcohol, Cetylpyridinium Chloride, D&C Red 27, FD&C Red 30, D&C Red 33, Ethylcellulose, FD&C Green 3, FD&C Red 40, FD&C Yellow 6, Gelatin, Hydrogenated Castor Oil, Silicon Dioxide, Sodium Lauryl Sulfate, Starch, Sucrose, and trace amounts of other inactive ingredients. Store at controlled room temperature (59°–86°F).

How Supplied: Maximum Strength 12 mg. Timed-Release capsules in packages of 12, 24 and 48 capsules.
Shown in Product Identification Guide, page 426

THROAT DISCS® Throat Lozenges

Description: Each lozenge contains sucrose, starch (may contain cornstarch), acacia, glycyrrhiza extract (licorice), gum tragacanth, anethole, linseed, cubeb oleoresin, anise oil, peppermint oil, capsicum, and mineral oil.

Indications: Effective for soothing, temporary relief of minor throat irritations from hoarseness and coughs due to colds.

Precautions: For severe or persistent cough or sore throat, or sore throat accompanied by high fever, headache, nausea, and vomiting, consult physician promptly. Not recommended for children under 3 years of age.

Directions: Allow lozenge to dissolve slowly in mouth. One or two should give the desired relief.

How Supplied: Boxes of 60 lozenges.
Shown in Product Identification Guide, page 426

TUMS® Antacid Tablets
TUMS E–X® Antacid Tablets

Description: Tums: Active Ingredient: Calcium Carbonate, precipitated U.S.P. 500 mg.
Tums Original Flavor: Inactive Ingredients: Flavor, mineral oil, sodium polyphosphate, starch, sucrose, talc.
Tums Assorted Flavors: Inactive Ingredients: Adipic acid, FD&C Blue 1, D&C Red 27, D&C Red 30, FD&C Yellow No. 6, flavors, mineral oil, sodium polyphosphate, starch, sucrose, talc.
An antacid composition providing liquid effectiveness in a low-cost, pleasant-tasting tablet. Tums tablets are free of the chalky aftertaste usually associated with calcium carbonate therapy and remain pleasant tasting even during long-term therapy. Each TUMS tablet contains not more than 2 mg of sodium and is considered to be dietetically sodium free. Non-laxative/ non-constipating.
Tums E-X: Active Ingredient: Calcium Carbonate, 750 mg.
Tums E-X Wintergreen Flavor Inactive Ingredients: FD&C Blue 1, D&C Yellow 10, FD&C Yellow No. 6, flavor, mineral oil, sodium polyphosphate, starch, sucrose, talc.
Tums E-X Cherry Flavor Inactive Ingredients: Adipic acid, D&C Red 27, D&C Red 30, flavor, mineral oil, sodium polyphosphate, starch sucrose, talc.
Tums E-X Peppermint Flavor Inactive Ingredients: Flavor, mineral oil, sodium polyphosphate, starch, sucrose, talc.
Tums E-X Assorted Flavors Inactive Ingredients: Adipic acid, FD&C Blue 1, D&C Red 27, D&C Red 30, FD&C Yellow

No. 6, flavors, mineral oil sodium polyphosphate, starch, sucrose, talc.
Each tablet contains not more than 2 mg of sodium and is considered to be dietetically sodium free. Non-laxative/non-constipating.

Indications: For fast relief of acid indigestion, heartburn, sour stomach and upset stomach associated with these symptoms.

Actions: Tums lowers the upper limit of the pH range without affecting the innate antacid efficiency of calcium carbonate. One tablet, when tested *in vitro* according to the *Federal Register* procedure (*Fed. Reg.* 39-19862, June 4, 1974), neutralizes 10 mEq of 0.1N HCl. This high neutralization capacity combined with a rapid rate of reaction makes Tums an ideal antacid for management of conditions associated with hyperacidity. It effectively neutralizes free acid yet does not cause systemic alkalosis in the presence of normal renal function. A double-blind placebo-controlled clinical study demonstrated that calcium carbonate taken at a dosage of 16 Tums tablets daily for a two-week period was non-constipating/non-laxative.

Warnings: Tums: Do not take more than 16 tablets in a 24-hour period or use the maximum dosage of this product for more than 2 weeks, except under the advice and supervision of a physician. If symptoms persist for 2 weeks, stop using this product and see a physician. Keep this and all drugs out of the reach of children.
Tums E-X: Do not take more than 10 tablets in a 24-hour period or use the maximum dosage of this product for more than two weeks, except under the advice and supervision of a physician. If symptoms persist for two weeks, stop using this product and see a physician. Keep this and all drugs out of the reach of children.

Drug Interaction Precaution: Antacids may interact with certain prescription drugs. If you are presently taking a prescription drug, do not take this product without checking with your physician or other health professional.

Dosage and Administration: Chew 1 or 2 TUMS tablets as symptoms occur. Repeat hourly if symptoms return, or as directed by a physician. No water is required. Simulated Drip Method: The pleasant-tasting TUMS tablet may be kept between the gum and cheek and allowed to dissolve gradually by continuous sucking to prolong the effective relief time.

Important Dietary Information—As a Source of Extra Calcium—Chew 1 or 2 tablets after meals or as directed by a physician.
Tums Original and Assorted Flavors: The 500 mg of calcium carbonate in each tablet provide 200 mg of elemental calcium which is 20% of the adult U.S. RDA for calcium. Five tablets provide 100% of the daily calcium needs for adults. When

used as a calcium supplement, do not exceed 9 tablets per day.
Tums E-X: The 750 mg of calcium carbonate in each tablet provide 300 mg of elemental calcium which is 30% of the adult U.S. RDA for calcium. Four tablets provide 120% of the daily calcium needs for adults. When used as a calcium supplement, do not exceed 6 tablets per day.

Professional Labeling: Indicated for the symptomatic relief of hyperacidity associated with the diagnosis of peptic ulcer, gastritis, peptic esophagitis, gastric hyperacidity, and hiatal hernia.

How Supplied: Tums: Peppermint and Assorted Flavors of Cherry, Lemon, Orange and Lime are available in 12-tablet rolls, 3-roll wraps, and bottles of 75 and 150 tablets. **Tums E-X Wintergreen, E-X Cherry, E-X Peppermint, and Assorted Flavors of Cherry, Lemon, Lime and Orange:** 8-tablet rolls, 3-roll wraps and bottles of 48 and 96 tablets.
Shown in Product Identification Guide, page 426

TUMS Anti-gas /Antacid Formula

Active Ingredients: 500 mg of calcium carbonate and 20 mg of simethicone per tablet.
Tums Anti-gas/Antacid formula Assorted Fruit Flavor Inactive Ingredients: Adipic Acid, Corn Syrup, D&C Red 27, D&C Red 30, D&C Yellow 10, FD&C Blue 1, FD&C Yellow 6, Flavors, Microcrystalline Cellulose, Mineral Oil, Sodium Polyphosphate, Starch, Sucrose, Talc, Triglycerol Monooleate.
Each tablet contains not more than 2 mg of sodium and is considered dietetically sodium free.
The 500 mg of calcium carbonate in each tablet provide 200 mg of elemental calcium.
Non-laxative/non-constipating.

Indications: For fast relief of acid indigestion, heartburn, and sour stomach accompanied by gas and upset stomach associated with these symptoms.

Actions: Calcium carbonate in Tums anti-gas/antacid formula lowers the upper limit of the pH range without affecting the innate antacid efficiency of calcium carbonate. Calcium carbonate, when tested in vitro according to the Federal Register procedure (Fed. Reg. 39-19862, June 4, 1974), neutralizes 10 mEq of 0.1N HCl. This high neutralization capacity combined with a rapid rate of reaction makes calcium carbonate an ideal antacid for management of conditions associated with hyperacidity. It effectively neutralizes free acid yet does not cause systemic alkalosis in the presence of normal renal function.

Warnings: Do not take more than 16 tablets in a 24-hour period or use the maximum dosage of this product for more than 2 weeks, except under the advice and supervision of a doctor. Keep

this and all drugs out of the reach of children.

Drug Interaction Precaution: Antacids may interact with certain prescription drugs. If you are presently taking a prescription drug, do not take this product without checking with your physician or other health professional.

Dosage and Administration: Chew 1 or 2 tablets as symptoms occur. Repeat hourly if symptoms return, or as directed by a doctor. No water is required. Simulated Drip Method: The pleasant-tasting Tums Anti-gas/Antacid formula tablets may be kept between the gum and cheek and allowed to dissolve gradually by continually sucking to prolong the effective relief time.

Professional Labeling: Indicated for the symptomatic relief of hyperacidity associated with the diagnosis of peptic ulcer, gastritis, peptic esophagitis, gastric hyperacidity, and hiatal hernia.

How Supplied: 60 tablet bottles 4770D
Shown in Product Identification Guide, page 427

VIVARIN® Stimulant Tablets and Caplets
[*vi 'va-rin*]

Active Ingredient: Each tablet/caplet contains 200 mg. Caffeine Alkaloid.

Inactive Ingredients Tablets: Dextrose, Magnesium Stearate, Microcrystalline Cellulose, Silicon Dioxide, Starch, FD&C Yellow #6, D&C Yellow #10.

Inactive Ingredients Caplets: Dextrose, Hydroxypropyl Methylcellulose, Magnesium Stearate, Microcrystalline Cellulose, Polyethylene Glycol, Polysorbate 80, Silicon Dioxide, Starch, Titanium Dioxide, FD&C Yellow #6, D&C Yellow #10.

Indications: Helps restore mental alertness or wakefulness when experiencing fatigue or drowsiness.

Actions: Stimulates cerebrocortical areas involved with active mental processes.

Directions: Adults and children 12 years of age and over: Oral dosage is 1 tablet or caplet (200 mg) not more often than every 3 to 4 hours.

Warnings: The recommended dose of this product contains about as much caffeine as two cups of coffee. Limit the use of caffeine containing medications, foods, or beverages while taking this product because too much caffeine may cause nervousness, irritability, sleeplessness, and, occasionally, rapid heart beat. For occasional use only. Not intended for use as a substitute for sleep. If fatigue or drowsiness persists or continues to recur, consult a doctor. Do not give to children under 12 years of age. As with any drug,

Continued on next page

SmithKline Beecham—Cont.

if you are pregnant or nursing a baby, seek the advice of a health professional before using this product. In case of accidental overdose, seek professional assistance or contact a poison control center immediately. Keep this and all drugs out of the reach of children.

Drug Interaction: Use of caffeine should be lowered or avoided if drugs are being used to treat cardiovascular ailments, psychological problems, or kidney trouble.

Precaution: Higher blood glucose levels may result from caffeine use.

Symptoms and Treatment of Oral Overdosage: Convulsions may occur if caffeine is consumed in doses larger than 10 g. Emesis should be induced to empty the stomach. In case of accidental overdose, seek professional assistance by contacting your physician, the local poison control center, or the Rocky Mt. Poison Control Center at 303-592-1710 (Collect), 24 hours a day.

How Supplied Tablets: Available in packages of 16, 40 and 80 tablets.

How Supplied Caplets: Available in packages of 24 and 48.

EDUCATIONAL MATERIAL

Booklets:
"A Personal Guide to Feminine Freshness"
A 16 page illustrated booklet on vaginal infections, feminine hygiene and douching. Free to physicians, pharmacists and patients in limited quantities by writing SmithKline Beecham Consumer Healthcare, L.P. or calling 800-233-2426.
"The Facts About Vaginal Infections and STDs: An Easy Guide For Women"
A 16 page booklet on the common types of STDs and prevention. Free to physicians, pharmacists and patients in limited quantities by sending a SASE to: SmithKline Beecham Consumer Healthcare, L.P. or calling 800-233-2426.
Film, Video:
"Feminine Hygiene and You"
This 14 minute color film begins with a simple explanation of how a woman's body works (reproductive system, menstrual cycle, and vaginal secretions) then explains douching. Free loan to physicians, pharmacists and clinics. Available in 16mm, and VHS by writing SmithKline Beecham Consumer Healthcare, L.P. or calling 800-233-2426.

Standard Homeopathic Company
210 WEST 131st STREET
BOX 61067
LOS ANGELES, CA 90061

HYLAND'S ARNICAID™ TABLETS
100% natural temporary relief of symptoms of pain and soreness from muscle overexertion or injury.

Indications: Hyland's Arnicaid Tablets are a homeopathic product indicated for the control and symptomatic relief of acute bruising and soreness due to falls, blows, and muscle strain. Arnicaid provides a 100% natural relief for children and adults. Use after minor accidents or after sports workouts. Arnicaid contains no sucrose, dextrose or fillers. Like all homeopathic products, Arnicaid has no known contraindications or side effects.

Directions: Adults—1–2 tablets every 4 hours, or as needed.
Children over 3 years of age—½ adult dose.

Active Ingredients: Arnica Montana 30X HPUS in a base of lactose USP.

Warnings: Do not use if cap band is broken or missing. If symptoms persist for more than seven days or worsen, contact a licensed health care professional. Do not use in children under three years of age without consulting a licensed health care professional. As with any drug, if you are pregnant or nursing a baby, seek the advice of a licensed health care professional before using this product. Keep this and all medications out of reach of children. In case of accidental overdose, contact a poison control center or the manufacturer at the number provided below.
P&S Laboratories
Los Angeles, CA 90061
Questions? Call us: 800/624-9659
MADE IN USA
Arnicaid and Hyland's are trademarks of Standard Homeopathic Co.

HYLAND'S BED WETTING TABLETS

Active Ingredients: *Equisetum hyemale* (Scouring Rush) 2X HPUS, *Rhus aromatica* (Fragrant Sumac) 3X HPUS, *Belladonna* 3X HPUS (0.0003% Alkaloids).

Inactive Ingredients: Lactose USP.

Indications: A homeopathic combination for the temporary relief of involuntary urination (common bed wetting) in children.

Directions: Children 3 to 12 years: 2 to 3 tablets before meals and at bedtime, or as directed by a licensed health care practitioner. Children over 12 years: double the above recommended dose.

Warnings: If symptoms persist for more than seven days or worsen, consult a Health Care Professional. As with any drug, if you are pregnant or nursing a baby, seek the advice of a health professional before using this product. Keep this and all medication out of the reach of children.

How Supplied: Bottles of 125—one grain sublingual tablets (NDC 54973-7501-01). Store at room temperature.

HYLAND'S CALMS FORTÉ TABLETS

Active Ingredients: *Passiflora* (Passion Flower) 1X triple strength HPUS, *Avena sativa* (Oat) 1X triple strength HPUS, *Humulus lupulus* (Hops) 1X double strength HPUS, *Chamomilla* (Chamomile) 2X HPUS, *Calcarea Phosphorica* (Calcium Phosphate) 3X HPUS, *Ferrum Phosphorica* (Iron Phosphate) 3X HPUS, *Kali Phosphoricum* (Potassium Phosphate) 3X HPUS, *Natrum Phosphoricum* (Sodium Phosphate) 3X HPUS, *Magnesia Phosphoricum* (Magnesium Phosphate) 3X HPUS.

Inactive Ingredients: Lactose USP.

Indications: Temporary symptomatic relief of simple nervous tension and insomnia.

Directions: Adults, As a relaxant: 1 to 2 tablets as needed or 3 times daily between meals. In insomnia: 1 to 3 tablets ½ to 1 hour before retiring. Repeat as needed without danger of side effects. Children, As a relaxant: 1 tablet as needed or 3 times daily before meals. In insomnia: 1 to 2 tablets 1 hour before retiring. Non-habit-forming.

Warnings: If symptoms persist for more than seven days or worsen, consult a Health Care Professional. As with any drug, if you are pregnant or nursing a baby, seek the advice of a health professional before using this product. Keep this and all medication out of the reach of children.

How Supplied: Bottles of 100 four grain tablets (NDC 54973-1121-02). Store at room temperature. Bottles of 50 four grain tablets (NDC 54973-1121-01). Store at room temperature.

HYLAND'S CLEARAC™ TABLETS
All natural ClearAc helps clear up acne, pimples, and acne blemishes.

Indications: Hyland's ClearAc Tablets are a homeopathic combination indicated for the management and symptomatic relief of symptoms of pimples, blackheads, and blemishes associated with common acne (acne vulgaris). ClearAc Tablets provide a 100% natural approach. Like all homeopathic products, ClearAc Tablets have no known contraindications or side effects. Use in conjunction with a high-quality skin cleanser, such as 100% Natural Hyland's ClearAc Cleanser with Calendula.

Directions: Adults—2–3 tablets every 4 hours, or as needed.

Active Ingredients: Echinacea Ang. 6X HPUS, Berberis Vulg. 6X HPUS, Sulphur Iod. 6X HPUS, Hepar Sulph. 6X HPUS in a base of lactose USP.

Warnings: Do not use if cap band is broken or missing. If symptoms persist or worsen, contact a licensed health care professional. As with any drug, if you are pregnant or nursing a baby, seek the advice of a licensed health care professional before using this product. Keep this and all medications out of reach of children. In case of accidental overdose, contact a poison control center or the manufacturer at the number provided below.
P&S Laboratories
Los Angeles, CA 90061
Questions? Call us: 800/624-9659
MADE IN USA
ClearAc and Hyland's are trademarks of Standard Homeopathic Co.

HYLAND'S COLIC TABLETS

Active Ingredients: *Disocorea* (Wild Yam) 2X HPUS, *Chamomilla* (Chamomile) 3X HPUS, *Colocynth* (Bitter Apple) 3X HPUS.

Inactive Ingredients: Lactose USP.

Indications: A homeopathic combination for the temporary relief of colic and gas pains caused by irritating food, feeding too quickly, swallowing air and similar conditions during teething, colds and other minor upset periods in children.

Directions: For children to 2 years of age: administer 2 tablets dissolved in a teaspoon of water or on the tongue every 15 minutes until relieved; then every 2 hours as required. Children over 2 years: 3 tablets dissolved on the tongue as above; or as recommended by a licensed health care practitioner.

Warnings: If symptoms persist for more than seven days or worsen, consult a Health Care Professional. Keep this and all medication out of the reach of children.

How Supplied: Bottles of 125—one grain sublingual tablets (NDC 54973-7502-01). Store at room temperature.

HYLAND'S COUGH SYRUP WITH HONEY™

Active Ingredients: Each fluid ounce contains: *Ipecacuanha* (Ipecac) 3X HPUS, *Aconitum napellus* (Aconite) 3X HPUS, *Spongia Tosta* (Sponge) 3X HPUS, *Antimonium Tartaricum* (Potassium Antimony Tartrate) 6X HPUS.

Inactive Ingredients: Simple syrup and honey.

Indications: A homeopathic combination for the temporary relief of symptoms of simple, dry, tight or tickling coughs due to colds in children.

Directions: Children 1 to 12 years: 1 to 3 teaspoonfuls as required. Children over

12 years and adults: 3 to 4 teaspoonfuls as required. May be taken with or without water. Repeat as often as necessary to relieve symptoms. For children under 1 year of age, consult a licensed health care practitioner.

Warnings: Do not use this product for persistent or chronic cough such as occurs with asthma, smoking or emphysema; or if cough is accompanied with excessive mucus, unless directed by a licensed health care practitioner. If symptoms persist for more than seven days, tend to recur, or are accompanied by a high fever, rash, or persistent headache, consult a Health Care Professional. As with any drug, if you are pregnant or nursing a baby, seek the advice of a health professional before using this product. Keep this and all medication out of the reach of children.

How Supplied: Bottles of 4 fluid ounces (120 ml) (NDC 54973-7503-02). Store at room temperature.

HYLAND'S C–PLUS™ COLD TABLETS

Active Ingredients: *Eupatorium perfoliatum* (Boneset) 2X HPUS, *Euphrasia officinalis* (Eyebright) 2X HPUS, *Gelsemium sempervirens* (Yellow Jasmine) 3X HPUS, *Kali Iodatum* (Potassium Iodide) 3X HPUS.

Inactive Ingredients: Lactose USP, Natural Raspberry Flavor.

Indications: A homeopathic combination for the temporary relief of symptoms of runny nose and sneezing due to common head colds in children.

Directions: Children 1 to 3 years: 2 tablets every 15 minutes for 4 doses, then hourly until relieved. For children 3 to 6 years: 3 tablets as above; for children 6 and older: 6 tablets as above or as directed by a licensed health care practitioner.

Warnings: If symptoms persist for more than seven days or worsen, consult a Health Care Professional. As with any drug, if you are pregnant or nursing a baby, seek the advice of a health professional before using this product. Keep this and all medication out of the reach of children.

How Supplied: Bottles of 125—one grain sublingual tablets (NDC 54973-7505-01). Store at room temperature.

HYLAND'S DIARREX™ TABLETS
100% natural temporary relief of symptoms of acute gastrointestinal distress associated with nonspecific diarrhea.

Indications: Hyland's Diarrex Tablets are a homeopathic combination indicated for the temporary control and symptomatic relief of acute nonspecific diarrhea. Diarrex provides a 100% natural approach which aids in relief of symp-

toms of loose stools and associated gastric symptoms. Like all homeopathic products, Diarrex has no known contraindications or side effects.

Directions: Adults—2-3 tablets every 4 hours, or as needed. Children over 3 years of age—½ adult dose.

Active Ingredients: Arsenicum Alb. 6X HPUS, Podophyllum Pelt. 6X HPUS, Chamomilla 6X HPUS, Phosphorus 6X HPUS, Mercurius Viv. 6X HPUS in a base of lactose USP.

Warnings: Do not use if cap band is broken or missing. If symptoms persist for more than two days or worsen, contact a licensed health care professional. Do not use in children under three years of age without consulting a licensed health care professional. Discontinue use if diarrhea is accompanied by a high fever (greater than 101°F), or if blood is present in the stool and contact a licensed health care professional. As with any drug, if you are pregnant or nursing a baby, seek the advice of a licensed health care professional before using this product. Keep this and all medication out of reach of children. In case of accidental overdose, contact a poison control center or the manufacturer at the number provided below.
P&S Laboratories
Los Angeles, CA 90061
Questions? Call us: 800/624-9659
MADE IN USA
Diarrex and Hyland's are trademarks of Standard Homeopathic Co.

HYLAND'S ENURAID™ TABLETS
100% natural temporary relief of symptoms of common incontinence in adults.

Indications: Hyland's EnurAid Tablets are a homeopathic combination indicated for the control and symptomatic relief of involuntary urination (common incontinence) in adults. EnurAid provides a 100% natural approach which aids in relief of symptoms of bladder control and related symptoms. Like all homeopathic products, EnurAid has no known contraindications or side effects.

Directions: Adults—2-3 tablets every 4 hours, or as needed.

Active Ingredients: Belladonna 6X HPUS, Cantharis 6X HPUS, Apis Mell. 6X HPUS, Arnica Mont. 6X HPUS, Allium Cepa 6X HPUS, Rhus Arom. 6X HPUS, Equisetum Hyem. 6X HPUS in a base of lactose USP.

Warnings: Do not use if cap band is broken or missing. If symptoms persist for more than seven days or worsen, contact a licensed health care professional. Discontinue use if symptoms are accompanied by a high fever (greater than 101°F), or if blood is present in urine and contact a licensed health care professional. As with any drug, if you are preg-

Continued on next page

Standard Homeopathic—Cont.

nant or nursing a baby, seek the advice of a licensed health care professional before using this product. Keep this and all medications out of reach of children. In case of accidental overdose, contact a poison control center or the manufacturer at the number provided below.
P&S Laboratories
Los Angeles, CA 90061
Questions? Call us: 800/624-9659
MADE IN USA
EnurAid and Hyland's are trademarks of Standard Homeopathic Co.

HYLAND'S TEETHING TABLETS

Active Ingredients: *Calcarea Phosphorica* (Calcium Phosphate) 3X HPUS, *Chamomilla* (Chamomile) 3X HPUS, *Coffea Cruda* (Coffee) 3X HPUS, *Belladonna* 3X HPUS (Alkaloids 0.0003%).

Inactive Ingredients: Lactose USP.

Indications: A homeopathic combination for the temporary relief of symptoms of simple restlessness and wakeful irritability due to cutting of teeth.

Directions: 2 to 3 tablets in a teaspoon of water or on the tongue, 4 times per day. If the child is restless or wakeful, 2 tablets every hour for 6 doses or as directed by a licensed health care practitioner.

Warnings: If symptoms persist for more than seven days or worsen, consult a Health Care Professional. As with any drug, if you are pregnant or nursing a baby, seek the advice of a health professional before using this product. Keep this and all medication out of the reach of children.

How Supplied: Bottles of 125—one grain sublingual tablets (NDC 54973-7504-01). Store at room temperature.

HYLAND'S VITAMIN C FOR CHILDREN™

Active Ingredients: 25 mg Vitamin C as Sodium Ascorbate (30 mg).

Inactive Ingredients: Lactose USP, Natural Lemon Flavor.

Indications: Each tablet provides children with 55% of the daily recommended requirement of Vitamin C. Sodium Ascorbate is preferred to Ascorbic Acid when gastric irritation may result from free acid.

Directions: Children 2 years and older: 1 to 2 tablets on the tongue or as directed by a licensed health care practitioner.

Warning: Keep this and all medication out of the reach of children.

How Supplied: Bottles of 125—one grain sublingual tablets (NDC 54973-7506-01). Store at room temperature.

Tablets may turn brown in color with exposure to light. Color change does not affect potency.

Stellar Pharmacal Corp.
Div./Star Pharmaceuticals, Inc.
1990 N.W. 44TH STREET
POMPANO BEACH, FL
33064-8712

STAR–OPTIC® EYE WASH
[*star op'tik*]
STERILE, ISOTONIC, BUFFERED SOLUTION

Description: STAR-OPTIC Eye Wash is specially formulated to soothe irritating 'Swimmers Eye'™ by bathing (washing) the eye providing cooling, refreshing relief. STAR-OPTIC Eye Wash is a sterile, isotonic buffered solution containing sodium chloride, sodium phosphate monobasic and sodium phosphate dibasic, preserved with edetate disodium and benzalkonium chloride in purified water, USP. CONTAINS NO BORIC ACID or THIMEROSAL (MERCURY).

Indications: For irrigating the eye to help relieve irritation, discomfort, burning, stinging or itching by removing loose foreign material, air pollutants (smog or pollen) or CHLORINATED WATER.

Directions: If eye cup is used, rinse cup with STAR-OPTIC Eye Wash or clean water immediately before and after each use. Avoid contamination of rim and inside surfaces of cup. Fill cup one-half full with STAR-OPTIC Eye Wash. Apply cup tightly to the affected eye to prevent leakage and tilt head backward. Open eyelids wide and rotate eyeball to ensure thorough bathing with the wash.
Note: Enclosed eye cup is sterile if package is intact. If cup is not used, flush affected eye by controlling the rate of flow of solution by pressure on the bottle.

Warnings: To avoid contamination, do not touch tip of container to any surface. Replace cap after using. If you experience eye pain, changes in vision, continued redness or irritation of the eye or if the condition worsens or persists, consult a physician. Obtain immediate medical treatment for all open wounds in or near the eyes. If solution changes color or becomes cloudy, do not use.
Keep out of the reach of children. Not for use with contact lenses. DO NOT USE IF IMPRINTED SAFETY SEAL ON CAP

IS BROKEN OR MISSING AT TIME OF PURCHASE.
Store at room temperature. Use before expiration date marked on bottle and carton.

How Supplied: Bottles of 4 fl. oz. (118 ml) with eye cup.

STAR–OTIC® EAR SOLUTION
Antibacterial, Antifungal, Nonaqueous Ear Solution

Active Ingredients: Acetic acid nonaqueous, Burow's solution, Boric acid, in a propylene glycol vehicle, with an acid pH and a low surface tension.

Indications: For the prevention of otitis externa, commonly called "Swimmer's Ear". To inhibit bacterial and fungal growth and maintain the external ear canal's normal acid mantle following swimming or showering.

Actions: Star-Otic Ear Solution is antibacterial, antifungal, hydrophilic, has an acid pH and a low surface tension. Acetic acid and boric acid inhibit the rapid multiplication of microorganisms and help maintain the lining mantle of the ear canal in its normal acid state. Burow's solution (aluminum acetate) is a mild astringent. Propylene glycol reduces moisture in the ear canal.

Warning: Do not use in ear if tympanic membrane (ear drum) is perforated or punctured.

Symptoms and Treatment of Overdosage: Discontinue use if undue irritation or sensitivity occurs.

Dosage and Administration: Adults and Children: To help restore normal pH to the outer ear canal. In susceptible persons, instill 3–5 drops of Star-Otic Ear Solution in each ear before and after swimming or bathing, or as directed by physician.

Professional Labeling: Same as those outlined under Indications.

How Supplied: Available in ½ oz measured drop, safety tip, plastic bottle.

Sterling Health
Division of Sterling Winthrop Inc.
90 PARK AVENUE
NEW YORK, NY 10016

BAYER® BUFFERED
Buffered Aspirin

Active Ingredients: Each Bayer Buffered contains Aspirin (325 mg), in a formulation buffered with Calcium Carbonate, Magnesium Carbonate, and Magnesium Oxide.

Inactive Ingredients: Corn Starch, Ethylcellulose, FD&C Blue #2, Hydroxypropyl Methylcellulose, Microcrystalline Cellulose, Pharmaceutical Glaze, Sodium Starch Glycolate, Talc, Zinc Stearate.

Indications: Analgesic, antipyretic, anti-inflammatory. For relief of headache; painful discomfort and fever of colds and flu; muscular aches and pains; temporary relief of minor pains of arthritis, rheumatism, bursitis, lumbago, sciatica; toothache, and pain following dental procedures; neuralgia and neuritic pain; functional menstrual pain; painful discomfort and fever accompanying immunizations.

Directions: The following dosages are those provided in the packaging, as appropriate for self-medication. Larger or more frequent dosage may be necessary as appropriate to the condition or needs of the patient. The addition of buffering agents makes Bayer® Buffered particularly appropriate for those who must take frequent doses of aspirin. The hydroxypropyl methylcellulose coating benefits aspirin users who have difficulty in swallowing uncoated tablets and caplets.
Usual Adult Dose: One or two tablets with water. May be repeated every four hours as necessary up to 12 tablets a day or as directed by a doctor. Do not give to children under 12 unless directed by a doctor.

Warnings: Children and teenagers should not use this medicine for chicken pox or flu symptoms before a doctor is consulted about Reye syndrome, a rare but serious illness reported to be associated with aspirin. Do not take for pain for more than 10 days or for fever for more than 3 days unless directed by a doctor. If pain or fever persists or gets worse, if new symptoms occur, or if redness or swelling is present consult a doctor because these could be signs of a serious condition. Do not take this product if you are allergic to aspirin, have asthma, stomach problems that persist or recur, gastric ulcers or bleeding problems unless directed by a doctor. If ringing in the ears or loss of hearing occurs, consult a doctor before taking any more of this product. Keep this and all drugs out of the reach of children. In case of accidental overdose, seek professional assistance or contact a poison control center immediately. As with any drug, if you are pregnant or nursing a baby, seek the advice of a health professional before using this product. **IT IS ESPECIALLY IMPORTANT NOT TO USE ASPIRIN DURING THE LAST 3 MONTHS OF PREGNANCY UNLESS SPECIFICALLY DIRECTED TO DO SO BY A DOCTOR BECAUSE IT MAY CAUSE PROBLEMS IN THE UNBORN CHILD OR COMPLICATIONS DURING DELIVERY.**

Drug Interaction Precaution: Do not take this product if you are taking a prescription drug for anticoagulation (thinning of the blood), diabetes, gout, or arthritis unless directed by a doctor.

Professional Labeling
ANTIARTHRITIC EFFECT

Indication: Conditions requiring chronic or long-term aspirin therapy for pain and/or inflammation, e.g., rheumatoid arthritis, juvenile rheumatoid arthritis, systemic lupus erythematosus, osteoarthritis (degenerative joint disease), ankylosing spondylitis, psoriatic arthritis, Reiter's syndrome, and fibrositis.

ANTIPLATELET EFFECT

In MI Prophylaxis:

Indication: Aspirin is indicated to reduce the risk of death and/or nonfatal myocardial infarction in patients with a previous infarction or unstable angina pectoris.

Clinical Trials: The indication is supported by the results of six large randomized, multicenter, placebo-controlled studies.[1–7] involving 10,816 predominantly male post-myocardial infarction (MI) patients and one randomized placebo-controlled study of 1,266 men with unstable angina. Therapy with aspirin was begun at intervals after the onset of acute MI varying from less than three days to more than five years and continuing for periods of from less than one year to four years. In the unstable angina study, treatment was started within one month after the onset of unstable angina and continued for 12 weeks, and complicating conditions, such as congestive heart failure, were not included in the study. Aspirin therapy in MI patients was associated with about a 20% reduction in the risk of subsequent death and/or nonfatal reinfarction, a median absolute decrease of 3% from the 12% to 22% event rates in the placebo groups. In the aspirin-treated unstable angina patients, the reduction in risk was about 50%, a reduction in the event rate of 5% from the 10% rate in the placebo group over the 12 weeks of the study.
Daily dosage of aspirin in the postmyocardial infarction studies was 300 mg in one study and 900–1,500 mg in five studies. A dose of 325 mg was used in the study of unstable angina.

Adverse Reactions: Gastrointestinal reactions: Doses of 1,000 mg per day of aspirin caused gastrointestinal symptoms and bleeding that, in some cases, were clinically significant. In the largest postinfarction study (the Aspirin Myocardial Infarction Study [AMIS] with 4,500 people), the percentage of incidences of gastrointestinal symptoms for the aspirin (1,000 mg of a standard, solid-tablet formulation) and placebo-treated subjects, respectively, were stomach pain (14.5%, 4.4%), heartburn (11.9%, 4.8%), nausea and/or vomiting (7.6%, 2.1%), and hospitalization for GI disorder (4.9%, 3.5%). In the AMIS and other trials, aspirin-treated patients had increased rates of gross gastrointestinal bleeding., Symptoms and signs of gastrointestinal irritation were not significantly increased in subjects treated for unstable angina with buffered aspirin in solution.

Cardiovascular and Biochemical: In the AMIS trial, the dosage of 1,000 mg per day of aspirin was associated with small increases in systolic blood pressure (BP) (average 1.5 to 2.1 mm) and diastolic BP (0.5 to 0.6 mm), depending upon whether maximal or last available readings were used. Blood urea nitrogen and uric acid levels were also increased but by less than 1.0 mg percent. Subjects with marked hypertension or renal insufficiency had been excluded from the trial so that the clinical importance of these observations for such subjects or for any subjects treated over more prolonged periods is not known. It is recommended that patients placed on long-term aspirin treatment, even at doses of 300 mg per day, be seen at regular intervals to assess changes in these measurements.

Dosage and Administration: Although most of the studies used dosages exceeding 300 mg, two trials used only 300 mg daily and pharmacologic data indicate that this dose inhibits platelet function fully. Therefore, 300 mg or a conventional 325 mg aspirin dose daily is a reasonable routine dose that would minimize gastrointestinal adverse reactions. This use of aspirin applies to both solid oral dosage forms (buffered and plain aspirin) and buffered aspirin in solution.

In Transient Ischemic Attacks:

Indication: Aspirin is indicated for reducing the risk of recurrent transient ischemic attacks (TIAs) or stroke in men who have transient ischemia of the brain due to fibrin emboli. There is no evidence that aspirin is effective in reducing TIAs in women, or is of benefit in the treatment of completed strokes in men or women.

Clinical Trials: The indication is supported by the results of a Canadian study[8] in which 585 patients with threatened stroke were followed in a randomized clinical trial for an average of 28 months to determine whether aspirin or sulfinpyrazone, singly or in combination,

Continued on next page

This product information was effective as of November 1, 1993. Current information may be obtained directly from Sterling Health, by writing to 90 Park Avenue, New York, NY 10016.

Sterling Health—Cont.

was superior to placebo in preventing transient ischemic attacks, stroke, or death. The study showed that, although sulfinpyrazone had no statistically significant effect, aspirin reduced the risk of continuing transient ischemic attacks, stroke, or death by 19 percent and reduced the risk of stroke or death by 31 percent. Another aspirin study carried out in the United States with 178 patients showed a statistically significant number of "favorable outcomes," including reduced transient ischemic attacks, stroke, and death.[9]

Precautions: Patients presenting with signs and/or symptoms of TIAs should have a complete medical and neurologic evaluation. Consideration should be given to other disorders which may resemble TIAs. It is important to evaluate and treat, if appropriate, diseases associated with TIAs and stroke, such as hypertension and diabetes.

Dosage: The recommended dosage for this new indication is 1,300 mg per day (650 mg b.i.d. or 325 mg q.i.d.).

References: 1. Elwood PC, et al: A randomized controlled trial of acetylsalicylic acid in the secondary prevention of mortality from myocardial infarction. *Br Med J* 1974;1:436-440. 2. The Coronary Drug Project Research Group: Aspirin in coronary heart disease. *J Chronic Dis* 1976;29:625–642. 3. Breddin K, et al: Secondary prevention of myocardial infarction: A comparison of acetylsalicylic acid, phenprocoumon or placebo. *Homeostasis* 1979;470:263–268. 4. Aspirin Myocardial Infarction Study Research Group: A randomized, controlled trial of aspirin in persons recovered from myocardial infarction. *JAMA* 1980;245:661–669. 5. Elwood PC, Sweetnam PM: Aspirin and secondary mortality after myocardial infarction. *Lancet*, December 22–29, 1979, pp 1313–1315. 6. The Persantine-Aspirin Reinfarction Study Research Group: Persantine and aspirin in coronary heart disease. *Circulation* 1980;62:449–460. 7. Lewis HD, et al: Protective effects of aspirin against acute myocardial infarction and death in men with unstable angina: Results of a Veterans Administration Cooperative Study. *N. Engl J Med* 1983;309:396–403. 8. The Canadian Cooperative Study Group: A randomized trial of aspirin and sulfinpyrazone in threatened stroke. *N. Engl J Med* 1978;299:53–59. 9. Fields WS, et al: Controlled trial of aspirin in cerebral ischemia. *Stroke* 1977;8:301–316.

How Supplied: Bayer® Buffered Aspirin (325 mg) is available in bottles of 24, 50, and 100 tablets.
Child resistant closures on 24s and 50s tablets. Bottles of 100s tablets available without safety closure for households without young children.

Shown in Product Identification Guide, page 427

BAYER® Children's Chewable Aspirin
Aspirin (Acetylsalicylic Acid)

Active Ingredients: Bayer Children's Chewable Aspirin—Aspirin 1¼ grains (81 mg) per orange flavored chewable tablet. Also available in cherry flavor.

Inactive Ingredients: Orange Flavored: Dextrose Excipient, FD&C Yellow #6, Flavor, Saccharin Sodium, Starch. Cherry Flavored: D&C Red #27, Dextrose Excipient, FD&C Red #40, Flavor, Saccharin Sodium, Starch.

Indications: For the temporary relief of minor aches, pains and headaches, and to reduce fever associated with colds, sore throats and teething.

Directions: The following dosages are those provided in the packaging, as appropriate for self-medication.
Children's Dose: To be administered only under adult supervision.

Age (Years)	Weight (lb)	Dosage
2 to under 4	32 to 35	2 tablets
4 to under 6	36 to 45	3 tablets
6 to under 9	46 to 65	4 tablets
9 to under 11	66 to 76	4–5 tablets
11 to under 12	77 to 83	4–6 tablets
12 and over	84 and over	5–8 tablets

Indicated dosage may be repeated every four hours up to a maximum of five doses per 24 hours or as directed by a doctor. For larger or more frequent doses or for children under 2, consult your doctor before taking.
Ways to Administer: CHEW, then follow with a half a glass of water, milk or fruit juice.
SWALLOW WHOLE with a half a glass of water, milk or fruit juice.
DISSOLVE ON TONGUE, followed with a half a glass of water, milk or fruit juice.
DISSOLVE TABLET in a little water, milk or fruit juice and drink the solution.
CRUSH in a teaspoonful of water—followed with a half a glass of water.

Warnings: Children and teenagers should not use this medicine for chicken pox or flu symptoms before a doctor is consulted about Reye syndrome, a rare but serious illness reported to be associated with aspirin. Do not take for pain for more than 10 days (for adults) or 5 days (for children), and do not take for fever for more than 3 days unless directed by a doctor. If pain or fever persists or gets worse, if new symptoms occur, or if redness or swelling is present, consult a doctor because these could be signs of a serious condition. Do not give this product to children for the pain of arthritis unless directed by a doctor. If sore throat is severe, persists for more than 2 days, is accompanied or followed by fever, headache, rash, nausea, or vomiting, consult a doctor promptly. Do not take this product for at least 7 days after tonsillectomy or oral surgery unless directed by a doctor. Do not take this product if you are allergic to aspirin, have asthma, have stomach problems (such as heartburn, upset stomach or

stomach pain) that persist or recur or have gastric ulcers or bleeding problems unless directed by a doctor. If ringing in the ears or loss of hearing occurs, consult a doctor before taking any more of this product.
KEEP THIS OUT OF THE REACH OF CHILDREN. IN CASE OF ACCIDENTAL OVERDOSE, CONTACT A DOCTOR IMMEDIATELY. AS WITH ANY DRUG, IF YOU ARE PREGNANT OR NURSING A BABY, SEEK THE ADVICE OF A HEALTH PROFESSIONAL BEFORE USING THIS PRODUCT. **IT IS ESPECIALLY IMPORTANT NOT TO USE ASPIRIN DURING THE LAST 3 MONTHS OF PREGNANCY UNLESS SPECIFICALLY DIRECTED TO DO SO BY A DOCTOR BECAUSE IT MAY CAUSE PROBLEMS IN THE UNBORN CHILD OR COMPLICATIONS DURING DELIVERY.**

Drug Interaction Precaution: Do not take this product if taking a prescription drug for anticoagulation (thinning of the blood), diabetes, gout or arthritis unless directed by a doctor.

How Supplied: Bayer Children's Chewable Aspirin 1¼ grains (81 mg) is available in orange and cherry flavors in bottles of 36 tablets with child-resistant safety closure.
Store at room temperature.
Shown in Product Identification Guide, page 427

Genuine BAYER® Aspirin
Aspirin (Acetylsalicylic Acid)
Tablets and Caplets

Active Ingredients: Each Genuine Bayer Aspirin contains aspirin 5 grains (325 mg) in a thin, inert, hydroxypropyl methylcellulose coating for easier swallowing. This is not an enteric coating and does not alter the onset of action of Genuine Bayer Aspirin.

Inactive Ingredients: Starch and Triacetin. May contain FD&C Blue #2 Lake, Potassium Sorbate, Titanium Dioxide, Xanthan Gum.

Indications: Analgesic, antipyretic, anti-inflammatory. For relief of headache; painful discomfort and fever of colds and flu; sore throats; muscular aches and pains; temporary relief of minor pains of arthritis, rheumatism, bursitis, lumbago, sciatica; toothache; and pain following dental procedures; neuralgia and neuritic pain; functional menstrual pain; painful discomfort and fever accompanying immunizations.

Directions: The following dosages are those provided in the packaging, as appropriate for self-medication. Larger or more frequent dosage may be necessary as appropriate to the condition or needs of the patient. The hydroxypropyl methylcellulose coating makes Genuine Bayer Aspirin particularly appropriate for those who have difficulty in swallowing uncoated tablets and caplets.

Usual Adult Dose: One or two tablets/caplets with water. May be repeated every four hours as necessary up to 12 tablets/caplets a day or as directed by a doctor. Do not give to children under 12 unless directed by a doctor.

Warnings: Children and teenagers should not use this medicine for chicken pox or flu symptoms before a doctor is consulted about Reye syndrome, a rare but serious illness reported to be associated with aspirin. Do not take for pain for more than 10 days or for fever for more than 3 days unless directed by a doctor. If pain or fever persists or gets worse, if new symptoms occur, or if redness or swelling is present consult a doctor because these could be signs of a serious condition. Do not take this product if you are allergic to aspirin, have asthma, stomach problems that persist or recur, gastric ulcers or bleeding problems unless directed by a doctor. If ringing in the ears or loss of hearing occurs, consult a doctor before taking any more of this product. Keep this and all drugs out of the reach of children. In case of accidental overdose, seek professional assistance or contact a poison control center immediately. As with any drug, if you are pregnant or nursing a baby, seek the advice of a health professional before using this product. **IT IS ESPECIALLY IMPORTANT NOT TO USE ASPIRIN DURING THE LAST 3 MONTHS OF PREGNANCY UNLESS SPECIFICALLY DIRECTED TO DO SO BY A DOCTOR BECAUSE IT MAY CAUSE PROBLEMS IN THE UNBORN CHILD OR COMPLICATIONS DURING DELIVERY.**

Drug Interaction Precaution: Do not take this product if you are taking a prescription drug for anticoagulation (thinning of the blood), diabetes, gout, or arthritis unless directed by doctor.

Professional Labeling:

ANTIARTHRITIC EFFECT

Indication: Conditions requiring chronic or long-term aspirin therapy for pain and/or inflammation, e.g., rheumatoid arthritis, juvenile rheumatoid arthritis, systemic lupus erythematosus, osteoarthritis (degenerative joint disease), ankylosing spondylitis, psoriatic arthritis, Reiter's syndrome, and fibrositis.

ANTIPLATELET EFFECT

In MI Prophylaxis:

Indication: Aspirin is indicated to reduce the risk of death and/or nonfatal myocardial infarction in patients with a previous infarction or unstable angina pectoris.

Clinical Trials: The indication is supported by the results of six large randomized, multicenter, placebo-controlled studies[1-7] involving 10,816 predominantly male post-myocardial infarction (MI) patients and one randomized placebo-controlled study of 1,266 men with unstable angina. Therapy with aspirin was begun at intervals after the onset of acute MI varying from less than three days to more than five years and continuing for periods of from less than one year to four years. In the unstable angina study, treatment was started within one month after the onset of unstable angina and continued for 12 weeks, and complicating conditions, such as congestive heart failure, were not included in the study. Aspirin therapy in MI patients was associated with about a 20% reduction in the risk of subsequent death and/or nonfatal reinfarction, a median absolute decrease of 3% from the 12% to 22% event rates in the placebo groups. In the aspirin-treated unstable angina patients, the reduction in risk was about 50%, a reduction in the event rate of 5% from the 10% rate in the placebo group over the 12 weeks of study.

Daily dosage of aspirin in the post-myocardial infarction studies was 300 mg in one study and 900–1,500 mg in five studies. A dose of 325 mg was used in the study of unstable angina.

Adverse Reactions: Gastrointestinal reactions: Doses of 1,000 mg per day of aspirin caused gastrointestinal symptoms and bleeding that, in some cases, were clinically significant. In the largest postinfarction study (the Aspirin Myocardial Infarction Study [AMIS] with 4,500 people), the percentage of incidences of gastrointestinal symptoms for the aspirin (1,000 mg of a standard, solid-tablet formulation) and placebo-treated subjects, respectively, were stomach pain (14.5%, 4.4%), heartburn (11.9%, 4.8%), nausea and/or vomiting (7.6%, 2.1%), hospitalization for GI disorder (4.9%, 3.5%). In the AMIS and other trials, aspirin-treated patients had increased rates of gross gastrointestinal bleeding. Symptoms and signs of gastrointestinal irritation were not significantly increased in subjects treated for unstable angina with buffered aspirin in solution.

Cardiovascular and Biochemical: In the AMIS trial, the dosage of 1,000 mg per day of aspirin was associated with small increases in systolic blood pressure (BP) (average 1.5 to 2.1 mm) and diastolic BP (0.5 to 0.6 mm), depending upon whether maximal or last available readings were used. Blood urea nitrogen and uric acid levels were also increased but by less than 1.0 mg percent. Subjects with marked hypertension or renal insufficiency had been excluded from the trial so that the clinical importance of these observations for such subjects or for any subjects treated over more prolonged periods is not known. It is recommended that patients placed on long-term aspirin treatment, even at doses of 300 mg per day, be seen at regular intervals to assess changes in these measurements.

Dosage and Administration: Although most of the studies used dosages exceeding 300 mg, two trials used only 300 mg daily and pharmacologic data indicate that this dose inhibits platelet function fully. Therefore, 300 mg or a conventional 325 mg aspirin dose daily is a reasonable routine dose that would minimize gastrointestinal adverse reactions. This use of aspirin applies to both solid oral dosage forms (buffered and plain aspirin) and buffered aspirin in solution.

In Transient Ischemic Attacks:

Indication: Aspirin is indicated for reducing the risk of recurrent transient ischemic attacks (TIAs) or stroke in men who have transient ischemia of the brain due to fibrin emboli. There is no evidence that aspirin is effective in reducing TIAs in women, or is of benefit in the treatment of completed strokes in men or women.

Clinical Trials: The indication is supported by the results of a Canadian study[8] in which 585 patients with threatened stroke were followed in a randomized clinical trial for an average of 28 months to determine whether aspirin or sulfinpyrazone, singly or in combination, was superior to placebo in preventing transient ischemic attacks, stroke, or death. The study showed that, although sulfinpyrazone had no statistically significant effect, aspirin reduced the risk of continuing transient ischemic attacks, stroke, or death by 19 percent and reduced the risk of stroke or death by 31 percent. Another aspirin study carried out in the United States with 178 patients showed a statistically significant number of "favorable outcomes," including reduced transient ischemic attacks, stroke, and death.[9]

Precautions: Patients presenting with signs and/or symptoms of TIAs should have a complete medical and neurologic evaluation. Consideration should be given to other disorders which may resemble TIAs. It is important to evaluate and treat, if appropriate, diseases associated with TIAs and stroke, such as hypertension and diabetes.

Dosage: The recommended dosage for this new indication is 1,300 mg per day (650 mg b.i.d. or 325 mg q.i.d.).

References: 1. Elwood PC, et al: A randomized controlled trial of acetylsalicylic acid in the secondary prevention of mortality from myocardial infarction. *Br Med J* 1974;1:436–440. 2. The Coronary Drug Project Research Group: Aspirin in coronary heart disease. *J Chronic Dis* 1976;29:625–642. 3. Breddin K, et al: Secondary prevention of myocardial infarction: A comparison of acetylsalicylic acid, phenprocoumon or placebo. *Homeostasis* 1979;470:263–268. 4. Aspirin Myocardial Infarction Study Research Group: A randomized, controlled trial of aspirin in persons recovered from myocardial infarction. *JAMA* 1980;245:661–669. 5. Elwood PC, Sweetnam PM: Aspirin and secondary mortality after myocardial

Continued on next page

Sterling Health—Cont.

infarction. *Lancet*, December 22–29, 1979, pp 1313–1315. 6. The Persantine-Aspirin Reinfarction Study Research Group: Persantine and aspirin in coronary heart disease. *Circulation* 1980;62:449–460. 7. Lewis, HD, et al: Protective effects of aspirin against acute myocardial infarction and death in men with unstable angina: Results of a Veterans Administration Cooperative Study. *N Engl J Med* 1983;309:396–403. 8. The Canadian Cooperative Study Group: A randomized trial of aspirin and sulfinpyrazone in threatened stroke. *N Engl J Med* 1978;299:53–59. 9. Fields WS, et al: Controlled trial of aspirin in cerebral ischemia. *Stroke* 1977;8:301–316.

How Supplied:
Genuine Bayer Aspirin 5 grains (325 mg) is supplied in packs of 12 tablets, bottles of 24, 50, 100, 200 and 300 tablets, and bottles of 50, 100 and 200 caplets.
Child-resistant safety closures on 12s, 24s, 50s, 200s, 300s tablets and 50s and 200s caplets. Bottles of 100s tablets and caplets available without safety closure for households without small children.
Shown in Product Identification Guide, page 427

Maximum BAYER® Aspirin
Aspirin (Acetylsalicylic Acid)
Tablets and Caplets

Active Ingredients: Maximum Bayer Aspirin—Aspirin 500 mg (7.7 grains) contains a thin, inert, Hydroxypropyl Methylcellulose coating for easier swallowing. This is not an enteric coating and does not alter the onset of action of Bayer Aspirin.

Inactive Ingredients: Starch and Triacetin.

Indications: Analgesic, antipyretic, anti-inflammatory. For relief of headache; painful discomfort and fever of colds and flu; sore throats; muscular aches and pains; temporary relief of minor pains of arthritis, rheumatism, bursitis, lumbago, sciatica; toothache, and pain following dental procedures; neuralgia and neuritic pain; functional menstrual pain; painful discomfort and fever accompanying immunizations.

Directions: The following dosages are those provided on the packaging, as appropriate for self- medication. Larger or more frequent dosage may be necessary as appropriate for the condition or needs of the patient. The hydroxypropyl methylcellulose coating makes Maximum Bayer Aspirin particularly appropriate for those who have difficulty in swallowing uncoated tablets/caplets.
Maximum Bayer Aspirin—500 mg (7.7 grains) tablets/caplets.
Usual Adult Dose: One or two tablets/caplets with water. May be repeated every four hours as necessary up to 8 tablets/caplets a day. Do not give to children under 12 unless directed by a doctor.

Warnings: Children and teenagers should not use this medicine for chicken pox or flu symptoms before a doctor is consulted about Reye syndrome, a rare but serious illness reported to be associated with aspirin. Do not take for pain for more than 10 days or for fever for more than 3 days unless directed by a doctor. If pain or fever persists or gets worse, if new symptoms occur, or if redness or swelling is present consult a doctor because these could be signs of a serious condition. Do not take this product if you are allergic to aspirin, have asthma, stomach problems that persist or recur, gastric ulcers or bleeding problems unless directed by a doctor. If ringing in the ears or loss of hearing occurs, consult a doctor before taking any more of this product. Keep this and all drugs out of the reach of children. In case of accidental overdose, seek professional assistance or contact a poison control center immediately. As with any drug, if you are pregnant or nursing a baby, seek the advice of a health professional before using this product. **IT IS ESPECIALLY IMPORTANT NOT TO USE ASPIRIN DURING THE LAST 3 MONTHS OF PREGNANCY UNLESS SPECIFICALLY DIRECTED TO DO SO BY A DOCTOR BECAUSE IT MAY CAUSE PROBLEMS IN THE UNBORN CHILD OR COMPLICATIONS DURING DELIVERY.**

Drug Interaction Precaution: Do not take this product if you are taking a prescription drug for anticoagulation (thinning of the blood), diabetes, gout, or arthritis unless directed by a doctor.

How Supplied:
Maximum Bayer Aspirin 500 mg (7.7 grains) is available in bottles of 30, 60 and 100 tablets, and bottles of 30 and 60 caplets.
Child-resistant safety closures on 30s bottles of tablets and caplets, 60s, bottles of caplets, and 100s bottles of tablets. Bottle of 60s tablets available without safety closure for households without young children.
Shown in Product Identification Guide, page 427

Extended-Release
BAYER® 8-Hour Aspirin
Aspirin (acetylsalicylic acid)

Active Ingredients: Each oblong white scored caplet contains 10 grains (650 mg) of aspirin in microencapsulated form.

Inactive Ingredients: Guar Gum, Microcrystalline Cellulose, Starch and other ingredients.

Indications: Extended-Release BAYER 8-Hour Aspirin is indicated for the temporary relief of low-grade pain amenable to relief with salicylates, such as in rheumatoid arthritis, osteoarthritis, spondylitis, bursitis and other forms of rheumatism, as well as in many common musculoskeletal disorders. It possesses the same advantages for other types of prolonged aches and pains, such as minor injuries, dental pain and dysmenorrhea. Its long-lasting effectiveness should also make it valuable as an analgesic in simple headache, colds, grippe, flu and other similar conditions in which aspirin is indicated for symptomatic relief, either by itself or as an adjunct to specific therapy.

Directions: Two Extended-Release BAYER 8-Hour Aspirin caplets q. 8 h. provide effective long-lasting pain relief. This two-caplet (20 grain or 1300 mg) dose of extended-release aspirin promptly produces salicylate blood levels greater than those achieved by a 10-grain (650 mg) dose of regular aspirin, and in the second 4-hour period produces a salicylate blood level curve which approximates that of two successive 10-grain (650 mg) doses of regular aspirin at 4-hour intervals. The 10-grain (650 mg) scored Extended-Release BAYER 8-Hour Aspirin caplets permit administration of aspirin in multiples of 5 grains (325 mg) allowing individualization of dosage to meet the specific needs of the patient. For the convenience of patients on a regular aspirin dosage schedule, two 10-grain (650 mg) Extended-Release BAYER 8-Hour Aspirin caplets may be administered with water every 8 hours. Whenever necessary, two caplets (20 grains or 1300 mg) should be given before retiring to provide effective analgesic and anti-inflammatory action—for relief of pain throughout the night and lessening of stiffness upon arising. Do not exceed 6 caplets in 24 hours. Extended-Release BAYER 8-Hour Aspirin has been made in a special caplet to permit easy swallowing. However, for patients who do have difficulty, Extended-Release BAYER 8-Hour Aspirin caplets may be gently crumbled in the mouth and swallowed with water without loss of timed-release effect. There is no bitter "aspirin" taste. For children under 12, consult physician.

Warnings: Children and teenagers should not use this medicine for chicken pox or flu symptoms before a doctor is consulted about Reye syndrome, a rare but serious illness reported to be associated with aspirin. Do not take for pain for more than 10 days or for fever for more than 3 days unless directed by a doctor. If pain or fever persists or gets worse, if new symptoms occur, or if redness or swelling is present consult a doctor because these could be signs of a serious condition. Do not take this product if you are allergic to aspirin, have asthma, stomach problems that persist or recur, gastric ulcers or bleeding problems unless directed by a doctor. If ringing in the ears or loss of hearing occurs, consult a doctor before taking any more of this product. Keep this and all drugs out of the reach of children. In case of accidental overdose, seek professional assistance or contact a poison control center immediately. As with any drug, if you are pregnant or nursing a baby, seek the advice of a health professional before using this product. **IT IS ESPECIALLY IMPORTANT NOT TO USE ASPIRIN DURING THE LAST 3 MONTHS OF PREGNANCY UNLESS SPECIFICALLY DIRECTED TO DO SO BY A DOCTOR BECAUSE IT MAY CAUSE PROBLEMS IN THE UNBORN CHILD OR COMPLICATIONS DURING DELIVERY.**

Drug Interaction Precaution: Do not take this product if you are taking a prescription drug for anticoagulation (thinning of the blood), diabetes, gout, or arthritis unless directed by a doctor.

How Supplied: Extended-Release Bayer 8-Hour Aspirin 650 mg (10 grains) is supplied in bottles of 72 and 125 caplets.
The 72s size, without a child-resistant safety closure, is recommended for households without young children.

BAYER® ENTERIC Aspirin
Delayed Release Enteric Aspirin
Extra Strength 500 mg and
Regular Strength 325 mg Caplets and
Adult Low Strength 81 mg Tablets

Composition: Active Ingredient: BAYER® ENTERIC is an enteric-coated aspirin available in 500 mg and 325 mg caplet and 81 mg tablet forms. The enteric coating prevents disintegration in the stomach and promotes dissolution in the duodenum, where there is a more neutral to alkaline environment. This action aids in protecting the stomach against injuries that may occur as a result of ingesting non-enteric coated aspirin.

Safety: The safety of enteric-coated aspirin has been demonstrated in a number of endoscopic studies comparing enteric-coated aspirin and plain aspirin, as well as buffered aspirin and "arthritis strength" preparations. In these studies, endoscopies were performed in healthy volunteers before and after either 2-day or 14-day administration of aspirin doses of 3,900 or 4,000 mg per day. Compared to all the other preparations, the enteric-coated aspirin produced signficantly less damage to the gastric mucosa. There was also statistically less duodenal damage when compared with the plain, i.e., non-enteric-coated aspirin.

Bioavailability: The bioavailability of aspirin from **BAYER® ENTERIC** has been confirmed. In single-dose studies[1] in which plasma acetylsalicylic acid and salicylic acid levels were measured, maximum concentrations were achieved at approximately 5 hours postdosing. **BAYER® ENTERIC,** when compared with plain aspirin, achieves maximum plasma salicylate levels not significantly different from plain, i.e., non-enteric-coated, aspirin. Dissolution of the enteric

coating occurs at a neutral to basic pH and is therefore dependent on gastric emptying into the duodenum. With continued dosing, appropriate therapeutic plasma levels are maintained.

Inactive Ingredients: Extra Strength 500mg—Acetylated Monoglycerides, D&C Yellow #10, FD&C Yellow #6, Hydroxypropyl Methylcellulose, Hydroxypropyl Methylcellulose Phthalate, Iron Oxides, Microcrystalline Cellulose, Polyethylene Glycol, Sodium Starch Glycolate, Starch, Titanium Dioxide.
Regular Strength 325mg—D&C Yellow #10, FD&C Yellow #6, Hydroxypropyl Methylcellulose, Methacrylic Acid Copolymer, Starch, Titanium Dioxide, Triacetin.
Adult Low Strength 81mg—Croscarmellose Sodium, D&C Yellow #10, FD&C Yellow #6, Hydroxypropyl Methylcellulose, Iron Oxides, Lactose, Methacrylic Acid, Microcrystalline Cellulose, Polysorbate 80, Sodium Lauryl Sulfate, Starch, Titanium Dioxide, Triacetin.

Indications: BAYER® ENTERIC is an anti-inflammatory, analgesic, and antiplatelet agent indicated for the relief of painful discomfort and muscular aches and pains associated with conditions requiring long-term aspirin therapy, e.g., arthritis or rheumatism, and for situations where compliance with aspirin usage may be hindered by gastrointestinal side effects of non-enteric-coated or buffered aspirin. For additional **Anti-inflammatory, Antiarthritic,** and **Antiplatelet** indications, see the **PROFESSIONAL LABELING** section.

Directions: The following dosages are provided as appropriate for self-medication:
For analgesic indications the maximum adult nonprescription dosage of aspirin is 4,000 mg per day in divided doses, i.e., two 500 mg caplets every six hours or two 325 mg caplets or eight 81 mg tablets every 4 hours or three 325 mg caplets or twelve 81 mg tablets every 6 hours. Under a physician's recommendation, the dosage or frequency may be modified as appropriate for the clinical situation.

Consumer Warnings: Children and teenagers should not use this medicine for chicken pox or flu symptoms before a doctor is consulted about Reye Syndrome, a rare but serious illness reported to be associated with aspirin. Do not take for pain for more than 10 days or for fever for more than 3 days unless directed by a doctor. If pain or fever persists or gets worse, if new symptoms occur, or if redness or swelling is present, consult a doctor because these could be signs of a serious condition. Do not take this product if you are allergic to aspirin, have asthma, have stomach problems (such as heartburn, upset stomach or stomach pain) that persist or recur, or have gastric ulcers or bleeding problems unless directed by a doctor. If ringing in the ears or loss of hearing occurs, consult a doctor before taking any more of this product. Keep out of reach of children. In case of

accidental overdose, contact a doctor immediately. As with any drug, if you are pregnant or nursing a baby, seek the advice of a health professional before using this product. **IT IS ESPECIALLY IMPORTANT NOT TO USE ASPIRIN DURING THE LAST 3 MONTHS OF PREGNANCY UNLESS SPECIFICALLY DIRECTED TO DO SO BY A DOCTOR BECAUSE IT MAY CAUSE PROBLEMS IN THE UNBORN CHILD OR COMPLICATIONS DURING DELIVERY.**

Drug Interaction Precaution: Do not take this product if you are taking a prescription drug for anticoagulation (thinning of the blood), diabetes, gout, or arthritis unless directed by a doctor.

Professional Labeling:

Antiarthritic and Anti-inflammatory Effect

Indications: For conditions requiring chronic or long-term aspirin therapy for pain and/or inflammation, e.g., rheumatoid arthritis, juvenile rheumatoid arthritis, systemic lupus erythematosus, osteoarthritis (degenerative joint disease), ankylosing spondylitis, psoriatic arthritis, Reiter's syndrome, and fibrositis.

Antiplatelet Effect
Aspirin for Myocardial Infarction

Indication: Aspirin is indicated to reduce the risk of death and/or nonfatal myocardial infarction in patients with a previous infarction or unstable angina pectoris.

Clinical Trials: The indication is supported by the results of six large, randomized, multicenter, placebo-controlled studies involving 10,816 predominantly male, post-myocardial infarction (MI) patients and one randomized placebo-controlled study of 1,266 men with unstable angina.[2,8] Therapy wih aspirin was begun at intervals after the onset of acute MI varying from less than 3 days to more than 5 years and continued for periods of from less than 1 year to 4 years. In the unstable angina study, treatment was started within 1 month after onset of unstable angina and continued for 12 weeks, and patients with complicating conditions, such as congestive heart failure, were not included in the study.
Aspirin therapy in MI patients was associated with about a 20 percent reduction in the risk of subsequent death and/or nonfatal reinfarction, a median absolute decrease of 3 percent from the 12 to 22 percent event rates in the placebo groups. In aspirin-treated unstable angina patients, the reduction in risk was

Continued on next page

This product information was effective as of November 1, 1993. Current information may be obtained directly from Sterling Health, by writing to 90 Park Avenue, New York, NY 10016.

Sterling Health—Cont.

about 50 percent, a reduction in the event rate of 5 percent from the 10 percent rate in the placebo group over the 12 weeks of the study.

Daily dosage of aspirin in the post-myocardial infarction studies was 300 mg in one study and 900 to 1,500 mg in five studies. A dose of 325 mg was used in the study of unstable angina.

Dosage and Administration: Although most of the studies used dosages exceeding 300 mg, two trials used only 300 mg and pharmacological data indicate that this dose inhibits platelet function fully. Therefore, 300 mg or a conventional 325 mg aspirin dose is a reasonable, routine dose that would minimize gastrointestinal adverse reactions. This use of aspirin applies to both solid oral dosage forms (buffered and plain aspirin) and buffered aspirin in solution.

Aspirin for Transient Ischemic Attacks

Indications: For reducing the risk of recurrent Transient Ischemic Attacks (TIAs) or storke in men who have transient ischemia of the brain due to fibrin emboli. There is inadequate evidence that aspirin or buffered aspirin is effective in reducing TIAs in women at the recommended dosage. There is no evidence that aspirin or buffered aspirin is of benefit in the treatment of completed strokes in men or women.

Clinical Trials: The indication is supported by the result of a Canadian study[9] in which 585 patients with threatened stroke followed in a randomized clinical trial for an average of 28 months to determine whether aspirin or sulfinpyrazone, singly or in combination, was superior to placebo in preventing transient ischemic attacks, stroke, or death. The study showed that although sulfinpyrazone had no statistically significant effect, aspirin reduced the risk of continuing transient ischemic attacks, stroke or death by 19 percent and reduced the risk of stroke or death by 31 percent. Another aspirin study trial carried out in the United States with 178 patients showed a statiscally significant number of "favorable outcomes" including reduced transient ischemic attacks, stroke, and death.[10]

Precautions: Patients presenting with signs and symptoms of a TIA should have a complete medical and neurological evaluation. Consideration should be given to other disorders that resemble TIAs. Attention should be given to risk factors; it is important to evaluate and treat, if appropriate, other diseases associated with TIAs and stroke, such as hypertension and diabetes.

Dosage and Administration: Adult oral dosage for men is 1,300 mg a day, in divided doses of 650 mg twice a day or 325 mg four times daily.

Adverse Reactions: Gastrointestinal Reactions: Doses of 1,000 mg per day of aspirin caused gastrointestinal symptoms and bleeding that in some cases were clinically significant. In the largest post-infarction study (the Aspirin Myocardial Infarction Study [AMIS] with 4,500 people), the percentage incidence of gastrointestinal symptoms for the aspirin- (1,000 mg of a standard, solid tablet formulation) and placebo-treated subjects, respectively, were: stomach pain (14.5 percent, 4.4 percent); heartburn (11.9 percent, 4.8 percent), nausea and/or vomiting (7.6 percent, 2.1 percent); hospitalization for gastrointestinal disorder (4.8 percent, 3.5 percent). In the AMIS and other trials, aspirin-treated patients had increased rates of gross gastrointestinal bleeding. Symptoms and signs of gastrointestinal irritation were not significantly increased in subjects treated for unstable angina with buffered aspirin in solution.

Cardiovascular and Biochemical: In the AMIS trial the dosage of 1,000 mg per day of aspirin was associated with small increases in systolic blood pressure (BP) (average 1.5 to 2.1 mm) and diastolic BP (0.5 to 2.1 mm), depending upon whether maximal or last available readings were used. Blood urea nitrogen and uric acid levels were also increased, but by less than 1.0 mg%. Subjects with marked hypertension or renal insufficiency had been excluded from trial so that the clinical importance of these observations for such subjects or for any subject treated over more prolonged periods is not known. It is recommended that patients placed on long-term aspirin treatment, even at doses of 300 mg per day, be seen at regular intervals to assess changes in these measurements.

Other Precautions: Concurrent administration of absorbable antacids at therapeutic doses may increase the clearance of salicylates in some individuals. The concurrent administration of nonabsorbable antacids may alter the rate of absorption of aspirin, resulting in a decreased acetylsalicylic acid/salicylate ratio in plasma. The clinical significance of these decreases in available aspirin is unknown.

Occasional reports have documented individuals with impaired gastric emptying in whom there may be retention of one or more enteric-coated tablets over time. This phenomenon may occur as a result of outlet obstruction from ulcer disease alone or combined with hypotonic gastric peristalsis. Because of the integrity of the enteric coating in an acidic environment, these tablets may accumulate and form a bezoar in the stomach. Individuals with this condition may present with complaints of early satiety or of vague upper abdominal distress. Diagnosis may be made by endoscopy or by abdominal films, which show opacities suggestive of a mass of small tablets.[11] Management may vary according to the condition of the patient. Options include gastrotomy and alternating slightly basic and neutral lavage.[12] While there have been no clinical reports, it has been suggested that such individuals may also be treated with parenteral cimetidine (to reduce acid secretion) and then given sips of slightly basic liquids to effect gradual dissolution of the enteric coating. Progress may be followed with plasma salicylate levels or via recognition of tinnitus by the patient. **It should be kept in mind that individuals with a history of partial or complete gastrectomy may produce reduced amounts of acid and therefore have less acidic gastric pH. Under these circumstances, the benefits offered by the acid-resistant enteric coating may not exist.**

References: 1. Data on file, Sterling Health. 2. Elwood PC, et al: A randomized controlled trial of acetylsalicylic acid in the secondary preventive of mortality from myocardial infarction. *Br Med J* 1974;1:436–440. 3. The Coronary Drug Project Research Group: Aspirin in coronary heart disease. *J Chronic Dis* 1976;29:625–642. 4. Breddin K, et al: Secondary prevention of myocardial infarction: A comparison of acetylsalicylic acid, phenprocoumon or placebo. *Homeostasis* 1979;470:263–268. 5. Aspirin Myocardial Infarction Study Research Group: A randomized, controlled trial of aspirin in persons recovered from myocardial infarction. *JAMA* 1980;245:661–669. 6. Elwood PC, Sweetnam PM: Aspirin and secondary mortality after myocardial infarction. *Lancet*, December 22–29, 1979, pp 1313–1315. 7. The Persantine-Aspirin Reinfarction Study Research Group: Persantine and aspirin in coronary heart disease. *Circulation* 1980;62:449–460. 8. Lewis HD, et al: Protective effects of aspirin against acute myocardial infarction and death in men with unstable angina: Results of a Veterans Administration Cooperative Study. *N Engl J Med* 1983;309:396–403. 9. The Canadian Cooperative Study Group: A randomized trial of aspirin and sulfinpyrazone in threatened stroke. *N Eng J Med* 1978;299:53–59. 10. Fields WS, et al: Controlled trial of aspirin in cerebral ischemia. *Stroke* 1977;8:301–316. 11. Bogacz K, Caldron P: Enteric-coated aspirin bezoar: Elevation of serum salicylate level by barium study. *Am J Med* 1987;83:783–786. 12. Baum J: Enteric-coated aspirin and the problem of gastric retention. *J Rheumatol* 1984;11:250–251.

How Supplied: Extra Strength BAYER Enteric 500 mg caplets in bottles of 60 with child-resistant safety closure. Regular Strength BAYER Enteric 325 mg caplets in bottles of 50, 100. Child-resistant safety closure on 50s caplets. Bottles of 100 caplets available without safety closure for households without small children.

Adult Low Strenth BAYER Enteric 81 mg tablets in bottles of 120 with child-resistant safety closure.

REV. 10/93

Shown in Product Identification Guide, page 427

Extra Strength BAYER® PLUS
Buffered Aspirin

Active Ingredients: Each Extra Strength Bayer Plus contains Aspirin (500 mg), in a formulation buffered with Calcium Carbonate, Magnesium Carbonate, and Magnesium Oxide.

Inactive Ingredients: Corn Starch, FD&C Blue #2, Hydroxypropyl Cellulose, Hydroxypropyl Methylcellulose, Methylparaben, Microcrystalline Cellulose, Propylene Glycol, Propylparaben, Sodium Starch Glycolate, Zinc Stearate.

Indications: Analgesic, antipyretic, anti-inflammatory. For relief of headache; painful discomfort and fever of colds and flu; muscular aches and pains; temporary relief of minor pains of arthritis, rheumatism, bursitis, lumbago, sciatica; toothache, and pain following dental procedures; neuralgia and neuritic pain; functional menstrual pain; painful discomfort and fever accompanying immunizations.

Directions: The following dosages are those provided in the packaging, as appropriate for self-medication. Larger or more frequent dosage may be necessary as appropriate to the condition or needs of the patient. The addition of buffering agents makes Extra Strength Bayer® Plus particularly appropriate for those who must take frequent doses of aspirin. The hydroxypropyl methylcellulose coating benefits aspirin users who have difficulty in swallowing uncoated tablets and caplets.
Usual Adult Dose: One or two caplets with water. May be repeated every four to 6 hours as necessary up to 8 caplets a day, or as directed by a doctor. Do not give to children under 12 unless directed by a doctor.

Warnings: Children and teenagers should not use this medicine for chicken pox or flu symptoms before a doctor is consulted about Reye syndrome, a rare but serious illness reported to be associated with aspirin. Do not take for pain for more than 10 days or for fever for more than 3 days unless directed by a doctor. If pain or fever persists or gets worse, if new symptoms occur, or if redness or swelling is present consult a doctor because these could be signs of a serious condition. Do not take this product if you are allergic to aspirin, have asthma, stomach problems that persist or recur, gastric ulcers or bleeding problems unless directed by a doctor. If ringing in the ears or loss of hearing occurs, consult a doctor before taking any more of this product. Keep this and all drugs out of the reach of children. In case of accidental overdose, seek professional assistance or contact a poison control center immediately. As with any drug, if you are pregnant or nursing a baby, seek the advice of a health professional before using this product. **IT IS ESPECIALLY IMPORTANT NOT TO USE ASPIRIN DURING THE LAST 3 MONTHS OF PREGNANCY UNLESS SPECIFICALLY DIRECTED TO DO SO BY A DOCTOR BECAUSE IT MAY CAUSE PROBLEMS IN THE UNBORN CHILD OR COMPLICATIONS DURING DELIVERY.**

Drug Interaction Precaution: Do not take this product if you are taking a prescription drug for anticoagulation (thinning of the blood), diabetes, gout, or arthritis unless directed by a doctor.

How Supplied: Extra Strength Bayer® Plus Aspirin (500 mg) is available in bottles of 30 and 60 caplets. Child resistant closure on 30s caplets. Bottles of 60s caplets available without safety closure for households without young children.
Shown in Product Identification Guide, page 428

BAYER® SELECT™ CHEST COLD
Cough Suppressant, Pain Reliever

Active Ingredients: 500mg Acetaminophen and 15mg Dextromethorphan HBr per caplet

Inactive Ingredients: Croscarmellose Sodium, D&C Red #27 Lake, FD&C Blue #1 Lake, FD&C Blue #2 Lake, Hydroxypropyl Methylcellulose, Iron Oxide, Magnesium Stearate, Microcrystalline Cellulose, Polyethylene Glycol, Polysorbate 80, Providone, Starch, Titanium Dioxide.

Indications: Temporarily calms and controls cough without narcotic side effects; temporarily relieves minor sore throat pain and body aches and pains.

Directions: Adults: Take 2 caplets with water every 6 hours up to a maximum of 8 caplets per 24 hours or as directed by a doctor. Children under 12 years of age: Consult your doctor.

Warnings: Do not take this product for more than 7 days. A persistent cough may be a sign of a serious condition. If cough persists for more than 7 days, tends to recur, or is accompanied by rash, persistent headache or fever that lasts for more than 3 days, or if new symptoms occur, consult a doctor. If sore throat is severe, persists for more than 2 days, is accompanied or followed by fever, headache, rash, nausea, or vomiting, consult a doctor promptly. Do not take this product for persistent or chronic cough such as occurs with smoking, asthma, or emphysema, or where cough is accompanied by excessive phlegm (mucus) unless directed by a doctor. Keep this and all drugs out of reach of children. In case of accidental overdose, seek professional assistance or contact a poison control center. Prompt medical attention is essential for adults as well as for children even if you do not notice any signs or symptoms. As with any drug, if you are pregnant or nursing a baby, seek the advice of a health professional before using this product.

Drug Interaction Precaution: Do not use this product if you are taking a prescription drug containing a monoamine oxidase inhibitor (MAOI) (certain drugs for depression or psychiatric or emotional conditions) without first consulting a doctor. If you are uncertain whether your prescription drug contains an MAOI, consult a health professional before taking this product.

How Supplied: Bayer Select Chest Cold is packaged in child resistant blister packages containing 16 caplets.
Shown in Product Identification Guide, page 427

BAYER® SELECT™ FLU RELIEF
Pain Reliever/Fever Reducer, Nasal Decongestant, Cough Suppressant, Antihistamine

Active Ingredients: 500 mg Acetaminophen, 30 mg Pseudoephedrine HCl, 15 mg Dextromethorphan HBr and 2 mg Chlorpheniramine Maleate per caplet.

Inactive Ingredients: Croscarmellose Sodium, D&C Red #27 Lake, FD&C Blue #2 Lake, FD&C Yellow #6 Lake, Hydroxypropyl Methylcellulose, Iron Oxide, Magnesium Stearate, Microcrystalline Cellulose, Polyethylene Glycol, Polysorbate 80, Starch, Titanium Dioxide.

Indications: Temporarily relieves body aches and pains, headache, fever and minor sore throat pain; temporarily relieves nasal congestion and reduces swollen nasal passages; temporarily calms and controls your tough cough; temporarily dries runny nose and relieves sneezing.

Directions: Adults: Take 2 caplets with water every 6 hours up to a maximum of 8 caplets per 24 hours or as directed by a doctor. Children under 12 years of age: Consult your doctor.

Warnings: Do not exceed recommended dosage because at higher doses nervousness, dizziness or sleeplessness may occur. May cause marked drowsiness; alcohol, sedatives, and tranquilizers may increase the drowsiness effect. Avoid alcoholic beverages while taking this product. Do not take this product if you are taking sedatives or tranquilizers without first consulting a doctor. Use caution when driving a motor vehicle or operating machinery. May cause excitability especially in children. Do not take this product, unless directed by a doctor, if you have breathing problems such as emphysema, or chronic bronchitis or if you have glaucoma or difficulty in urination due to enlargement of the prostate gland. Do not take this product for more than 7 days. If symptoms do not improve or are accompanied by fever that lasts for more than 3 days, or if new symptoms occur, consult a doctor. If sore throat is

Continued on next page

This product information was effective as of November 1, 1993. Current information may be obtained directly from Sterling Health, by writing to 90 Park Avenue, New York, NY 10016.

Sterling Health—Cont.

severe, persists for more than 2 days, is accompanied or followed by fever, headache, rash, nausea, or vomiting, consult a doctor promptly. Do not take this product for persistent or chronic cough such as occurs with smoking, asthma, or emphysema, or where cough is accompanied by excessive phlegm (mucus) unless directed by a doctor. A persistent cough may be a sign of a serious condition. If cough persists for more than 1 week, tends to recur, or is accompanied by fever, rash, or persistent headache, consult a doctor. Keep this and all drugs out of reach of children. In case of accidental overdose, seek professional assistance or contact a poison control center. Prompt medical attention is essential for adults as well as for children even if you do not notice any signs or symptoms. As with any drug, if you are pregnant or nursing a baby, seek the advice of a health professional before using this product.

Drug Interaction Precaution: Do not use this product if you are taking a prescription drug containing a monoamine oxidase inhibitor (MAOI) (certain drugs for depression or psychiatric or emotional conditions) without first consulting a doctor. If you are uncertain whether your prescription drug contains an MAOI, consult a health professional before taking this product.

How Supplied: Bayer Select Flu Relief is packaged in child resistant blister packages containing 16 caplets.
Shown in Product Identification Guide, page 427

BAYER® SELECT™ HEAD & CHEST COLD
Nasal Decongestant, Cough Suppressant, Expectorant, Pain Reliever

Active Ingredients: 325mg Acetaminophen, 100mg Guaifenesin, 30mg Pseudoephedrine HCl and 10mg Dextromethorphan HBr per caplet.

Inactive Ingredients: FD&C Blue #2 Lake, FD&C Yellow #6 Lake, Hydroxypropyl Methylcellulose, Iron Oxide, Magnesium Stearate, Microcrystalline Cellulose, Polyethylene Glycol, Polysorbate 80, Povidone, Sodium Starch Glycolate, Sodium Stearyl Fumarate, Starch, Titanium Dioxide.

Indications: Temporarily relieves nasal congestion and reduces swollen nasal passages; temporarily calms and controls your tough cough; helps loosen phlegm (mucus) and thin bronchial secretions to clear chest congestion; temporarily relieves headache, minor sore throat pain and body aches and pains.

Warnings: Do not exceed recommended dosage because at higher doses nervousness, dizziness or sleeplessness may occur. Do not take this product for more than 7 days. If symptoms do not improve or are accompanied by fever that lasts for more than 3 days, or if new

symptoms occur, consult a doctor. If sore throat is severe, persists for more than 2 days, is accompanied or followed by fever, headache, rash, nausea, or vomiting, consult a doctor promptly. Do not take this product if you have heart disease, high blood pressure, thyroid disease, diabetes or difficulty in urination due to enlargement of the prostate gland unless directed by a doctor. Do not take this product for persistent or chronic cough such as occurs with smoking, asthma, chronic bronchitis or emphysema, or where cough is accompanied by excessive phlegm (mucus) unless directed by a doctor. A persistent cough may be a sign of a serious condition. If cough persists for more than 7 days, tends to recur, or is accompanied by fever, rash, or persistent headache, consult a doctor. Keep this and all drugs out of reach of children. In case of accidental overdose, seek professional assistance or contact a poison control center. Prompt medical attention is essential for adults as well as for children even if you do not notice any signs or symptoms. As with any drug, if you are pregnant or nursing a baby, seek the advice of a health professional before using this product.

Drug Interaction Precaution: Do not use this product if you are taking a prescription drug containing a monoamine oxidase inhibitor (MAO)(certain drugs for depression or psychiatric or emotional conditions) without first consulting a doctor. If you are uncertain whether your prescription drug contains an MAOI, consult a health professional before taking this product.

How Supplied: Bayer Select Head and Chest Cold is packaged in child resistant blister packages containing 16 caplets.
Shown in Product Identification Guide, page 427

BAYER® SELECT™ HEAD COLD
Nasal Decongestant, Pain Reliever

Active Ingredients: 500mg Acetaminophen and 30mg Pseudoephedrine HCl per caplet.

Inactive Ingredients: Colloidal Silicon Dioxide, D&C Yellow #10 Lake, FD&C Blue #1 Lake, FD&C Blue #2 Lake, FD&C Yellow #6 Lake, Hydroxypropyl Methylcellulose, Iron Oxide, Magnesium Stearate, Microcrystalline Cellulose, Polyethylene Glycol, Polysorbate 80, Povidone, Starch, Titanium Dioxide

Indications: Temporarily relieves nasal congestion and sinus pressure and reduces swollen nasal passages; temporarily relieves headache, minor sore throat pain and body aches and pains.

Directions: Adults: Take 2 caplets with water every 6 hours up to a maximum of 8 caplets per 24 hours or as directed by a doctor. Children under 12 years of age: Consult your doctor.

Warnings: Do not exceed recommended dosage because at higher doses nervousness, dizziness or sleeplessness may occur. Do not take this product for

more than 7 days. If symptoms do not improve or are accompanied by fever that lasts for more than 3 days, or if new symptoms occur, consult a doctor. If sore throat is severe, persists for more than 2 days, is accompanied or followed by fever, headache, rash, nausea, or vomiting, consult a doctor promptly. Do not take this product if you have heart disease, high blood pressure, thyroid disease, diabetes or difficulty in urination due to enlargement of the prostate gland unless directed by a doctor. Keep this and all drugs out of reach of children. In case of accidental overdose, seek professional assistance or contact a poison control center immediately. Prompt medical attention is essential for adults as well as for children even if you do not notice any signs or symptoms. As with any drug, if you are pregnant or nursing a baby, seek the advice of a health professional before using this product.

Drug Interaction Precaution: Do not use this product if you are taking a prescription drug containing a monoamine oxidase inhibitor (MAOI)(certain drugs for depression or psychiatric or emotional conditions) without first consulting a doctor. If you are uncertain whether your prescription drug contains an MAOI, consult a health professional before taking this product.

How Supplied: Bayer Select Head Cold is packaged in child resistant blister packages containing 16 caplets.
Shown in Product Identification Guide, page 427

BAYER® SELECT™ IBUPROFEN
Pain Relief Formula
Pain Reliever/Fever Reducer

Warning: ASPIRIN SENSITIVE PATIENTS. Do not take this product if you have had a severe allergic reaction to aspirin, e.g.-asthma, swelling, shock or hives, because even though this product contains no aspirin or salicylates, cross-reactions may occur in patients allergic to aspirin.

Active Ingredient: 200 mg Ibuprofen USP per caplet

Inactive Ingredients: Colloidal Silicon Dioxide, Dibasic Calcium Phosphate, Hydroxypropyl Methylcellulose, Magnesium Stearate, Microcrystalline Cellulose, Polyethylene Glycol, Polysorbate 80, Sodium Lauryl Sulfate, Sodium Starch Glycolate, Stearic Acid, Titanium Dioxide.

Indications: For the temporary relief of minor aches and pains associated with the common cold, headache, toothache, muscular aches, backache, for the minor pain of arthritis, for the pain of menstrual cramps and for reduction of fever.

Directions: ADULTS: Take 1 caplet every 4 to 6 hours while symptoms persist. If pain or fever does not respond to 1 caplet, 2 caplets may be used but do not exceed 6 caplets in 24 hours, unless directed by a doctor. The smallest effective dose should be used. Take with food or milk if occasional and mild heartburn, upset stomach, or stomach pain occurs with use. Consult a doctor if these symptoms are more than mild or if they persist. CHILDREN: Do not give this product to children under 12 except under the advice and supervision of a doctor.

Warnings: Do not take for pain for more than 10 days or for fever for more than 3 days unless directed by a doctor. If pain or fever persists or gets worse, if new symptoms occur, or if the painful area is red or swollen, consult a doctor. These could be signs of a serious illness. If you are under a doctor's care for any serious condition, consult a doctor before taking this product. As with aspirin and acetaminophen, if you have any condition which requires you to take prescription drugs or if you have had any problems or serious side effects from taking any non-prescription pain reliever, do not take this product without first discussing it with your doctor. If you experience any symptoms which are unusual or seem unrelated to the condition for which you took ibuprofen, consult a doctor before taking any more of it. Although ibuprofen is indicated for the same conditions as aspirin and acetaminophen, it should not be taken with them except under a doctor's direction. Do not combine this product with any other ibuprofen containing product. As with any drug if you are pregnant or nursing a baby, seek the advice of a health professional before using this product. IT IS ESPECIALLY IMPORTANT NOT TO USE IBUPROFEN DURING THE LAST 3 MONTHS OF PREGNANCY UNLESS SPECIFICALLY DIRECTED TO DO SO BY A DOCTOR BECAUSE IT MAY CAUSE PROBLEMS IN THE UNBORN CHILD OR COMPLICATIONS DURING DELIVERY. Keep this and all drugs out of the reach of children. In case of accidental overdose, seek professional assistance or contact a poison control center immediately.

How Supplied: BAYER® SELECT™ IBUPROFEN Pain Relief Formula is available in 24, 50 and 100 count bottles.
Shown in Product Identification Guide, page 427

BAYER® SELECT™
Maximum Strength HEADACHE
Pain Relief Formula
Aspirin-Free

Active Ingredients: Acetaminophen 500 mg and Caffeine 65 mg per caplet.

Inactive Ingredients: Croscarmellose Sodium, FD&C Blue #2, Hydroxypropyl Methylcellulose, Magnesium Stearate, Microcrystalline Cellulose, Polyethylene Glycol, Potassium Sorbate, Starch, Titanium Dioxide, Xanthan Gum.

Indications: BAYER® SELECT™ HEADACHE Pain Relief Formula contains a specially chosen combination of safe, aspirin-free ingredients in a maxi-mum dosage form for strong, fast, temporary relief of HEADACHES.

Directions: Adults: Take 2 caplets with water every 4 hours, as needed, up to a maximum of 8 caplets per 24 hours. **Children under 12 years of age:** Consult a doctor.

Warnings: Do not take this product for pain for more than 10 days or fever for more than 3 days unless directed by a doctor. If pain is severe or recurrent, or fever persists or gets worse, if new symptoms occur, or if redness or swelling is present, consult a doctor because these could be signs of a serious condition. The recommended dose of this product contains about as much caffeine as a cup of coffee. Limit use of caffeine containing medications, foods, or beverages while taking this product because too much caffeine may cause nervousness, irritability, sleeplessness, and occasionally rapid heart beat. Keep out of reach of children. In case of accidental overdose, prompt medical attention is essential for adults as well as for children even if you do not notice any signs or symptoms. Contact a doctor immediately. As with any drug, if you are pregnant or nursing a baby, seek the advice of a health professional before using this product.

How Supplied: BAYER® SELECT™ Maximum Strength HEADACHE Pain Relief Formula is available in 24, 50 and 100 count bottles.
Shown in Product Identification Guide, page 427

BAYER® SELECT™
Maximum Strength MENSTRUAL
Multi-Symptom Formula
Aspirin-Free

Active Ingredients: Acetaminophen 500 mg and Pamabrom 25 mg per caplet.

Inactive Ingredients: Croscarmellose Sodium, D&C Red #27, Hydroxypropyl Methylcellulose, Iron Oxide, Magnesium Stearate, Microcrystalline Cellulose, Polyethylene Glycol, Polysorbate 80, Starch, Titanium Dioxide.

Indications: BAYER® SELECT™ MENSTRUAL Multi-Symptom Formula contains a specially chosen combination of safe, aspirin-free, caffeine-free ingredients that is not found in any ordinary pain reliever to provide temporary relief of the following symptoms associated with PREMENSTRUAL and MENSTRUAL pain and discomfort:
- Cramps
- Bloating
- Backache
- Water-weight gain
- Headache
- Muscular aches and pains

Directions: Adults: Take 2 caplets with water every 4 hours, as needed, up to a maximum of 8 caplets per 24 hours. **Children under 12 years of age:** Consult a doctor.

Warnings: Do not take for pain for more than 10 days unless directed by a doctor. Consult a doctor if pain is severe or recurrent, as this may be a sign of serious illness. Keep out of reach of children. In case of accidental overdose, prompt medical attention is essential for adults as well as for children even if you do not notice any signs or symptoms. As with any drug, if you are pregnant or nursing a baby, seek the advice of a health professional before using this product.

How Supplied: BAYER® SELECT™ Maximum Strength MENSTRUAL Multi-Symptom Formula is available in 24 and 50 count bottles.
Shown in Product Identification Guide, page 427

BAYER® SELECT™
Maximum Strength
NIGHT TIME PAIN RELIEF
Analgesic/Sleep Aid Formula for Pain with Sleeplessness
Aspirin-Free

Active Ingredients: Acetaminophen 500 mg and Diphenhydramine HCl 25 mg per caplet.

Inactive Ingredients: FD&C Blue #1 and #2, Hydroxypropyl Methylcellulose, Polyethylene Glycol, Polysorbate 80, Potassium Sorbate, Povidone, Starch, Stearic Acid, Talc, Titanium Dioxide.

Indications: BAYER® SELECT™ NIGHT TIME PAIN RELIEF Formula contains a specially chosen combination of safe, aspirin-free, caffeine-free ingredients in a maximum dosage form to provide temporary relief of minor aches and NIGHT TIME PAIN while helping you fall asleep safely and gently.

Directions: Adults: Take 2 caplets at bedtime if needed or as directed by a doctor. Do not exceed recommended dosage.

Warnings: Do not give this product to children under 12 years of age or use for more than 10 days unless directed by a doctor. Consult a doctor if pain is severe, recurrent, persists or gets worse, if new symptoms occur, or if sleeplessness persists continuously for more than 2 weeks. These may be symptoms of a serious underlying medical illness. Do not take this product, unless directed by a doctor, if you have breathing problems such as emphysema or chronic bronchitis or if you have glaucoma, or difficulty in urination due to enlargement of the prostate gland. Avoid alcoholic beverages while taking this product. Do not take this product if

Continued on next page

This product information was effective as of November 1, 1993. Current information may be obtained directly from Sterling Health, by writing to 90 Park Avenue, New York, NY 10016.

Sterling Health—Cont.

you are taking sedatives or tranquilizers without first consulting your doctor. Keep out of reach of children. In case of accidental overdose, prompt medical attention is essential for adults as well as for children even if you do not notice any signs or symptoms. Contact a doctor immediately. As with any drug, if you are pregnant or nursing a baby, seek the advice of a health professional before using this product.

How Supplied: BAYER® SELECT™ Maximum Strength NIGHT TIME PAIN RELIEF FORMULA is available in 24 and 50 count bottles.

Shown in Product Identification Guide, page 427

BAYER® SELECT™
Maximum Strength
SINUS PAIN RELIEF
Analgesic/Decongestant Formula
Aspirin-Free

Active Ingredients: Acetaminophen 500 mg and Pseudoephedrine HCl 30 mg per caplet.

Inactive Ingredients: Colloidal Silicon Dioxide, D&C Yellow #10, FD&C Blue #1, FD&C Yellow #6, Hydroxypropyl Methylcellulose, Iron Oxide, Magnesium Stearate, Microcrystalline Cellulose, Polyethylene Glycol, Polysorbate 80, Povidone, Starch, Titanium Dioxide.

Indications: BAYER® SELECT™ SINUS PAIN RELIEF Formula contains a specially chosen combination of safe, aspirin-free, caffeine-free ingredients in a maximum dosage to provide temporary relief of the following SINUS symptoms without making you drowsy:
- Sinus headache pain and pressure
- Swollen nasal passages
- Nasal congestion due to the common cold, hay fever, other respiratory allergies or associated with sinusitis.

Directions: Adults: Take 2 caplets with water every 4-6 hours, up to a maximum of 8 caplets per 24 hours. **Children under 12 years of age:** Consult your doctor.

Warnings: Do not exceed recommended dosage because at higher doses nervousness, dizziness, or sleeplessness may occur. Do not take this product for more than 7 days unless directed by a doctor. If symptoms do not improve, are severe or recurrent, or are accompanied by fever, consult a doctor. Do not take this product if you have heart disease, high blood pressure, thyroid disease, diabetes, or difficulty in urination due to enlargement of the prostate gland unless directed by a doctor. Keep out of reach of children. In case of accidental overdose, prompt medical attention is essential for adults as well as for children even if you do not notice any signs or symptoms. Contact a doctor immediately. As with any drug, if you are pregnant or nursing

a baby, seek the advice of a health professional before using this product.

Drug Interaction Precaution: Do not take this product if you are presently taking a prescription drug for high blood pressure or depression without first consulting your doctor.

How Supplied: BAYER® SELECT™ Maximum Strength SINUS PAIN RELIEF FORMULA is available in 24 and 50 count bottles.

Shown in Product Identification Guide, page 427

BAYER® SELECT™ NIGHT TIME COLD
Nasal Decongestant, Cough Suppressant, Pain Reliever, Antihistamine

Active Ingredients: 500mg Acetaminophen, 30mg Pseudoephedrine HCl, 15mg Dextromethorphan HBr and 1.25mg Triprolidine HCl per caplet.

Inactive Ingredients: Croscarmellose Sodium, FD&C Blue #1 Lake, FD&C Blue #2 Lake, Hydroxypropyl Methylcellulose, Iron Oxide, Magnesium Stearate, Microcrystalline Cellulose, Polyethylene Glycol, Polysorbate 80, Starch, Titanium Dioxide.

Directions: Adults: Take 2 caplets with water at bedtime. If cold symptoms keep you confined to bed or at home, dosage may be repeated every 6 hours up to a maximum of 8 caplets per 24 hours or as directed by a doctor. Children under 12 years of age: Consult your doctor.

Indications: Temporarily relieves nasal congestion and reduces swollen nasal passages; temporarily calms and controls your tough cough; temporarily relieves night time aches and pains, headache and minor sore throat pain; temporarily dries runny nose and relieves sneezing.

Warnings: Do not exceed recommended dosage because at higher doses nervousness, dizziness or sleeplessness may occur. May cause marked drowsiness; alcohol, sedatives, and tranquilizers may increase the drowsiness effect. Avoid alcoholic beverages while taking this product. Do not take this product if you are taking sedatives or tranquilizers without first consulting a doctor. Use caution when driving a motor vehicle or operating machinery. May cause excitability especially in children. Do not take this product if you have asthma, glaucoma, emphysema, chronic pulmonary disease, shortness of breath, difficulty in breathing, or difficulty in urination due to enlargement of the prostate gland unless directed by a doctor. Do not take this product for more than 7 days. If symptoms do not improve or are accompanied by fever that lasts for more than 3 days, or if new symptoms occur, consult a doctor. If sore throat is severe, persists for more than 2 days, is accompanied or followed by fever, headache, rash, nausea, or vomiting, consult a doctor promptly.

Do not take this product if you have heart disease, high blood pressure, thyroid disease, or diabetes unless directed by a doctor. Do not take this product for persistent or chronic cough such as occurs with smoking, asthma, or emphysema, or where cough is accompanied by excessive phlegm (mucus) unless directed by a doctor. A persistent cough may be a sign of a serious condition. If cough persists for more than 1 week, tends to recur, or is accompanied by fever, rash, or persistent headache, consult a doctor. Keep this and all drugs out of reach of children. In case of accidental overdose, seek professional assistance or contact a poison control center. Prompt medical attention is essential for adults as well as for children even if you do not notice any signs or symptoms. As with any drug, if you are pregnant or nursing a baby, seek the advice of a health professional before using this product, unless directed by a doctor, if you have breathing problems such as emphysema or chronic bronchitis or if you have glaucoma or difficulty in urination due to enlargement of the prostate gland.

Drug Interaction Precaution: Do not use this product if you are taking a prescription drug containing a monoamine oxidase inhibitor (MAOI) (certain drugs for depression or psychiatric or emotional conditions) without first consulting a doctor. If you are uncertain whether your prescription drug contains an MAOI, consult a health professional before taking this product.

How Supplied: Bayer Select Night Time Cold is packaged in child resistant blister packages containing 16 caplets.

Shown in Product Identification Guide, page 427

BRONKAID® MIST
EPINEPHRINE INHALATION
AEROSOL
BRONCHODILATOR
FOR ORAL INHALATION ONLY

Active Ingredient: Epinephrine USP 0.5% (w/w), (as nitrate and hydrochloride salts). Each spray delivers 0.25 mg epinephrine.

Inactive Ingredients: Alcohol 33% (w/w), Ascorbic acid, Dichlorodifluoromethane, Dichlorotetrafluoroethane, Purified water. Contains no sulfites.

Indications: For temporary relief of shortness of breath, tightness of chest and wheezing due to bronchial asthma.

Directions: Adults and children 4 years of age and older: Start with one inhalation, then wait at least one (1) minute. If symptoms not relieved, use once more. Do not use again for at least 3 hours. The use of this product by children should be supervised by an adult. **Children under 4 years of age:** Consult a doctor. Each spray delivers 0.25 mg epinephrine.
1. Remove cap and mouthpiece from bottle.

2. Remove cap from mouthpiece and check to see that mouthpiece opening is clean and free from foreign objects.
3. Turn mouthpiece sideways and fit metal stem of nebulizer into hole in flattened end of mouthpiece.
4. Exhale, as completely as possible. Now, hold bottle **upside down** between thumb and forefinger and close lips loosely around end of mouthpiece.
5. Inhale deeply while pressing down firmly on bottle, once only.
6. Remove mouthpiece and hold your breath a moment to allow for maximum absorption of medication. Then exhale slowly through nearly closed lips.
7. After use, remove mouthpiece from bottle and replace cap. When possible, rinse mouthpiece with tap water immediately after use. Soap and water will not hurt it. A clean mouthpiece always works better. Slide mouthpiece over bottle for protection.

Warning: Contains CFC-12, and CFC-114, substances which harm public health and environment by destroying ozone in the upper atmosphere.

Warnings: FOR ORAL INHALATION ONLY. Avoid spraying in eyes. Do not use this product unless a diagnosis of asthma has been made by a doctor. Do not use this product if you have heart disease, high blood pressure, thyroid disease, diabetes, or difficulty in urination due to enlargement of the prostate gland unless directed by a doctor. Do not use this product if you have ever been hospitalized for asthma or if you are taking any prescription drug for asthma. **Do not use this product more frequently or at higher doses than recommended, unless directed by a doctor.** Excessive use may cause nervousness and rapid heart beat, and possibly, adverse effects on the heart. **Do not continue to use this product, but seek medical assistance immediately if symptoms are not relieved within 20 minutes or become worse.** As with any drug, if you are pregnant or nursing a baby, seek the advice of a health professional before using this medication. Keep this and all drugs out of the reach of children. In case of accidental overdose, seek professional assistance or contact a poison control center immediately.

DRUG INTERACTION PRECAUTION: Do not use this product if you are presently taking a prescription drug for high blood pressure or depression, including those containing a monoamine oxidase inhibitor (MAOI), without first consulting your doctor.

Storage and Handling: Store at controlled room temperature 59°F–86°F (15°C–30°C). Contents under pressure. Do not puncture or incinerate. Using or storing near open flame or heating above 120°F may cause bursting.

How Supplied: Bottles of ½ fl oz (15 mL) with actuator. Also available–refills (no mouthpiece) in ½ fl oz (15 mL) and ¾ fl oz (22.5 mL).

Shown in Product Identification Guide, page 428

BRONKAID® MIST SUSPENSION EPINEPHRINE BITARTRATE INHALATION AEROSOL BRONCHODILATOR FOR ORAL INHALATION ONLY

Active Ingredient: Epinephrine Bitartrate 7.0 mg per ml. Each spray delivers 0.3 mg epinephrine bitartrate equivalent to 0.16 mg epinephrine base. Contains 200 metered inhalations per canister.

Inactive Ingredients: Cetylpyridinium Chloride, dichlorodifluoromethane, dichlorotetrafluoroethane, sorbitan trioleate, trichloromonofluoromethane. Contains no sulfites.

Indications: For temporary relief of shortness of breath, tightness of chest and wheezing due to bronchial asthma.

Directions: Adults and children 4 years of age and older: Start with one inhalation, then wait one (1) minute. If symptoms not relieved, use once more. Do not use again for at least 3 hours. The use of this product by children should be supervised by an adult. **Children under 4 years of age:** Consult a doctor. Each spray delivers 0.3 mg epinephrine bitartrate equivalent to 0.16 mg epinephrine base.
1. **SHAKE WELL.** Remove dust cap and inspect to see that nozzle is clean and free from foreign objects.
2. Hold inhaler with nozzle down while using.
3. Exhale, as completely as possible. Purse the lips as in saying the letter "O" and hold the nozzle up to the lips, keeping the tongue flat. As you start to take a deep breath, squeeze the nozzle and can together, releasing one full application. Complete taking deep breath, drawing medication into your lungs.
4. Hold breath for as long as comfortable. This distributes the medication in the lungs. Then exhale slowly keeping the lips nearly closed.
5. Replace dust cap after each use.
6. Rinse nozzle daily with soap and warm water after removing from vial. Dry with clean cloth.

Warning: Contains CFC-11, CFC-12 and CFC-114, substances which harm public health and environment by destroying ozone in the upper atmosphere.

Warnings: FOR ORAL INHALATION ONLY. Avoid spraying in eyes. Do not use this product unless a diagnosis of asthma has been made by a doctor. Do not use this product if you have heart disease, high blood pressure, thyroid disease, diabetes, or difficulty in urination due to enlargement of the prostate gland. Do not use this product if you have ever been hospitalized for asthma or if you are taking any prescription drug for asthma. **Do not use this product more frequently or at higher doses than recommended, unless directed by a doctor.** Excessive use may cause nervousness and rapid heart beat, and possibly, adverse effects on the heart. **Do not**

continue to use this product, but seek medical assistance immediately if symptoms are not relieved within 20 minutes or become worse. As with any drug, if you are pregnant or nursing a baby, seek the advice of a health professional before using this medication. Keep this and all drugs out of the reach of children. In case of accidental overdose, seek professional assistance or contact a poison control center immediately.

Drug Interaction Precaution: Do not use this product if you are presently taking a prescription drug for high blood pressure or depression, including those containing a monoamine oxidase inhibitor (MAOI), without first consulting your doctor.

Storage and Handling: Store at controlled room temperature 59°F–86°F (15°C –30°C). Contents under pressure. Do not puncture or incinerate. Using or storing near open flame or heating above 120°F may cause bursting.

How Supplied: ⅓ fl. oz. (10cc) pocket size inhaler, with actuator.

BRONKAID® CAPLETS BRONCHODILATOR AND EXPECTORANT
*New Formula

Active Ingredients: Ephedrine Sulfate 25 mg and Guaifenesin 400 mg per caplet.

Inactive Ingredients: Croscarmellose Sodium, Hydroxypropyl Methylcellulose, Magnesium Stearate, Magnesium Trisilicate, Microcrystalline Cellulose, Polyethylene Glycol, Povidone, and Starch.

Indications: For the temporary relief of shortness of breath, tightness in chest, wheezing and cough associated with bronchial asthma. Helps loosen phlegm (mucus) and thin bronchial secretions to rid the bronchial passageways of bothersome mucus and drain bronchial tubes.

Directions: Adults and Children 12 years and over: 1 caplet every 4 hours, not to exceed 6 caplets in 24 hours, or as directed by a doctor. Do not exceed recommended dose unless directed by a doctor. **Children under 12 years of age:** Consult a doctor.

Warnings: Do not use this product unless a diagnosis of asthma has been made by a doctor. Do not use this product if you have heart disease, high blood pressure, thyroid disease, diabetes, or difficulty in urination due to enlargement of the prostate gland unless directed by a doctor. Do not use this product if you have ever been

Continued on next page

This product information was effective as of November 1, 1993. Current information may be obtained directly from Sterling Health, by writing to 90 Park Avenue, New York, NY 10016.

Sterling Health—Cont.

hospitalized for asthma or if you are taking any prescription drug for asthma unless directed by a doctor. **Do not continue to use this product, but seek medical assistance immediately if symptoms are not relieved within 1 hour or become worse.** Some users of this product may experience nervousness, tremor, sleeplessness, nausea, and loss of appetite. If these symptoms persist or become worse, consult a doctor. Do not take this product for persistent or chronic cough such as occurs with smoking, asthma, chronic bronchitis, or emphysema, or where cough is accompanied by excessive phlegm (mucus) unless directed by a doctor. A persistent cough may be a sign of a serious condition. If cough persists for more than 1 week, tends to recur, or is accompanied by a fever, rash, or persistent headache, consult a doctor. Keep this and all drugs out of the reach of children. In case of accidental overdose, seek professional assistance or contact a poison control center immediately. As with any drug, if you are pregnant or nursing a baby, seek the advice of a health professional before using this medication.

Drug Interaction Precaution: Do not take this product if you are presently taking a prescription drug for high blood pressure or depression, including those containing a Monoamine Oxidase Inhibitor (MAOI), without first consulting your doctor.

How Supplied: Boxes of 24 and 60.
Shown in Product Identification Guide, page 428

CAMPHO-PHENIQUE®
ANTISEPTIC GEL
[kam 'fo-finēk]
First Aid Antiseptic/Pain Reliever

Active Ingredient: Camphorated Phenol (Camphor 10.8% and Phenol 4.7% in light mineral oil).

Inactive Ingredients: Colloidal Silicon Dioxide, Eucalyptus Oil, Glycerin, Light Mineral Oil.

Indications: For the temporary relief of pain and itching associated with minor burns, sunburn, minor cuts, scrapes, insect bites or minor skin irritation. Protects against the risk of infection in minor cuts, scrapes and burns.

Directions: Clean the affected area. Apply with cotton 1 to 3 times daily.

Warnings: For External Use Only. Do not use in or near the eyes or apply over large areas of the body. If product gets into the eyes, flush thoroughly with water and obtain medical attention. In case of deep or puncture wounds, animal bites, or serious burns, consult a doctor. Stop use and consult a doctor if condition worsens or if symptoms persist for more than 7 days or clear up and occur again within a few days. Do not use longer than 1 week unless directed by a doctor. Do

not bandage. Keep this and all drugs out of the reach of children. In case of accidental ingestion seek professional assistance or contact a poison control center immediately.
DO NOT INDUCE VOMITING before contacting a doctor or poison control center.

How Supplied: 0.5 oz (14g) Tube.
Shown in Product Identification Guide, page 428

CAMPHO-PHENIQUE®
[kam 'fo-finēk]
COLD SORE GEL

Active Ingredient: Camphorated Phenol (Camphor 10.8% and Phenol 4.7% in a light mineral oil).

Inactive Ingredients: Colloidal Silicon Dioxide, Eucalyptus Oil, Glycerin, Light Mineral Oil.

Indications: For the temporary relief of pain and discomfort associated with cold sores/fever blisters.

Directions: Clean the affected area. Apply directly to cold sore or fever blister 1 to 3 times daily.

Warnings: For External Use Only. Do not use in or near the eyes or apply over large areas of the body. If product gets into the eyes, flush thoroughly with water and obtain medical attention. Stop use and consult a doctor if condition worsens or if symptoms persist for more than 7 days or clear up and occur again within a few days. Do not use longer than 1 week unless directed by a doctor. Do not bandage. Keep this and all drugs out of the reach of children. In case of accidental ingestion seek professional assistance or contact a poison control center immediately. DO NOT INDUCE VOMITING before contacting a doctor or poison control center.

How Supplied: 0.23 oz (6.5 g) Tube
Shown in Product Identification Guide, page 428

CAMPHO-PHENIQUE®
[kam 'fo-finēk]
Pain Relieving Antiseptic Liquid

Active Ingredient: Camphorated Phenol (Camphor 10.8% and Phenol 4.7% in light mineral oil).

Inactive Ingredients: Eucalyptus Oil, Light Mineral Oil.

Indications: For the temporary relief of pain and itching associated with minor burns, sunburn, minor cuts, scrapes, insect bites or minor skin irritation. Protects against the risk of infection in minor cuts, scrapes and burns.

Directions: Clean the affected area. Apply with cotton 1 to 3 times daily.

Warnings: For External Use Only. Do not use in or near the eyes or apply over large areas of the body. If product gets into the eyes, flush thoroughly with water and obtain medical attention. In case of deep or puncture wounds, animal bites, or serious burns, consult a doctor.

Stop use and consult a doctor if condition worsens or if symptoms persist for more than 7 days or clear up and occur again within a few days. Do not use longer than 1 week unless directed by a doctor. Do not bandage. Keep this and all drugs out of the reach of children. In case of accidental ingestion seek professional assistance or contact a poison control center immediately. DO NOT INDUCE VOMITING before contacting a poison control center.

How Supplied: Bottles of .75, 1.5, and 4.0 fl oz.
Shown in Product Identification Guide, page 428

CAMPHO-PHENIQUE®
[kam 'fo-finēk]
First Aid Antibiotic plus Pain Reliever NEW! Maximum Strength

Active Ingredients: Each gram contains: Bacitracin Zinc 500 units, Neomycin Sulfate 5 mg (equiv. to 3.5 mg Neomycin Base), Polymyxin B Sulfate 10,000 units, Lidocaine HCl 40 mg (Pain Reliever).

Inactive Ingredient: White Petrolatum

Indications: First aid ointment both for temporary relief of pain and to help prevent infection of minor cuts, scrapes and burns.

Directions: Clean the affected area. Apply a small amount (an amount equal to the surface area of the tip of a finger) on the area 1 to 3 times daily. Do not apply more than 3 times daily. May be covered with a sterile bandage. Children under 2 years of age: consult a doctor.

Warnings: For External Use Only. Do not use in or near the eyes or apply over large areas of the body. If product gets into the eyes, flush thoroughly with water and obtain medical attention. In case of deep or puncture wounds, animal bites, or serious burns, consult a doctor. Stop use and consult a doctor if the condition worsens or if symptoms persist for more than 7 days or clear up and occur again within a few days, or if a rash or other allergic reaction develops. Do not use this product if you are allergic to any of the listed ingredients. Do not use longer than 1 week unless directed by a doctor. Do not use in large quantities, particularly over raw surfaces or blistered areas. Keep this and all drugs out of the reach of children. In case of accidental ingestion seek professional assistance or contact a poison control center immediately.
Store at 15°–30°C (59°–86°F).

How Supplied: 0.50 oz (14 g) Tube
Shown in Product Identification Guide, page 428

DAIRY EASE® Tablets/Caplets
Natural Lactase Enzyme Supplement

Ingredients: Each Tablet/Caplet contains 3000 FCC Lactase units (derived from Aspergillus Oryzae). Other ingredients are: (Tablets) Dibasic Calcium Phosphate, Mannitol, Colloidal Silicon Dioxide, Magnesium Stearate. (Caplets): Colloidal Silicon Dioxide, Dibasic Calcium Phosphate, Magnesium Stearate, Microcrystalline Cellulose, Pregelatinized Starch.

Indications: Lactase insufficiency, suspected from gastrointestinal disturbances after consumption of milk or milk-containing products (i.e., Gas, Bloating, Flatulence, Cramps and Diarrhea) or identified by a lactose intolerance test.

Action: Lactase enzyme converts, by hydrolysis, the lactose into its simple sugar components: glucose and galactose.

Product Uses: Dairy Ease is a natural lactase enzyme which supplements the natural level of lactase in the body and helps make lactose more easily digestible. The most common products where lactose can be found are milk, cheese, ice cream & chocolate and it is also found in some vitamins and medications. Dairy Ease can be used with all foods which contain lactose such as pizza, hot dogs, pancakes, creamed salad dressings and soups, instant cocoa mix, puddings and other foods where milk, milk solids, whey, whey protein concentrate, casein or cheese are listed on the ingredient panel.

Dosage: Recommended dosage is 2–3 chewable tablets/swallowable caplets along with or immediately following dairy food consumption. However, since natural lactase levels vary, actual dosage may differ from person to person.

Toxicity: None.

Drug Interactions: None. Dairy Ease tablets and caplets are classified as food products.

Warnings: Do not use if you have had an allergic reaction to products containing lactase enzyme. If symptoms persist consult a doctor about a possible food allergy or other digestive disorder.

Precautions: Diabetics should be aware that the milk sugar will now be metabolically available and must be taken into account (17.5 gm glucose and 17.5 gm galactose per quart at 70% hydrolysis). No reports received of any diabetics' reactions. Galactosemics may not have milk in any form, lactase enzyme modified or not.

Note: Possible adverse reactions are mainly gastrointestinal in nature, sometimes mimicking the symptoms of lactose intolerance and sometimes involving vomiting. Skin rashes possibly due to allergic reactions have been reported. Persons sensitive to penicillin and other molds may be particularly susceptible. Discontinue use of tablets/caplets immediately and consult a physician.

How Supplied: Dairy Ease Chewable Tablets are available in 36, 60 and 100 counts. Dairy Ease Swallowable Caplets are available in a 40 count bottle.
Shown in Product Identification Guide, page 428

DAIRY EASE® Drops
Natural Lactase Enzyme

Ingredients: Water, Glycerol, Lactase Enzyme (derived from Kluyveromyces Lactis). One ml contains no less than 5400 Neutral Lactase units.

Indications: Lactase insufficiency, suspected from gastrointestinal disturbances after consumption of milk or milk-containing products (i.e., Gas, Bloating, Flatulence, Cramps and Diarrhea) or identified by a lactose tolerance test.

Product Uses: Dairy Ease drops are a natural lactase enzyme in liquid form which when added to milk, make it more easily digestible. Dairy Ease drops can be used in any kind of milk including: whole, 1%, 2%, nonfat, canned, powdered and chocolate. Also, cream, baby formulas containing milk and high protein diet formulas. The treated milk can be used for cooking, on cereal or directly from the carton.

Action: Lactase enzyme converts, by hydrolysis, the lactose into its simple sugar components: glucose and galactose.

Dosage: Add Dairy Ease drops to a quart of milk, shake gently and refrigerate for 24 hours. Five drops will remove 70% of the lactose, 10 drops, 90% and 15 drops, 97+%. Since the degree of natural lactase levels varies, each person may have to adjust the number of drops that work best.

Toxicity: None.

Drug Interactions: None. Dairy Ease drops are classified as food products.

Warnings: Do not use if you have had an allergic reaction to products containing lactase enzyme. If symptoms persist consult a doctor about a possible food allergy or other digestive disorder.

Precautions: Diabetics should be aware that the milk sugar will now be metabolically available and must be taken into account (17.5 gm glucose and 17.5 gm galactose per quart at 70% hydrolysis). No reports received of any diabetics' reactions. Galactosemics may not have milk in any form, lactase enzyme modified or not.

Adverse Reactions: No reactions of any kind have been observed from Dairy Ease liquid drops.

How Supplied: Dairy Ease drops are available in a 7ml bottle which will treat up to 32 quarts of milk.
Shown in Product Identification Guide, page 428

DAIRY EASE® Real Milk
Lactose Reduced Milk

Dairy Ease is also available in Real Milk which is 70% lactose reduced and contains vitamins A & D. A one quart size in three varieties is available: Nonfat, 1% lowfat, and 2% lowfat. Dairy Ease Real Milk can be used for cooking, on cereal or directly from the carton.
Shown in Product Identification Guide, page 428

FERGON® Iron Supplement Tablets
[fur-gone]
brand of ferrous gluconate

Each FERGON Iron Supplement tablet contains 320 mg (5 grains) Ferrous Gluconate equal to approximately 36 mg elemental iron. Also contains: Acacia, Carnauba Wax, Dextrose Excipient, FD&C Red #40, D&C Yellow #10, FD&C Blue #1 as color additives. Gelatin, Kaolin, Magnesium Stearate, Parabens, Pharmaceutical Glaze, Povidone, Precipitated Calcium Carbonate, Sodium Benzoate, Starch, Sucrose, Talc, Titanium Dioxide, Yellow Wax.

Action and Uses: For use as a dietary supplement.

Warnings: CLOSE TIGHTLY AND KEEP OUT OF THE REACH OF CHILDREN. Contains iron, which can be harmful or fatal to children in large doses. In case of accidental overdose, seek professional assistance or contact a poison control center immediately. If you are pregnant or nursing a baby, seek the advice of a health professional before using this product.
AVOID EXCESSIVE HEAT

Dosage and Administration: Adults —One FERGON tablet daily.

How Supplied: FERGON Tablets of 320 mg (5 grains) bottle of 100.
Shown in Product Identification Guide, page 428

PMS
Multi-Symptom Formula
MIDOL®
Physical Symptom Relief

Active Ingredients: Each caplet contains Acetaminophen 500 mg, Pamabrom 25 mg and Pyrilamine Maleate 15 mg.

Inactive Ingredients: Croscarmellose Sodium, D&C Red #30, D&C Yellow #10, Hydroxypropyl Methylcellulose, Magnesium Stearate, Microcrystalline

Continued on next page

This product information was effective as of November 1, 1993. Current information may be obtained directly from Sterling Health, by writing to 90 Park Avenue, New York, NY 10016.

Sterling Health—Cont.

Cellulose, Pregelatinized Starch and Triacetin.

Indications: Contains maximum strength medication for all these PMS symptoms: bloating, water-weight gain, cramps, headaches and backaches.
- Provides maximum strength relief of the physical symptoms of Premenstrual Syndrome so you can feel like yourself again.
- Contains a combination of aspirin-free ingredients which is not found in any ordinary pain reliever: a diuretic to alleviate water retention and an analgesic for pain.

Directions: Adults and children 12 years and over: Take 2 caplets with water. Repeat every 4 hours, as needed, up to a maximum of 8 caplets per day. Under age 12: Consult your doctor.

Warnings: If pain persists for more than 10 days, consult a doctor immediately. May cause drowsiness. Use caution when driving or operating machinery. Alcohol, sedatives or tranquilizers may increase drowsiness. Do not take this product, unless directed by a doctor, if you have a breathing problem such as emphysema or chronic bronchitis or if you have glaucoma or difficulty in urination due to enlargement of the prostate gland. Keep out of reach of children. In case of accidental overdose, immediate medical attention is essential for adults as well as for children even if you do not notice any signs or symptoms. As with any drug, if you are pregnant or nursing a baby, seek the advice of a health professional before using this product.

How Supplied: White capsule-shaped caplets available in packages of 2 blisters of 8 caplets each and bottles of 32 caplets. Child-resistant safety closure on bottles of 32 caplets.
Shown in Product Identification Guide, page 428

CRAMP RELIEF FORMULA
MIDOL ® IB
Ibuprofen Tablets, USP 200 mg
Menstrual Pain/Cramp Reliever

Warning: Aspirin-Sensitive Patients —Do not take this product if you have had a severe allergic reaction to aspirin, eg, asthma, swelling, shock or hives, because even though this product contains no aspirin or salicylates, cross-reactions may occur in patients allergic to aspirin.

Indications: For the temporary relief of painful menstrual cramps (dysmenorrhea); also headaches, backaches and muscular aches and pains associated with Premenstrual Syndrome.

Directions:
Adults: Take 1 tablet every 4 to 6 hours at the onset of menstrual symptoms and while pain persists. If pain does not respond to 1 tablet, 2 tablets may be used but do not exceed 6 tablets in 24 hours, unless directed by a doctor. The smallest effective dose should be used. Take with food or milk if occasional and mild heartburn, upset stomach, or stomach pain occurs with use. Consult a doctor if these symptoms are more than mild or if they persist. *Children:* Do not give this product to children under 12 except under the advice and supervision of a doctor.

Warnings: Do not take for pain for more than 10 days unless directed by a doctor. If pain persists or gets worse, or if new symptoms occur, consult a doctor. These could be signs of serious illness. If you are under a doctor's care for any serious condition, consult a doctor before taking this product. As with aspirin and acetaminophen, if you have any condition which requires you to take prescription drugs or if you have had any problems or serious side effects from taking any nonprescription pain reliever, do not take this product without first discussing it with your doctor. If you experience any symptoms which are unusual or seem unrelated to the condition for which you took ibuprofen, consult a doctor before taking any more of it. Although ibuprofen is indicated for the same conditions as aspirin and acetaminophen, it should not be taken with them except under a doctor's direction. Do not combine this product with any other ibuprofen-containing product. As with any drug, if you are pregnant or nursing a baby, seek the advice of a health professional before using this product. **IT IS ESPECIALLY IMPORTANT NOT TO USE IBUPROFEN DURING THE LAST 3 MONTHS OF PREGNANCY UNLESS SPECIFICALLY DIRECTED TO DO SO BY A DOCTOR BECAUSE IT MAY CAUSE PROBLEMS IN THE UNBORN CHILD OR COMPLICATIONS DURING DELIVERY.** Keep this and all drugs out of the reach of children. In case of accidental overdose, seek professional assistance or contact a poison control center immediately.

Action and Uses: Ibuprofen is used for the relief of painful menstrual cramps and the pain associated with Premenstrual Syndrome. Ibuprofen has been proven more effective in relieving menstrual pain and cramps than aspirin and is gentler on the stomach. Ibuprofen had been widely prescribed for years and is now available in nonprescription strength.

Active Ingredient: Each tablet contains ibuprofen USP 200 mg.

Inactive Ingredients: Calcium phosphate, cellulose, magnesium stearate, silicon dioxide, sodium lauryl sulfate, sodium starch glycolate, stearic acid, titanium dioxide.
Store at room temperature; avoid excessive heat 40°C (104°F).

How Supplied:
White tablets in bottles of 16 and 32 tablets.

Child-resistant safety closure on bottles of 32 tablets.
Shown in Product Identification Guide, page 428

Maximum Strength
Multi-Symptom Formula
MIDOL®
Menstrual Formula

Active Ingredients: Each caplet contains Acetaminophen 500 mg, Caffeine 60 mg and Pyrilamine Maleate 15 mg.

Inactive Ingredients: Croscarmellose Sodium, FD&C Blue #2 Hydroxypropyl Methylcellulose, Magnesium Stearate, Microcrystalline Cellulose, Pregelatinized Starch and Triacetin.

Indications: Relieves all of these physical menstrual symptoms: cramps, bloating, water-weight gain, headaches, backaches, muscular aches and fatigue.
- Provides maximum strength relief of painful physical symptoms suffered during your menstrual cycle.
- Contains a combination of maximum strength, aspirin-free ingredients which is not found in any ordinary pain reliever.

Directions: Adults and children 12 years and over: Take 2 caplets with water. Repeat every 4 hours, as needed, up to a maximum of 8 caplets per day. Under age 12: Consult your doctor.

Warnings: If pain persists for more than 10 days, consult a doctor immediately. May cause drowsiness. Use caution when driving or operating machinery. Alcohol, sedatives or tranquilizers may increase drowsiness. The recommended dose of this product contains about as much caffeine as a cup of coffee. Limit the use of caffeine-containing medications, foods, or beverages while taking this product because too much caffeine may cause nervousness, irritability, sleeplessness, and occasionally, rapid heartbeat. Do not take this product, unless directed by a doctor, if you have a breathing problem such as emphysema or chronic bronchitis or if you have glaucoma or difficulty in urination due to enlargement of the prostate gland. Keep out of reach of children. In case of accidental overdose, immediate medical attention is essential for adults as well as for children even if you do not notice any signs or symptoms. As with any drug, if you are pregnant or nursing a baby, seek the advice of a health professional before using this product.

How Supplied: White capsule-shaped caplets available in 2-caplet packets for sample use, bottles of 8 and 32 caplets, and packages of 2 blisters of 8 caplets each. Child-resistant safety closures on bottles of 8 and 32 caplets.
Shown in Product Identification Guide, page 428

Teen
Multi-Symptom Formula
MIDOL®
Menstrual Formula

Active Ingredients: Each caplet contains Acetaminophen 400 mg and Pamabrom 25 mg.

Inactive Ingredients: Croscarmellose Sodium, D&C Red #7 Lake, FD&C Blue #2 Lake, Hydroxpropyl Methylcellulose, Magnesium Stearate, Microcrystaline Cellulose, Pregelatinized Starch and Triacetin.

Indications: Relieves cramps, bloating, water-weight gain, headaches, backaches and muscular aches and pains.
• Provides effective relief of painful menstrual symptoms so you can get on with your life.
• Contains a special combination of safe, aspirin-free, caffeine-free ingredients which is not found in any ordinary pain reliever.
• Non-drowsy formula won't slow you down!

Directions: Adults and children 12 years and over: Take 2 caplets with water. Repeat every 4 hours, as needed, up to a maximum of 8 caplets per day. Under age 12: Consult your doctor.

Warnings: If pain persists for more than 10 days, consult a doctor immediately. Keep out of reach of children. In case of accidental overdose, immediate medical attention is essential for adults as well as for children even if you do not notice any signs or symptoms. As with any drug, if you are pregnant or nursing a baby, seek the advice of a health professional before using this product.

How Supplied: White capsule-shaped caplets available in packages of 2 blisters of 8 caplets each and bottles of 32 caplets. Child-resistant safety closure on bottles of 32 caplets.
Shown in Product Identification Guide, page 428

NaSal™ Moisturizer AF
Saline (buffered)
0.65% Sodium chloride
Nasal Spray and Drops

Description: The nasal spray and nose drops contain Sodium Chloride 0.65%. Also contains: Benzalkonium Chloride and Thimerosal 0.001% as preservative, Mono- and Dibasic Sodium Phosphates as buffers, Purified Water.
Contains No Alcohol.

Actions: Immediate relief for dry nose. Formulated to match the pH of normal nasal secretions to help prevent stinging or burning.

Indications: Provides gentle relief for dry, irritated nasal passages due to colds, low humidity, air travel, allergies, minor nose bleeds, crusting, overuse of decongestant sprays/drops and other nasal irritations. As an ideal moisturizer, it can be used with cold, allergy, and sinus medications.

Adverse Reactions: No associated side effects.

Dosage and Administration: Spray: Spray twice in each nostril as often as needed or as directed by doctor.
Drops: For infants, children and adults, 2 to 6 drops in each nostril as often as needed or as directed by doctor.

How Supplied: Nasal Spray—plastic squeeze bottles of 30 mL (1 fl. oz.).
Nose Drops—MonoDrop® bottles of 15 mL (½ fl. oz.).
Shown in Product Identification Guide, page 428

NEO-SYNEPHRINE®
Pediatric Formula, Mild Formula,
Regular Strength, and
Extra Strength.
phenylephrine hydrochloride

Description: This line of Nasal Sprays, Drops and Spray Pumps contains Phenylephrine Hydrochloride in strengths ranging from 0.125% (drops only) to 1%. Also contains: Benzalkonium Chloride and Thimerosal 0.001% as preservatives, Citric Acid, Purified Water, Sodium Chloride, Sodium Citrate.

Action: Rapid-acting nasal decongestant.

Directions: Adults and children 12 years and over: May use 0.25%, 0.5% or 1.0%
Adults and children 6 years and over: May use 0.25%
Children 2 to under 6 years: Use 0.125%

2 or 3 sprays (drops) in each nostril not more often than every 4 hours.

Indications: For temporary relief of nasal congestion due to common cold, hay fever, sinusitis, or other upper respiratory allergies.

Warnings: Do not exceed recommended dosage because symptoms may occur such as burning, stinging, sneezing or increased nasal discharge. Do not use this product for more than 3 days. If symptoms persist, consult a doctor. Frequent and continued usage of the higher concentrations (especially the 1% solution) occasionally may cause a rebound congestion of the nose. Therefore, long-term or frequent use of this solution is not recommended without the advice of a physician.
Prolonged exposure to air or strong light will cause oxidation and some loss of potency. Do not use if brown in color or contains a precipitate.
Keep these and all drugs out of the reach of children. In case of accidental ingestion seek professional assistance or contact a poison control center immediately. The use of the dispenser by more than one person may spread infection.
Do not use this product if you have heart disease, high blood pressure, thyroid disease, diabetes, or difficulty in urination due to enlargement of the prostate gland unless directed by a doctor.

Adverse Reactions: Generally very well tolerated; systemic side effects such as tremor, insomnia, or palpitation rarely occur at recommended dosages.

How Supplied: Pediatric Formula (0.125%) in 15 mL drops. Mild Formula (0.25%) in 15 mL drops and spray. Regular Strength (0.5%) in 15 mL drops and spray. Extra Strength (1.0%) in 15 mL drops and spray.
Shown in Product Identification Guide, page 428

NEO-SYNEPHRINE®
Maximum Strength 12 Hour
oxymetazoline hydrochloride
Nasal Spray 0.05%

Description: *Adult Strength Nasal Spray* and *Nasal Spray Pump* contain: Oxymetazoline Hydrochloride 0.05%. Also contain: Benzalkonium Chloride and Phenylmercuric Acetate 0.002% as preservatives, Glycine, Purified Water, Sorbitol, may also contain Sodium Chloride.

Action: 12 HOUR Nasal Decongestant.

Indications: Provides temporary relief, for up to 12 HOURS, of nasal congestion due to colds, hay fever, sinusitis, or other upper respiratory allergies. NEO-SYNEPHRINE MAXIMUM STRENGTH 12-HOUR Nasal Spray and Pump contain oxymetazoline which provides the longest-lasting relief of nasal congestion available.

Warnings: Do not exceed recommended dosage because symptoms may occur such as burning, stinging, sneezing, or increase of nasal discharge. Do not use these products for more than 3 days. If symptoms persist, consult a doctor. The use of the dispenser by more than one person may spread infection.
Do not use this product if you have heart disease, high blood pressure, thyroid disease, diabetes, or difficulty in urination due to enlargement of the prostate gland unless directed by a doctor.
Keep this and all drugs out of the reach of children. In case of accidental ingestion, seek professional assistance or contact a poison control center immediately.

Directions: *Adult Strength Nasal Spray* —For adults and children 6 years of age and over (with adult supervision): 2 or 3 sprays in each nostril not more often than every 10 to 12 hours. Do not exceed 2 applications in any 24-hour period. Children under 6 years of age:

Continued on next page

This product information was effective as of November 1, 1993. Current information may be obtained directly from Sterling Health, by writing to 90 Park Avenue, New York, NY 10016.

Sterling Health—Cont.

consult a doctor. To administer, hold head upright, spray 2 or 3 times in each nostril twice daily—morning and evening. To spray, squeeze bottle quickly and firmly.

Nasal Spray Pump —For adults and children 6 years of age and over (with adult supervision): 2 or 3 sprays in each nostril not more often than every 10–12 hours. Do not exceed 2 applications in any 24 hour period. Children under 6 years of age: consult a doctor. Hold bottle with thumb at base and nozzle between first and second fingers. To administer, hold head upright and insert spray nozzle in nostril. Depress pump 2 or 3 times, all the way down, with a firm even stroke and sniff deeply. Repeat in other nostril. Do not tilt head backward while spraying.

How Supplied: *Nasal Spray Adult Strength* — plastic squeeze bottles of 15 ml (½ fl. oz.); *Nasal Spray Pump* —15 ml bottle (½ fl. oz.).

Shown in Product Identification Guide, page 428

NTZ®
Long Acting
Oxymetazoline hydrochloride
Nasal Spray 0.05%
Nose Drops 0.05%

Description: Both the nasal spray and nose drops contain Oxymetazoline Hydrochloride 0.05%. Also contain: Benzalkonium Chloride and Phenylmercuric Acetate 0.002% as preservatives, Glycine, Purified Water, Sorbitol, and may also contain Sodium Chloride.

Actions: 12 Hour Nasal Decongestant.

Indications: Provides temporary relief, for up to 12 hours, of nasal congestion due to colds, hay fever, sinusitis, or allergies. Oxymetazoline hydrochloride provides the longest-lasting relief of nasal congestion available. It decongests nasal passages up to 12 hours, reduces swelling of nasal passages, and temporarily restores freer breathing through the nose.

Warnings: Not recommended for children under six. Do not exceed recommended dosage because symptoms may occur such as burning, stinging, sneezing, or increase of nasal discharge. Do not use these products for more than 3 days. If symptoms persist, consult a physician. The use of the dispenser by more than one person may spread infection. Do not use this product if you have heart disease, high blood pressure, thyroid disease, diabetes, or difficulty in urination due to enlargement of the prostate gland unless directed by a doctor. Keep these and all drugs out of the reach of children. In case of accidental ingestion seek professional assistance or contact a poison control center immediately.

Directions: Intranasally by spray and dropper. *Nasal Spray* —For adults and children 6 years of age and over: With head upright, spray 2 or 3 times in each nostril twice daily—morning and evening. To spray, squeeze bottle quickly and firmly. *Nose Drops* —For adults and children 6 years of age and over: 2 or 3 drops in each nostril twice daily—morning and evening.

How Supplied: *Nasal Spray* —plastic squeeze bottles of 15 ml (½ fl. oz.). *Nose Drops* —bottles of 15 ml (½ fl. oz.) with dropper.

Children's PANADOL®
Acetaminophen Chewable Tablets, Liquid, Drops

Description: Each Children's PANADOL Chewable Tablet contains 80 mg acetaminophen in a fruit-flavored sugar-free tablet. Children's PANADOL Acetaminophen Liquid is fruit-flavored, red in color, and is alcohol-free, sugar-free and aspirin-free. Each ½ teaspoonful contains 80 mg of acetaminophen. Infant's PANADOL Drops are fruit-flavored, red in color, and are alcohol-free, sugar-free and aspirin-free. Each 0.8 mL (one calibrated dropperful) contains 80 mg acetaminophen.

Indications: Acetaminophen, the active ingredient in Children's PANADOL, is the analgesic/antipyretic most widely recommended by pediatricians for fast, effective relief of children's fevers. It also relieves the aches and pains of colds and flu, earaches, headaches, teething, immunizations, tonsillectomy, and childhood illnesses.
Children's PANADOL Tablets, Liquid, and Drops are aspirin-free and contain no alcohol or sugar. The pleasant-tasting formulations are not likely to upset or irritate children's stomachs.

Usual Dosage: Dosing is based on single doses in the range of 10–15 mg/kg body weight. Doses may be repeated every four hours up to 4 or 5 times daily, but not to exceed 5 doses in 24 hours. To be administered to children under 2 years only on advice of a physician.
Children's PANADOL Chewable Tablets: 2–3 yr, 24–35 lb, 2 tablets; 4–5 yr, 36–47 lb, 3 tablets; 6–8 yr, 48–59 lb, 4 tablets; 9–10 yr, 60–71 lb, 5 tablets; 11 yr, 72–95 lb, 6 tablets. May be repeated every 4 hours, up to 5 times in a 24-hour period.
Children's PANADOL Liquid: 0–3 mo, 6–11 lb, ¼ teaspoonful; 4–11 mo, 12–17 lb, ½ teaspoonful; 12–23 mo, 18–23 lb, ¾ teaspoonful; 2–3 yr, 24–35 lb, 1 teaspoonful; 4–5 yr, 36–47 lb, 1½ teaspoonfuls; 6–8 yr, 48–59 lb, 2 teaspoonfuls; 9–10 yr, 60–71 lb, 2½ teaspoonfuls; 11 yr, 72–95 lb, 3 teaspoonfuls. May be repeated every 4 hours up to 5 times in a 24-hour period. May be administered alone or mixed with formula, milk, juice, cereal, etc.

Infant's PANADOL Drops: 0–3 mo, 6–11 lb, ½ dropperful (0.4 mL); 4–11 mo, 12–17 lb, 1 dropperful (0.8 mL); 12–23 mo, 18–23 lb, 1½ dropperfuls (1.2 mL); 2–3 yr, 24–35 lb, 2 dropperfuls (1.6 mL); 4–5 yr, 36–47 lb, 3 dropperfuls (2.4 mL); 6–8 yr, 48–59 lb, 4 dropperfuls (3.2 mL). May be repeated every 4 hours, up to 5 times in a 24-hour period. May be administered alone or mixed with formula, milk, juice, cereal, etc.

WARNINGS: Do not give this product for pain for more than 5 days or for fever for more than 3 days unless directed by a doctor. If symptoms persist or new ones occur, consult a doctor. Keep this and all drugs out of the reach of children. In case of accidental overdose, immediate medical attention is essential even if you do not notice any sign or symptoms.

Composition:
Tablets: Active Ingredient: Acetaminophen. Inactive Ingredients: FD&C Red No. 28, FD&C Red No. 40, flavor, Mannitol, Saccharin Sodium, Starch, Stearic Acid and other ingredients.
Liquid: Active Ingredient: Acetaminophen. Inactive Ingredients: Benzoic acid, FD&C Red No. 40, Flavor, Glycerin, Polyethylene Glycol, Potassium Sorbate, Propylene Glycol, Purified Water, Saccharin Sodium, Sorbitol solution. May also contain Sodium Chloride or Sodium Hydroxide.
Drops: Active Ingredient: Acetaminophen. Inactive Ingredients: Citric Acid, FD&C Red No. 40, Flavors, Glycerin, Parabens, Polyethylene Glycol, Propylene Glycol, Purified Water, Saccharin Sodium, Sodium Chloride, Sodium Citrate.

How Supplied: Chewable Tablets (colored pink and scored)—bottles of 30. Liquid (colored red)—bottles of 2 fl. oz. and 4 fl. oz. Drops (colored red)—bottles of ½ oz. (15 mL).
All packages listed above have child-resistant safety caps and tamper-resistant features.

Shown in Product Identification Guide, page 428

Junior Strength PANADOL®
Acetaminophen Caplets

Description: Each Junior Strength PANADOL® Caplet contains 160 mg of acetaminophen.

Indications: Acetaminophen, the active ingredient in Junior Strength PANADOL®, is the analgesic/antipyretic most widely recommended by pediatricians for fast, effective relief of children's fevers. It also relieves the aches and pains of colds and flu, earaches, headaches, teething, immunizations, tonsillectomy, menstrual discomfort, and childhood illness.
Junior Strength PANADOL® Caplets are aspirin-free, sugar-free.

Usual Dosage: Dosing is based on single doses in the range of 10–15 mg/kg body weight. Doses may be repeated every 4 hours up to 4 or 5 times daily, but not to exceed 5 doses in 24 hours. To be administered to children under 2 years only on the advice of a physician.

2–3 yr, 24–35 lb, 1 caplet; 4–5 yr, 36–47 lb, 1½ caplets; 6–8 yr, 48–59 lb, 2 caplets; 9–10 yr, 60–71 lb, 2½ caplets; 11 yr, 72–95 lb, 3 caplets. 12 yr and over, 96 lb and over, 4 caplets. Dosage may be repeated every 4 hours, up to 5 times in a 24-hour period.

Inactive Ingredients: Hydroxypropyl Methylcellulose, Potassium Sorbate, Povidone, Pregelatinized Starch, Starch, Stearic Acid, Talc, Triacetin.

Warnings: Do not give this product for pain for more than 5 days or for fever for more than 3 days unless directed by a doctor. If symptoms persist or new ones occur, consult a doctor. As with any drug, if you are pregnant or nursing a baby, seek the advice of a health professional before using this product. Keep this and all drugs out of the reach of children. In case of accidental overdose, immediate medical attention is essential even if you do not notice any sign or symptoms.

How Supplied: Swallowable caplets (white)—blister-pack of 30. Package has child-resistant and tamper-resistant features.

Shown in Product Identification Guide, page 428

PHILLIPS'® GELCAPS
Laxative plus Stool Softener

Active Ingredients: A combination of phenolphthalein (90 mg) and docusate sodium (83 mg) per gelcap.

Inactive Ingredients: FD&C Blue # 2, gelatin, glycerin, PEG 400 and 3350, propylene glycol, sorbitol, and titanium dioxide.

Indications: For relief of occasional constipation (irregularity). This product generally produces bowel movement in 6 to 12 hours.

Action: Phenolphthalein is a stimulant laxative which increases the peristaltic activity of the intestine. Docusate sodium is a stool softener which allows easier passage of the stool.

Directions: Adults and children 12 and over take one (1) or two (2) gelcaps daily with a full glass (8 oz) of liquid, or as directed by a doctor. For children under 12, consult your doctor.

Warnings: Do not take any laxative if abdominal pain, nausea, vomiting, change in bowel habits persisting for over 2 weeks, rectal bleeding or kidney disease is present. Laxative products should not be used for a period longer than one week, unless directed by a physician. If there is a failure to have a bowel movement after use, discontinue and consult your doctor. If a skin rash appears do not take this or any other preparation which contains phenolphthalein. Keep this and all drugs out of the reach

of children. In case of accidental overdose, seek professional assistance or contact a poison control center immediately. As with any drug, if you are pregnant or nursing a baby, seek the advice of a health professional before using this product.

How Supplied: Blister packs of 30 and 60 gelcaps.

Shown in Product Identification Guide, page 428

PHILLIPS'® MILK OF MAGNESIA
Laxative/Antacid

Active Ingredients: A suspension of magnesium hydroxide in purified water meeting all USP specifications. Phillips' Milk of Magnesia contains 400 mg per teaspoon (5 mL) of magnesium hydroxide.

Inactive Ingredients: Original—Purified water. Mint—Carboxymethylcellulose Sodium, Citric Acid, Flavor, Glycerin, Microcrystalline Cellulose, Propylene Glycol, Purified water, Sorbitol, Sucrose, Xanthan Gum.
Cherry—(same as mint), D&C Red #28.

Indications: For relief of occasional constipation (irregularity), relief of acid indigestion, sour stomach and heartburn. The laxative dosage generally produces bowel movement in ½ to 6 hours.

Action at Laxative Dosage: Phillips' Milk of Magnesia is a mild saline laxative which acts by drawing water into the gut, increasing intraluminal pressure, and increasing intestinal motility.

Action at Antacid Dosage: Phillips' Milk of Magnesia is an effective acid neutralizer.

Directions: As a laxative, adults and children 12 years and older, 2–4 tbsp; children 6–11 years, 1–2 tbsp; children 2–5 years, 1–3 tsp followed by a full glass (8 oz) of liquid. Children under 2, consult a doctor.
As an antacid, adults & children 12 & older, 1–3 tsp with a little water, up to four times a day, or as directed by your doctor.

Drug Interaction Precaution: Antacids may interact with certain prescription drugs. If you are presently taking a prescription drug do not take this product without checking with your doctor or other health professional.

Laxative Warnings: Do not take any laxative if abdominal pain, nausea, vomiting, change in bowel habits persisting for over 2 weeks, rectal bleeding, or kidney disease is present. Laxative products should not be used for a period longer than 1 week, unless directed by a doctor. If there is a failure to have a bowel movement after use, discontinue and consult your doctor.

Antacid Warnings: Do not take more than the maximum recommended daily dosage in a 24-hour period (see Directions), or use the maximum dosage of this

product for more than two weeks, or use this product if you have kidney disease, except under the advice and supervision of a doctor. May have laxative effect.

General Warnings: As with any drug, if you are pregnant or nursing a baby, seek the advice of a health professional before using this product. Keep this and all drugs out of reach of children. In case of accidental overdose, seek professional assistance or contact a poison control center immediately.

How Supplied: Phillips' Milk of Magnesia is available in original, mint and cherry flavor in 4, 12 and 26 fl oz bottles. Also available in tablet form and concentrated liquid form.

Shown in Product Identification Guide, page 428

STRI-DEX®
[Strī-dex]
CLEAR GEL ACNE MEDICATION

Active Ingredient: Salicylic Acid 2.0%.

Inactive Ingredients: Carbomer 940, Citric Acid, DMDM Hydantoin, Glycerin, Phenoxyethanol, Polyglycerylmethacrylate, Propylene Glycol, Purified Water, SD Alcohol 9.3% (w/w), Tetrasodium EDTA, Triethanolamine.

Indications: For the treatment of acne. Reduces the number of blackheads and allows the skin to heal. Helps prevent new acne pimples from forming.

Directions: Clean the skin thoroughly before use. Apply a thin layer to acne pimple areas of face, neck and body 1 to 3 times daily. Because excessive drying of the skin may occur, start with one application daily, then gradually increase to two or three times daily if needed or as directed by a doctor. If bothersome dryness or peeling occurs, reduce application to once a day or every other day.

Warnings: FOR EXTERNAL USE ONLY. Using other topical acne medications at the same time or immediately following use of this product may increase dryness or irritation of the skin. If this occurs, only one medication should be used unless directed by a doctor. Persons who are sensitive to or have a known allergy to salicylic acid should not use this medication. If excessive itching, dryness, redness or swelling occurs, discontinue use. If these symptoms persist, consult a doctor promptly. Keep away from eyes, lips and other mucous membranes. Keep this and all drugs out of the reach of children. In case of accidental

Continued on next page

This product information was effective as of November 1, 1993. Current information may be obtained directly from Sterling Health, by writing to 90 Park Avenue, New York, NY 10016.

Sterling Health—Cont.

ingestion, seek professional assistance or contact a poison control center immediately.

How Supplied: 1oz Tube.
Shown in Product Identification Guide, page 428

STRI–DEX® DUAL TEXTURED PADS
Regular Strength
STRI–DEX® DUAL TEXTURED PADS
Maximum Strength
STRI–DEX® DUAL TEXTURED PADS
Sensitive Skin
STRI–DEX® SUPER SCRUB PADS
Oil Fighting Formula
STRI–DEX® SINGLE TEXTURED PADS
Maximum Strength
STRI–DEX® ANTIBACTERIAL CLEANSING BAR

Active Ingredients:
Stri-Dex® Regular Strength: Salicylic Acid 0.5%.
Stri-Dex® Maximum Strength: Salicylic Acid 2.0%.
Stri-Dex® Sensitive Skin: Salicylic Acid 0.5%.
Stri-Dex® Super Scrub: Salicylic Acid 2.0%.
Stri-Dex® Single Textured Maximum Strength: Salicylic Acid 2.0%.
Stri-Dex® Antibacterial Cleansing Bar: Triclosan 1%.

Inactive Ingredients:
Stri-Dex® Regular Strength: Purified Water, SD Alcohol 28%, Sodium Xylenesulfonate, Sodium Dodecylbenzenesulfonate, Citric Acid, Sodium Carbonate, Fragrance, Menthol, Simethicone Emulsion.
Stri-Dex® Maximum Strength: Purified Water, SD Alcohol 44%, Ammonium Xylenesulfonate, Sodium Dodecylbenzenesulfonate, Citric Acid, Sodium Carbonate, Fragrance, Menthol, Simethicone Emulsion.
Stri-Dex® Sensitive Skin: Purified Water, SD Alcohol 28%, Aloe Vera Gel, Sodium Xylenesulfonate, Sodium Dodecylbenzenesulfonate, Citric Acid, Sodium Carbonate, Fragrance, Menthol, Simethicone Emulsion.
Stri-Dex® Super Scrub: SD Alcohol 54%, Purified Water, Ammonium Xylenesulfonate, Sodium Dodecylbenzenesulfonate, Citric Acid, Sodium Lauroyl Sarcosinate, Sodium Carbonate, Menthol, Fragrance, Simethicone Emulsion.
Stri-Dex® Single Textured: Purified Water, SD Alcohol 44%, Ammonium Xylenesulfonate, Sodium Dodecylbenzenesulfonate, Citric Acid, Sodium Carbonate, Fragrance, Simethicone Emulsion.
Stri-Dex® Antibacterial Cleansing Bar: Sodium Tallowate, Sodium Cocoate and/or Sodium Palm Kernelate, Water, Glycerin, Sucrose, Potassium Cy-

clocarboxypropyloleate, Bentonite, Cetyl Acetate, Acetylated Lanolin Alcohol, Pentasodium Pentetate, Tetrasodium Etidronate, D&C Yellow #10, D&C Orange #4.

Indications: Stri-Dex® Pads for the treatment of acne. Reduces the number of acne pimples and blackheads, and allows the skin to heal. Helps prevent new acne pimples from forming.
Stri-Dex® Antibacterial Cleansing Bar: Antibacterial Soap.

Directions:
Stri-Dex® Pads. Cleanse the skin thoroughly before using all varieties of Stri-Dex medicated pads. Use the pad to open pores and loosen the oil and dirt that can clog them. Then wipe away oil and dirt and leave behind a tough pimple fighting medicine that will treat pimples and help prevent new ones from forming. Use the pad to wipe the entire affected area one to three times daily. Because excessive drying of the skin may occur, start with one application daily, then gradually increase to two or three times daily if needed or as directed by a doctor.
Stri-Dex Bar. Use Stri-Dex® Antibacterial Cleansing Bar in place of ordinary soap. For best results use three times daily. Work up an abundant lather with warm water and massage into the skin. Rinse thoroughly and pat dry with a towel. Use Stri-Dex® Antibacterial Cleansing Bar for facial cleansing as well as in the bath.
After deep cleaning the skin with Stri-Dex® Antibacterial Cleansing Bar, continue on acne treatment program with Stri-Dex® Medicated Acne Pads.

Warnings: Stri-Dex Pads : FOR EXTERNAL USE ONLY: Using other topical acne medications at the same time or immediately following use of this product may increase dryness or irritation of the skin. If this occurs, only one medication should be used unless directed by a doctor. Persons with very sensitive skin or known allergy to salicylic acid should not use this medication. If irritation or excessive dryness and/or peeling occurs, reduce frequency of use or dosage. If excessive itching, dryness, redness, or swelling occurs, discontinue use. If these symptoms persist, consult a physician promptly. Keep away from eyes, lips, and other mucous membranes. Keep this and all drugs out of reach of children. In the case of accidental ingestion, seek professional assistance or contact a Poison control center immediately.
Stri-Dex Antibacterial Cleansing Bar: Do not use this product on infants under 6 months of age. For external use only. Do not get in eyes.

How Supplied:
Stri-Dex Regular Strength is available in packages of 32 and 50 pads.
Stri-Dex Maximum Strength is available in packages of 32 and 50 pads.
Stri-Dex Sensitive Skin is available in a package of 32 pads.
Stri-Dex Super Scrub is available in a package of 32 pads.

Stri-Dex Single Textured is available in a package of 55 pads.
Stri-Dex Antibacterial Cleansing Bar is available in a 3.5 ounce package.
Shown in Product Identification Guide, page 428

VANQUISH® Analgesic Caplets

Active Ingredients: Each caplet contains aspirin 227 mg, acetaminophen 194 mg, caffeine 33 mg, dried aluminum hydroxide gel 25 mg, magnesium hydroxide 50 mg in a thin, inert hydroxypropyl methylcellulose coating for easier swallowing.

Inactive Ingredients: Microcrystalline Cellulose, Polyethylene Glycol, Polysorbate 80, Silicon Dioxide, Starch, Titanium Dioxide, Zinc Stearate.

Indications: A buffered analgesic, antipyretic for relief of headache; muscular aches and pains; neuralgia and neuritic pain; toothache; pain following dental procedures; for painful discomforts and fever of colds and flu; functional menstrual pain, headache and pain due to cramps; temporary relief from minor pains of arthritis, rheumatism, bursitis, lumbago, sciatica.

Directions: Adults and children 12 years and over: Two caplets with water. May be repeated every four hours if necessary up to 12 caplets per day. Larger or more frequent doses may be prescribed by doctor if necessary.

Warnings: Children and teenagers should not use this medicine for chicken pox or flu symptoms before a doctor is consulted about Reye syndrome, a rare but serious illness reported to be associated with aspirin. Do not take for pain for more than 10 days or for fever for more than 3 days unless directed by a doctor. If pain or fever persists or gets worse, if new symptoms occur, or if redness or swelling is present consult a doctor immediately. Do not take this product if you are allergic to aspirin, have asthma, stomach problems that persist or recur, gastric ulcers or bleeding problems unless directed by a doctor. If ringing in the ears or loss of hearing occurs, consult a doctor before taking any more of this product. Keep this and all drugs out of the reach of children. In case of accidental overdose, immediate medical attention is essential for adults as well as for children even if you do not notice any sign or symptoms. As with any drug, if you are pregnant or nursing a baby, seek the advice of a health professional before using this product. **IT IS ESPECIALLY IMPORTANT NOT TO USE ASPIRIN DURING THE LAST 3 MONTHS OF PREGNANCY UNLESS SPECIFICALLY DIRECTED TO DO SO BY A DOCTOR BECAUSE IT MAY CAUSE PROBLEMS IN THE UNBORN CHILD OR COMPLICATIONS DURING DELIVERY.**

Drug Interaction Precaution: Do not take this product if you are taking a prescription drug for anticoagulation (thinning of the blood), diabetes, gout, or arthritis unless directed by a doctor.

How Supplied:
White, capsule-shaped caplets in bottles of 30, 60 and 100 caplets.

Shown in Product Identification Guide, page 429

Thompson Medical Company, Inc.
**222 LAKEVIEW AVENUE
WEST PALM BEACH
FLORIDA 33401**

ASPERCREME®
[ăs-per-crēme]
External Analgesic Rub With Aloe

Description: ASPERCREME® is available as an odor-free creme and lotion for use as a topical massage rub that temporarily relieves minor muscle aches and pains without stomach upset. **Aspercreme does not contain aspirin.**

Active Ingredients: Salycin® 10% (Thompson Medical's brand of Trolamine Salicylate).

Other Ingredients: Creme: Aloe Vera Gel, Cetyl Alcohol, Glycerin, Methylparaben, Mineral Oil, Potassium Phosphate, Propylparaben, Stearic Acid, Triethanolamine, Water. Lotion: Aloe Vera Gel, Cetyl Alcohol, Fragrance, Glyceryl Stearate, Isopropyl Palmitate, Lanolin, Methylparaben, Potassium Phosphate, Propylene Glycol, Propylparaben, Sodium Lauryl Sulfate, Stearic Acid, Water.

Actions: External analgesic rub.

Indications: Analgesic rub for temporary relief of minor aches and pains of muscles associated with simple strains and sprains. **Aspercreme contains no aspirin.**

Warnings: Use only as directed. If prone to allergic reaction from aspirin or salicylate, consult your doctor before using. If redness is present or condition worsens, or if pain persists for more than 7 days or clears up and occurs again within a few days, discontinue use and consult a doctor. Do not use on children under 10 years of age. Do not apply if skin is irritated or if irritation develops. As with any drug, if you are pregnant or nursing a baby, seek the advice of a health professional before using this product. For external use only. Avoid contact with eyes. **KEEP THIS AND ALL MEDICINES OUT OF THE REACH OF CHILDREN.**
In case of accidental ingestion seek professional assistance or contact a Poison Control Center immediately.

Dosage and Administration: Apply generously directly to affected area. Massage into painful area until thoroughly

absorbed into skin, repeat as necessary, especially before retiring but not more than 4 times daily.

How to Store: Store at controlled room temperature 59°–86°F (15°–30°C).

How Supplied: Creme: 1¼ oz., 3 oz. and 5 oz. tubes. Lotion: 6 oz. bottle.

CORTIZONE–5®
Cream and Ointment
CORTIZONE FOR KIDS™ Cream
**Anti-itch
(0.5% hydrocortisone)**

Description: CORTIZONE-5® cream and ointment are topical anti-itch preparations.

Active Ingredient: Hydrocortisone 0.5%.

Other Ingredients: Cream: Aluminum Sulfate, Calcium Acetate, Glycerin, Light Mineral Oil, Methylparaben, Potato Dextrin, Purified Water, Sodium Lauryl Sulfate, White Petrolatum. May Also Contain: Cetearyl Alcohol, Propylparaben, Sodium C₁₂₋₁₅ Alcohols Sulfate, Synthetic Beeswax, White Wax. CORTIZONE for Kids additionally contains Aloe Vera gel.
Ointment: White Petrolatum.

Indications: CORTIZONE-5® is recommended for the temporary relief of itching associated with minor skin irritations, inflammations and rashes due to: eczema, insect bites, poison ivy, oak, sumac, soaps, detergents, cosmetics, jewelry, seborrheic dermatitis, psoriasis, external anal and genital itching. Other uses of this product should be only under the advice and supervision of a physician.

Warnings: For external use only. Avoid contact with the eyes. If condition worsens, or if symptoms persist for more than 7 days or clear up and occur again within a few days, stop use of this product and do not begin use of any hydrocortisone product unless you have consulted a physician. Do not use in genital area if you have a vaginal discharge. Consult a physician. Do not use for the treatment of diaper rash. Consult a physician.
Warnings For External Anal Itching Users: Do not exceed the recommended daily dosage unless directed by a physician. In case of bleeding, consult a physician promptly. Do not put this product into the rectum by using fingers or any mechanical device or applicator.
KEEP THIS AND ALL MEDICINES OUT OF THE REACH OF CHILDREN. In case of accidental ingestion, seek professional assistance or contact a Poison Control Center immediately.

Dosage and Administration: Adults and children 2 years of age and older: Apply to affected area not more than 3 to 4 times daily. Children under 2 years of age: Do not use, consult a physician.
Directions For External Anal Itching Users: Adults: When practical, cleanse

the affected area with mild soap and warm water and rinse thoroughly. Gently dry by patting or blotting with toilet tissue or a soft cloth before application of this product. Children under 12 years of age: Consult a physician.

How to Store: Store at controlled room temperature 15°–30°C (59°–86°F).

How Supplied: CORTIZONE-5 cream: 1 oz. and 2 oz. tubes. CORTIZONE for Kids™ cream: ½ oz. and 1 oz. tubes. CORTIZONE-5 ointment: 1 oz. tube.

Shown in Product Identification Guide, page 429

CORTIZONE–10™
Cream and Ointment
CORTIZONE-10™ EXTERNAL ANAL ITCH RELIEF Cream
CORTIZONE-10™ SCALP ITCH FORMULA™ Liquid
**Anti-itch
(1.0% hydrocortisone)**

Description: CORTIZONE-10™ cream, ointment and liquid are topical anti-itch preparations. Maximum Strength available without a prescription.

Active Ingredient: Hydrocortisone 1.0%.

Other Ingredients: Cream: Aluminum Sulfate, Calcium Acetate, Cetearyl Alcohol, Glycerin, Light Mineral Oil, Methylparaben, Potato Dextrin, Sodium Lauryl Sulfate, Water, White Petrolatum, White Wax. **May Also Contain:** Aloe Vera Gel, Sodium C12–15 Alcohols Sulfate, Propylparaben.
Ointment: White Petrolatum.
Liquid: Benzyl Alcohol, Propylene Glycol, Purified Water, SD Alcohol 40-2 (60% v/v)

Indications: Cortizone-10™ is recommended for the temporary relief of itching associated with minor skin irritations, inflammation and rashes due to: eczema, insect bites, poison ivy, oak, sumac, soaps, detergents, cosmetics, jewelry, seborrheic dermatitis, psoriasis, external anal and genital itching. Other uses of this product should be only under the advice and supervision of a physician.

Warnings: For external use only. Avoid contact with the eyes. If condition worsens, or if symptoms persist for more than 7 days or clear up and occur again within a few days, stop use of this product and do not begin use of any hydrocortisone product unless you have consulted a physician. Do not use in genital area if you have a vaginal discharge. Consult a physician. Do not use for the treatment of diaper rash. Consult a physician.
Warnings For External Anal Itching Users: Do not exceed the recommended daily dosage unless directed by a physician. In case of bleeding, consult a physician promptly. Do not put this product

Continued on next page

Thompson Medical—Cont.

into the rectum by using fingers or any mechanical device or applicator.
KEEP THIS AND ALL MEDICINES OUT OF THE REACH OF CHILDREN. In case of accidental ingestion, seek professional assistance or contact a Poison Control Center immediately.

Dosage and Administration: Adults and children 2 years of age and older: Apply to affected area not more than 3 to 4 times daily. Children under 2 years of age: Do not use, consult a physician.

Directions For External Anal Itching Users: Adults: When practical, cleanse the affected area with mild soap and warm water. Rinse thoroughly. Gently dry by patting or blotting with tissue or a soft cloth before application of this product. Children under 12 years of age: consult a physician.

How to Store: Store at controlled room temperature 15°–30°C (59°–86°F).

How Supplied: CORTIZONE-10™ cream: 1 oz. and 2 oz. tubes. CORTIZONE-10™ ointment: 1 oz. tube. CORTIZONE-10™ External Anal Itch Relief cream: 1 oz. tube. CORTIZONE-10™ Scalp Itch Formula™ liquid: 1.5 fl. oz.
Shown in Product Identification Guide, page 429

DEXATRIM® Caplets and Tablets
[dĕx-a-trĭm]
Prolonged action anorectic for weight control

DEXATRIM® Maximum Strength Plus Vitamin C/Caplets and Caffeine-Free Caplets
phenylpropanolamine HCl   75mg
(time release)
(180 mg Vitamin C, immediate release, added for nutritional supplementation)

DEXATRIM® Maximum Strength Extended Duration Time Tablets
phenylpropanolamine HCl   75mg
(time release)

Indication: DEXATRIM® is an aid for effective appetite control to assist weight reduction. It is available in a time release dosage form.

Directions: Adult oral dosage is **one caplet** at mid-morning with a full glass of water. **Exceeding the recommended dose has not been shown to result in greater weight loss.** (This product's effectiveness is directly related to the degree to which you reduce your usual daily food intake.) The use of this product should be limited to periods not exceeding 3 months, because this should be enough time to establish new eating habits. Read and follow the important Diet Plan enclosed.

Warnings: FOR ADULT USE ONLY. DO NOT TAKE MORE THAN 1 CAPLET PER DAY (24 HOURS). **Exceeding the recommended dose may cause**

serious health problems. Do not give this product to children under 12 years of age. Persons between 12 and 18 are advised to consult their physician before using this product. If nervousness, dizziness, sleeplessness, palpitations or headache occurs stop taking this medication and consult your physician. If you are being treated for depression, an eating disorder or have heart disease, diabetes, thyroid or any other disease, do not take this product except under the supervision of a physician. Check your blood pressure regularly. If you have high blood pressure, do not use this product and consult your physician. As with any drug, if your are pregnant or nursing a baby seek the advice of a health professional before using this product.

Drug Interaction Precaution: If you are taking a cough/cold or allergy medication containing any form of phenylpropanolamine, or any oral nasal decongestant, do not take this product. Do not use this product if you are taking any prescription drug, except under the advice and supervision of a physician. Do not use this product if you are presently taking a prescription monoamine oxidase inhibitor (MAOI) for depression or for two weeks after stopping use of an MAOI without first consulting a physician.
KEEP THIS AND ALL MEDICATION OUT OF THE REACH OF CHILDREN. In case of accidental overdose, seek professional assistance or contact a Poison Control Center immediately.

Dosage and Administration:
Caplet Dosage Forms: DEXATRIM® Maximum Strength Plus Vitamin C, DEXATRIM® Maximum Strength/Caffeine-Free.
Tablet Dosage Form: DEXATRIM® Maximum Strength Extended Duration Time Tablets.
Administration: One caplet or tablet at midmorning with a full glass of water.

How Supplied: All Dexatrim products are supplied in tamper-evident blister packages. Do not use if individual seals are broken.
DEXATRIM® Maximum Strength Plus Vitamin C/Caffeine-Free Caplets: Packages of 20 and 40 with 1250 calorie DEXATRIM Diet Plan.
DEXATRIM® Maximum Strength Extended Duration Time Tablets: Packages of 20 and 40 with 1250 calorie DEXATRIM Diet Plan.

References: Altschuler, S., et. al., *Int J Obesity*, 1982;6:549–556.
Atkinson, RL, Dannels SA, Marlin RL; AM J Clin Nutr, 56 (4); 755; Oct. 1992.
Blackburn, G.L., et. al., *JAMA*, 1989; 261:3267–3272.
Morgan, J.P., et. al., *J Clin Psychopharm*, 1989:9(1):33–38.
Lasagna, L., *Phenylpropanolamine—A Review*, New York, John Wiley and Sons, 1988.
All referenced materials available on request.
Shown in Product Identification Guide, page 429

ENCARE®
[en'kar]
Vaginal Contraceptive Suppositories

Description: Encare is a safe and effective contraceptive in a convenient vaginal suppository form available without a prescription. Encare is reliable because it offers two-way protection: (1) Encare kills sperm on contact by releasing a precise dose of nonoxynol 9, the spermicide most recommended by doctors. (2) Encare gently disperses a physical barrier of protection against the cervix to help prevent pregnancy.
Encare is colorless and odorless; it is as pleasant to use as it is effective.
Encare is an effective contraceptive in vaginal suppository form.

Active Ingredient: Each Suppository contains 100 mg Nonoxynol 9.

Other Ingredients: Polyethylene Glycols, Sodium Bicarbonate, Sodium Citrate, Tartaric Acid.

Indications: Encare is effective in the prevention of pregnancy.

Action: Encare is 100% free of hormones and free of the serious side effects associated with oral contraceptives.
Encare is convenient and easy to use. Women like Encare because each insert is individually wrapped and can be easily carried in a pocket or purse. Encare is approximately as effective as vaginal foam contraceptives in actual use, yet there is no applicator, so there is nothing to fill, remove, or clean. In addition, women may find Encare convenient to use in conjunction with other contraceptive methods, such as a condom or as a second application with a diaphragm.
Because Encare can be inserted as much as an hour before intercourse, it does not interfere with spontaneity or ruin the mood. Many men are not even aware a woman is using Encare. Encare has been used successfully by millions of women throughout Europe and America.

Special Warning: Spermicidal contraceptives should not be used during pregnancy. Some experts believe that there may be an increased risk of birth defects occurring in children whose mothers used a spermicidal contraceptive at the time of conception or during pregnancy. If you have used a spermicidal contraceptive after becoming pregnant, or used a spermicidal contraceptive when you became pregnant, discuss this issue with your doctor.

Cautions: If your doctor has told you that you should not become pregnant, consult your doctor as to which method, including Encare, is best for you.
If you or your partner experience irritation, discontinue use. If irritation persists, consult your doctor. This product has not been shown to protect against HIV (AIDS) and other sexually transmitted diseases.
Do not take orally. **KEEP THIS AND ALL DRUGS OUT OF THE REACH OF CHILDREN.** In case of accidental in-

gestion, call a Poison Control Center, emergency medical facility or a doctor immediately.

Keep away from excessive heat and moisture. Store at controlled room temperature: 15°C–30°C (59°–86°F).

Dosage and Administration: For best protection against pregnancy, it is essential to follow package instructions. At least 10 minutes before intercourse, place one Encare insert with your fingertip as far as possible into the vagina, towards the small of your back. Best protection will occur when Encare is placed deep into the vagina. You may feel a pleasant sensation of warmth as Encare effervesces and distributes the spermicide, nonoxynol 9, within the vagina. This is a natural attribute of the active ingredient.

IMPORTANT: It is essential to insert Encare at least 10 minutes before intercourse. If one chooses, Encare can be inserted up to one hour before intercourse. If intercourse has not taken place within one hour after insertion, use a new Encare insert. Use a new Encare insert each time intercourse is repeated. Encare can be used safely as frequently as needed. Douching after use of Encare is not required; however, should you desire to do so, wait at least six hours after intercourse.

How Supplied: Boxes of 12.

References: Barwin, B., *Contraceptive Delivery System*, 4, 331–334, 1983. Masters, W., et. al. *Fertility and Sterility*, 32, 161–165, 1979.

Dimpfl J., et. al. sexualmedizin 1984; 2: 95-8. Schill WB, Wolff HH. Andrologia 1981; 13(1): 42-9. Stone SC, Cardinale F. AM J Obstet Gynecol 1979; 133: 635-8.

SLEEPINAL®
Night-time Sleep Aid Capsules and Softgels
(Diphenhydramine HCl)

Description: SLEEPINAL is a nighttime sleep aid. When taken prior to bedtime, it helps to relieve sleeplessness and aids in falling asleep.

Active Ingredient: Diphenhydramine HCl 50 mg.

Other Ingredients: Capsules: FD&C Blue No. 1, Gelatin, Lactose, Magnesium Stearate, Povidone, Talc.
Softgels: D&C Yellow No. 10, FD&C Blue No. 1, Gelatin, Glycerin, Polyethylene Glycol 400, Povidone 30, Propylene Glycol, Sorbitol, Water.

Indications: For relief of occasional sleeplessness.

Action: SLEEPINAL is an antihistamine with anticholinergic and sedative action.

Warnings: Read before using. Do not exceed recommended dosage. Do not give to children under 12 years of age. If sleeplessness persists continuously for more than 2 weeks, consult a physician. Insom-

nia may be a symptom of serious underlying medical illness. Do not take this product if you have asthma, glaucoma, emphysema, chronic pulmonary disease, shortness of breath, difficulty in breathing, or difficulty in urination due to enlargement of the prostate gland unless directed by a physician. Avoid alcoholic beverages while taking this product. Do not take this product if you are taking sedatives or tranquilizers, without first consulting your physician. As with any drug, if you are pregnant or nursing a baby, seek the advice of a health professional before using this product.

KEEP THIS AND ALL MEDICATIONS OUT OF THE REACH OF CHILDREN. In the case of accidental overdose, seek professional assistance or contact a Poison Control Center immediately.

Dosage and Administration: Capsules and Softgels: Adults and children 12 years of age and over: Oral dosage, one at bedtime if needed, or as directed by a physician.

How to Store: Store in a dry place at controlled room temperature 15° C–30° C (59° F–86° F). Protect softgels from light, retain product in box until administered.

How Supplied: Capsules and Softgels: Sleepinal is supplied in tamper-evident blister packages. Do not use if individual seals are broken. Packages of 16 and 32 capsules and 8 and 16 softgels.
Shown in Product Identification Guide, page 429

SPORTSCREME
[*spōrts-crēme*]
External Analgesic Rub Products

Description: Sportscreme External Analgesic Rub Products are available in a fresh scent, 10% Trolamine Salicylate lotion and cream formulation, as well as a 2% Menthol ice.

Actions and Uses: These products were formulated for hours of relief of aches, strains, and minor muscle pain of the arms, legs, shoulders, and back. The ice formulation also provides temporary relief of minor arthritis pain.

Directions: Apply generously. Massage into painful area until completely absorbed into skin. Repeat as needed not more than 4 times daily.

Warnings: For external use only as directed. Avoid contact with eyes. Do not apply if skin is irritated. Keep this and all medicines out of the reach of children. In case of accidental ingestion, seek professional assistance or contact a Poison Control Center immediately. If redness is present or condition worsens, or if pain persists for more than 7 days or clears up and occurs again within a few days, discontinue use and consult a doctor.
Cream and lotion: If prone to allergic reaction from aspirin or salicylate, consult your doctor before using. Do not use on children under 10 years of age. Do not apply if skin is irritated or if irritation

develops. As with any drug, if you are pregnant or nursing a baby, seek the advice of a health professional before using this product.
Ice: Avoid contact with mucous membranes, broken or irritated skin. Do not bandage tightly. Do not use on children under 2 years of age except under the advice and supervision of a doctor.

How to Store: Store at controlled room temperature 59°–86°F (15°–30°C).

How Supplied: Cream: 1¼ oz., 3 oz., and 5 oz tubes. Lotion: 6 oz bottle. Ice: 8 oz jar.
Shown in Product Identification Guide, page 429

TEMPO
[*tem-pō*]
Soft Antacid

Description: Tempo is a unique, chewable soft antacid that provides fast, effective relief from acid indigestion, heartburn, and gas. Tempo has 75% more acid relieving medicine than the leading tablet, so you need just one. Tempo is pleasant tasting, not chalky or gritty.

Active Ingredients: Each drop contains Calcium Carbonate 414 mg., Aluminum Hydroxide 133 mg., Magnesium Hydroxide 81 mg., Simethicone 20 mg.

Other Ingredients: Corn Syrup, Deionized Water, FD&C Blue No. 1, Flavor, Sorbitol, Soy Protein, Starch, Titanium Dioxide, 3.0 mg. Sodium per drop (dietetically sodium free).

Indication: For the relief of heartburn, sour stomach, acid indigestion, gas, and upset stomach associated with these symptoms.

Warnings: Do not take more than 12 drops in a 24-hour period or use the maximum dosage for more than two weeks except under the advice and supervision of a doctor. **KEEP THIS AND ALL DRUGS OUT OF THE REACH OF CHILDREN.**

Drug Interaction Precaution: Antacids may interact with certain prescription drugs. If you are presently taking a prescription drug, do not take this product without checking with your physician or other health professional.

Dosage and Administration: One tablet dosage. Not to exceed more than 12 tablets in a 24-hour period.

How to Store: Store at controlled room temperature 15°–30°C (59°–86°F).

How Supplied: 10, 30, and 60 Pieces
Shown in Product Identification Guide, page 429

TRASK Industries
163 FARRELL STREET
SOMERSET, NJ 08873

Fibro Malic®
Malic Acid and
Magnesium Hydroxide

Ingredients: Fibro Malic® tablets are free from alar, animal products, sugar, starch, corn antigens, dairy products, wheat products, yeast products, fish oil, kelp, artificial colors, artificial flavors, or preservatives.

	% U.S. R.D.A.*
Six tablets provide:	
Magnesium (hydroxide) 300 mg	75

Other ingredients: Malic Acid (1,200 mg per 6 tablets). Pharmaceutical grade excipients.
*Percentage United States recommended daily allowance for adults and children over 4 years of age.

Indications And Usage: Relieves the pain and other symptoms caused by fibromyalagia and Chronic fatigue syndrome. And as a source of magnesium and malic acid, ingest three (3) tablets with a glass of water one hour before breakfast and at bedtime, or as directed by a physician.

Side Effects: Gastrointestinal disturbances such as diarrhea and loose stool may occur in some individuals at doses greater than 6 tablets a day. If you experience any of these side effects, decrease the amount used and consult your physician.

Warnings: If you are under medical care and receiving medication for a medical problem, consult with your physician prior to use.
STORE IN A COOL DRY PLACE
Dietary Supplement: Keep out of reach of children. Pregnant and Lactating Mothers should consult Physician before taken.

READ BROCHURE INSIDE BOTTLE BEFORE USE
TRASK Industries
Somerset N.J.

Triton Consumer Products, Inc.
561 W. GOLF ROAD
ARLINGTON HEIGHTS, IL 60005

MG 217® PSORIASIS/DANDRUFF MEDICATION
Skin Care: Ointment and Lotion
Scalp: Shampoo

Active Ingredients: Ointment—Coal Tar Solution USP 10%. **Lotion**—Coal Tar Solution USP 5%. **Tar Shampoo**—Coal Tar Solution USP 15%. **Tar-Free Shampoo**—Sulfur 5% and salicylic acid 3%.

Action/Uses: Relief for itching, scaling and flaking of psoriasis, seborrheic dermatitis and/or dandruff.

Warnings: For external use only. Keep out of the reach of children. Avoid contact with eyes. If undue skin irritation occurs, discontinue use.

Administration: Ointment or Lotion —Apply to affected area one to four times daily. **Shampoo**—Shake well before using. Wet hair, then massage liberal amount of MG 217 into scalp and leave on for several minutes. Rinse thoroughly. For best results, use at least twice a week or as directed by a physician.

How Supplied: Ointment—3.8 oz. jars. **Lotion**—4 oz. bottles. **Shampoo**—4 oz. and 8 oz. bottles.

Wakunaga of America Co., Ltd.
Subsidiary of Wakunaga
Pharmaceutical Co., Ltd.
23501 MADERO
MISSION VIEJO, CA 92691

KYOLIC®
Odor Modified Garlic

Active Ingredient: Aged Garlic Extract.™

Indications: Dietary Supplement.

Suggested Use: Average serving, four capsules or tablets a day during or after meals.

How Supplied: Liquid—Kyolic-Aged Garlic Extract Flavor and Odor Modified Enriched with Vitamin B_1 and B_{12} (and empty gelatine capsules) 2 fl oz (62 capsules) and 4 fl oz (124 capsules). Kyolic-Aged Garlic Extract Flavor and Odor Modified Plain (and empty gelatine capsules) 2 fl oz (62 capsules) and 4 fl oz (124 capsules).
Tablets and Capsules—Ingredients per Tablet or Capsule:
Kyolic—Super Formula 100 Tablets: Aged Garlic Extract Powder (300 mg), Whey (168 mg) blended with natural vegetable sources: Cellulose and Algin, bottles of 100 and 200 tablets.
Kyolic—Super Formula 100 Capsules: Aged Garlic Extract Powder (300 mg), Whey (168 mg), bottles of 100 and 200 capsules.
Kyolic—Super Formula 101 Garlic Plus® Tablets: Aged Garlic Extract Powder (270 mg) blended with Brewer's Yeast (27 mg), Kelp (9 mg), bottles of 100 and 200 tablets.
Kyolic—Super Formula 101 Garlic Plus® Capsules: Aged Garlic Extract Powder (270 mg) blended with Brewer's Yeast (27 mg), Kelp (9 mg), bottles of 50, 100 and 200 capsules.
Kyolic—Super Formula 102 Tablets: Aged Garlic Extract Powder (350 mg), "Kyolic Enzyme Complex™" [Amylase, Protease, Cellulase and Lipase] (30 mg), bottles of 100 and 200 tablets.

Kyolic—Super Formula 102 Capsules: Aged Garlic Extract Powder (350 mg), "Kyolic Enzyme Complex™" [Amylase, Protease, Cellulase and Lipase] (30 mg), bottles of 100 and 200 tablets.
Kyolic—Super Formula 103 Capsules: Aged Garlic Extract Powder (220 mg), Ester C® [Calcium Ascorbate] (150 mg), Astragulus membranaceous (100 mg), Calcium citrate (80 mg), bottles of 100 and 200 capsules.
Kyolic—Super Formula 104 Capsules: Aged Garlic Extract Powder (300 mg), Lecithin (200 mg), bottles of 100 and 200 capsules.
Kyolic—Super Formula 105 Capsules: Aged Garlic Extract Powder (250 mg), Beta-Carotene (37.5 mg) d-Alpha-Tocopheryl Acid Succinate [Vitamin E] (50 mg) in a base of Alfalfa and Parsley, bottles of 100 capsules.
Kyolic—Super Formula 106 Capsules: Aged Garlic Extract Powder (300 mg), d-Alpha Tocopheryl Succinate [Vitamin E] (90 mg), Hawthorn Berry (50 mg), Cayenne Pepper (10 mg), bottles of 50 and 100 capsules.

Professional label "SGP" is available in Aged Garlic Extract powder forms.
Shown in Product Identification Guide, page 429

EDUCATIONAL MATERIAL

From Soil to Shelf
Brochure describing our company, garlic fields, aging tanks and factory, plus our product line.

Wallace Laboratories
P.O. BOX 1001
HALF ACRE ROAD
CRANBURY, NJ 08512

MALTSUPEX®
(malt soup extract)
Powder, Liquid, Tablets

Composition: MALTSUPEX is a nondiastatic extract from barley malt, which is available in powder, liquid, and tablet form. MALTSUPEX has a gentle laxative action and promotes soft, easily passed stools. Each Tablet contains 750 mg of MALTSUPEX and approximately 0.15 to 0.25 mEq of potassium. Tablet Ingredients: D&C Yellow No. 10, FD&C Red No. 40, flavor (artificial), hydroxypropyl methylcellulose, methylparaben, polyethylene glycol, propylparaben, povidone, simethicone emulsion, stearic acid, talc, titanium dioxide.
Powder: Each level scoop provides approximately 8 g of Malt Soup Extract.
Liquid: Each tablespoonful (½ fl. oz.) contains approximately the equivalent of 16 g Malt Soup Extract Powder. Other ingredients: Sodium propionate and potassium sorbate.

EFFECTIVE, NON-HABIT FORMING

Indications: For relief of occasional constipation. This product generally produces bowel movement in 12 to 72 hours.

Warnings: Do not use laxative products when abdominal pain, nausea or vomiting are present unless directed by a physician. If constipation persists, consult a physician.

If you have noticed a sudden change in bowel habits that persists over a period of 2 weeks, consult a physician before using a laxative.

Keep this and all medications out of the reach of children.

Laxative products should not be used for a period longer than one week unless directed by a physician. Rectal bleeding or failure to have a bowel movement after use of a laxative may indicate a serious condition. Discontinue use and consult with a physician.

MALTSUPEX Powder and Liquid only—Do not use these products except under the advice and supervision of a physician if you have kidney disease.

As with any drug, if you are pregnant or nursing a baby, seek the advice of a health professional before using this product.

Precautions: Allow for carbohydrate content in diabetic diets and infant formulas.

Liquid: (67%, 14 g/tablespoon, or 56 calories/tablespoon)

Powder: (83%, 6 g or 24 calories per scoop)

Tablets: 0.6 g per tablet or 3 calories. MALTSUPEX Liquid contains approximately 23 mg of sodium per tablespoonful. Each scoop of **Powder** contains the equivalent of 8 g of Malt Soup Extract Powder and 1.5 to 2.75 mEq of potassium.

Directions: General—Drink a full glass (8 ounces) of liquid with each dose.

AGE	CORRECTIVE*	MAINTENANCE
12 years to ADULTS	Up to 4 scoops twice a day (Take a full glass [8 oz.] of liquid with each dose.)	2 to 4 scoops at bedtime
CHILDREN 6–12 years of age	Up to 2 scoops twice a day (Take a full glass [8 oz.] of liquid with each dose.)	
CHILDREN 2–6 years of age	1 scoop twice a day (Take a full glass [8 oz.] of liquid with each dose.)	
BOTTLE FED INFANTS (Over 1 month)	1 to 2 scoops per day in formula	½ to 1 scoop per day in formula
BREAST FED INFANTS (Over 1 month)	½ scoop in 2–4 oz. of water or fruit juice twice a day	

* Full corrective dosage should be used for 3 or 4 days or until relief is noted. Then continue on maintenance dosage as needed. Use a clean, dry scoop to remove powder. Replace cover tightly to keep out moisture.

The recommended daily dosage of MALTSUPEX may vary. Use the smallest dose that is effective and lower dosage as improvement occurs.

MALTSUPEX Powder—Each bottle contains a scoop. Each scoopful (which is the equivalent to a standard measuring tablespoon) should be levelled with a knife.

Usual Dosage—Powder:
[See table above.]
Usual Dosage—Liquid:
[See table below.]
MALTSUPEX Tablets: Adult Dosage: The recommended daily dosage of MALTSUPEX may vary from 12 to 64 g. Start with four tablets (3 g) four times daily (with meals and at bedtime) and adjust dosage according to response. Drink a full glass of (8 oz.) of liquid with each dose.

Preparation Tips: Powder—Add dosage to milk, water, or fruit juice and stir until dissolved. Mixing is easier if added to warm milk or warm water. May be flavored with vanilla or cocoa to make "malteds."

Excellent with hot milk at bedtime. Also available in tablet and liquid forms.

Note: Although shade, texture, taste, and height of contents may vary between bottles, action remains the same.

Liquid: Mixing is easier if MALTSUPEX Liquid is added to an ounce or two of warm water and stirred. Then add milk, water, or fruit juice and stir until dissolved. May be flavored with vanilla or cocoa to make "malteds." Excellent with hot milk at bedtime. Also available in tablet and powder forms.

How Supplied: MALTSUPEX is supplied in 8 ounce (NDC 0037-9101-12) and 16 ounce (NDC 0037-9101-08) jars of MALTSUPEX Powder; 8 fluid ounce (NDC 0037-9051-12) and 1 pint (NDC 0037-9051-08) bottles of MALTSUPEX Liquid; and in bottles of 100 MALTSUPEX Tablets (NDC 0037-9201-01).

MALTSUPEX **Powder** and **Liquid** are Distributed by
WALLACE LABORATORIES
Division of
CARTER-WALLACE, INC.
Cranbury, New Jersey 08512
MALTSUPEX **Tablets** are Manufactured by
WALLACE LABORATORIES
Division of
CARTER-WALLACE, INC.
Cranbury, New Jersey 08512
Rev. 9/92

Shown in Product Identification Guide, page 429

AGE	CORRECTIVE*	MAINTENANCE
12 years to ADULTS	2 tablespoonfuls twice a day (Take a full glass [8 oz.] of liquid with each dose.)	1 to 2 tablespoonfuls at bedtime
CHILDREN 6–12 years of age	1 to 2 tablespoonfuls once or twice a day (Take a full glass [8 oz.] of liquid with each dose.)	
CHILDREN 2–6 years of age	½ tablespoonful twice a day (Take a full glass [8 oz.] of liquid with each dose.)	
BOTTLE FED INFANTS (Over 1 month)	½ to 2 tablespoonfuls per day in formula	1 to 2 teaspoonfuls per day in formula
BREAST FED INFANTS (Over 1 month)	1 to 2 teaspoonfuls in 2 to 4 oz. water or fruit juice once or twice a day	

* Full corrective dosage should be used for 3 or 4 days or until relief is noted. Then continue on maintenance dosage as needed. Use a clean, dry scoop to remove the liquid. Replace cover tightly after use.

Continued on next page

Wallace—Cont.

RYNA®
(Liquid)
RYNA-C® ℂ
(Liquid)
RYNA-CX® ℂ
(Liquid)

Description:
RYNA Liquid—Each 5 mL (one teaspoonful) contains:
Chlorpheniramine maleate .... 2 mg
Pseudoephedrine hydrochloride....30 mg
Other ingredients: flavor (artificial), glycerin, malic acid, purified water, sodium benzoate, sorbitol, in a clear, colorless to slightly yellow colored, lemon-vanilla flavored demulcent base containing no sugar, dyes, or alcohol.
RYNA-C Liquid—Each 5 mL (one teaspoonful) contains, in addition:
Codeine phosphate ....10 mg
 (WARNING: May be habit-forming)
Other ingredients: flavor (artificial), glycerin, malic acid, purified water, saccharin sodium, sodium benzoate, sorbitol, in a clear, colorless to slightly yellow, cinnamon-flavored, demulcent base containing no sugar, dyes, or alcohol.
RYNA-CX Liquid—Each 5 mL (one teaspoonful) contains:
Codeine phosphate ....10 mg
 (WARNING: May be habit-forming)
Pseudoephedrine hydrochloride....30 mg
Guaifenesin ....100 mg
Other ingredients: flavors (artificial), glycerin, glycine, malic acid, povidone, propylene glycol, purified water, saccharin sodium, sorbitol, in a clear, colorless to slightly yellow or straw colored, cherry-vanilla-menthol flavored demulcent base containing no sugar, dyes, or alcohol.

Actions:
Chlorpheniramine maleate in RYNA and RYNA-C is an antihistamine that antagonizes the effects of histamine.
Codeine phosphate in RYNA-C and RYNA-CX is a centrally-acting antitussive that relieves cough.
Pseudoephedrine hydrochloride in RYNA, RYNA-C and RYNA-CX is a sympathomimetic nasal decongestant that acts to shrink swollen mucosa of the respiratory tract.
Guaifenesin in RYNA-CX is an expectorant that increases mucus flow to help prevent dryness and relieve irritated respiratory tract membranes.

Indications:
RYNA: For the temporary relief of nasal congestion due to the common cold, hay fever or other upper respiratory allergies. Temporarily relieves runny nose, sneezing, itching of the nose or throat, and itchy, watery eyes due to hay fever or other respiratory allergies such as allergic rhinitis.
RYNA-C: Temporarily relieves cough, nasal congestion, runny nose and sneezing as may occur with the common cold.
RYNA-CX: Temporarily relieves cough and nasal congestion as may occur with

the common cold. Relieves irritated membranes in the respiratory passageways by preventing dryness through increased mucus flow.

Warnings:
For RYNA:
Do not give this product to children taking other medication or to children under 6 years except under the advice and supervision of a doctor. Do not exceed recommended dosage because nervousness, dizziness or sleeplessness may occur. Do not take this product for more than 7 days. If symptoms do not improve or are accompanied by fever, consult a doctor. Do not take this product except under the advice and supervision of a doctor if you have any of the following symptoms or conditions: high blood pressure; heart disease; thyroid disease; diabetes; asthma; glaucoma; emphysema; chronic pulmonary disease; shortness of breath; difficulty in breathing; or difficulty in urination due to enlargement of the prostate.
For RYNA-C and RYNA-CX:
Adults and children who have a chronic pulmonary disease or shortness of breath, or children who are taking other drugs, should not take these products unless directed by a doctor. Do not give these products to children under 6 years of age except under the advice and supervision of a doctor. A persistent cough may be a sign of a serious condition. If cough persists for more than one week, tends to recur, or is accompanied by fever, rash or persistent headache, consult a doctor. Do not take these products for persistent or chronic cough such as occurs with smoking, asthma, emphysema, or if cough is accompanied by excessive phlegm (mucus) unless directed by a doctor. Do not take these products if you have glaucoma, asthma, emphysema, difficulty in breathing, difficulty in urination due to enlargement of the prostate gland, heart disease, high blood pressure, thyroid disease, or diabetes unless directed by a doctor. May cause or aggravate constipation.
Do not take these products or give to children for more than 7 days. If symptoms do not improve or are accompanied by fever, consult a doctor. Unless directed by a doctor, do not exceed recommended dosage because nervousness, dizziness or sleeplessness may occur at higher doses.
For RYNA and RYNA-C:
These products contain an antihistamine which may cause excitability, especially in children, or may cause drowsiness. Alcohol may increase the drowsiness effect. Do not drive motor vehicles, operate machinery, or drink alcoholic beverages while taking these products.
As with any drug, if you are pregnant or nursing a baby, seek the advice of a health professional before using these products.

Drug Interaction Precaution: Do not use these products if you are presently taking a prescription drug for high blood pressure or depression without first consulting your doctor.

Dosage and Administration:
Adults: 2 teaspoonfuls every 6 hours
Children 6 to under 12 years: 1 teaspoonful every 6 hours.
Children under 6 years: Do not take except under the advice and supervision of a doctor.
DO NOT EXCEED 4 DOSES IN 24 HOURS.
Ryna-C and Ryna-CX:
A special measuring device should be used to give an accurate dose of these products to children under 6 years of age. Giving a higher dose than recommended by a doctor could result in serious side effects for the child.

How Supplied:
RYNA: bottles of 4 fl oz (NDC 0037-0638-66) and one pint (NDC 0037-0638-68).
RYNA-C: bottles of 4 fl oz (NDC 0037-0522-66) and one pint (NDC 0037-0522-68).
RYNA-CX: bottles of 4 fl oz (NDC 0037-0801-66) and one pint (NDC 0037-0801-68).
TAMPER-RESISTANT BAND ON CAP, PRINTED "WALLACE LABORATORIES". DO NOT USE IF BAND IS MISSING OR BROKEN.

Storage:
RYNA: Store at controlled room temperature 15°–30°C (59°–86°F).
RYNA-C and RYNA-CX: Store at controlled room temperature 15°–30°C (59°–86°F). Dispense in a tight, light-resistant container.
KEEP THESE AND ALL DRUGS OUT OF THE REACH OF CHILDREN. IN CASE OF ACCIDENTAL OVERDOSE, SEEK PROFESSIONAL ASSISTANCE OR CONTACT A POISON CONTROL CENTER IMMEDIATELY.
WALLACE LABORATORIES
Division of
CARTER-WALLACE, Inc.
Cranbury, New Jersey 08512
Rev. 8/92
Shown in Product Identification
Guide, page 429

SYLLACT®
(Psyllium Hydrophilic Mucilloid for Oral Suspension, U.S.P.)
(Powdered Psyllium Seed Husks)

Description: Each rounded teaspoonful of fruit-flavored SYLLACT contains approximately 3.3 g of powdered psyllium seed husks and an equal amount of dextrose as a dispersing agent, and provides about 14 calories. Potassium sorbate, methyl and propylparaben are added as preservatives. Other ingredients: citric acid, dextrose, FD&C Red #40, flavor (artificial), and saccharin sodium.

Actions: The active ingredient in SYLLACT is hydrophilic mucilloid, non-absorbable dietary fiber derived from the powdered husks of natural psyllium seed, which acts by increasing the water content and bulk volume of stools. It gives SYLLACT a bland, non-irritating, laxative action and promotes physiologic evacuation of the bowel.

Indications: SYLLACT is indicated for the relief of occasional constipation. This product generally produces bowel movement in 12 to 72 hours.

Warnings: Do not use laxative products when abdominal pain, nausea or vomiting are present unless directed by a physician. If you have noticed a sudden change in bowel habits that persists over a period of 2 weeks, consult a physician before using a laxative. Laxative products should not be used for a period longer than 1 week unless directed by a physician. Rectal bleeding or failure to have a bowel movement after use of a laxative may indicate a serious condition. Discontinue use and consult a physician. Bulk-forming agents should not be swallowed dry. They should not be used if impaction or gross intestinal pathology is present.

WARNING: MIX THIS PRODUCT WITH AT LEAST 8 OUNCES (A FULL GLASS) OF WATER OR OTHER FLUID. TAKING THIS PRODUCT WITHOUT ADEQUATE FLUID MAY CAUSE IT TO SWELL AND TO BLOCK YOUR THROAT OR ESOPHAGUS AND MAY CAUSE CHOKING. DO NOT TAKE THIS PRODUCT IF YOU HAVE EVER HAD DIFFICULTY IN SWALLOWING OR HAVE ANY THROAT PROBLEMS.

IF YOU EXPERIENCE CHEST PAIN, VOMITING, OR DIFFICULTY IN SWALLOWING OR BREATHING AFTER TAKING THIS PRODUCT, SEEK IMMEDIATE MEDICAL ATTENTION. Keep this and all medications out of the reach of children. This product may cause allergic reactions in people sensitive to inhaled or ingested psyllium powder. As with any drug, if you are pregnant or nursing a baby, seek the advice of a health professional before using this product.

Dosage and Administration: Drink a full glass (8 ounces) of liquid with each dose. Do not swallow dry. Use the smallest dose that is effective and lower the dosage as improvement occurs. Use a dry spoon to measure powder. Tighten lid to keep out moisture.
Adults and children 12 years of age and over: Oral dosage is 1 rounded teaspoonful in a full glass of liquid, one to three times daily, before or after meals.
Children 6 to under 12 years of age: ½ to 1 rounded teaspoonful in a full glass of liquid, one to three times daily.
Children under 6 years of age: Consult a physician.
For best results, place powder in a dry glass, add about ½ inch of liquid and stir briskly. Add remainder of liquid, stir and drink immediately. Follow with an additional glass of water if desired.

How Supplied: SYLLACT Powder —in 10 oz jars (NDC 0037-9501-13).
Rev. 2/91
WALLACE LABORATORIES
Division of
CARTER-WALLACE, INC.
Cranbury, New Jersey 08512
Shown in Product Identification Guide, page 429

Warner-Lambert Company

Consumer Health Products Group
201 TABOR ROAD
MORRIS PLAINS, NJ 07950

HALLS® MENTHO–LYPTUS®
Cough Suppressant Tablets

Active Ingredients: Each tablet contains eucalyptus oil and menthol.

Inactive Ingredients: Glucose Syrup, Flavoring, Sugar and Artificial Colors.

Indications: For temporary relief of minor throat irritation and coughs due to colds or inhaled irritants. Makes nasal passages feel clearer.

Warning: A persistent cough or sore throat may be a sign of a serious condition. If cough persists for more than 1 week, tends to recur, or is accompanied by fever, rash or persistent headache, or if sore throat is severe, persistent or accompanied by high fever, headache, nausea, and vomiting, consult a doctor. Do not take this product for sore throat lasting more than 2 days or persistent or chronic cough such as occurs with smoking, asthma, emphysema, or if cough is accompanied by excessive phlegm (mucus) unless directed by a doctor. Keep this and all drugs out of the reach of children.

Dosage and Administration: Adults and children 5 years and over: dissolve one tablet slowly in mouth. Repeat every hour as needed or as directed by a doctor. Children under 5 years: consult a doctor.

How Supplied: Halls Mentho-Lyptus Cough Suppressant Tablets are available in single sticks of 9 tablets each, and in bags of 30 and 60 tablets. They are available in five flavors: Regular Mentho-Lyptus, Cherry, Honey-Lemon, Ice Blue–Peppermint, and Spearmint.
Shown in Product Identification Guide, page 429

MAXIMUM STRENGTH HALLS® PLUS
Cough Suppressant Tablets

Active Ingredients: Menthol 10 mg. per centerfilled tablet.

Inactive Ingredients: Mentho-Lyptus: Corn Syrup, Flavoring, Glycerin, High Fructose Corn Syrup and Sucrose. Cherry: Corn Syrup, FD&C Blue No. 2, FD&C Red No. 40, Flavoring, Glycerin, High Fructose Corn Syrup and Sucrose. Honey-Lemon: Acesulfame Potassium, Corn Syrup, D&C Yellow No. 10, FD&C Yellow No. 6, Flavoring, Glycerin, High Fructose Corn Syrup, Honey and Sucrose.

Indications: For temporary relief of minor throat irritation and coughs due to colds or inhaled irritants. Makes nasal passages feel clearer.

Warnings: A persistent cough or sore throat may be a sign of a serious condition. If cough persists for more than 1 week, tends to recur, or is accompanied by fever, rash or persistent headache or if sore throat is severe, persistent or accompanied by high fever, headache, nausea, and vomiting, consult a doctor. Do not take this product for sore throat lasting more than 2 days or persistent or chronic cough such as occurs with smoking, asthma, emphysema, or if cough is accompanied by excessive phlegm (mucus) unless directed by a doctor. Keep this and all drugs out of the reach of children.

Dosage and Administration: Adults and children 5 years and over: for cough dissolve 1 tablet slowly in mouth-repeat every hour as needed or as directed by a doctor; for sore throat dissolve either 1 tablet or 2 tablets (one at a time) slowly in mouth-repeat every 2 hours as needed or as directed by a doctor. Children under 5 years; consult a doctor.

How Supplied: Maximum Strength Halls Plus Cough Suppressant Tablets are available in single sticks of 10 tablets each and in bags of 25 tablets. They are available in three flavors: Regular Mentho-Lyptus, Cherry and Honey-Lemon.
Shown in Product Identification Guide, page 430

HALLS® Vitamin C Drops

Description: Halls Vitamin C Drops are a delicious way to get 100% of the U.S. Recommended Daily Allowance of Vitamin C. Each drop provides 60 mg. of Vitamin C (100% U.S. RDA).

Ingredients: Sugar, Glucose Syrup, Sodium Ascorbate, Citric Acid, Ascorbic Acid, Natural Flavoring and Artificial Color (Including Yellow 5 and Yellow 6).

Indication: Dietary Supplementation.

How Supplied: Halls Vitamin C Drops are available in single sticks of 9 drops each and in bags of 30 drops. They are available in an all-natural citrus flavor assortment: (lemon, sweet grapefruit and orange).
Shown in Product Identification Guide, page 430

LISTERINE® Antiseptic

Active Ingredients: Thymol .06%, Eucalyptol .09%, Methyl Salicylate .06% and Menthol .04%. Also contains: Water, Alcohol 26.9%, Benzoic Acid, Poloxamer 407 and Caramel.

Continued on next page

Warner-Lambert—Cont.

Indications: To help prevent and reduce supragingival plaque and gingivitis; for general oral hygiene and bad breath.

Actions: Listerine Antiseptic has been shown to help prevent and reduce supragingival plaque and gingivitis when used in a conscientiously applied program of daily oral hygiene and regular professional care. Its effect on periodontitis has not been determined. Listerine is the only leading nonprescription mouthrinse that has received the American Dental Association's Council on Dental Therapeutics Seal of Acceptance for helping to prevent and reduce plaque above the gumline and gingivitis.

Directions: Rinse full strength for 30 seconds with ⅔ ounce (4 teaspoonfuls) morning and night. If bad breath persists, see your dentist.

Warnings: Do not administer to children under twelve years of age. Keep this and all drugs out of the reach of children. Do not swallow. In case of accidental overdose, seek professional assistance or contact a poison control center immediately.

How Supplied: Listerine Antiseptic is supplied in 3, 6, 12, 18, 24, 32, 48, 58 fl. oz. bottles, and available to professionals in 3 and 48 fl. oz. bottles and in gallons.
Shown in Product Identification Guide, page 430

COOL MINT LISTERINE™

Active Ingredients: Thymol 0.06%, Eucalyptol 0.09%, Methyl Salicylate 0.06%, and Menthol 0.04%.

Inactive Ingredients: Water, Sorbitol Solution, Alcohol 21.6%, Poloxamer 407, Benzoic Acid, Flavoring, Sodium Saccharin, Sodium Citrate, Citric Acid and FD&C Green #3.

Indications: To help prevent and reduce supragingival plaque and gingivitis; for general oral hygiene and bad breath.

Actions: Cool Mint Listerine Antiseptic has been shown to help prevent and reduce supragingival plaque and gingivitis when used in a conscientiously applied program of daily oral hygiene and regular professional care. Its effect on periodontitis has not been determined. Listerine is the only leading nonprescription mouthrinse that has received the American Dental Association's Council on Dental Therapeutics Seal of Acceptance for helping to prevent and reduce plaque above the gumline and gingivitis.

Directions: Rinse full strength for 30 seconds with ⅔ ounce (4 teaspoonfuls) morning and night. If bad breath persists, see your dentist.

Warnings: Do not administer to children under twelve years of age. Keep this and all drugs out of the reach of children. Do not swallow. In case of accidental overdose, seek professional assistance or contact a poison control center immediately.

How Supplied: Cool Mint Listerine Antiseptic is supplied in 3, 6, 12, 18, 24, 32, 48, 58 fl. oz. bottles, and available to professionals in 3 and 48 fl. oz. bottles and in gallons.
Shown in Product Indentification Guide, page 430

LISTERMINT®
Mouthwash with Fluoride

Active Ingredient: Sodium Fluoride (0.02%). Also contains: Water, SD alcohol 38-B (6.65%), glycerin, poloxamer 407, sodium lauryl sulfate, sodium citrate, flavoring, sodium saccharin, zinc chloride, citric acid, D&C Yellow No. 10, FD&C Green No. 3.

Indications: Aids in prevention of dental cavities and freshens breath.

Directions: Adults and children 6 years of age and older: Use twice a day after brushing teeth with toothpaste. Vigorously swish 10 ml. (2 teaspoonfuls) of rinse between teeth for 1 minute and spit out. Do not swallow the rinse. Do not eat or drink for 30 minutes after rinsing.

Warnings: Children under 12 years of age should be supervised in the use of this product. Consult a dentist or physician for use in children under 6 years of age. Developing teeth of children under 6 years of age may become permanently discolored if excessive amounts of fluoride are repeatedly swallowed. This is not a dentifrice and should not be used as a substitute for regular toothbrushing. Keep this and all drugs out of reach of children. In case of accidental overdose, seek professional assistance or contact a poison control center immediately.

How Supplied: Listermint with Fluoride is supplied to consumers in 6, 12, 18, 24 and 32 fl. oz. bottles and available to professionals in 3 fl. oz. bottles and in gallons.
Shown in Product Identification Guide, page 430

LUBRIDERM® LOTION
Skin Lubricant Moisturizer

Composition:
Scented—Contains Water, Mineral Oil, Petrolatum, Sorbitol, Lanolin, Lanolin Alcohol, Stearic Acid, Triethanolamine, Cetyl Alcohol, Fragrance, Butylparaben, Methylparaben, Propylparaben, Sodium Chloride.
Fragrance Free—Contains Water, Mineral Oil, Petrolatum, Sorbitol, Lanolin, Lanolin Alcohol, Stearic Acid, Triethanolamine, Cetyl Alcohol, Butylparaben, Methylparaben, Propylparaben, Sodium Chloride.

Actions and Uses: Lubriderm Lotion is an oil-in-water emulsion indicated for use in softening, soothing and moisturizing dry chapped skin. Lubriderm relieves the roughness, tightness and discomfort associated with dry or chapped skin and helps protect the skin from further drying.
Lubriderm's formula smoothes easily into skin without leaving a greasy feeling.

Administration and Dosage: Apply as often as needed to hands and body to restore and maintain the skin's natural suppleness.

Precautions: For external use only.

How Supplied:
Scented: Available in 1, 6, 10 and 16 fl. oz. plastic bottles, and a 2.5 ounce tube.
Fragrance Free: Available in 1, 6, 10 and 16 fl. oz. plastic bottles, and a 2.5 ounce tube.
Shown in Product Identification Guide, page 430

LUBRIDERM® BATH AND SHOWER OIL

Composition: Contains Mineral Oil, PPG-15 Stearyl Ether, Oleth-2, Nonoxynol-5, Fragrance, D&C Green No. 6.

Actions and Uses: Lubriderm Bath and Shower Oil is a lanolin-free, mineral oil–based, bath oil designed for softening and soothing dry skin during the bath. The formula disperses into countless droplets of oil that coat the skin and help lubricate and soften. It is equally effective in hard or soft water and provides an excellent way to moisturize the skin and help counterbalance the drying effects of harsh soaps and hot water.

Administration and Dosage: One to two capfuls in bath, or apply with hand or moistened cloth in shower and rinse. For use as a skin cleanser, rub into wet skin and rinse.

Precautions: Avoid getting in eyes; if this occurs, flush with clear water. When using any bath oil, take precautions against slipping. For external use only.

How Supplied: Available in 8 fl. oz. plastic bottles.

ROLAIDS® Antacid Tablets
Original Flavor and Spearmint

Active Ingredient: Calcium Carbonate 412 mg. and Magnesium Hydroxide 80 mg.

Inactive Ingredients: Flavoring, Light Mineral Oil, Magnesium Stearate, Mannitol, Microcrystalline Cellulose, Polyethylene Glycol, Pregelatinized Starch, Silicon Dioxide and Sucrose.

Indications: For the relief of heartburn, sour stomach or acid indigestion and upset stomach associated with these symptoms.

Actions: Rolaids® provides rapid neutralization of stomach acid. Each tablet has acid-neutralizing capacity of 11 mEq and the ability to maintain the pH of stomach contents to 3.5 or greater for a significant period of time. Each tablet provides 16% of the nutritional Daily Value for calcium and 8% of the nutritional Daily Value for magnesium and contains less than 0.4 mg. of sodium.

Warnings: Do not take more than 14 tablets in a 24-hour period or use the maximum dosage of this product for more than 2 weeks except under the advice and supervision of a physician. Keep this and all drugs out of the reach of children.

Drug Interaction Precaution: Antacids may interact with certain prescription drugs. If you are presently taking a prescription drug, do not take this product without checking with your physician or other health professional.

Dosage and Administration: Chew 1 or 2 tablets as symptoms occur. Repeat hourly if symptoms return or as directed by a physician.

How Supplied: One roll contains 12 tablets; 3-pack contains three 12-tablet rolls; one bottle contains 75 tablets; one bottle contains 150 tablets.
Shown in Product Identification Guide, page 430

CALCIUM RICH/SODIUM FREE ROLAIDS® Antacid Tablets
Cherry and Assorted Fruit Flavors

Active Ingredient: Calcium Carbonate 550 mg. per tablet.

Inactive Ingredients:
Cherry Flavor: Colors (Red 27 and Titanium Dioxide), Corn Starch, Flavoring, Light Mineral Oil, Magnesium Stearate, Mannitol, Pregelatinized Starch, Silicon Dioxide and Sucrose.
Assorted Fruit Flavors: Colors (Blue 1, Red 27, Red 40, Titanium Dioxide, Yellow 5 [Tartrazine] and Yellow 6), Corn Starch, Flavoring, Light Mineral Oil, Magnesium Stearate, Mannitol, Pregelatinized Starch, Silicon Dioxide and Sucrose.

Indications: For the relief of heartburn, sour stomach or acid indigestion and upset stomach associated with these symptoms.

Actions: Calcium Rich/Sodium Free Rolaids provides rapid neutralization of stomach acid. Each tablet has an acid-neutralizing capacity of 11 mEq and the ability to maintain the pH of stomach contents at 3.5 or greater for a significant period of time. Each tablet provides 22% of the nutritional Daily Value for calcium and contains less than 0.4 mg. of sodium.

Warnings: Do not take more than 14 tablets in a 24-hour period or use the maximum dosage of this product for

more than 2 weeks except under the advice and supervision of a physician. Keep this and all drugs out of the reach of children.

Drug Interaction Precaution: Antacids may interact with certain prescription drugs. If you are presently taking a prescription drug, do not take this product without checking with your physician or other health professional.

Dosage and Administration: Chew 1 or 2 tablets as symptoms occur. Repeat hourly if symptoms return or as directed by a physician.

How Supplied: One roll contains 12 tablets; 3-pack contains three 12-tablet rolls; one bottle contains 75 tablets; one bottle contains 150 tablets.
Shown in Product Identification Guide, page 430

EXTRA STRENGTH ROLAIDS®Antacid Tablets
Wintergreen Flavor

Active Ingredient: Calcium Carbonate 1000 mg. per tablet.

Inactive Ingredients: Acesulfame Potassium, Colors (Blue 1, Titanium Dioxide), and Yellow 5 [Tartrazine]), Corn Syrup, Dextrose, Flavoring, Glyceryl Monostearate, Pregelatinized Starch, Simethicone, Sucrose and Triglycerol Monooleate.

Indications: For the relief of heartburn, sour stomach or acid indigestion and upset stomach associate with these symptoms.

Actions: Extra Strength Rolaids provides rapid neutralization of stomach acid. Each tablet has an acid-neutralizing capacity of 20 mEq and the ability to maintain the pH of stomach contents at 3.5 or greater for a significant period of time. Each tablet provides 40% of the nutritional Daily Value for calcium and contains less than 0.4 mg. of sodium.

Warnings: Do not take more than 8 tablets in a 24-hour period or use the maximum dosage of this product for more than 2 weeks except under the advice and supervision of a physician. Keep this and all drugs out of the reach of children.

Drug Interaction Precaution: Antacids may interact with certain prescription drugs. If you are presently taking a prescription drug, do not take this product without checking with your physician or other health professional.

Dosage and Administration: Chew 1 or 2 tablets as symptoms occur. Repeat hourly if symptoms return or as directed by a physician.

How Supplied: One roll contains 10 tablets; 3-pack contains three 10-tablet rolls; one bottle contains 55 tablets; one bottle contains 110 tablets.
Shown in Product Identification Guide, page 430

SOOTHERS® Throat Drops
From the makers of Halls

Active Ingredient: Each centerfilled tablet contains menthol 2 mg.

Inactive Ingredients: Colors (Including Yellow 6), Corn Syrup, Flavoring, Glycerin, High Fructose Corn Syrup, Honey and Sugar.

Indications: For temporary relief of occasional minor irritation, pain, sore mouth, and sore throat or pain associated with canker sores.

Warnings: If sore throat is severe, persists for more than 2 days, is accompanied or followed by fever, headache, rash, nausea, or vomiting, consult a doctor promptly. If sore mouth symptoms do not improve in 7 days, see your dentist or doctor promptly. Keep this and all drugs out of the reach of children.

Dosage and Administration: Adults and children 5 years of age and older: dissolve 1 drop slowly in mouth. May be repeated every 2 hours as needed or as directed by a dentist or doctor. Children under 5 years of age: consult a dentist or doctor.

How Supplied: Soothers Throat Drops are available in bags of 25 tablets. They are available in cherry and orange flavors.
Shown in Product Identification Guide, page 430

Water-Jel Technologies, Inc.
243 VETERANS BLVD.
CARLSTADT, NJ 07072

WATER–JEL® Sterile Burn Dressings
One-Step Emergency Burn Care
Product for all types of burns

WATER-JEL® Burn Jel®
Topical for minor burns

WATER-JEL® UnBurn
Topical for fast relief
of sunburn pain.

Key Facts: Water-Jel is a unique, patented one-step product ideal for emergency first aid burn care. The scientifically formulated gel combines with a special carrier material to: Ease pain, prevent burn progression, cool the skin and stabilize skin temperature, protect the covered wound from contamination, facilitate removal of burnt clothing or jewelry; Won't harm skin or eyes, does not require a water source to continue cooling, and is non-allergenic.
Water-Jel Burn Jel is a new topical for minor burns that works fast and provides lasting relief. It contains the active ingre-

Continued on next page

Water-Jel Tech. Inc. —Cont.

dient, lidocaine, thereby offering the pain relief capabilities of lidocaine, and in combination with the Water-Jel gel, also cools and soothes. It is water-based, dissipates heat and is easily removed.

Major Uses: Water-Jel Sterile Burn Dressings are used as Emergency First Aid for all types of burns... Fire, steam, heat, electrical, boiling water.
Water-Jel Burn Jel is a topical used for long-lasting relief of minor burns.
Water-Jel UnBurn is used for the fast relief of sunburn pain.

Safety Information: Chemical burns must be thoroughly flushed before applying Water-Jel. Consult a physician if the burn is severe, covers an area larger than your palm, or involves your face.

Description: Each Sterile Burn Dressing packet contains a gel-soaked polyester fabric.
The gel is an off-white translucent color. It has a characteristic odor. It is sterile. A freezing point of −15°C and a boiling point of +92°C. The gel is a proprietary formulation of natural gums and oils in a preserved, sterile, easily washed-off aqueous base.
Water-Jel Burn Jel is available in a 4 oz. squeeze bottle or in single dose, foil packets each ⅛ oz (25 packets per dispenser box).
Water-Jel UnBurn is available in 12 unit and 5 unit sizes (for first-aid kits and boxes) or in a 3-unit personal pack. Each unit is a 6-gram dose. UnBurn is also available in 2 oz. and 4 oz. squeeze bottles for first-aid stations.

Indications: Water-Jel Sterile Burn Dressings provide Emergency First Aid for all burns. The Burn Dressings provide fast relief of pain due to burns. It soothes and cools the burned area and protects the covered wound from contamination. It stops burn progress and is easily removed without re-injuring the wound. It is non-allergenic.
Water-Jel Burn Jel is a topical that offers the same benefits as the Water-Jel dressings plus lidocaine for fast, lasting pain relief of minor burns.
Water-Jel UnBurn is a topical specifically designed for the fast relief of sunburn pain. It includes pain relieving lidocaine, is not sticky and non-staining. UnBurn cools and soothes while moisturizing the skin to help prevent peeling.

Application: Simply open the Water-Jel Sterile Dressing package and apply the dressing to the burned area. Pour the excess gel from the package onto the dressing. Keep in place for approximately 15 to 20 minutes.
Water-Jel Burn Jel is applied directly to the wound. Simply squeeze the gel out or open the packet & pour.
Water-Jel UnBurn (for adults and children over 2 years of age); Spread an even and generous layer of UnBurn over the effected area(s).

Warning: In the case of chemical burns, the wound must be thoroughly flushed before applying Water-Jel. Consult a physician if the burn is severe, covers an area larger than your palm, or involves the face.

How Supplied: Water-Jel Sterile Burn Dressings are available in several sizes for use on different size burns—2″×2″; 2″×6″; 4″×4″; 4″×16″; and 8″×18″. Water-Jel is contained in heat-sealed foil packets.
Water-Jel Burn Jel is available in a 4 oz squeeze bottle and in single-dose ⅛ oz foil packets. The single-dose packets are packaged 25 to a dispenser box. Squeeze bottle and dispenser box are designed to fit first aid kits and medicine cabinets.

EDUCATIONAL MATERIAL

"Since the Dawn of Civilization ..."
4-page, full color brochure.
Descriptive use and application of all Water-Jel® Burn Care Products.
"At Last ... A Burn Topical that Measures up ..."
2-page, full-color brochure. Descriptive use and application of Water-Jel Burn Jel, a 'topical' for minor burns.
"Technical Specifications"
2-page, in-depth specifications of all Water-Jel® products.
"Presentation Video"
13-minute video on the use of Water-Jel® products.
"For First Aid Burn Care..."
8 page information brochure covering burns and burn care.

Wellness Pharmaceutical, Inc.
**3840 S. 103 E. AVE, STE 200
TULSA, OK 74146
(918) 622-1226**

PHYSICIAN'S HEALTH & DIET PROGRAM™ MEAL REPLACEMENT NUTRITIONAL DRINK

NuTriLean Nutritional Drink is scientifically designed for effective weight management which promotes the loss of body fat, while maintaining lean body mass (muscle, bone, internal organs). NuTriLean Nutritional Drink is recommended as part of a dietary plan to achieve low fat, low cholesterol, low sodium, high fiber diet.
NuTriLean Nutritional Drink is a delicious limited calorie drink containing unique blends of high quality protein, carbohydrates, dietary fiber, vitamins, minerals and amino acids with the ideal ratios for the ultimate approach for stress related and dietary deficiencies of today's lifestyle.

High P.E.R. Protein

Protein efficiency ration (P.E.R.) is a measure of protein quality and depends on a complete spectrum of essential amino acids with a P.E.R. of 2.5 as a standard of high quality protein. NuTriLean Nutritional Drink, with its unique protein blend, has a P.E.R. of 2.5.

*Essential Amino Acids
  Alanine
  Arginine
  Aspartic Acid
  Cysteine
  Glutamic Acid
  Glycine
  *Histidine
  *Isoleucine
  *Leucine
  *Lysine
  *Methionine
  *Phenylalanine
  Proline
  Serine
  *Threonine
  *Tyrosine
  *Valine

Recommended Use: Add contents of one packet of NuTriLean Nutritional Drink to 8 ounces of water, juice or nonfat milk. Add 2–3 ice cubes and mix thoroughly with a hand or power blender. For added flavor, blend in a banana and/or other favorite fruit. (Optional: sweeten to taste with a low calorie sweetener.)

Ingredients: Carbohydrate blend (sugar, fructose, dextrose, maltodextrin), protein blend (calcium caseinate, soy protein isolate, whey protein concentrate, dl-methionine, chickpea protein), vitamin/mineral and amino acid blend (magnesium oxide, potassium phosphate, dicalcium phosphate, l-carnitine hydrochloride, calcium ascorbate, beta carotene, choline bitartrate, inositol, niacin, d-calcium pantothenate, vitamin A palmitate, vitamin E acetate, ferrous fumarate, zinc oxide, l-glutamine, pyridoxine hydrochloride, riboflavin, l-phenylalanine, thiamine hydrochloride, l-methionine, vitamin D3, glycine, folic acid, biotin, potassium iodide, cyanocobalamin, chromium picolinate, and sodium selenite), citric acid, natural flavor, fiber blend (oat fiber, guar gum, cellulose, carrageenan, apple fiber, pectin) lecithin, bromelain, papain, bee pollen, beet powder and carrot powder.

ALSO PROVIDES per serving:
Chromium	50 mcg
Selenium	20 mcg
Choline	50 mg
Inositol	50 mg
Bioflavonoids	25 mg
L-phenylalanine	830 mcg
Glycine	250 mcg

NUTRITIONAL FACTS:
SERVING SIZE—APPROX. 1 PACKET, 46.35 GRAMS
1 CUP AS PREPARED
SERVINGS PER CONTAINER—1

AMOUNT PER SERVING:

		DAILY VALUE
Calories	160	
Total Fat	0 gm	0%
Sodium	70 mg	14%
Potassium	200 mg	6%
Total Carbohydrate	28 gm	8%
Fiber	3 gm	12%
Sugars	14 gm	
Protein	9	18%

Vitamin A–100%, Vitamin C–200%, Calcium–35%, Iron–10%, Vitamin D–200%, Vitamin E–200%, Thiamine–100%, Riboflavin–100%, Niacin–200%, Vitamin B6–200%, Folic Acid–200%, Vitamin B12–200%, Biotin–100%, Pantothenic Acid–100%, Phosphorous–20%, Iodine–50%, Magnesium–150%, Zinc–60%

Other Nutrients:

Bee Pollen	100 mg
Papain	50 mg
Bromelain	50 mg
Chromium	50 mcg
Selenium	20 mcg
Choline	50 mg
Inositol	50 mg
Bioflavonoids	25 mg
L-phenylalanine	830 mcg
Glycine	250 mcg

Caution: It is advisable to consult with a physician before beginning any weight loss program. Pregnant and lactating women and individuals in poor health or with known medical conditions should diet only under the supervision of a physician.

Manufactured Exclusively for
Wellness Pharmaceutical Inc.
Tulsa, OK 74146
(918) 622-1226

EDUCATIONAL MATERIAL

PHD Information Pamphlet
Audio Cassette by Stephen Langer, MD
Video Cassette by Stephen Langer, MD

Whitehall Laboratories
**American Home
Products Corporation
FIVE GIRALDA FARMS
MADISON, NJ 07940-0871**

ADVIL®
[ad 'vil]
**Ibuprofen Tablets, USP
Ibuprofen Caplets*
Pain Reliever/Fever Reducer
*Oval-Shaped Tablets**

WARNING: ASPIRIN-SENSITIVE PATIENTS. Do not take this product if you have had a severe allergic reaction to aspirin, e.g.—asthma, swelling, shock or hives, because even though this product contains no aspirin or salicylates, cross-reactions may occur in patients allergic to aspirin.

Active Ingredient: Each tablet or caplet contains Ibuprofen 200 mg.

Inactive Ingredients: Acetylated Monoglyceride, Beeswax and/or Carnauba Wax, Croscarmellose Sodium, Iron Oxides, Lecithin, Methylparaben, Microcrystalline Cellulose, Pharmaceutical Glaze, Povidone, Propylparaben, Silicon Dioxide, Simethicone, Sodium Benzoate, Sodium Lauryl Sulfate, Starch, Stearic Acid, Sucrose, Titanium Dioxide.

Indications: For the temporary relief of minor aches and pains associated with the common cold, headache, toothache, muscular aches, backache, for the minor pain of arthritis, for the pain of menstrual cramps and for reduction of fever.

Dosage and Administration: Adults: Take one tablet or caplet every 4 to 6 hours while symptoms persist. If pain or fever does not respond to one tablet or caplet, two tablets or caplets may be used but do not exceed six tablets or caplets in 24 hours unless directed by a doctor. The smallest effective dose should be used. Take with food or milk if occasional and mild heartburn, upset stomach, or stomach pain occurs with use. Consult a doctor if these symptoms are more than mild or if they persist. Children: Do not give this product to children under 12 except under the advice and supervision of a doctor.

Warnings: Do not take for pain for more than 10 days or for fever for more than 3 days unless directed by a doctor. If pain or fever persists or gets worse, if new symptoms occur, or if the painful area is red or swollen, consult a doctor. These could be signs of serious illness. If you are under a doctor's care for any serious condition, consult a doctor before taking this product. As with aspirin and acetaminophen, if you have any condition which requires you to take prescription drugs or if you have had any problems or serious side effects from taking any nonprescription pain reliever, do not take this product without first discussing it with your doctor. **IF YOU EXPERIENCE ANY SYMPTOMS WHICH ARE UNUSUAL OR SEEM UNRELATED TO THE CONDITION FOR WHICH YOU TOOK IBUPROFEN, CONSULT A DOCTOR BEFORE TAKING ANY MORE OF IT.** Although ibuprofen is indicated for the same conditions as aspirin and acetaminophen, it should not be taken with them except under a doctor's direction. Do not combine this product with any other ibuprofen-containing product. As with any drug, if you are pregnant or nursing a baby, seek the advice of a health professional before using this product. **IT IS ESPECIALLY IMPORTANT NOT TO USE IBUPROFEN DURING THE LAST 3 MONTHS OF PREGNANCY UNLESS SPECIFICALLY DIRECTED TO DO SO BY A DOCTOR BECAUSE IT MAY CAUSE PROBLEMS IN THE UNBORN CHILD OR COMPLICA-**

TIONS DURING DELIVERY. Keep this and all drugs out of the reach of children. In case of accidental overdose, seek professional assistance or contact a poison control center immediately.

How Supplied: Coated tablets in bottles of 4, 8, 24, 50 (non-child resistant size), 100, 165 and 250. Coated caplets in bottles of 24, 50 (non-child resistant size), 100, 165, and 250. Coated tablets in thermoform packaging of 8.

Storage: Store at room temperature; avoid excessive heat 40°C (104°F).
*Shown in Product Identification
Guide, page 430*

ADVIL® Cold and Sinus
**Ibuprofen/Pseudoephedrine Caplets*
Pain Reliever/Fever Reducer/Nasal Decongestant**

*Oval-Shaped tablets

WARNING: ASPIRIN-SENSITIVE PATIENTS. Do not take this product if you have had a severe allergic reaction to aspirin, eg, asthma, swelling, shock or hives, because even though this product contains no aspirin or salicylates, cross-reactions may occur in patients allergic to aspirin.

Indications: For temporary relief of symptoms associated with the common cold, sinusitis or flu, including nasal congestion, headache, fever, body aches, and pains.

Directions: *Adults:* Take 1 caplet every 4 to 6 hours while symptoms persist. If symptoms do not respond to 1 caplet, 2 caplets may be used, but do not exceed 6 caplets in 24 hours unless directed by a doctor. The smallest effective dose should be used. Take with food or milk if occasional and mild heartburn, upset stomach, or stomach pain occurs with use. Consult a doctor if these symptoms are more than mild or if they persist. *Children:* Do not give this product to children under 12 years of age except under the advice and supervision of a doctor.

Warnings: Do not take for colds for more than 7 days or for fever for more than 3 days unless directed by a doctor. If the cold or fever persists or gets worse, or if new symptoms occur, consult a doctor. These could be signs of serious illness. As with aspirin and acetaminophen, if you have any condition which requires you to take prescription drugs or if you have had any problems or serious side effects from taking any nonprescription pain reliever, do not take this product without first discussing it with your doctor. IF YOU EXPERIENCE ANY SYMPTOMS WHICH ARE UNUSUAL OR SEEM UNRELATED TO THE CONDITION FOR WHICH YOU TOOK THIS PRODUCT, CONSULT A DOCTOR BEFORE TAKING ANY MORE OF IT. If you are under a doctor's care for any serious con-

Continued on next page

Whitehall—Cont.

dition, consult a doctor before taking this product.

Do not exceed recommended dosage because at higher doses nervousness, dizziness, or sleeplessness may occur. Do not take this product if you have high blood pressure, heart disease, diabetes, thyroid disease or difficulty in urination due to enlargement of the prostate gland, except under the advice and supervision of a doctor.

Drug Interaction Precaution: Do not take this product if you are presently taking a prescription drug for high blood pressure or depression without first consulting your doctor. Do not combine this product with other nonprescription pain relievers. Do not combine this product with any other ibuprofen-containing product. As with any drug, if you are pregnant or nursing a baby, seek the advice of a health professional before using this product.

IT IS ESPECIALLY IMPORTANT NOT TO USE THIS PRODUCT DURING THE LAST 3 MONTHS OF PREGNANCY UNLESS SPECIFICALLY DIRECTED TO DO SO BY A DOCTOR BECAUSE IT MAY CAUSE PROBLEMS IN THE UNBORN CHILD OR COMPLICATIONS DURING DELIVERY. Keep this and all drugs out of the reach of children. In case of accidental overdose, seek professional assistance or contact a poison control center immediately.

Active Ingredients: Each caplet contains Ibuprofen 200 mg and Pseudoephedrine HCl 30 mg.

Inactive Ingredients: Carnauba or Equivalent Wax, Croscarmellose Sodium, Iron Oxides, Methylparaben, Microcrystalline Cellulose, Propylparaben, Silicon Dioxide, Sodium Benzoate, Sodium Lauryl Sulfate, Starch, Stearic Acid, Sucrose, Titanium Dioxide.

How Supplied: Advil® Cold and Sinus is an oval-shaped tan-colored caplet supplied in consumer bottles of 40 and blister packs of 20. Medical samples are available in a 2's pouch dispenser.

Storage: Store at room temperature; avoid excessive heat (40°C, 104°F).

Shown in Product Identification Guide, page 430

PREPARATION H®
[prep-e 'rä-shen-āch]
Hemorrhoidal Ointment and Cream
PREPARATION H®
Hemorrhoidal Suppositories

Description: Preparation H is available in ointment, cream and suppository product forms. The **Ointment** contains Live Yeast Cell Derivative, supplying 2,000 units Skin Respiratory Factor per ounce of Ointment, and Shark Liver Oil 3.0% in a specially prepared Rectal Petrolatum Base.

The **Cream** contains Live Yeast Cell Derivative, supplying 2,000 units Skin Respiratory Factor per ounce of Cream, and Shark Liver Oil 3.0% in a specially prepared Rectal Cream Base containing Petrolatum.

The **Suppositories** contain Live Yeast Cell Derivative, supplying 2,000 units Skin Respiratory Factor per ounce of Cocoa Butter Suppository Base, and Shark Liver Oil 3.0%.

Indications: Preparation H helps shrink swelling of hemorrhoidal tissues caused by inflammation and gives prompt, temporary relief in many cases from pain and itching in tissues.

Precautions: In case of bleeding, or if your condition persists, see your physician. Keep this and all drugs out of the reach of children. In case of accidental ingestion, seek professional assistance or contact a poison control center immediately.

Dosage and Administration: **Ointment/Cream:** Before applying, remove protective cover from applicator. Lubricate applicator before each application and thoroughly cleanse after use. It is recommended that Preparation H Hemorrhoidal ointment/cream be applied freely to the affected rectal area whenever symptoms occur, from three to five times per day, especially at night, in the morning, and after each bowel movement. Frequent application and lubrication with Preparation H ointment/cream provide continual therapy which leads to more rapid improvement of rectal conditions. For best results, squeeze tube from bottom and flatten it as you go up.

Suppositories: Whenever symptoms occur, remove wrapper, insert one suppository rectally from three to five times per day, especially at night, in the morning, and after each bowel movement. Frequent application and lubrication with Preparation H suppositories provides continual therapy which leads to more rapid improvement of rectal conditions .

Inactive Ingredients*: **Ointment—** Beeswax, Glycerin, Lanolin, Lanolin Alcohol, Mineral Oil, Paraffin, Phenylmercuric Nitrate 1:10,000 (as a preservative), Thyme Oil.
Cream— BHA, Cellulose Gum, Cetyl Alcohol, Citric Acid, Disodium EDTA, Glycerin, Glyceryl Stearate, Lanolin, Methylparaben, Phenylmercuric Nitrate, 1:10,000 (as a preservative), Propyl Gallate, Propylene Glycol, Propylparaben, Simethicone, Sodium Lauryl Sulfate, Stearyl Alcohol, Water, Xanthan Gum. May also contain Glyceryl Oleate and/or Polysorbate 80.
Suppositories — Beeswax, Glycerin, Phenylmercuric Nitrate 1:10,000 (as a preservative), Polyethylene Glycol 600 Dilaurate, Water.

How Supplied: **Ointment:** Net Wt. 1 oz. and 2 oz. **Cream:** Net wt. 0.9 oz. and 1.8 oz. **Suppositories:** 12's, 24's, 36's and 48's.

Store at room temperature in cool place but not over 80° F.
*The preservative and inactive ingredients differ slightly in California.

Shown in Product Identification Guide, page 430

PREPARATION H®
HYDROCORTISONE 1%
[prep-e 'ra-shen-ach]
Anti-Itch Cream

Description: Preparation H® Hydrocortisone 1% is an antipruritic external analgesic cream containing 1% Hydrocortisone.

Indications: For the temporary relief of external anal itch and itching associated with minor skin irritations and rashes. Other uses of this product should be only under the advice and supervision of a doctor.

Warnings: For external use only. Avoid contact with the eyes. If condition worsens, or if symptoms persist for more than 7 days or clear up and occur again within a few days, stop use of this product and do not begin use of any other hydrocortisone product unless you have consulted a doctor. Do not exceed the recommended daily dosage unless directed by a doctor. In case of bleeding, consult a doctor promptly. Do not put this product into the rectum by using fingers or any mechanical device or applicator. Do not use for the treatment of diaper rash; consult a doctor. Keep this and all drugs out of the reach of children. In case of accidental ingestion, seek professional assistance or contact a poison control center immediately.

Directions: Adults: When practical, cleanse the affected area by patting or blotting with an appropriate cleansing tissue, such as Preparation H Cleansing Tissues. Gently dry by patting or blotting with toilet tissue or soft cloth before application of this product. Apply to affected area not more than 3 to 4 times daily.
Children under 12 years of age: consult a doctor.

Inactive Ingredients: BHA, Cellulose Gum, Cetyl Alcohol, Citric Acid, Disodium EDTA, Glycerin, Glyceryl Oleate, Glyceryl Stearate, Lanolin, Methylparaben, Petrolatum, Propyl Gallate, Propylene Glycol, Propylparaben, Simethicone, Sodium Benzoate, Sodium Lauryl Sulfate, Stearyl Alcohol, Water, Xanthan Gum.

How Supplied: Available in Net Wt. 0.9 oz. tube. Store at room temperature or in cool place not over 80°F.

Shown in Product Identification Section, page 430

PRIMATENE® Dual Action Formula
[prīm ′a-tēn]
Tablets

Description: Primatene Dual Action Tablets contain Theophylline Anhydrous 60 mg, Ephedrine Hydrochloride 12.5 mg, and Guaifenesin 100 mg.

Indications: For temporary relief of shortness of breath, tightness of chest, and wheezing due to bronchial asthma. Eases breathing by reducing spasms of bronchial muscles and helps loosen phlegm and thin bronchial secretions to rid bronchial passageways of mucus and make coughs more productive.

Warnings: Do not use this product unless a diagnosis of asthma has been made by a doctor. Do not use this product if you have heart disease, high blood pressure, thyroid disease, or difficulty in urination due to enlargement of the prostate gland unless directed by a doctor. Do not use this product if you have ever been hospitalized for asthma or if you are taking any prescription drug for asthma unless directed by a doctor. Do not continue to use this product, but seek medical assistance immediately if symptoms are not relieved within 1 hour or become worse. Some users of this product may experience nervousness, tremor, sleeplessness, nausea, and loss of appetite. If these symptoms persist or become worse, consult your doctor. Do not take this product for persistent chronic cough such as occurs with smoking, chronic bronchitis, or emphysema unless directed by a doctor. A persistent cough may be a sign of a serious condition. If cough persists for more than one week, tends to recur, or is accompanied by a fever, rash, or persistent headache, consult a doctor. As with any drug, if you are pregnant or nursing a baby, seek the advice of a health professional before using this product. Keep this and all drugs out of the reach of children. In case of accidental overdose, seek professional assistance or contact a poison control center immediately.

Drug Interaction Precaution: DO NOT USE THIS PRODUCT IF YOU ARE PRESENTLY TAKING A PRESCRIPTION DRUG FOR HIGH BLOOD PRESSURE OR DEPRESSION, OR A MONOAMINE OXIDASE INHIBITOR, WITHOUT FIRST CONSULTING YOUR DOCTOR.

Directions: Adults and children 12 years of age and over, 2 tablets initially, then two every 4 hours, as needed, not to exceed 12 tablets in 24 hours. Do not exceed recommended dosage unless directed by a doctor. Children (under 12)—consult a doctor.

Inactive Ingredients: Calcium Stearate, Hydrogenated Vegetable Oil, Microcrystalline Cellulose

How Supplied: Available in 24 and 60 tablet thermoform blister cartons.
Shown in Product Identification Guide, page 431

PRIMATENE®
[prīm ′a-tēn]
Mist
(Epinephrine Inhalation Aerosol Bronchodilator)

Description: Primatene Mist contains Epinephrine 5.5 mg/mL.

Indications: For temporary relief of shortness of breath, tightness of chest, and wheezing due to bronchial asthma. Eases breathing for asthma patients by reducing spasms of bronchial muscles.

Directions: Inhalation dosage for adults and children 4 years of age and older: Start with one inhalation, then wait at least 1 minute. If not relieved, use once more. Do not use again for at least 3 hours. The use of this product by children should be supervised by an adult. Children under 4 years of age: Consult a doctor. Each inhalation delivers 0.22 mg. of epinephrine.

Warnings: Do not use this product unless a diagnosis of asthma has been made by a doctor. Do not use this product if you have heart disease, high blood pressure, thyroid disease, diabetes, or difficulty in urination due to enlargement of the prostate gland unless directed by a physician. As with any drug, if you are pregnant or nursing a baby, seek the advice of a health professional before using this product. Do not use this product if you have ever been hospitalized for asthma or if you are taking any prescription drug for asthma unless directed by a doctor. Keep this and all drugs out of the reach of children. In case of accidental overdose, seek professional assistance or contact a poison control center immediately.

Drug Interaction Precaution: Do not use this product if you are presently taking a prescription drug for high blood pressure or depression, without first consulting your doctor. DO NOT CONTINUE TO USE THIS PRODUCT, BUT SEEK MEDICAL ASSISTANCE IMMEDIATELY IF SYMPTOMS ARE NOT RELIEVED WITHIN 20 MINUTES OR BECOME WORSE. DO NOT USE THIS PRODUCT MORE FREQUENTLY OR AT HIGHER DOSES THAN RECOMMENDED UNLESS DIRECTED BY A DOCTOR. EXCESSIVE USE MAY CAUSE NERVOUSNESS AND RAPID HEART BEAT AND POSSIBLY, ADVERSE EFFECTS ON THE HEART.

Caution: Contents under pressure. Do not puncture or throw container into incinerator. Using or storing near open flame or heating above 120° F (49° C) may cause bursting. Store at room temperature 59° F–86° F (15° C–30° C).

Directions For Use of The Mist:
The Primatene Mist mouthpiece, which is enclosed in the Primatene Mist 15mL size (not the refill size), should be used for inhalation only with Primatene Mist.
1. Take plastic cap off mouthpiece. (For refills, use mouthpiece from previous purchase.)
2. Take plastic mouthpiece off bottle.
3. Place other end of mouthpiece on bottle.
4. Turn bottle upside down. Place thumb on bottom of mouthpiece over circular button and forefinger on top of vial. Empty the lungs as completely as possible by exhaling.
5. Place mouthpiece in mouth with lips closed around opening. Inhale deeply while squeezing mouthpiece and bottle together. Release immediately and remove unit from mouth. Complete taking the deep breath, drawing the medication into your lungs and holding breath as long as comfortable.
6. Then exhale slowly keeping lips nearly closed. This distributes the medication in the lungs.
7. Replace plastic cap on mouthpiece.
Care of the Mouthpiece:
The Primatene Mist mouthpiece should be washed once daily with soap and hot water, and rinsed thoroughly. Then it should be dried with a clean, lint-free cloth.
If the unit becomes clogged and fails to spray, please send the clogged unit to:
Whitehall Laboratories
5 Giralda Farms
Madison, N.J. 07940

Inactive Ingredients: Alcohol 34%, Ascorbic Acid, Fluorocarbons (Propellant), Water. Contains No Sulfites.

Warning: Contains CFC 12, 114, substances which harm public health and environment by destroying ozone in the upper atmosphere.

How Supplied:
½ Fl. oz. (15 mL) With Mouthpiece.
½ Fl. oz. (15 mL) Refill
¾ Fl. oz. (22.5 mL) Refill
Shown in Product Identification Guide, page 431

PRIMATENE®
[prīm ′a-tēn]
Mist Suspension
(Epinephrine Bitartrate Inhalation Aerosol Bronchodilator)

Description: Primatene Mist Suspension contains Epinephrine Bitartrate 7.0 mg/mL.

Indications: For temporary relief of shortness of breath, tightness of chest, and wheezing due to bronchial asthma. Eases breathing for asthma patients by reducing spasms of bronchial muscles.

Directions: Shake before using. Inhalation dosage for adults and children 4 years of age and older: Start with one inhalation, then wait at least 1 minute. If not relieved, use once more. Do not use again for at least 3 hours. The use of this product by children should be supervised by an adult. Children under 4 years of age: Consult a doctor. Each inhalation delivers 0.3 mg. Epinephrine Bitartrate equivalent to 0.16 mg. Epinephrine Base.

Continued on next page

Whitehall—Cont.

Warnings: Do not use this product unless a diagnosis of asthma has been made by a doctor. Do not use this product if you have heart disease, high blood pressure, thyroid disease, diabetes, or difficulty in urination due to enlargement of the prostate gland unless directed by a physician. As with any drug, if you are pregnant or nursing a baby, seek the advice of a health professional before using this product. Do not use this product if you have ever been hospitalized for asthma or if you are taking any prescription drug for asthma unless directed by a doctor. Keep this and all drugs out of the reach of children. In case of accidental overdose, seek professional assistance or contact a poison control center immediately. **Drug Interaction Precaution:** Do not use this product if you are presently taking a prescription drug for high blood pressure or depression, without first consulting your doctor. DO NOT CONTINUE TO USE THIS PRODUCT, BUT SEEK MEDICAL ASSISTANCE IMMEDIATELY, IF SYMPTOMS ARE NOT RELIEVED WITHIN 20 MINUTES OR BECOME WORSE. DO NOT USE THIS PRODUCT MORE FREQUENTLY OR AT HIGHER DOSES THAN RECOMMENDED UNLESS DIRECTED BY A DOCTOR. EXCESSIVE USE MAY CAUSE NERVOUSNESS AND RAPID HEART BEAT AND POSSIBLY, ADVERSE EFFECTS ON THE HEART.

Caution: Contents under pressure. Do not puncture or throw container into incinerator. Using or storing near open flame or heating above 120° F (49° C) may cause bursting. Store at room temperature 59° F–86° F (15° C–30° C).

Directions For Use of Mist Suspension
1. SHAKE WELL BEFORE USING.
2. HOLD INHALER WITH NOZZLE DOWN WHILE USING. Empty the lungs as completely as possible by exhaling.
3. Purse the lips as in saying "O" and hold the nozzle up to the lips keeping the tongue flat. As you start to take a deep breath, squeeze nozzle and can together, releasing one full application. Complete taking a deep breath, drawing medication into your lungs.
4. Hold breath for as long as comfortable. Then exhale slowly, keeping the lips nearly closed. This distributes the medication in the lungs.
Care of the Pocket Size Spray:
The Primatene Mist Suspension nozzle should be washed once daily. After removing the nozzle from the vial, wash it with soap and hot water, and rinse thoroughly. Then it should be dried with a clean, lint-free cloth.
If the unit becomes clogged and fails to spray, please send the clogged unit to:

Whitehall Laboratories
5 Giralda Farms
Madison, N.J. 07940

Warning: Contains CFC 12, 114, substances which harm public health and environment by destroying ozone in the upper environment.

Inactive Ingredients: Fluorocarbons (Propellant), Sorbitan Trioleate. Contains No Sulfites.

Warning: Contains CFC 12, 114, substances which harm public health and environment by destroying ozone in the upper environment.

How Supplied: ⅓ Fl. oz. (10 mL) pocket-size aerosol inhaler.
Shown in Product Identification Guide, page 431

PRIMATENE®
[prīm'a-tēn]
Tablets

Description: Primatene Tablets contain Theophylline Anhydrous 130 mg and Ephedrine Hydrochloride 24 mg.

Indications: For temporary relief of shortness of breath, tightness of chest, and wheezing due to bronchial asthma. Eases breathing for asthma patients by reducing spasms of bronchial muscles.

Warnings: Do not use this product unless a diagnosis of asthma has been made by a doctor. Do not use this product if you have heart disease, high blood pressure, thyroid disease, diabetes or difficulty in urination due to enlargement of the prostate gland unless directed by a doctor. Do not use this product if you have ever been hospitalized for asthma or if you are taking any prescription drug for asthma unless directed by a doctor. **DRUG INTERACTION PRECAUTION:** DO NOT TAKE THIS PRODUCT IF YOU ARE PRESENTLY TAKING A PRESCRIPTION DRUG FOR HIGH BLOOD PRESSURE OR DEPRESSION. IF YOU ARE PRESENTLY TAKING A MONOAMINE OXIDASE INHIBITOR, FIRST CONSULT YOUR DOCTOR. Do not continue to use this product but seek medical assistance immediately if symptoms are not relieved within 1 hour or become worse. Some users of this product may experience nervousness, tremor, sleeplessness, nausea, and loss of appetite. If these symptoms persist or become worse, consult your doctor. As with any drug, if you are pregnant or nursing a baby, seek the advice of a health professional before using this product. Keep this and all drugs out of the reach of children. In case of accidental overdose, seek professional assistance or contact a poison control center immediately.

Directions: Adults and children 12 years of age and over: 1 or 2 tablets initially and then one every 4 hours, as needed, not to exceed 6 tablets in 24 hours. For children under 12, consult a doctor.

Inactive Ingredients: Croscarmellose Sodium, D&C Yellow No. 10 Lake, FD&C Yellow No. 6 Lake, Magnesium Stearate, Microcrystalline Cellulose, Silica, Starch, Stearic Acid.

How Supplied: Available in 24 and 60 tablet thermoform blister cartons.
Shown in Product Identification Guide, page 431

SEMICID®
[sĕm'ē-sĭd]
Vaginal Contraceptive Inserts

Indication: For the prevention of pregnancy.

Warnings: DO NOT INSERT SEMICID IN URINARY OPENING (urethra). If you accidentally insert Semicid into the urinary opening, you may have increased burning when urinating, difficulty in starting to urinate, you may also notice a pink color of your urine or have abdominal pain. If these symptoms occur, drink large amounts of water in order to urinate as frequently as possible (even if urinating causes discomfort), and consult your doctor or clinic immediately. If you accidentally insert Semicid into the urinary opening and become aware of this before intercourse, do not proceed with sexual activity. If your doctor has told you that you should not become pregnant, ask your doctor if you can use this product for contraception. Any delay in your menstrual period may be an early sign of pregnancy. If this happens, consult your doctor or clinic as soon as possible. If you or your partner think you have had an allergic reaction to the spermicide (nonoxynol-9) in this product, do not use Semicid. A small number of men and women may be sensitive to nonoxynol-9. Therefore, if you or your partner experience irritation, burning or itching in the genital area, discontinue use. If these symptoms persist, consult your doctor or clinic. If douching is desired, always wait at least 6 hours after intercourse before douching. Keep this and all drugs out of the reach of children. In case of accidental ingestion, seek professional assistance or contact a poison control center immediately.

Directions for use: BEFORE using Semicid, it is important that you read the package insert carefully for complete instructions and warnings.
FOR USE ALONE OR WITH A CONDOM.
EACH INSERT IS INDIVIDUALLY SEALED FOR YOUR PROTECTION. IF SEAL ON IMPRINTED STRIP IS OPENED WHEN PURCHASED, DO NOT USE.
To use, just unwrap one insert. Use the forefinger and thumb to position the unwrapped insert as deeply as possible into the VAGINAL OPENING, the same opening from which the menstrual flow leaves the body (and where a tampon is placed). EXTREME CARE SHOULD BE TAKEN NOT TO INSERT SEMICID INTO THE URINARY OPENING (URE-

THRA), the opening from which urine passes out of the body.

It is ESSENTIAL that Semicid be inserted at least 15 minutes before intercourse so it can dissolve in the vagina. If intercourse is delayed for more than one (1) hour after insertion or if intercourse is repeated at any time, another insert must be used. It is safe to use Semicid as frequently as needed, however, "directions for use" should be carefully followed each time.

Active Ingredients: Each insert contains Nonoxynol-9, 100 mg.

Inactive Ingredients: Benzethonium Chloride, Citric Acid, D&C Red #21 Lake, D&C Red #33 Lake, Methylparaben, Polyethylene Glycol, Water.

How Supplied: Strip Packaging of 9's and 18's.

Keep Semicid at room temperature (not over 86°F or 30°C).

Shown in Product Identification Guide page 431

TODAY®
[*tü-dā*]
Vaginal Contraceptive Sponge

Description: Today Vaginal Contraceptive Sponge is a soft polyurethane foam sponge containing nonoxynol-9, a spermicide used by millions of women for over 25 years.

Today Sponge is effective, safe, and convenient. Today Sponge provides 24-hour contraceptive protection without hormones, allowing spontaneity. Today Sponge is easy to use, nonmessy and disposable.

Active Ingredient: Each Today Sponge contains nonoxynol-9, one gram.

Inactive Ingredients: Benzoic acid, citric acid, sodium dihydrogen citrate, sodium metabisulfite, sorbic acid, water in a polyurethane foam sponge.

Indication: For the prevention of pregnancy.

Actions: Used as directed, Today Vaginal Contraceptive Sponge prevents pregnancy in three ways: 1) the spermicide nonoxynol-9 kills sperm before they can reach the egg; 2) Today Sponge traps and absorbs sperm; 3) Today Sponge blocks the cervix so that sperm cannot enter. Today Sponge is designed for easy insertion into the vagina. It is positioned against the cervix, and while in place provides protection against pregnancy for 24 hours. The soft polyurethane foam sponge is formulated to feel like normal vaginal tissue and has a specially designed ribbon loop attached to an interior web for maximum strength.

In clinical trials of Today Sponge in over 1,800 women worldwide who completed over 12,000 cycles of use, the method-effectiveness, i.e., the level of effectiveness seen in women who followed the printed instructions exactly and who used Today Sponge every time that they had intercourse, was 89 to 91%. In women who did not use Today Sponge consistently and properly, the effectiveness was 84 to 87%.

Instructions: Remove one Today Sponge from airtight inner pack, wet thoroughly with clean tap water, and squeeze gently several times until it becomes very sudsy. The water activates the spermicide. Fold the sides of Today Sponge upward until it looks long and narrow and then insert it deeply into the vagina with the string loop dangling below. Protection begins immediately and continues for 24 hours. It is not necessary to add creams, jellies, foams, or any other additional spermicide as long as Today Sponge is in place, no matter how many acts of intercourse may occur during a 24-hour period. Always wait 6 hours after your last act of intercourse before removing Today Sponge. If you have intercourse when Today Sponge has been in place for 24 hours, it must be left in place an additional 6 hours after intercourse before removing it. It is unlikely that Today Sponge will fall out. During a bowel movement or other form of internal straining, it may be pushed down to the opening of the vagina and perhaps fall out. If you suspect this is happening, simply insert a finger into your vagina and push the sponge back. If it should fall into the toilet, moisten a new sponge and insert it immediately.

To remove Today Sponge, place a finger in the vagina and reach up and back to find the string loop. Hook a finger around the loop. Slowly and gently pull the Sponge out. Some women, especially first-time users, may have difficulty removing the Sponge. This situation may be due to tension or unusually strong muscular pressure. Simple relaxation of the vaginal muscles and bearing down should make it possible to remove the Sponge without difficulty. See User Instruction Booklet (Section 8) for details on removing Today Sponge or call the Today TalkLine 1-800-223-2329.

Warnings: Some cases of Toxic Shock Syndrome (TSS) have been reported in women using barrier contraceptives including the diaphragm, cervical cap and Today Sponge. Although the occurrence of TSS is uncommon, some studies indicate that there is an increased risk of non-menstrual TSS with the use of barrier contraceptives, including Today Sponge. Today Sponge should not be left in place for more than 30 hours after insertion. If you experience two or more of the warning signs of TSS including fever, vomiting, diarrhea, muscular pain, dizziness, and rash similar to sunburn, consult your physician or clinic immediately. If you have difficulty removing the sponge from your vagina or you remove only a portion of the sponge, contact the Today TalkLine or consult your physician or clinic immediately. Today Sponge should not be used during the menstrual period. After childbirth, miscarriage or other termination of pregnancy, it is important to consult your physician or clinic before using this product. If you have ever had Toxic Shock Syndrome do not use Today Sponge.

A small number of men and women may be sensitive to the spermicide in this product (nonoxynol-9) and should not use this product if irritation occurs and persists. If you or your partner have ever experienced an allergic reaction to the spermicide used in this product, it is best to consult a physician before using Today Vaginal Contraceptive Sponge. If either you or your partner develops burning or itching in the genital area, stop using this product and contact your physician.

A higher degree of protection against pregnancy will be afforded by using another method of contraception in addition to a spermicidal contraceptive. This is especially true during the first few months, until you become familiar with the method. In our clinical studies, approximately one-half of all accidental pregnancies occurred during the first three months of use. Where avoidance of pregnancy is essential, the choice of contraceptive should be made in consultation with a doctor or a family planning clinic. Any delay in your menstrual period may be an early sign of pregnancy. If this happens, consult your physician or clinic as soon as possible. Keep this and all drugs out of reach of children. In case of accidental ingestion of Today Sponge, call a poison control center, emergency medical facility or doctor. (For most people ingestion of small amounts of the spermicide alone should not be harmful.) As with any drug, if you are pregnant or nursing a baby, seek professional advice before using this product.

How To Store: Store at normal room temperature.

How Supplied: Packages of 3s, 6s, and 12s.

Wyeth-Ayerst Laboratories
Division of American Home Products Corporation
P.O. BOX 8299
PHILADELPHIA, PA 19101

Wyeth-Ayerst Tamper-Resistant/Evident Packaging

Statements alerting consumers to the specific type of Tamper-Resistant/Evident Packaging appear on the bottle labels and cartons of all Wyeth-Ayerst over-the-counter products. This includes plastic cap seals on bottles, individually wrapped tablets or suppositories, and sealed cartons. This packaging has been developed to better protect the consumer.

Continued on next page

Wyeth-Ayerst—Cont.

ALUDROX®
[al 'ū-drox]
Antacid
(alumina and magnesia)
ORAL SUSPENSION

Composition: *Suspension* —each 5 ml teaspoonful contains 307 mg aluminum hydroxide [Al(OH)₃] as a gel and 103 mg of magnesium hydroxide. The inactive ingredients present are artificial and natural flavors, benzoic acid, butylparaben, glycerin, hydroxypropyl methylcellulose, methylparaben, propylparaben, saccharin, simethicone, sorbitol solution, and water. Sodium content is 0.10 mEq per 5 ml suspension.

Indications: For temporary relief of heartburn, upset stomach, sour stomach, and/or acid indigestion.

Directions: *Suspension* —Two teaspoonfuls (10 ml) every 4 hours or as directed by a physician. Medication may be followed by a sip of water if desired.

Warnings: Do not take more than 12 teaspoonfuls (60 ml) of suspension in a 24-hour period or use maximum dosage for more than two weeks except under the advice and supervision of a physician. Prolonged use of aluminum-containing antacids in patients with renal failure may result in or worsen dialysis osteomalacia. Elevated tissue aluminum levels contribute to the development of dialysis encephalopathy and osteomalacia syndromes. Also, a number of cases of dialysis encephalopathy have been associated with elevated aluminum levels in the dialysate water. Small amounts of aluminum are absorbed from the gastro-intestinal tract and renal excretion of aluminum is impaired in renal failure. Prolonged use of aluminum-containing antacids in such patients may contribute to increased plasma levels of aluminum. Aluminum is not well removed by dialysis because it is bound to albumin and transferrin, which do not cross dialysis membranes. As a result, aluminum is deposited in bone, and dialysis osteomalacia may develop when large amounts of aluminum are ingested orally by patients with impaired renal function. As with any drug, if you are pregnant or nursing a baby, seek the advice of a health professional before using this product.

Drug Interaction Precautions: Do not take this product if you are presently taking a prescription antibiotic drug containing any form of tetracycline.
Keep at Room Temperature, Approx. 77°F (25°C).
Suspension should be kept tightly closed and shaken well before use. Avoid freezing.
Keep this and all drugs out of the reach of children.

How Supplied: *Oral Suspension* —bottles of 12 fluidounces.
Shown in Product Identification Guide, page 431

Professional Labeling: Consult *1994 Physicians' Desk Reference.*

AMPHOJEL®
[am 'fo-jel]
Antacid
(aluminum hydroxide gel)
ORAL SUSPENSION • TABLETS

Composition: *Suspension—Peppermint flavored* —Each teaspoonful (5 mL) contains 320 mg aluminum hydroxide [Al(OH)₃] as a gel, and not more than 0.10 mEq of sodium. The inactive ingredients present are calcium benzoate, glycerin, hydroxypropyl methylcellulose, menthol, peppermint oil, potassium butylparaben, potassium propylparaben, saccharin, simethicone, sorbitol solution, and water. *Suspension—Without flavor* —Each teaspoonful (5 mL) contains 320 mg of aluminum hydroxide [Al (OH)₃] as a gel. The inactive ingredients present are butylparaben, calcium benzoate, glycerin, hydroxypropyl methylcellulose, methylparaben, propylparaben, saccharin, simethicone, sorbitol solution, and water. *Tablets* are available in 0.3 and 0.6 g strengths. Each contains, respectively, the equivalent of 300 mg and 600 mg aluminum hydroxide as a dried gel. The inactive ingredients present are artificial and natural flavors, cellulose, hydrogenated vegetable oil, magnesium stearate, polacrilin potassium, saccharin, starch, and talc. The 0.3 g (5 grain) strength is equivalent to about 1 teaspoonful of the suspension and the 0.6 g (10 grain) strength is equivalent to about 2 teaspoonfuls. Each 0.3 g tablet contains 0.08 mEq of sodium and each 0.6 g tablet contains 0.13 mEq of sodium.

Indications: For temporary relief of heartburn, upset stomach, sour stomach, and/or acid indigestion.

Directions: *Suspension* —Two teaspoonfuls (10 ml) to be taken five or six times daily, between meals and on retiring or as directed by a physician. Medication may be followed by a sip of water if desired. *Tablets* —Two tablets of the 0.3 g strength, or one tablet of the 0.6 g strength, five or six times daily, between meals and on retiring or as directed by a physician. It is unnecessary to chew the 0.3 g tablet before swallowing with water. After chewing the 0.6 g tablet, sip about one-half glass of water.

Warnings: Do not take more than 12 teaspoonfuls (60 ml) of suspension, or more than twelve (12) 0.3 g tablets, or more than six (6) 0.6 g tablets in a 24-hour period or use this maximum dosage for more than two weeks except under the advice and supervision of a physician. May cause constipation. Prolonged use of aluminum-containing antacids in patients with renal failure may result in or worsen dialysis osteomalacia. Elevated tissue aluminum levels contribute

to the development of dialysis encephalopathy and osteomalacia syndromes. Also, a number of cases of dialysis encephalopathy have been associated with elevated aluminum levels in the dialysate water. Small amounts of aluminum are absorbed from the gastrointestinal tract and renal excretion of aluminum is impaired in renal failure. Prolonged use of aluminum-containing antacids in such patients may contribute to increased plasma levels of aluminum. Aluminum is not well removed by dialysis because it is bound to albumin and transferrin, which do not cross dialysis membranes. As a result, aluminum is deposited in bone, and dialysis osteomalacia may develop when large amounts of aluminum are ingested orally by patients with impaired renal function. As with any drug, if you are pregnant or nursing a baby, seek the advice of a health professional before using this product.

Drug Interaction Precaution: Antacids may interact with certain prescription drugs. Do not use this product if you are presently taking a prescription antibiotic containing any form of tetracycline. If you are presently taking a prescription drug, do not take this product without checking with your physician.
Keep tightly closed and store at room temperature, Approx. 77°F (25°C).
Suspension should be shaken well before use. Avoid freezing.
Keep this and all drugs out of the reach of children.

How Supplied: *Suspension* —Peppermint flavored; without flavor—bottles of 12 fluidounces. *Tablets* —a convenient auxiliary dosage form—0.3 g (5 grain) bottles of 100; 0.6 g (10 grain), boxes of 100.
Shown in Product Identification Guide, page 431

Professional Labeling: Consult *1994 Physicians' Desk Reference.*

BASALJEL®
[bā 'sel-jel]
(basic aluminum carbonate gel)
ORAL SUSPENSION • CAPSULES • TABLETS

Composition: *Suspension* —each 5 mL teaspoonful contains basic aluminum carbonate gel equivalent to 400 mg aluminum hydroxide [Al(OH)₃]. The inactive ingredients present are artificial and natural flavors, butylparaben, calcium benzoate, glycerin, hydroxypropyl methylcellulose, methylparaben, mineral oil, propylparaben, saccharin, simethicone, sorbitol solution, and water. *Capsule* contains dried basic aluminum carbonate gel equivalent to 608 mg of dried aluminum hydroxide gel or 500 mg aluminum hydroxide [Al(OH)₃]. The inactive ingredients present are D&C Yellow 10, FD&C Blue 1, FD&C Red 40, FD&C Yellow 6, gelatin, polacrilin potassium, polyethylene glycol, talc, and titanium dioxide. *Tablet* contains dried basic aluminum carbonate gel equivalent to

608 mg of dried aluminum hydroxide gel or 500 mg aluminum hydroxide. The inactive ingredients present are cellulose, hydrogenated vegetable oil, magnesium stearate, polacrilin potassium, starch, and talc.

Indications: For the symptomatic relief of hyperacidity, associated with the diagnosis of peptic ulcer, gastritis, peptic esophagitis, gastric hyperacidity, and hiatal hernia.

Warnings: Do not take more than 24 tablets/capsules/teaspoonsful of BASALJEL in a 24-hour period, or use this maximum dosage for more than two weeks except under the advice and supervision of a physician. Dosage should be carefully supervised since continued overdosage, in conjunction with restriction of dietary phosphorus and calcium, may produce a persistently lowered serum phosphate and a mildly elevated alkaline phosphatase. A usually transient hypercalciuria of mild degree may be associated with the early weeks of therapy. Prolonged use of aluminum-containing antacids in patients with renal failure may result in or worsen dialysis osteomalacia. Elevated tissue aluminum levels contribute to the development of dialysis encephalopathy and osteomalacia syndromes. Also, a number of cases of dialysis encephalopathy have been associated with elevated aluminum levels in the dialysate water. Small amounts of aluminum are absorbed from the gastrointestinal tract and renal excretion of aluminum is impaired in renal failure. Prolonged use of aluminum-containing antacids in such patients may contribute to increased plasma levels of aluminum. Aluminum is not well removed by dialysis because it is bound to albumin and transferrin, which do not cross dialysis membranes. As a result, aluminum is deposited in bone, and dialysis osteomalacia may develop when large amounts of aluminum are ingested orally by patients with impaired renal function. As with any drug, if you are pregnant or nursing a baby, seek the advice of a health professional before using this product.

Dosage and Administration: *Suspension* —two teaspoonsful (10 mL) in water or fruit juice taken as often as every two hours up to twelve times daily. Two teaspoonsful have the capacity to neutralize 23 mEq of acid. *Capsules* —two capsules as often as every two hours up to twelve times daily. Two capsules have the capacity to neutralize 24 mEq of acid. *Tablets* —two tablets as often as every two hours up to twelve times daily. Two tablets have the capacity to neutralize 25 mEq of acid. The sodium content of each dosage form is as follows: 0.13 mEq/5 mL for the suspension, 0.12 mEq per capsule, and 0.12 mEq per tablet.

Precautions: May cause constipation. Adequate fluid intake should be maintained in addition to the specific medical or surgical management indicated by the patient's condition.

Drug Interaction Precaution: Alumina-containing antacids should not be used concomitantly with any form of tetracycline therapy.

How Supplied: Suspension—bottles of 12 fluidounces.
Capsules—bottles of 100 and 500.
Tablets (scored)—bottles of 100.
Shown in Product Identification Guide, page 431

Professional Labeling: Consult *1994 Physicians' Desk Reference.*

CEROSE®DM
[se-ros 'DM]
Antihistamine/Nasal Decongestant/Cough Suppressant

Description: Each teaspoonful (5 mL) contains 15 mg dextromethorphan hydrobromide, 4 mg chlorpheniramine maleate, and 10 mg phenylephrine hydrochloride. Alcohol 2.4%. The inactive ingredients present are artificial flavors, citric acid, edetate disodium, FD&C Yellow 6, glycerin, saccharin sodium, sodium benzoate, sodium citrate, sodium propionate, and water.

Indications: For the temporary relief of cough due to minor throat and bronchial irritation as may occur with the common cold or with inhaled irritants. Temporarily relieves nasal congestion, runny nose, and sneezing due to the common cold, hay fever, or other upper respiratory allergies.

Directions: Adults and children 12 years of age and over: One teaspoonful every four hours as needed. Children 6 to under 12 years of age: One-half teaspoonful every four hours as needed. Do not exceed six doses in a 24-hour period. For children under 6 years, consult a doctor.

Drug Interaction Precaution: Do not take this product if you are presently taking a prescription drug for high blood pressure or depression without first consulting your doctor.
Warnings: May cause marked drowsiness; alcohol may increase the drowsiness effect. Avoid alcoholic beverages while taking this product. Use caution when driving a motor vehicle or operating machinery. Do not take this product if you have heart disease, high blood pressure, thyroid disease, diabetes, asthma, glaucoma, emphysema, chronic pulmonary disease, shortness of breath, difficulty in breathing, or difficulty in urination due to enlargement of the prostate gland unless directed by a doctor. This product may cause excitability, especially in children. Do not exceed recommended dosage because at higher doses nervousness, dizziness, or sleeplessness may occur. Do not take this product for more than 7 days. A persistent cough may be a sign of a serious condition. If symptoms persist for more than one week, tend to recur, or are accompanied by fever, rash, or persistent headache,

consult a doctor. Do not take this product for persistent or chronic cough such as occurs with smoking, or if cough is accompanied by excessive phlegm (mucus) unless directed by a doctor. As with any drug, if you are pregnant or nursing a baby, seek the advice of a health professional before using this product.
Keep this and all drugs out of the reach of children. In case of accidental overdose, seek professional assistance or contact a Poison Control Center immediately.

How Supplied: Cases of 12 bottles of 4 fl. oz.; bottles of 1 pint.
Keep tightly closed—Store below 77° F (25° C).
Shown in Product Identification Guide, page 431

COLLYRIUM for FRESH EYES
[ko-lir 'e-um]
a neutral borate solution
EYE WASH

Description: Soothing Collyrium Eye Wash for Fresh Eyes is specially formulated to soothe, refresh, and cleanse irritated eyes. Collyrium Eye Wash is a neutral borate solution that contains boric acid, sodium borate, benzalkonium chloride (as a preservative), and water.

Indications: To cleanse the eye, loosen foreign material, air pollutants or chlorinated water.

Recommended Uses:
Home—For emergency flushing of foreign bodies or whenever a soothing eye rinse is necessary.
Hospitals, dispensaries and clinics— For emergency flushing of chemicals or foreign bodies from the eye.

Directions: Remove the eyecup from blister. Puncture bottle by twisting threaded eyecup down onto bottle; then remove it from the bottle. Rinse eyecup with clean water immediately before and after each use. Avoid contamination of rim and interior surface of eyecup. Fill eyecup one-half full with Collyrium Eye Wash. Apply cup tightly to the affected eye to prevent the escape of the liquid and tilt head backward. Open eyelid wide and rotate eyeball to thoroughly wash eye. Rinse cup with clean water after use and recap by twisting threaded eyecup on the bottle for storage.

Warnings: Do not use if solution changes color or becomes cloudy, or with a wetting solution for contact lenses or other eye care products containing polyvinyl alcohol.
This product contains benzalkonium chloride as a preservative. Do not use this product if you are sensitive to benzalkonium chloride.
To avoid contamination do not touch tip of container to any surface. Replace cap after using. If you experience eye pain, changes in vision, continued redness, irritation of the eye, or if the condition

Continued on next page

Wyeth-Ayerst—Cont.

worsens or persists, consult a doctor. Obtain immediate medical treatment for all open wounds in or near the eye.
The Collyrium for Fresh Eyes bottle is sealed for your protection. Prior to first use, remove cap and squeeze bottle. If bottle leaks, do not use.
Keep this and all medication out of the reach of children.
Keep bottle tightly closed at Room Temperature, Approx. 77°F (25°C).

How Supplied: Bottles of 4 fl. oz. (118 ml) with eyecup.
Shown in Product Identification Guide, page 431

COLLYRIUM FRESH™
[ko-lir'e-um]
Sterile Eye Drops
Lubricant
Redness Reliever

Description: Collyrium Fresh is a specially formulated sterile eye drop which can be used, up to 4 times daily, to relieve redness and discomfort due to minor eye irritations caused by dust, smoke, smog, swimming, or sun glare.
The active ingredients are tetrahydrozoline HCl (0.05%) and glycerin (1.0%). Other ingredients include benzalkonium chloride (0.01%) and edetate disodium (0.1%) as preservatives, boric acid, hydrochloric acid and sodium borate.

Indications: For the temporary relief of redness due to minor eye irritations or discomfort due to burning or exposure to wind or sun.

Directions: Tilt head back and squeeze 1 to 2 drops into each eye up to 4 times daily, or as directed by a physician.

Warnings: Do not use if solution changes color or becomes cloudy. Remove contact lenses before using. If you have glaucoma, do not use this product except under the advice and supervision of a physician. Overuse of this product may produce increased redness of the eye. To avoid contamination, do not touch tip of container to any surface. Replace cap after using. If you experience eye pain, changes in vision, continued redness or irritation of the eye, or if the condition worsens or persists for more than 72 hours, discontinue use and consult a physician.
Keep this and all medication out of the reach of children.

Retain carton for complete product information.
Keep bottle tightly closed at Room Temperature, Approx. 77°F (25°C).

How Supplied: Bottles of ½ fl. oz. (15 ml) with built-in eye dropper.
Shown in Product Identification Guide, page 431

DONNAGEL®
[don'nǎ-jel]
Liquid and Chewable Tablets

Each tablespoon (15 mL) of **Donnagel Liquid** contains: 600 mg Attapulgite, USP.

Inactive Ingredients: Alcohol 1.4%, Benzyl Alcohol, Carboxymethylcellulose Sodium, Citric Acid, FD&C Blue 1, Flavors, Magnesium Aluminum Silicate, Methylparaben, Phosphoric Acid, Propylene Glycol, Propylparaben, Saccharin Sodium, Sorbitol, Titanium Dioxide, Water, Xanthan Gum.

Each **Donnagel Chewable** Tablet contains: 600 mg Attapulgite, USP.

Inactive Ingredients: D&C Yellow 10 Aluminum Lake, FD&C Blue 1 Aluminum Lake, Flavors, Magnesium Stearate, Mannitol, Saccharin Sodium, Sorbitol, Water.

Indications: Donnagel is indicated for the symptomatic relief of diarrhea. It reduces the number of bowel movements, improves consistency of loose, watery bowel movements and relieves cramping.

Warnings: Patients are told that diarrhea may be serious. They are warned not to use this product for more than 2 days, or in the presence of fever, or in children under 3 years of age unless directed by a physician.
This product should not be taken by patients who are hypersensitive to any of the ingredients. As with any drug, women who are pregnant or nursing a baby should seek the advice of a health professional before using this product.

Dosage and Administration: Full recommended dose should be administered at the first sign of diarrhea and after each subsequent bowel movement, NOT TO EXCEED 7 DOSES IN A 24-HOUR PERIOD.
[See table below.]

How Supplied: Donnagel Liquid (green suspension) in 4 fl. oz. (NDC 0031-3017-12) and 8 fl. oz. (NDC 0031-3017-18). Donnagel Chewable Tablets (light-green, flat-faced, beveled-edged, round tablets

with darker green flecks; one side engraved AHR, obverse engraved Donnagel) in consumer blister packages of 18 (NDC 0031-3018-51).
Store at Controlled Room Temperature, between 15°C and 30°C (59°F and 86°F).
Shown in Product Identification Guide, page 431

NURSOY®
[nur-soy]
Soy protein isolate formula
READY–TO–FEED
CONCENTRATED LIQUID
POWDER

Breast milk is best for babies. NURSOY® milk-free, lactose-free formula is intended to meet the nutritional needs of infants and children who are not breast-fed and are allergic to cow's milk protein and/or intolerant to lactose. It should not be used in infants and children allergic to soybean protein.
NURSOY Ready-to-Feed and Concentrated Liquid are corn free and contain only sucrose as their carbohydrate. NURSOY Powder contains corn syrup solids and sucrose as its carbohydrate. Professional advice should be followed.
NURSOY's fat blend closely resembles the fatty acid composition of human milk and has physiologic levels of linoleic and linolenic acid.
NURSOY contains beta-carotene, a component of human milk. The estimated renal solute load of NURSOY is relatively low.

Ingredients (in normal dilution supplying 20 calories per fluidounce): 87% water; 6.7% sucrose; 3.4% oleo, coconut, oleic (safflower) and soybean oils; 2.0% soy protein isolate; and less than 1% of each of the following: potassium citrate; monobasic sodium phosphate; calcium carbonate; dibasic calcium phosphate; magnesium chloride; calcium chloride; soy lecithin; calcium carrageenan; calcium hydroxide; L-methionine; sodium chloride; potassium bicarbonate; taurine; ferrous, zinc, and cupric sulfates; L-carnitine; potassium iodide; ascorbic acid; choline chloride; alpha-tocopheryl acetate; niacinamide; calcium pantothenate; riboflavin; vitamin A palmitate; thiamine hydrochloride; pyridoxine hydrochloride; beta-carotene; phytonadione; folic acid; biotin; cholecalciferol; cyanocobalamin.

PROXIMATE ANALYSIS
at 20 calories per fluidounce
READY-TO-FEED, CONCENTRATED
LIQUID, and POWDER

	(W/V)
Protein	1.8 %
Fat	3.6 %
Carbohydrate	6.9 %
Water	87.0 %
Crude fiber ... not more than	0.01 %
Calories/fl. oz.	20

DONNAGEL®

	Liquid	Chewable Tablets
Adults	2 Tablespoons	2 Tablets
Children		
12 years and over	2 Tablespoons	2 Tablets
6 through 11 years	1 Tablespoon	1 Tablet
3 through 5 years	½ Tablespoon	½ Tablet
Under 3 years	Consult Physician	

Liquid should be shaken well. Tablets should be chewed thoroughly and swallowed.

Vitamins, Minerals: In normal dilution, each liter contains:

A	2,000	IU
D_3	400	IU
E	9.5	IU
K_1	100	mcg
C (ascorbic acid)	55	mg
B_1 (thiamine)	670	mcg
B_2 (riboflavin)	1000	mcg
B_6	420	mcg
B_{12}	2	mcg
Niacin	5000	mcg
Pantothenic acid	3000	mcg
Folic acid (folacin)	50	mcg
Choline	85	mg
Inositol	27	mg
Biotin	35	mcg
Calcium	600	mg
Phosphorus	420	mg
Sodium	200	mg
Potassium	700	mg
Chloride	375	mg
Magnesium	67	mg
Manganese	200	mcg
Iron	12.0	mg
Copper	470	mcg
Zinc	5	mg
Iodine	60	mcg

Preparation: *Ready-to-Feed* (32 fl. oz. cans of 20 calories per fluidounce formula)—shake can, open and pour into previously sterilized nursing bottle; attach nipple and feed. Cover opened can and immediately store in refrigerator. Use contents of can within 48 hours of opening.
Prolonged storage of can at excessive temperatures should be avoided.
Expiration date is on top of can.
WARNING: DO NOT USE A MICROWAVE TO PREPARE OR WARM FORMULA. SERIOUS BURNS MAY OCCUR.
Concentrated Liquid—For normal dilution supplying 20 calories per fluidounce, use equal amounts of NURSOY® liquid and cooled, previously boiled water.
Note: Prepared formula should be used within 24 hours.
Prolonged storage of can at excessive temperatures should be avoided.
Expiration date is on top of can.
WARNING: DO NOT USE A MICROWAVE TO PREPARE OR WARM FORMULA. SERIOUS BURNS MAY OCCUR.
Powder—For normal dilution supplying 20 calories per fluidounce, add 1 level measuring scoop to 2 fluidounces of water.
Note: Prepared formula should be used within 24 hours.
Prolonged storage of can at excessive temperatures should be avoided.
Expiration date is on bottom of can.
WARNING: DO NOT USE A MICROWAVE TO PREPARE OR WARM FORMULA. SERIOUS BURNS MAY OCCUR.

How Supplied: *Ready-to-Feed*—presterilized and premixed, 32 fluidounce (1 quart) cans, cases of 6 cans;
Concentrated Liquid—13 fluidounce cans, cases of 12 cans;
Powder—1 pound cans, cases of 6 cans.

Questions or Comments regarding NURSOY: 1-800-99-WYETH.
Shown in Product Identification Guide, page 431

SMA®
Iron fortified
Infant formula
READY–TO–FEED
CONCENTRATED LIQUID
POWDER

Breast milk is best for babies. Infant formula is intended to replace or supplement breast milk when breast feeding is not possible or is insufficient, or when mothers elect not to breast feed.
Good maternal nutrition is important for the preparation and maintenance of breast feeding. Extensive or prolonged use of partial bottle feeding, before breast feeding has been well established, could make breast feeding difficult to maintain. A decision not to breast feed could be difficult to reverse.
Professional advice should be followed on all matters of infant feeding. Infant formula should always be prepared and used as directed. Unnecessary or improper use of infant formula could present a health hazard. Social and financial implications should be considered when selecting the method of infant feeding.
SMA® is close in nutrient composition to human milk with its physiologic fat blend, whey-dominated protein composition, and inclusion of beta-carotene and nucleotides.
SMA, utilizing a hybridized safflower (oleic) oil, became the first infant formula offering fat and calcium absorption closest to that of human milk, with physiologic levels of linoleic acid and linolenic acid. Thus, the fat blend in SMA provides a ready source of energy, helps protect infants against neonatal tetany and produces a ratio of vitamin E to polyunsaturated fatty acids (linoleic acid) more than adequate to prevent hemolytic anemia and yields a serum lipid profile close to that of the breast-fed infant.
By combining reduced minerals whey with skimmed cow's milk, SMA reduces the protein content to fall within the range of human milk, adjusts the whey-protein to casein ratio to that of human milk, and subsequently reduces the mineral content to a physiologic level.
The resultant 60:40 whey-protein to casein ratio provides protein nutrition superior to a casein-dominated formula. In addition, the essential amino acids, including cystine, are present in amounts close to those of human milk. So the protein in SMA is of high biologic value.
Five nucleotides found in higher amounts in human milk compared to infant formula have been added to SMA at the levels found in breast milk.
The physiologic mineral content makes possible a low renal solute load which helps protect the functionally immature infant kidney, increases expendable water reserves and helps protect against dehydration.

Use of lactose as the carbohydrate results in a physiologic stool flora and a low stool pH, decreasing the incidence of perianal dermatitis.

Ingredients: SMA Concentrated Liquid or Ready-to-Feed. Water; nonfat milk; reduced minerals whey; oleo, coconut, oleic (safflower or sunflower), and soybean oils; lactose; soy lecithin; taurine; cytidine-5'-monophosphate; calcium carrageenan; adenosine-5'-monophosphate; disodium uridine-5'-monophosphate; disodium inosine-5'-monophosphate; disodium guanosine-5'-monophosphate; *Minerals:* Potassium bicarbonate and chloride; calcium chloride and citrate; sodium bicarbonate and citrate; ferrous, zinc, cupric, and manganese sulfates. *Vitamins:* ascorbic acid, alpha tocopheryl acetate, niacinamide, vitamin A palmitate, calcium pantothenate, thiamine hydrochloride, riboflavin, pyridoxine hydrochloride, beta-carotene, folic acid, phytonadione, biotin, cholecalciferol, cyanocobalamin.
SMA Powder. Lactose; oleo, coconut, oleic (safflower or sunflower), and soybean oils; nonfat milk; whey protein concentrate; soy lecithin; taurine; cytidine-5'-monophosphate; adenosine-5'-monophosphate; disodium uridine-5'-monophosphate; disodium inosine-5'-monophosphate; disodium guanosine-5'-monophosphate. *Minerals:* Potassium phosphate; calcium hydroxide; magnesium chloride; calcium chloride; sodium bicarbonate; ferrous sulfate; potassium hydroxide; potassium bicarbonate; zinc, cupric, and manganese sulfates; potassium iodide. *Vitamins:* Ascorbic acid, choline chloride, inositol, alpha tocopheryl acetate, niacinamide, calcium pantothenate, vitamin A palmitate, riboflavin, thiamine hydrochloride, pyridoxine hydrochloride, beta-carotene, folic acid, phytonadione, biotin, cholecalciferol, cyanocobalamin.

PROXIMATE ANALYSIS
at 20 calories per fluidounce
READY-TO-FEED, POWDER, and
CONCENTRATED LIQUID:

	(W/V)
Fat	3.6 %
Carbohydrate	7.2 %
Protein	1.5 %
60% Lactalbumin (whey protein)	0.9 %
40% Casein	0.6 %
Crude Fiber	None
Total Solids	12.6 %
Calories/fl. oz.	20

Vitamins, Minerals: In normal dilution, each liter contains:
[See table on top of next column]

Preparation: *Ready-to-Feed* (8 and 32 fl. oz. cans of 20 calories per fluidounce formula)—shake can, open and pour into previously sterilized nursing bottle; attach nipple and feed immediately. Cover opened can and immediately store in refrigerator. Use contents of can within 48 hours of opening.

Continued on next page

Wyeth-Ayerst—Cont.

A	2000	IU
D₃	400	IU
E	9.5	IU
K₁	55	mcg
C (ascorbic acid)	55	mg
B₁ (thiamine)	670	mcg
B₂ (riboflavin)	1000	mcg
B₆	420	mcg
(pyridoxine hydrochloride)		
B₁₂	1.3	mcg
Niacin	5000	mcg
Pantothenic Acid	2100	mcg
Folic Acid (folacin)	50	mcg
Choline	100	mg
Biotin	15	mcg
Calcium	420	mg
Phosphorus	280	mg
Sodium	150	mg
Potassium	560	mg
Chloride	375	mg
Magnesium	45	mg
Manganese	100	mcg
Iron	12	mg
Copper	470	mcg
Zinc	5	mg
Iodine	60	mcg

Prolonged storage of can at excessive temperatures should be avoided. Expiration date is on top of can. WARNING: DO NOT USE A MICROWAVE TO PREPARE OR WARM FORMULA. SERIOUS BURNS MAY OCCUR.
Powder —(1 pound can)—For normal dilution supplying 20 calories per fluidounce, use 1 level measuring scoop to 2 fluidounces of cooled, previously boiled water.
Prolonged storage of can of powder at excessive temperatures should be avoided. Expiration date is on bottom of can. WARNING: DO NOT USE A MICROWAVE TO PREPARE OR WARM FORMULA. SERIOUS BURNS MAY OCCUR.
Concentrated Liquid —For normal dilution supplying 20 calories per fluidounce, use equal amounts of SMA® liquid and cooled, previously boiled water. Prolonged storage of can at excessive temperatures should be avoided. Expiration date is on top of can. WARNING: DO NOT USE A MICROWAVE TO PREPARE OR WARM FORMULA. SERIOUS BURNS MAY OCCUR.
Note: Prepared formula should be used within 24 hours.

How Supplied: *Ready-to-Feed* —presterilized and premixed, 32 fluidounce (1 quart) cans, cases of 6 cans; 8 fluidounce cans, cases of 24 (4 carriers of 6 cans). *Powder* —1 pound and 2 pound 3 ounce cans with measuring scoop, cases of 6 cans. *Concentrated Liquid* —13 fluidounce cans, cases of 24 cans.

Also Available: SMA® lo-iron. Those who appreciate the particular advantages of SMA® infant formula, close in nutrient composition to mother's milk,

sometimes need or wish to recommend a formula that does not contain a high level of iron. SMA® lo-iron has all the benefits of regular SMA® but with a reduced level of iron of 1.4 mg per quart. Infants should receive supplemental dietary iron from an outside source to meet daily requirements.
Concentrated Liquid —13 fl. oz. cans, cases of 12 cans. *Powder* —1 pound cans with measuring scoop, cases of 6 cans. *Ready-to-Feed* —32 fl. oz. cans, cases of 6 cans.
Preparation of the standard 20 calories per fluidounce formula of SMA® lo-iron is the same as SMA® iron fortified given above.
Questions or Comments regarding SMA: 1-800-99-WYETH.
Shown in Product Identification Guide, page 431

STUART PRENATAL® Tablets
Multivitamin/Multimineral Supplement

One Tablet Daily Provides
VITAMINS

A*	4,000 IU
D	400 IU
E	11 mg
C	100 mg
Folic Acid	0.8 mg
B₁	1.5 mg
(thiamin)	
B₂	1.7 mg
(riboflavin)	
Niacin	18 mg
B₆	2.6 mg
(pyridoxine hydrochloride)	
B₁₂	4 mcg
(cyanocobalamin)	

MINERALS

Calcium	200 mg
Iron	60 mg
Zinc	25 mg

*Input as vitamin A acetate and beta carotene.

Ingredients
Each tablet contains:
Active: calcium sulfate, ferrous fumarate, ascorbic acid, dl-alpha tocopheryl acetate, zinc oxide, niacinamide, vitamin A acetate, beta carotene, pyridoxine hydrochloride, riboflavin, thiamin mononitrate, folic acid, cholecalciferol, cyanocobalamin. Inactive: croscarmellose sodium, hydroxypropyl methylcellulose, microcrystalline cellulose, pregelatinized starch, red iron oxide, titanium dioxide.

Indications: STUART PRENATAL is a nonprescription multivitamin/multimineral supplement for use before, during, and after pregnancy. It provides essential vitamins and minerals, including 60 mg of elemental iron as well-tolerated ferrous fumarate, and 200 mg of elemental calcium (nonalkalizing and phosphorus-free), and 25 mg zinc. STUART PRENATAL also contains 0.8 mg folic acid.

Directions: Before, during and after pregnancy, one tablet daily, or as directed by a physician.

Warning: In case of accidental overdose, seek professional assistance or contact a Poison Control Center immediately. Keep out of the reach of children.

How Supplied: Bottles of 100 light pink tablets imprinted "Wyeth 794". A child-resistant safety cap is standard on 100 tablet bottles as a safeguard against accidental ingestion by children.
NDC 0008-0794-01.
Shown in Product Identification Guide, page 431

WYANOIDS® Relief Factor
[wi 'a-noids]
Hemorrhoidal Suppositories

Description: Active Ingredients: Live Yeast Cell Derivative, Supplying 2,000 units Skin Respiratory Factor Per Ounce of Cocoa Butter Suppository Base and Shark Liver Oil 3%. **Inactive Ingredients:** Beeswax, Glycerin, Phenylmercuric Nitrate 1:10,000 (as a preservative), Polyethylene Glycol 600 Dilaurate.

Indications: To help shrink swelling of hemorrhoidal tissues and provide prompt, temporary relief from pain and itching.

Usual Dosage: Use one suppository up to five times daily, especially in the morning, at night, and after bowel movements, or as directed by a physician.

Directions: Remove wrapper and insert one suppository rectally using gentle pressure. Frequent application and lubrication with Wyanoids® Relief Factor provide continual therapy which will lead to more rapid improvement of rectal conditions.

Caution: In case of bleeding or if the condition persists, the patient should consult a physician. Keep this and all medicines out of the reach of children. Do not store above 80°F.

How Supplied: Boxes of 12 and 24.
Shown in Product Identification Guide, page 431

EDUCATIONAL MATERIAL

Audiovisual Programs
The *Wyeth-Ayerst Audiovisual Catalog,* listing audiovisual programs available through the Wyeth-Ayerst Audiovisual Library or on loan through the local Wyeth-Ayerst representative, can be obtained by writing Professional Service, Wyeth-Ayerst Laboratories, P.O. Box 8299, Philadelphia, PA 19101.

Zila Pharmaceuticals, Inc.
5227 NORTH 7th STREET
PHOENIX, AZ 85014-2817

ZILACTIN® Medicated Gel
ZILACTIN®-L Liquid
DERMAFLEX® Topical Anesthetic
Gel Coating

Description: Zilactin Medicated Gel stops pain and speeds healing of canker sores, fever blisters and cold sores. Zilactin forms a tenacious, occlusive film which holds the medication in place while controlling pain. Intra-orally, the film can last up to six hours, usually allowing pain-free eating and drinking. Extra-orally, the film can last much longer.

Zilactin-L is a non film-forming liquid that treats and relieves the pain, itching and burning of developing and existing cold sores and fever blisters. Zilactin-L is specially formulated to treat the initial signs of tingling, itching or burning that signal an oncoming cold sore or fever blister. Zilactin-L can often prevent developing cold sores or fever blisters from breaking out. If a lesion does occur, Zilactin-L will significantly reduce the size of the outbreak.

DermaFlex is a topical anesthetic gel "bandage" that provides temporary relief and protection of minor skin irritations including the pain and itching associated with scrapes, minor cuts, insect bites and minor rashes. DermaFlex forms a flexible, invisible, waterproof bandage which holds the active ingredient (pain relieving lidocaine) in place for hours while protecting the affected skin.

Clinical studies on the effectiveness of Zila's products are available on request.

Active Ingredients: Zilactin—Benzyl Alcohol (10%); **Zilactin-L**—Lidocaine (2.5%); **DermaFlex**—Lidocaine (2.5%)

Application: Zilactin: FOR USE IN THE MOUTH AND ON LIPS. Apply every four hours for the first three days and then as needed. Dry the affected area. Apply a thin coat of Zilactin and allow 30-60 seconds for the gel to dry into a film. Outside the mouth, Zilactin forms a transparent film. Inside the mouth, the film is white.

Zilactin-L: FOR USE ON THE LIPS AND AROUND THE MOUTH. Apply every 1-2 hours for the first three days and then as needed. For maximum effectiveness use at first signs of tingling or itching. Moisten a cotton swab with several drops of Zilactin-L. Apply on lip area where symptoms are noted or directly on existing cold sore or fever blister and allow to dry for 15 seconds.

DermaFlex: FOR EXTERNAL USE. Apply as needed (not more than 3-4 times daily). Dry the affected area. Apply a coat of DermaFlex and allow 60 seconds for the gel to dry into a transparent film. Apply a second coat and allow it to dry. Additional coats are applied directly over existing film bandage.

Warning: A mild, temporary stinging sensation may be experienced when applying Zilactin, Zilactin-L or DermaFlex to an open cut, sore or blister. DO NOT USE IN OR NEAR EYES. In the event of accidental contact with the eye, flush with water immediately and continuously for ten minutes. Seek immediate medical attention if pain or irritation persists. For temporary relief only. As with all medications, keep out of the reach of children.

How Supplied: Zila products are non-prescription and carried by most drug wholesalers, retail chains and independent pharmacies. Each product is available to physicians and dentists directly from Zila in full size and single use packages.

For further information call or write:

Zila Pharmaceuticals, Inc.
5227 N. 7th Street, Phoenix, AZ 85014-2817, (602) 266-6700

U.S. patent numbers 4,285,934; 4,381,296; 5,081,157 and 5,081,158
Shown in Product Identification Guide, page 432

EDUCATIONAL MATERIAL

Samples and literature are available to medical professionals on request.

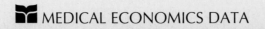
MEDICAL ECONOMICS DATA

DIAGNOSTICS, DEVICES, AND MEDICAL AIDS

This section provides information on testing kits and other medical products designed for home use by consumers. It is made possible through the courtesy of the manufacturers whose products appear on the following pages. The information concerning each product has been prepared, edited, and approved by the medical department, medical director, and/or medical counsel of each manufacturer.

The product descriptions in this section are designed to provide all information necessary for informed use, including, when applicable, active ingredients, indications, actions, warnings, cautions, directions for use, professional labeling, and how supplied.

The publisher has emphasized the necessity of describing products comprehensively in order to supply all information essential for sound and intelligent use.

The descriptions seen here include all information made available by the manufacturer. The publisher does not warrant or guarantee any product described here, and does not perform any independent analysis of the information provided. Inclusion of a product in this book does not represent an endorsement, and the publisher does not necessarily advocate the use of any product listed.

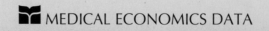
MEDICAL ECONOMICS DATA

Lavoptik Company, Inc.
661 WESTERN AVENUE N.
ST. PAUL, MN 55103

LAVOPTIK® Eye Cups

Description: Device—Sterile disposable eye cups.

How Supplied: Individually bagged eye cups are packed 12 per box, NDC 10651-01004.

Parke-Davis
Consumer Health Products Group
Division of Warner-Lambert
Company
201 TABOR ROAD
MORRIS PLAINS, NJ 07950

e·p·t® QUICK STICK™
Early Pregnancy Test

You can find out whether or not you're pregnant by testing any time of day and as early as the first day of your missed period.

With just one easy step, **e·p·t** gives you clear results in two minutes.

e·p·t Early Pregnancy Test. The name more women trust™.

Before You Begin The e·p·t Test

Please read the instructions carefully. Registered nurses are available to confidentially answer your calls regarding **e·p·t**.

If you have any questions, call toll-free 1-800-562-0266 or 1-800-223-0182, weekdays 9 a.m. to 5 p.m. EST.

[See table above.]

To Use e·p·t

Remove the test stick from the foil pouch and throw away the freshness sachet.

Slide back the clear splashguard to expose the absorbent tip and protect the results windows.

Hold the test stick by the thumb grip with the absorbent tip pointing downward and urinate on the absorbent tip for at least 5 seconds.

[See table below.]

To Read The Results

After 2 minutes you can read the results. A pink/purple line will form in the control window (small square) to tell you the test is working. The results window (large round) will show your test results.

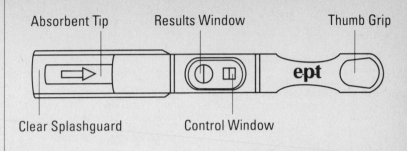

Absorbent Tip   Results Window   Thumb Grip

Clear Splashguard   Control Window

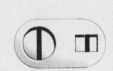

2 LINES— PREGNANT
If you see one pink/purple line in each window, the test has indicated that you are pregnant.

1 LINE—NOT PREGNANT
If you see a line in the small square window but no line in the large round window, the test has indicated that you are not pregnant.

The pink/purple lines do not have to match.

Invalid result—If no lines appear, or no pink/purple line appears in the small square window, do not read the results as they may be inaccurate. Please save the stick and box and call our toll-free number 1-800-562-0266 or 1-800-223-0182, weekdays 9 a.m. to 5 p.m. EST.

Frequently Asked Questions

How Does e·p·t Work?

When a woman becomes pregnant, her body produces a special hormone known as hCG (human Chorionic Gonadotrophin), which appears in the urine. **e·p·t** can detect this hormone as early as the first day you miss your period. The test utilizes monoclonal antibodies specific for hCG. If the test indicates you are pregnant, it is detecting hCG, and you should see your doctor.

Do I Have To Test In The Morning?
No. You can use **e·p·t** any time of day. You do not have to use first morning urine.

How Soon Can I Use e·p·t?
e·p·t can detect hCG hormone levels in your urine as early as the day your period should have started. **e·p·t** can be used on the day of your missed period as well as any day thereafter.

Can I Collect The Urine In A Cup Instead?
Yes, If the cup or container is clean and dry. Push back the splashguard and immerse the absorbent tip of the test stick into the urine for at least 5 seconds. Then remove the test stick from the urine and wait 2 minutes to read your results.

What If The Test Changes Color, But The Color Isn't The Same As The Picture In These Instructions?
If the test is positive, the round results window will retain a line of some shade of pink/purple color after the 2-minute waiting period. The line can be ANY SHADE of pink/purple and DOES NOT HAVE TO MATCH the color pictured or the color present in the square control window.

NOTE: e·p·t is so sensitive, it can detect pregnancy as early as the first day of a missed period. However, during pregnancy, each day after a missed period results in higher levels of hCG (the pregnancy hormone) in the urine. This is why testing a few days or a week after a missed period will result in a darker test color than the first day of a missed period.

What Do I Do If The Test Result Is Positive?
If the test result is positive, you should see your doctor to discuss your pregnancy and next steps. Early prenatal care is important to ensure the health of you and your baby.

What Do I Do If The Test Result Is Negative?
If the test result is negative, no pregnancy hormone (hCG) has been detected and you are probably not pregnant. However, you may have miscalculated when your period was due. If your period does

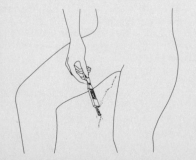

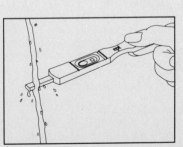

Continued on next page

768/DIAGNOSTICS, DEVICES, AND MEDICAL AIDS

Parke-Davis—Cont.

not start within a week, repeat the test. If you still get a negative result and your period has not started, you should see your doctor.

What If I Don't Wait The Full 2 Minutes Before Reading The Test Result?
If you read the test result before the full 2 minutes have passed, you may not give the test enough time to work, and the results may be inaccurate.

What If I Don't Think The Results Of The Test Are Correct?
If you follow the instructions carefully, you should not get a false result. Certain drugs and rare medical conditions may give a false result. Analgesics, antibiotics, and birth control pills should not affect the test result. If you repeat the test and continue to get an unexpected result, contact your doctor.

IF YOU HAVE FURTHER QUESTIONS ABOUT **e·p·t** CALL TOLL-FREE 1-800-562-0266 OR 1-800-223-0182, WEEKDAYS 9 AM to 5 PM EST.

e·p·t ENCOURAGES "EARLY PREGNANCY THINKING" 3 STEPS TO HEALTHIER BABIES
Today's habits make for tomorrow's healthier babies. That's why the makers of **e·p·t** feel that it is crucial for women who are thinking of becoming pregnant to begin practicing the "early pregnancy thinking" 3-step plan as soon as possible. This includes:

1. Preconception Care: To help prepare her body for pregnancy, a woman should remember that living a healthy lifestyle is vital to having a healthy baby. If the pregnancy test result is negative, a woman should continue to practice good health habits such as proper nutrition, regular exercise, and the avoidance of alcohol, cigarettes and other potentially harmful substances. During this preconception time, more physicians are recommending monthly use of home pregnancy tests to reinforce the importance of a healthy lifestyle routine.

2. Early Pregnancy Detection: Unfortunately, many women are unaware that they are pregnant until well into their first trimester. So early pregnancy detection can prove crucial given how quickly the fetus develops. The sooner a woman learns of her pregnancy, the sooner she can take the necessary steps to better her health and that of her baby.

3. Comprehensive Prenatal Care: If the test result is positive, it is essential to visit your doctor immediately. This visit marks the formal beginning of prenatal care, and the final early pregnancy thinking step.

Preconception care and early pregnancy detection make comprehensive prenatal care possible, and this represents an important advance for the health of both mother and child. Together, **e·p·t's** 3 "early pregnancy thinking" steps form the basis of a smooth and healthy pregnancy.

Notes:
For in-vitro diagnostic use. (Not for internal use.)
The test utilizes monoclonal antibodies specific for hCG.
Shown in Product Identification Guide, page 417

Whitehall Laboratories
**American Home Products Corporation
FIVE GIRALDA FARMS
MADISON, NJ 07940-0871**

CLEARBLUE EASY™
Pregnancy Test Kit

Clearblue Easy is one of the easiest and fastest pregnancy tests available because all a woman has to do is hold the absorbent tip in her urine stream and in 3 minutes she can read the result. A blue line appears in the small window to show that the test is complete and the large window shows the test result. If there is a blue line in the large window, the woman is pregnant. If there is no line, she is not pregnant.

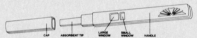

Clearblue Easy is a rapid, one-step pregnancy test for home use, which detects the pregnancy hormone HCG (human chorionic gonadotropin) in the urine. This hormone is produced in increasing amounts during the first part of pregnancy. Clearblue Easy uses sensitive monoclonal antibodies to detect the presence of this hormone from the first day of a missed period.

A negative result means that no pregnancy hormone was detected and the woman is probably not pregnant. If the menstrual period does not start within a week, she may have miscalculated the day her period was due. She should repeat the test using another Clearblue Easy test. If the second test still gives a negative result and she still has not menstruated, she should see her doctor. Clearblue Easy is specially designed for easy use at home. However, if there are any questions about the test or results, give the Clearblue Easy TalkLine a call at 1-800-883-EASY. A specially trained staff of advisors is available to answer your questions.

Manufactured by Unipath Ltd., Bedford, U.K. Unipath, Clearblue Easy and the fan device are trademarks.
Distributed by Whitehall Laboratories, Madison, NJ 07940-0871.
Shown in Product Identification Guide, page 430

CLEARPLAN EASY™
One-Step Ovulation Predictor

CLEARPLAN EASY is one of the easiest home ovulation predictor tests to use because of its unique technological design. It consists of just one piece and involves

only one step to get results. To use CLEARPLAN EASY, a woman simply holds the absorbent tip in her urine stream (a woman can test any time of day) for 5 seconds, and after 5 minutes, she can read the results. A blue line will appear in the small window to show her that the test has worked correctly. The large window indicates the presence of luteinizing hormone (LH) in her urine. If there is a line in the large window which is similar to or darker than the line in the small window, she has detected her LH surge.

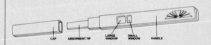

Laboratory tests confirm that CLEARPLAN EASY is over 98% accurate in detecting the LH surge as shown by radioimmunoassay (RIA).

CLEARPLAN EASY employs highly sensitive monoclonal antibody technology to accurately predict the onset of ovulation, and, consequently, the best time each month for a woman to try to become pregnant. The test monitors the amount of LH in a woman's urine. Small amounts of LH are present during most of the menstrual cycle, but the level normally rises sharply about 24 to 36 hours before ovulation (which is when an egg is released from the ovary). CLEARPLAN EASY detects this LH surge preceding ovulation so that a woman knows 24–36 hours beforehand the time she is most able to become pregnant.

A woman will be most fertile during the 2 to 3 days after an LH surge is detected. Sperm can fertilize an egg for many hours after sexual intercourse. So, if sexual intercourse occurs during the 2–3 days after a similar or darker line appears in the large window, the chances of getting pregnant are maximized.

CLEARPLAN EASY contains 5 days of tests. If, because a woman's cycles are irregular or if for any other reason a woman does not detect her LH surge after 5 days of testing, she should continue testing with a second CLEARPLAN EASY kit. CLEARPLAN EASY offers users the support of a TalkLine (1-800-883-EASY). This service is operated by trained advisors who are available to answer any questions about using the test or reading the results.

Produced by Unipath Ltd., Bedford, U.K. Unipath, CLEARPLAN EASY and the fan device are trademarks.

Distributed by Whitehall Laboratories, Madison, NJ 07940-0871.

Shown in Product Identification Guide, page 430

NOTES

NOTES